Medical Histology

**A Text-Atlas
with Introductory Pathology**

Medical Histology

A Text-Atlas
with Introductory Pathology

Robert L. Bacon, PH.D.
Professor Emeritus of Anatomy
School of Medicine
Oregon Health Sciences University

Nelson R. Niles, M.D.
Professor of Pathology
School of Medicine
Oregon Health Sciences University

Drawings by Joel Ito, M.S., Medical Illustrator
Oregon Regional Primate Research Center
Photographs by James T. Phillips

With 734 illustrations.

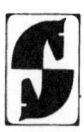

Springer-Verlag
New York   Heidelberg   Berlin

The quotation on page one is from *The Complete Sherlock Holmes* by Arthur Conan Doyle (Garden City, New York: Garden City Publishing Company), 1938. The quotation on page 76 is from *Classic Descriptions of Disease,* 3rd edition by Ralph H. Major, M.D. (Springfield, Illinois: Charles C Thomas, Publisher), 1945, page 587.

The photograph on the cover is a scanning electron micrograph of the inner surface of a small artery with a loop of suture through its wall. It is reproduced as Fig. 9.19 on page 165.

Library of Congress Cataloging in Publication Data

Bacon, Robert L. (Robert Lewis), 1918–
    Medical histology.

    Bibliography: p.
    Includes index.
    1. Histology.   2. Histology, Pathological.
I. Niles, Nelson R.   II. Title.   [DNLM: 1. Histology—
Atlases.   QS 517 B129m]
QM551.B216   1983   611'.018   83-384
ISBN-13: 978-1-4613-8201-0   e-ISBN-13: 978-1-4613-8199-0
DOl: 10.1007/978-1-4613-8199-0

Typeset by Kingsport Press
Printed and bound by Halliday Lithographers
Design by Caliber Design Planning Inc.

9 8 7 6 5 4 3 2 1

Contents

Contents

Preface

It is difficult for a teacher to accept the fact that not all of the information in his or her field is a necessary part of the armamentarium of the student. This holds for histologists, and for that matter, pathologists, biochemists, and ophthalmologists. It may especially hold for those who were trained during exciting periods in the history of their discipline. In the past two decades, information in every basic medical science has increased greatly, perhaps exponentially, and the basic science curriculum has been compressed to the point where the medical student can reasonably be expected to acquire only a superficial knowledge of any one of these sciences. Hence the information provided must be carefully selected, effectively presented in retainable doses, and useful for understanding material to be presented later in the curriculum and for the solution of clinical problems. In the compact courses of today, the presentation of only enough data to support basic working concepts of structure and function is appropriate. Additional factual information constitutes trivia, which in our opinion interferes with effective development, retention, and use of the concepts. This philosophy has been the basis for the preparation of this book.

Consistent with this philosophy, the text is brief, and the content has been carefully examined for its appropriateness to the needs of the medical student. Although there are many exciting areas under investigation in laboratories throughout the world, we have not included discussion or evaluation of unresolved "hot" controversies. We believe that it is the task of the teacher to evaluate such areas and to incorporate the best of the current literature into the lecture sequence. The material presented here should permit lecturers and discussion leaders in a variety of course structures to develop their own approaches and to build on this basic material.

Also consistent with our basic philosophy, a limited amount of pathologic material is included for most tissues and organs. No previous experience with pathology is required to teach or study this material. With careful observation of the photographs the student should be able to understand, and even predict, the impact of pathologic change on structure and function of the affected tissues. We do not intend to teach pathology, but we do believe that after students have studied normal structure they should be able to recognize when a tissue is not normal; that is, when it is outside the range of appearances which constitute normal. Furthermore, they will begin to learn how structure determines the development and course of disease.

This is basically a book of histology and organology. We assume the detailed organization and function of the cell are considered in a different course. There is a chapter on the cell, of course—indeed a fairly sizable one; but it does not provide all the material appropriate for a modern course in cell biology or cytology. In a given program, if the histology course is meant to include cell biology, an additional book covering that subject should probably be employed.

Since, as we have pointed out in Chapter 1, histology is a visual subject, we owe much to two people on whom we have depended for most of the illustrations. We acknowledge their contribution here because they were involved throughout the production of the book. Almost all of the drawings are from the hand of Joel Ito, M.S., Oregon Regional Primate Research Center. We feel most fortunate to have had the benefit of his artistic talent, practical know-how, and good-humored patience. James T. Phillips made most of the negatives and printed photographs and willingly enlarged and reduced them at our whim. But more importantly, he provided us with the critical eyes of a master with a lifetime of experience in scientific and medical photography.

Acknowledgments

Our first acknowledgment must go to the more than 4,000 medical students who have unwittingly guided us and shaped this book by their responses to the different methods and techniques we have employed over many years of teaching experience. They have in fact built this book.

Many others have also contributed. First among these is Kenneth Fletcher, who badgered us into undertaking this project and gave valuable advice from his long experience in the field of medical book publishing. Most of the remaining contributions were in the form of photomicrographs, microscopic preparations, tissue specimens or diagrams, and these sources are acknowledged where the images are printed.

We wish particularly to thank Dr. Catherine Smith for her help with the section on the ear. In addition to providing unique and beautiful photographic material she gave careful analysis and criticism of the text and made a major contribution far beyond our request. Drs. Rodney Beals, Howard Davis, Scott Goodnight, Jack Keyes, Howard Mason, and Richard Moore provided similar criticism of other chapters. Drs. Lesley Hallick, John Howard, Edward Keenan, and Alfred Lewy generously gave conceptual assistance in critical areas. Nick Roman, Ronald Sauter, Betty Sexton, and the histotechnologists of the Pathology Department, and Drs. Richard Anderson, Robert Brooks, Reid Connell, Anthony D'Agostino, Henner Fahrenbach, David Gunberg, David Johnson, William Montagna, Thomas Richards, and James Thliveris were extremely generous with their research materials, providing us with a large pool from which we could select items. Medical students Bradley Hindman, Craig Kennedy, Robert Kline, Euthym Kontaxis, John Wiley, Stephen Wilkinson, and Paul Zimmermann acted as student analysts and read many of our chapters. Their suggestions helped us make our writing more effective for student reading. For two years, the first-year medical students were issued some of the chapters as handouts to be returned with comments at the end of the course. These suggestions have also helped us greatly in making student-oriented modifications.

From the very beginning of our work we have been fortunate in having the continued interest and advice of Fred Harwin, whose artistic excellence, judgment, and experience in the preparation of published material have been invaluable.

Joanie Livermore and Suzanne Moody, both talented artists, were of great assistance in early stages of the work, providing drawings some of which persisted as the basis for some of the final versions. Geoffrey Sauncy provided the cartoons.

Many residents and student assistants in the Department of Pathology were alert to our needs and watched for instructive specimens from surgical and autopsy material.

Several individuals provided secretarial help over the years in which the book was being prepared. Especially helpful were Lanette Gepford and Elaine Jendritza in the Department of Anatomy, and Patricia Bessant and Carol Maxwell in the Department of Pathology. Beverly Cartwright arranged for typing of drafts of the manuscript.

The staff of Springer-Verlag, New York, specifically Larry Carter, Dr. Marie Low, Ute Bujard, Berta Steiner, and John Morgan gave freely of their time and expertise, answering our innumerable questions as well as providing other services. Berta Steiner and John Morgan also carried the major burden of converting our manuscript into a book.

Finally, but not by any means least, we wish to express our gratitude for the incredible patience and understanding of our families, especially our wives. They gave more than just psychotherapy; they gave sound, substantive advice.

A Message to the Student

Histologists have always been an ambivalent lot. On the one hand, their rigorous thinking has often been the key to major scientific advances, but on the other, they have manifested an interesting if not disturbing tendency to lose themselves in esthetic and intellectual attitudes that are philosophically diffuse if not actually vague. Complicating their lives further, medical science demands a practical application of their subject matter in its service to patients in a world short on time, money, and working space and in a society forever compelled to "get on with it."

The teaching of histology to students in biology and health science has both gained and lost from each of these three facets—the scientific, the esthetic, and the pragmatic (or perhaps more plainly, research, personal satisfaction, and service). The exactness of the scientific method may be effectively conveyed, and the excitement of scientific discovery dramatically demonstrated, in a field which lends itself to precision in dimension and spatial relationships. Considerable satisfaction of the human desire for order and visually pleasing patterns in nature can also be attained, and the ultimate demand of practical men for practical results can be clearly satisfied. But on the negative side, the very nature of the materials which histologists use in their work may suggest a conceptual rigidity which can dismay other disciplines that hold themselves to be more dynamic. And the microscopic structure which is so esthetically pleasing can all too easily become seductive, slowing progress in the assimilation of knowledge. The usefulness of the discipline in service to patients has its danger in the possible belief (undoubtedly held by many) that that is the only cause that it need recognize.

The all-important conclusion, then, is that histology is at once visual, precise, scientifically rigorous, esthetically satisfying, and highly useful to society. Each of these facets is important, and none should be pursued to the exclusion of the others.

You who use this book are not likely to dwell on these considerations for long, if at all, and you may wonder why they have been emphasized. There is a reason. Some understanding of the motivation of the histologist (and of his more pragmatic brother, the pathologist) is vital to acquiring that basic knowledge of microscopic structure which you must have in order to succeed in a health profession. Knowing where the faculty is coming from should serve to make the journey through the land of cells, tissues, and organs a more interesting and satisfying experience.

I would ask you to keep the foregoing considerations in mind as you use this volume as one tool in attaining mastery of the elements of microscopic structure. The fresh approach to the subject contained herein reflects with great effectiveness the three philosophically separable areas of concern that histology can present to those who would or must study it, while maintaining a coherence of approach that some other books achieve only at the expense of neglecting one area or another.

Since this is a *medical* histology text directed toward health science students, the emphasis on clinical and especially pathologic correlates should prove to be a very attractive feature. The clinical and functional correlates are well chosen, well placed and integrated into the text, and cogent. While they cannot be considered an innovation, they are so well done that they seem fresh and original. In their appropriateness, in their development as natural consequences of the histologic material, and in the breadth of their application, the pathologic correlates *do* constitute an innovative approach to the teaching of microscopic anatomy. They will make your transition from fundamental basic science to the study of disease states, and most especially to the complexities of the structure of diseased organs, a much easier one.

I must emphasize that this book's contribution to an orderly interface between normal and abnormal microscopic structure is not made at the sacrifice of any emphasis peculiar to histology, nor of any concept or detail important to a basic understanding of microscopic structure. The material on pathologic microscopic structure not only does not interfere with the primary purposes of the book, it also reinforces them in a way that is impressive. The careful selection of material, the natural flow of the text from consideration of the normal to the introduction of the abnormal, and the careful placement of pathologic material in the work as a whole have resulted in a marriage of viewpoints that will be highly beneficial to you not only while you are a student, but also throughout your professional career.

If the emphasis on the implications of normal structure for the understanding of pathologic change were all this volume had to offer, it would be enough in a new histology text; but there is more.

Since this text is designed neither as a reference work nor as a scientific review monograph, detailed citation of experimental evidence has been omitted. But while you will be spared much that is controversial and conjectural, this has not been done at the expense of a fair and valid assessment of important scientific issues. These have been presented in a fashion that imparts understanding, maintains a balance of current views in matters where interpretations vary, and avoids simplifications which might mislead.

Interestingly, if not most importantly, the esthetic and philosophic viewpoint of the histologist is mirrored in this book in a way that is not trivial on the one hand nor obtrusive on the other. The selection of the plates and the execution of the diagrams clearly reflect the authors' appreciation for the art and beauty in histologic material, as well as its instructive value and scientific merit. Even more important is their awareness of the world around them, our cultural heritage, and the involvement in wider areas of human concern of those elements of human biology which are of importance to the microscopist. This is discernible throughout the book but is most clearly evident in the final chapter, *Recapitulation with Variations*.

This book should make its subject exciting to some, interesting to many, and instructive to all. I wish you success as you travel through it.

W. Curtis Worthington, Jr., M.D.
Professor of Anatomy
Colleges of Medicine and Dental Medicine
Medical University of South Carolina
Charleston, South Carolina

1 Basic Principles: "What You See Is What You Get"

Introduction to Histology: Purposes and Methods of Study

". . . all I heard pointed in the one direction. The amazing strength, the skill in the use of the harpoon, the rum and water, the sealskin tobaccopouch with the coarse tobacco—all these pointed to a seaman, and one who had been a whaler. I'm convinced that the initials P.C. upon the pouch were a coincidence, and not those of Peter Carey, since he seldom smoked, and no pipe was found in his cabin. You remember that I asked whether whisky and brandy were in the cabin. You said they were. How many landsmen are there who would drink rum when they could get these other spirits? Yes, I was certain it was a seaman."

From The Adventure of Black Peter in The Complete Sherlock Holmes by A. Conan Doyle

    Histology is largely a visual discipline. Observation is vitally important. For most students, as for Sherlock Holmes, the attainment of this facility of observing and reasoning on the basis of observation requires training and practice. In microscopy, as in detective work, one must not simply look; one must look with a system and an objective. The essence of scientific study is to observe and record differences and similarities among a group of specimens or circumstances using reliable criteria to determine these characteristics. By distinguishing and identifying form, dimension, and substance one can develop a useful morphologic construct of cell, tissue, organ, or system. Also, by keeping in mind the physiologic capabilities of individual elements of entire organs and systems one can understand more easily the function of the whole.

    Microscopy is a single specialty of this art of combined observation and reasoning. If the student begins to look according to a plan, to compare microscopic sections and individual microscopic fields with illustrations and with each other, and perhaps to work with fellow students, he soon begins to succeed. Early familiarity with appearances of tissues in sections will facilitate progress in the entire course. In this regard competent use of the microscope assumes great importance. As a result, more of the responsibility lies with the student. Further, some students may have to work harder than others because not all have equivalent experience with the microscope.

Over recent years the rate of growth of information in the sciences basic to medicine has been increasing rapidly. This has added greatly to the academic burden traditionally placed on the student. It is our belief that this burden has reached a level where much valuable information is lost and is not easily retrieved when needed. In this book we have tried to make the learning of basic, useful histology less burdensome and more effective. Although in doing this we have departed somewhat from tradition, we have chosen an approach we believe is more practical and of

greater long-term value for the student. We have written this text with the needs of the student in mind.

Histology comprises more than a description of forms and includes functions of tissues as well. Consideration of some recent advances made with the aid of such tools as histochemistry, electron microscopy, radioautography, or immunofluorescence gives evidence that histology continues to offer great potential in medical research.

We urge students to retain and improve their skill with the light microscope after they complete the course. Hospitals now require pathologists to examine all tissues taken at surgery. Every specimen is described grossly, and almost every one is carefully dissected and examined histologically as well. Even mundane items such as warts, moles, hemorrhoids, and appendices deserve histopathologic diagnosis if only because their innocent appearance may belie a serious underlying disease.

Autopsies of patients who have died in hospitals are performed as another regular service and include microscopic and gross exami-

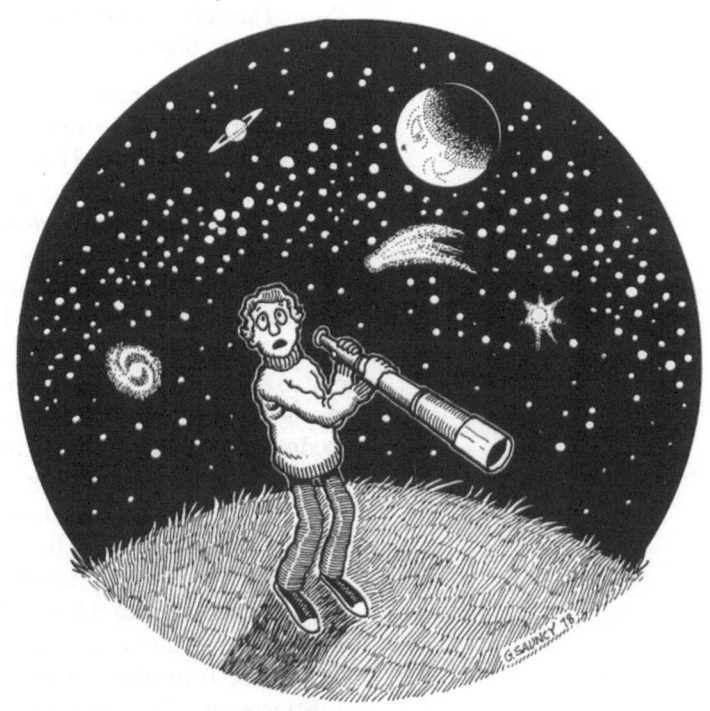

"Where do I start?"

nations. Biopsies for diagnosis constitute a more immediately important application of histology. The fund of anatomic and histologic material, and the information derived from it, obtained from current patients is a vital resource that serves for the continuing education of physicians and improvement in medical care.

Some people may question whether microscopy is as useful or as important as we claim it to be. Seldom are students required to examine histologic preparations in subsequent courses, and when they do it is always in the field of pathology. Most clinicians rarely or never examine microsections. What then is our reason for pushing this point so forcefully? The answer comes from the doctors who have actually acquired this talent. For one of these, a brief look at the sections may establish in his mind an accurate picture of the disease in that case, a picture that must help in treatment of the patient. Once this talent has been acquired it tends to remain with a person and require only a modicum of reinforcement. The lessons learned by this system are worth many formal courses.

Fields of biology necessary to the practice of medicine include anatomy, chemistry, and physiology as well as extensions and combinations of these such as genetics, cell biology, and psychology. Traditionally these subjects are taught either concurrently or in rapid succession, and most medical curriculum strategists feel that they should be effectively linked because each discipline encompasses one aspect of human biology and the subjects are not truly separate but support each other. Usually the study of one tissue, substance, or function by one of the basic methods necessarily soon extends to involve the other fields in spite of attempts to keep it restricted.

Nature, Purposes and Scope of This Book

The student is faced with the prospect of being required to learn "all" about the different tissues of the body in the histology course. In other courses one hopes to allow, but sometimes compels, him to complement and integrate this information with that from other areas. We cannot stress enough the importance to histology of a perspective of the interrelationships among different courses and for this reason try to make clear the basic functions of the various cells, tissues, and organs as well as systems.

This volume introduces a correlation that does not usually appear in histology textbooks: the presentation of examples of pathologic anatomy as supplement to the histologic demonstrations. We have two reasons for making this addition. The first is to supply the student with some view of the practical application of histology, which may be obscure until he sees the work put to use clinically. One important application is the subject, as well as the daily practice in clinical medicine, of anatomic pathology or, as the British say, morbid anatomy. We feel that including reactions to injury helps to define capabilities of different tissues.

The second reason for including examples of diseased tissues in this book is that these depict more accurately the range of findings in a standard population. Variations in form exist in all biological species, including the human. Experience has led us to the conclusion that the norms usually demonstrated in histology and anatomy texts and classes are overly idealized. The frequency of serious, potentially serious, and insignificant lesions renders the human body, like the sexual life of the camel, stranger than anyone thinks.

If one considers the number of parts in the body and the functions each can perform, one must wonder how such a small container can hold so much and work so efficiently. A great deal of the information about ourselves lies beyond present understanding. Some of what is known in histology has only recently been discovered; other matters have been established for ages. Even if we presented all the available information in this field our knowledge would be terribly incomplete and some of it would later be proved wrong. Therefore we have produced a volume that is briefer than most histology texts but that still contains the significant information medical students and physicians may be expected to retain and, later, to use. The book lacks some details available elsewhere. Although they may be important to some researchers or specialists, we question their value to physicians and surgeons in general.

We have tried to acquire clear, instructive, and representative sections for our photomicrographs. Most of the normal material has been taken from sections in the set used in the histology course. The aim of good microtechnique is the production of sections that resemble as nearly as possible the presumed condition of the living tissue. However, the required chemical and physical manipulations cannot help but leave their mark on the specimen. We have not attempted to eliminate all artifacts; indeed, in some instances we have made it a point to include them. They will be present, sometimes even prominent, in sections that students and physicians will see on conference room screens, in photomicrographs in journals, and in biopsy and autopsy specimens. Further, some particular artifacts are almost characteristic of certain tissues, as, for example, the "chatter" or fracture of colloid in the thyroid gland, the shrinkage in cross-sections of skeletal muscle that gives the characteristic "broken tile" mosaic appearance, and the tears produced when unexpected areas of calcification are encountered. Effective analysis of a section requires the ability to differentiate fact from artifact.

The student may find many new and unfamiliar terms in this book. Definitions are supplied for many of these, including all of the histologic ones. But terms from other basic disciplines and clinical sciences, require access to a modern medical dictionary. Habituation to looking things up is part of medicine.

Our policy is to avoid the use of eponyms in favor of descriptive terms. However, we acknowledge some of them as part of the language by including them parenthetically.

Finally, the illustrations in this book and their legends are basic material, not supplementary, and we have juxtaposed these with the related textual material. We emphasize: Do not neglect them. As we stated already, histology is a visual subject.

Basic Procedures in Histology

Histology is the study of the microscopic structure of organisms. The human body, like other zoologic organisms, is made up of *cells*, *tissues*, *organs*, and *systems*. The *cell* is the fundamental structural and functional unit of organisms. Hundreds of different types of cells exist in the human body. A *tissue* is an assemblage of cells and extracellular materials whose form, arrangement and biochemical differentiation enables it to carry out one or more specific functions. Bone and muscle are tissues. An *organ* is a localized assemblage of different tissues. The stomach is an organ; it contains muscle, connective tissue, nerve, and several types of epithelial cells, as well as blood vessels. A *system* is a functionally and structurally integrated series of organs. An example is the gastrointestinal system, which includes the oral cavity, esophagus, stomach, small bowel, colon, rectum, and anus as well as accessory organs—the salivary glands, liver, and pancreas.

Microtechnique

The specimen is examined as a *section*, i.e., a thin stained slice of tissue seen with transmitted light.

First it is necessary to treat the tissue with a reagent that will preserve as many structural characteristics as possible in a condition as similar to the living state as possible. This step is termed *fixation*. An important part of this process is the rapid and complete denaturation of the proteins and the precipitation in insoluble form of as many other components as possible. There is no true universal fixative and some of the solutions used in steps subsequent to fixation are strong solvents. Special solutions are necessary to preserve certain cell or tissue components so they will persist through later steps in processing.

The second part of tissue preparation is *dehydration*. All water is extracted and replaced, usually by a graded series of mixtures of alcohol and water. The alcohol is then replaced during *infiltration* by some liquid that subsequently can be polymerized or otherwise hardened. This may be paraffin, methacrylate, epoxy resins, or other *embedding materials*, depending upon whether a light or electron microscope is to be used. Embedding is necessary because the tissue must be made relatively firm to permit sectioning. Slices are cut from the now rigid but still soft tissue blocks. These measure 6–8 μm (micrometers) for general light microscopy and are as thin as 80 nm (nanometers) or less for transmission electron microscopy (TEM). These are then placed on glass slides and stained for examination with the light microscope (Fig. 1.1), or placed on copper grids and stained for TEM. In any case one examines a very thin two-dimensional section (Fig. 1.2). The relatively recent development of scanning electron microscopy (SEM) makes it possible to examine the three-dimensional surfaces of cells and tissues at high magnification.

A freezing microtome is extremely useful in cases where it is important not to adulterate the tissue with fixatives, embedding materials or other nonphysiologic chemicals. Biological activity is retained and sections can be histochemically tested for various delicate and complex chemicals, including enzymes.

A number of stains are in common use. These demonstrate or emphasize certain components of cells or tissues, but always at the expense of other components. The list of available staining methods may appear endless, but depending on the type of laboratory and its purposes, usually only one or two techniques are in routine use. A few or several techniques are available as needed in selected cases; many additional ones are applied only rarely.

Many stains are used in combinations. For example, hematoxylin (a dark blue or purple dye), being acidic, is *basophilic* ("base-loving"). It stains nuclear chromatin and nucleic acid generally. Hematoxylin is often used in combination with eosin, which is pink and *acidophilic;* eosin stains most cytoplasm and ground substance. This is the familiar H & E stain.

A few of the more common stains and categories of stains follow:

The Papanicolaou stain is applied to *exfoliated* or *free cells.* It gives very fine nuclear detail, thus being useful in the diagnosis of malignancy. Good results with this technique are particularly dependent on prompt fixation.

Wright's stain is used on smears of *cells of blood* and *bone marrow* because it provides excellent nuclear and cytoplasmic detail of these cells.

There are many different methods for demonstration of one or another type of *connective tissue fibers* and for distinguishing these from other elements. This group includes: Masson's and Mallory's trichrome and the Van Gieson stains, all basically for collagen; Weigert's elastic stain for elastic fibers; Bielschowsky stain and silver impregnation for reticulum; and Movat's pentachrome stain, which separately identifies nuclei, elastic fibers, collagen, ground substance, fibrinoid deposits, and muscle.

Periodic acid-Schiff reaction for aldehyde groups of polysarcharides.

Reactions for demonstration of *proteins,* based largely on identification of amino acids.

A group of reactions for precipitated *iron* in tissue; others for *calcium;* others for *argentaffin* ("attracted to silver") *substance.* (These are helpful in identifying certain very specific cell types.)

A group of stains for *triglycerides;* others for *phospholipids;* others for *cholesterol.* All of these require that solvents, which are usually used in processing of the tissue, be avoided.

A group of stains for *nucleic acids,* especially Feulgen's reaction for DNA and methylene or toluidine blue for RNA. Some of these are sufficiently reliable for quantitative measurement of these substances.

A group of stains for various *bacteria, fungi* or *protozoa.*

As the above listing implies, the use of several stains on one section can assist in the identification of structures that may be so delicate as to be practically invisible by the routine methods. Examples are small blood vessels, individual muscle fibers, and nerve filaments. This approach may be especially helpful in cases where a disease process has invaded or otherwise distorted the tissue.

The study and use of histologic stains extends into the domain of *histochemistry.* All staining methods are based on chemistry, but the older techniques are empirical. For example, the exact formula of the hematoxylin molecule is still unknown. Much of the knowledge of histology has been accumulated as the result of simple observation of form—stained and showing contrast, but giving little opportunity to assess function. Invention of modern techniques has allowed specific and even

Fig. 1.1. *Steps in producing a microscopic section from a gross specimen.* **A:** The specimen is a surgically removed eye. **B:** The specimen is made semifirm by fixation in formalin. It is infiltrated with melted paraffin, allowed to harden, and bisected. **C:** Section is cut by a microtome. **D:** The section is mounted on a slide and stained. The retinal detachment (arrows) is an artifact of preparation. (Courtesy of L. Christensen.) **E:** An enlargement of the area indicated in **D.** ×11.5.

Fig. 1.2. *Cutting a section for TEM.* At the left the chuck holding the block with tissue moves up and down and advances over the blade to cut sections of desired thickness. At the center the ribbon of sections is being floated on water and will be picked up on the surface of the copper grid shown on the right. The actual diameter of the grid is 3 mm.

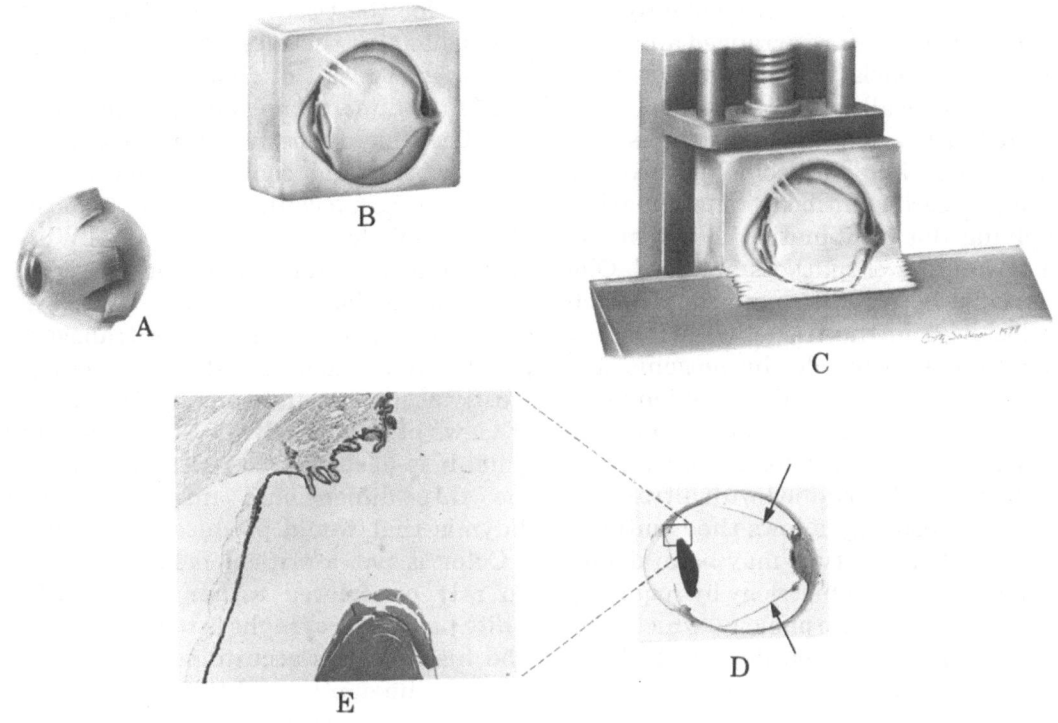

1.1

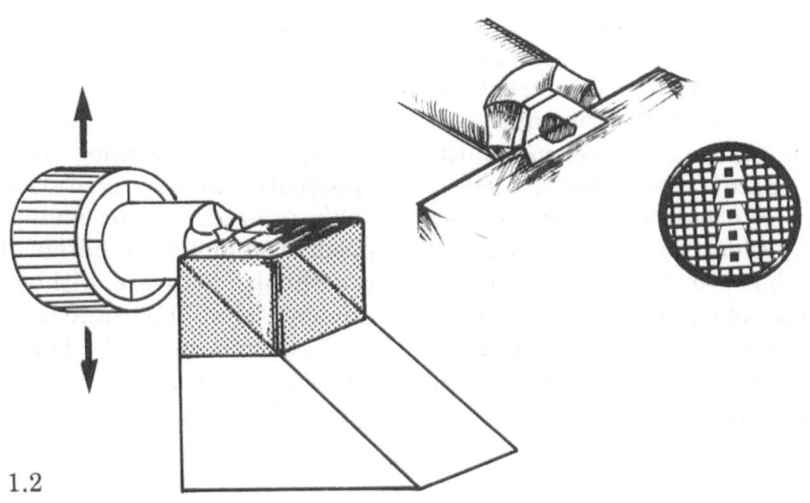

1.2

quantitative chemical determinations. Thus it has become possible to specify not only how the different cell parts are arranged and what materials these consist of, but also how they function metabolically and kinetically.

The subdivision immunohistology is just coming into its own. The technique involves combining a specific antibody with a marker and applying this combination to the micro-section. Two types of markers are used. One is the enzyme horseradish peroxidase which is then localized in the tissue by microscopy after addition of a suitable chromogenic substrate so as to produce a visible reaction product, as in histochemistry. The other marker that may be applied is a fluorescent dye, and the localization is determined with ultraviolet light. Immunohistology allows the identification of cells when the type may be in doubt. It adds more science to histology by requiring less reliance on pure morphology, which may be distorted. The cell is identified on the basis of its specific immunologic characteristics. The method is useful in embryology and studies of neoplasia.

Microscopy

The magnifying power of the microscope varies by factors of hundreds of thousands (Fig. 1.3). A special word of warning is in order here: it will assist the student's comprehension if he keeps a sense of the gross structures and the appearances at low magnification when examining tissues at higher magnifications. *Use the naked eye and the low power ("scanning") objective regularly.* A satisfactory zoom lens system would be helpful if it were available, but the standard microscope with three or four objective lenses can do almost as well and is more practical. Use the different magnifications to check details and their relative positions.

The picture one sees may sometimes be confusing, for the tissues themselves are three-dimensional structures. A good example of the strange result of a two-dimensional view of a three-dimensional world is shown in Fig. 1.4. The epididymis is simply a tube, but a very twisted and contorted one. (One may think of it as a bowlful of spaghetti consisting of one single long spaghetti noodle.) When we procure a slice from our tissue block, we cut different portions of the tube at many different angles—across its long axis (transversely), parallel to the long axis (longitudinally), and mostly at intermediate angles. Thus a variety of views of the epididymis is obtained on one slide. It is necessary to reconstruct mentally the three-dimensional image of the epididymis that would produce such a picture.

Color is not a critical factor in histology. To rely on colored rather than black-and-white photomicrographs is to have false trust. The histologist is accustomed to wide variations in the depths and tints of the colors in the slides he sees. These inconsistencies generally reflect slight differences in the methods or the reagents used in processing the tissue, or in the amount of fading afterward. One comes to know histologic structure by its form and texture, rather than by colors artificially applied. In our experience, color-blind students often acquire clearer concepts of tissue and organ morphology than do those with normal color vision. This book contains no color photos.

One of the problems for the beginner in histology is the variation that occurs among supposedly similar preparations. One section of skin or pancreas, for example, may at first appear completely different from another, even though both are without disease, from patients of similar age and habits, and stained by the same method. The most common causes for this variation are differences in the degree of postmortem autolysis and differ-

Fig. 1.3. a: *Table of useful equivalents.* **b:** *Relative sizes of some common biological units.*

Å ANGSTROMS		nm NANOMETERS		μm MICROMETERS		mm MILLIMETERS
1						
10	=	1				
100	=	10				
1,000	=	100				
10,000	=	1,000	=	1		
100,000	=	10,000	=	10		
1,000,000	=	100,000	=	100		
10,000,000	=	1,000,000	=	1,000	=	1

1 mm = 1,000 μm (micrometers) or μ (microns)
1 mm = 1,000,000 nm (nanometers) or mμ (millimicrons)
1 mm = 10,000,000 A (angstroms – now obsolescent)

1.3a

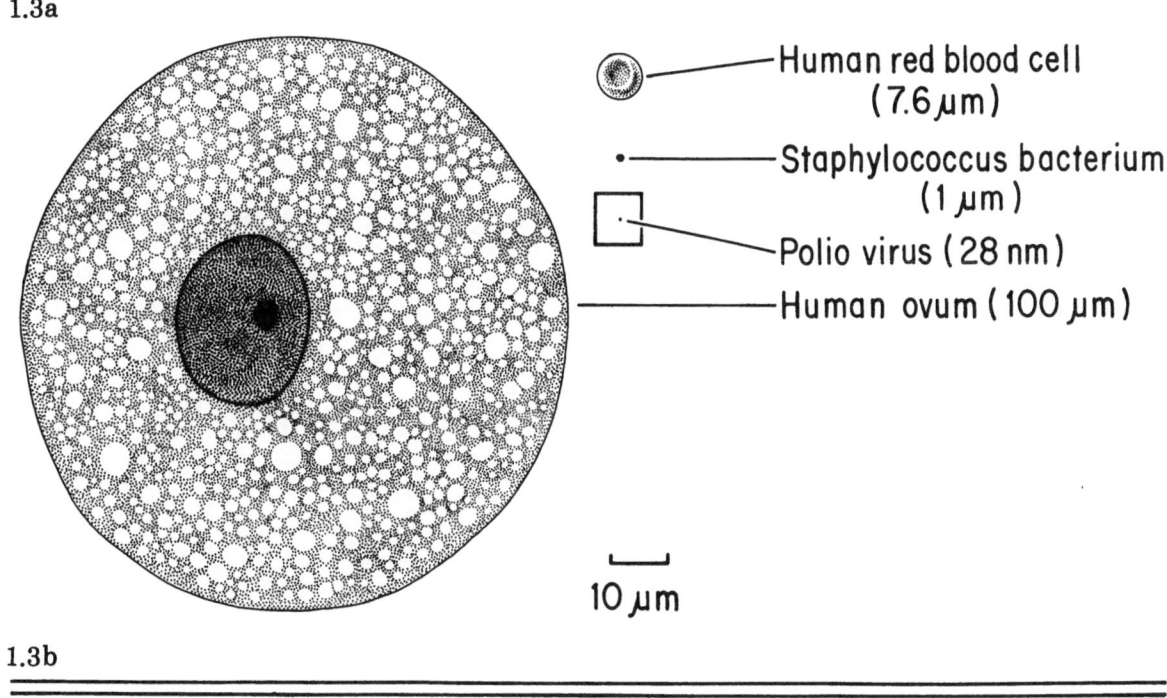

Human red blood cell
(7.6 μm)

Staphylococcus bacterium
(1 μm)

Polio virus (28 nm)

Human ovum (100 μm)

10 μm

1.3b

ences in the details of preparation. Histology technicians generally try to reduce these variables to the minimum but the student must realize that the world is not yet ideal and may have to look beyond the superficial aspects.

The appearance of the tissue will vary greatly depending on the technique used. Often a combination of methods will be astonishingly informative. Figure 1.5 indicates the results obtained by viewing the small intestine with four different methods.

Occasional use is made of polarizing, ultraviolet, dark field, and phase contrast microscopy. Cells may be taken from tissue surfaces or liquid suspensions and spread out on slides as smears or imprints. Microdissection, tissue culture, and other techniques are helpful adjunct disciplines.

Fig. 1.4. *Planes of sectioning.* **a:** Epididymis is a single, tightly contorted tubule of uniform diameter. **b:** A section shows this tubule cut at many angles. ×50.

Fig. 1.5. *Different views of the same tissue: small intestine.* **a:** Close-up photograph of the cut surface with the lining of the lumen at the top. ×7. (Courtesy of P. Stenzel.) **b:** Scanning electron micrograph, a surface view of the lining. ×100. (Courtesy of M. Webb.) **c:** Low-power photomicrograph of a section. ×8. **d:** Transmission electron micrograph of a section. ×2500. (Courtesy of R. S. Connell.)

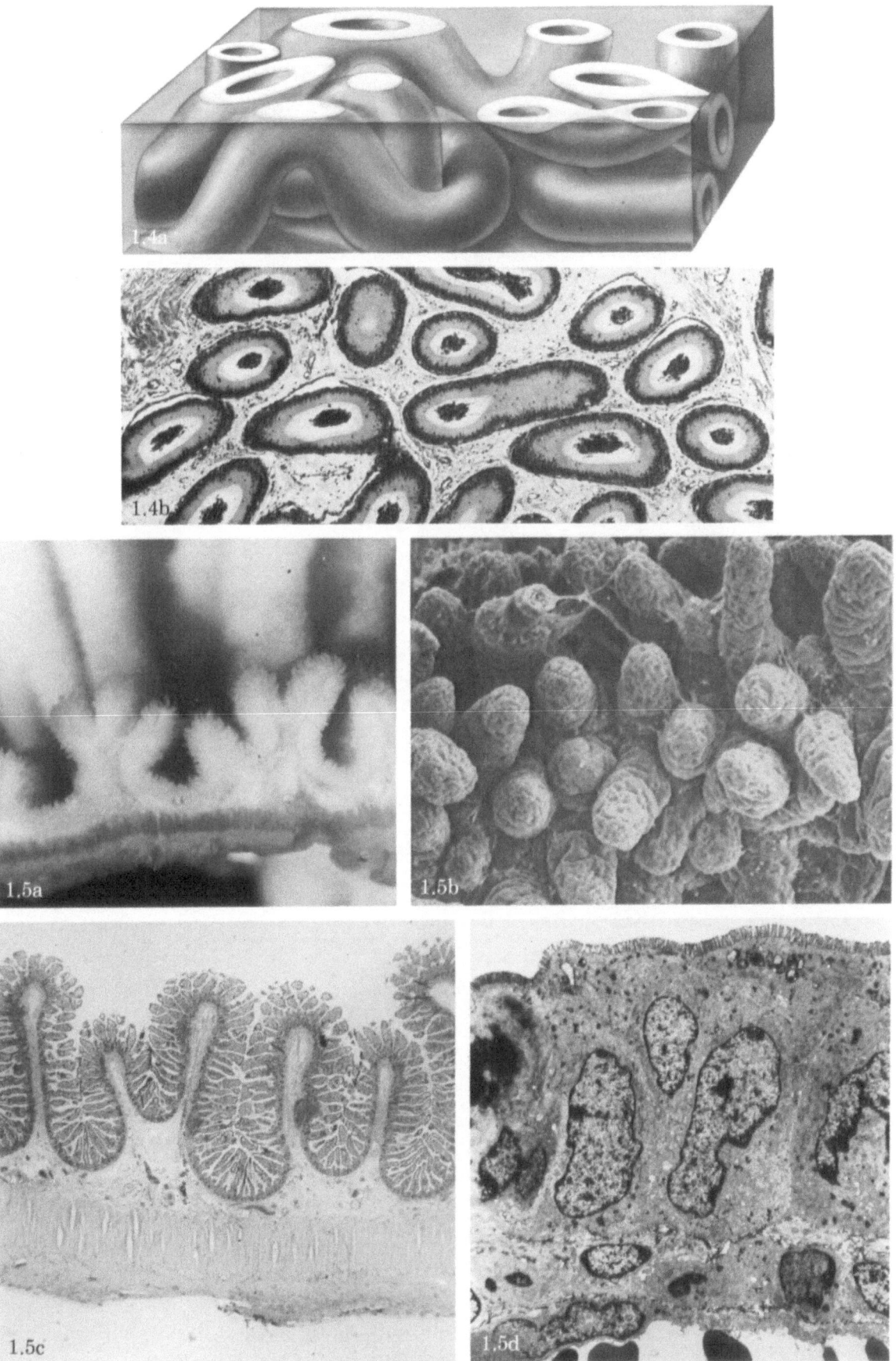

1.4a

1.4b

1.5a

1.5b

1.5c

1.5d

2 The Cell

Introduction

The fundamental structural and functional unit of every organism is the cell (Fig. 2.1). The human body is composed of cells and intercellular material formed by cells. In primitive organisms, as in primitive human societies, each individual cell (person) performs all of the several activities basic to survival and function. In more complex organisms (societies) different cells (persons) are responsible for performing one or a few of these basic functions for the entire organism (society). Through evolution, specialization and dependence on the specialization of others have reached a level such that it is difficult to find a cell (person) capable of surviving isolated from its organism (society). Thus it is probably impossible to find in the complex human body a generalized or typical cell whose description would fit a universal definition of *cell*, and no definition is general enough to include all cells.

The following description of each of the structural elements of "the" cell is intended to provide only the fundamentals of cell morphology and of its functional implications (Figs. 2.2 through 2.5).

Fig. 2.1. *Composite cell* containing the basic features of cells generally. The *plasma-lemma* is the cell boundary. *Nuclear envelope* is shown with pores. It encloses the nuclear content but permits passage of RNA and other materials. The *chromosome* is a portion of the linear coding system for genetic information. The *nucleolus* is the site of ribosome formation. *Ribosomes* assemble amino acids into polypeptides and proteins. *Microfilaments* and *microtubules,* the skeleton and the muscle of the cell, maintain and modify cell form. *Centrioles* guide the process of mitosis, direct the formation of cilia, and apparently control the assembly of microtubules. *Mitochondria* contain enzymes for the production of ATP. *Endoplasmic reticulum* synthesizes cell products for export. *Golgi* apparatus performs final assembly and packaging of cell products. *Lysosomes* carry out intracellular digestion. *Microvilli* increase cell surface area. *Cilia* cause movement of cell or of adjacent material. *Intercellular junctions* provide attachment and communication between cells.

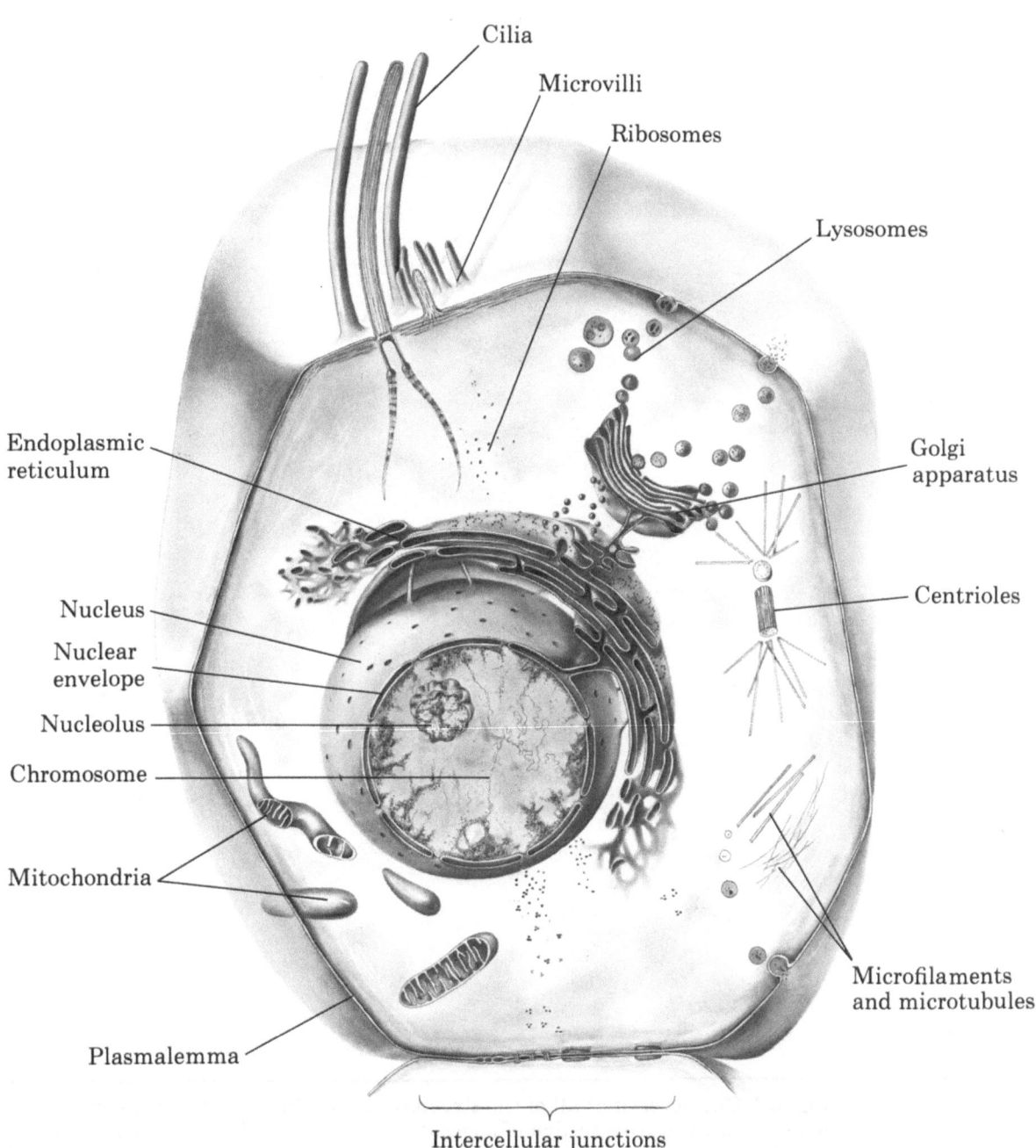

Cilia

Microvilli

Ribosomes

Lysosomes

Endoplasmic
reticulum

Golgi
apparatus

Nucleus

Centrioles

Nuclear
envelope

Nucleolus

Chromosome

Mitochondria

Microfilaments
and microtubules

Plasmalemma

Intercellular junctions

2.1

Fig. 2.2. One never finds all of the structures shown in Fig. 2.1 well demonstrated in any single cell. This section of a *smooth muscle cell* in the wall of a small blood vessel shows the *Golgi apparatus* and *centrioles*. Rectangle shows area enlarged for Fig. 2.3. ×3250. (Courtesy of M. Webb.)

Fig. 2.3. Further magnification of Fig. 2.2. G, *Golgi;* C, *centrioles;* N, *nucleus;* arrows, *pinocytotic vesicles.* ×13,000. (Courtesy of M. Webb.)

Fig. 2.4. Cells may have special functions that reflect the prominence of a particular organelle. This neutrophil has a bilobed nucleus (N) and many *lysosomes*. Rectangle shows area enlarged for Fig. 2.5. Approximately ×6500. (Courtesy of M. Webb.)

Fig. 2.5. The *lysosomes* vary in appearance depending on the stage of lysis of phago-cytosed particles. G, *Golgi*. Approximately ×15,000. (Courtesy of M. Webb.)

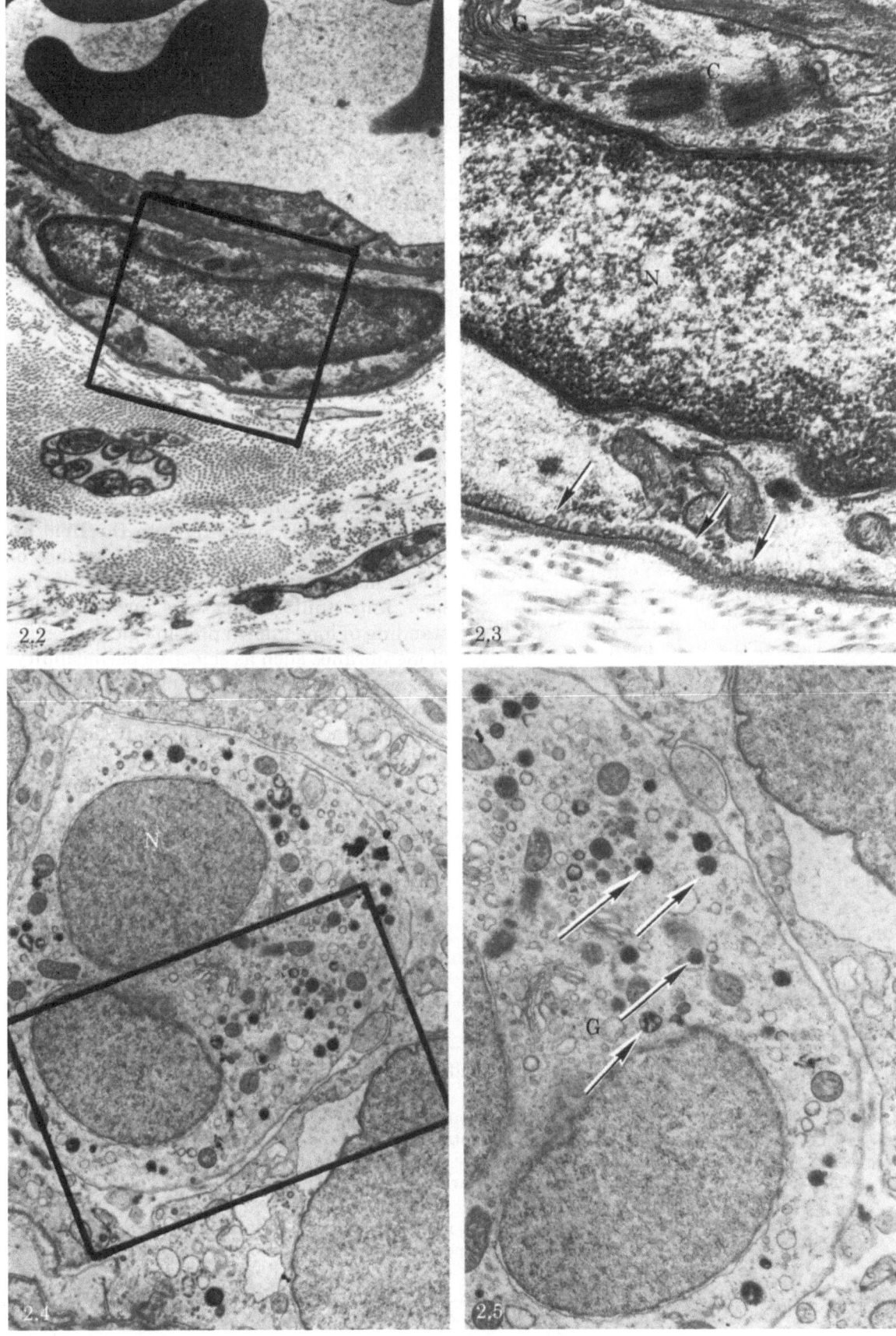

Plasmalemma (Cell Membrane, Plasma Membrane)

The structural organization of a eukaryotic cell is a function of its membranes. The membrane defines a cell's outer limits and delineates the characteristic form of several of the various organelles.

The cytoplasm is separated from the external environment by a metabolically active sheet, the plasmalemma (Fig. 2.6). The most adequately studied plasmalemma, that of the red blood cell, is found to be composed of lipid (20–30% of dry weight), protein (50–60%), and carbohydrate (about 15%).

Lipoprotein Bimolecular Layer

The basic structure of the plasmalemma and all other membranes is a phospholipid bilayer. Fatty acid portions of the two layers of phospholipid face one another to form an inner hydrophobic zone. The hydrophilic portions are exposed to the aqueous environment on each side of the lipid layer, forming the intracellular and extracellular surfaces of the membrane (Fig. 2.7). Electron micrographs show two dark lines representing the outward-facing sheets of phospholipid and an intervening clear layer representing the zone of fatty acid. This basic structure of all membranes is called the *unit membrane.*

Globular Proteins

The wide range of functional differentiation in membranes is related to quantitative and qualitative variations in their protein and polysaccharide components. The lipid bilayer is essentially a fluid containing 50 or more types of globular proteins. These proteins vary in number, size, and configuration among different areas of the same cell surface and among different cell types. One group, the peripheral proteins, may move about in the lipid bilayer, whereas others, the integral proteins, are key structural and functional elements so tightly bound to the membrane that they cannot be removed without destruction of the membrane. Others are easily removed experimentally, but with resulting alteration in physiologic properties of the membrane.

At least some, and perhaps many, of the proteins are enzymes; adenylate cyclase and ATPase are well known examples. Some proteins are large enough to protrude from both surfaces of the membrane; other, smaller, ones extend only partially into the lipid bilayer and protrude from only one surface of the membrane (Fig. 2.7). These arrangements have important implications for the understanding of long known physiologic properties of membranes such as selective permeability, passive diffusion, active transport, and enzymatic activity.

The passage of particles of small molecular size produces no visible changes in membrane morphology. However, large particulate material and droplets of solutions also may enter cells by a process known as *endocytosis.* The material or liquid is enclosed in bulbous invaginations of the plasmalemma that subsequently pinch off from the inner surface of the membrane to form vesicles or vacuoles in the cytoplasm. Ingestion of particulate matter such as bacteria is *phagocytosis;* that

---

Fig. 2.6. *Plasmalemma* (rectangle) as shown in Fig. 2.1.

Fig. 2.7. Model of the *plasmalemma* based on biochemical and morphological observations. Biochemical components are illustrated in foreground dissection, and at left and right the characteristic double lines of the unit membrane as seen with the electron microscope. The carbohydrate chains are on the external surface.

Fig. 2.8. The processes of *endo-* and *exocytosis.* Material may be completely (**a**) or partially digested. Indigestible portions may be retained (**b**) or excreted (**c**).

Fig. 2.9. *Cell surface* with *microvilli* demonstrating the polysaccharide "fuzz" known as glycocalyx (arrows). ×60,000. (Courtesy of M. Webb.)

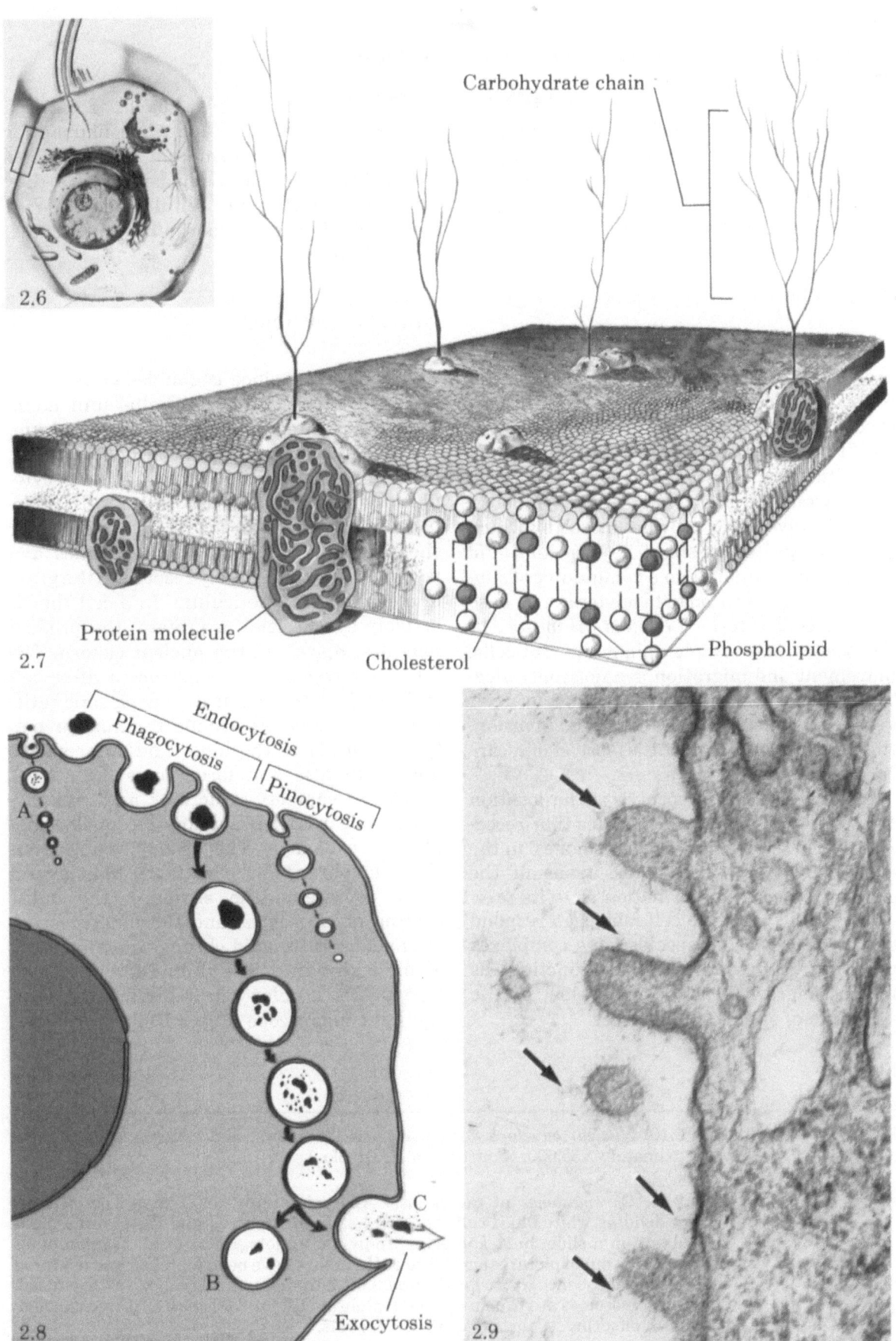

Carbohydrate chain

2.6

Protein molecule

2.7

Cholesterol

Phospholipid

Endocytosis

Phagocytosis

Pinocytosis

A

B

C

Exocytosis

2.8

2.9

involving water or solutions is *pinocytosis*. The converse of endocytosis, that is, the process by which visible materials are extruded from the cell, is termed *exocytosis* and involves fusion of internal vesicles and vacuoles with the inner surface of the membrane and the extrusion of their contents into the environment (Fig. 2.8).

Glycocalyx

Complex polysaccharides are attached to the protruding or external surface of many membrane proteins. Some of these are cell-type-specific carbohydrates and constitute the visible "fuzzy" surface coat or glycocalyx (Fig. 2.9) which is the first area of contact between the cell and its environment and neighbors. Thus the glycocalyx provides a code by which a cell recognizes others of its own kind and behaves appropriately in a community of similar cells. Modification of behavior in response to other cells is termed *contact inhibition*. In its absence, for example as in malignant cells, movement and migration are not controlled. Thus the structural organization of cell groups into tissues breaks down and invasion, the forerunner of metastasis (spread of a cancer to a different site), occurs.

In addition, the glycocalyx is the location of a variety of receptor molecules that recognize specific substances (e.g., hormones) in the environment. These receptors transmit the substance itself or information as to its presence into the cell. The cell may then respond by turning on or off specific gene complexes to bring about such important functions as increased growth rate, cell division, or the synthesis of specific products.

Nucleus

The nucleus is a membrane-enclosed package of genetic information and a mechanism for transcribing this information into messages for transport to the cytoplasm, where they may be translated into cellular action. With some notable exceptions the range of diameters is 5–10 μm.

Nuclear Envelope

The nuclear envelope is double-layered, that is, it is composed of two parallel unit membranes separated by a space of about 15 nm, the nuclear *cistern*. From the outer sheet, folds or invaginations extend into the cytoplasm where they are continuous with endoplasmic reticulum (*see later*). In fact, the outer sheet is often studded with ribosomes and polyribosomes and closely resembles the granular endoplasmic reticulum. In a cell that is actively synthesizing a protein, the product may first appear in the nuclear cistern. The nuclear envelope is reconstructed after cell division from fragments of endoplasmic reticulum that assemble around the nuclear materials. In places the inner and outer sheets appear to fuse and form pores (Fig. 2.10). Pores are complex structures and probably not simple passageways for free nucleocytoplasmic exchange. The clearly visible "nuclear membrane" seen with the light microscope represents the envelope, the outer coating of ribosomes, and the inner coating of envelope-associated chromatin, all seen as a single structure. The thinness of the envelope places it below the resolving power of the light microscope (Fig. 2.10).

Fig. 2.10. *Nuclear envelope* with pores (small arrows) and cistern (large arrow). Approximately ×35,000. (Courtesy of R. Brooks.)

Fig. 2.11. *Chromosomes* at metaphase. Approximately ×3800. **a:** *A complete set* from a dividing white blood cell. The cell has been ruptured and the chromosomes spread out on a slide. **b:** *A karyotype.* Individual photographs of all chromosomes have been cut out of pictures similar to **a.** Homologs have been matched and mounted in numerical sequence. **c:** *Translocation.* One chromosome 13 and one 14 are fused. These chromosomes are from a normal female at risk for a trisomy 13 (three chromosomes 13) offspring. (Courtesy of R. E. Magenis.)

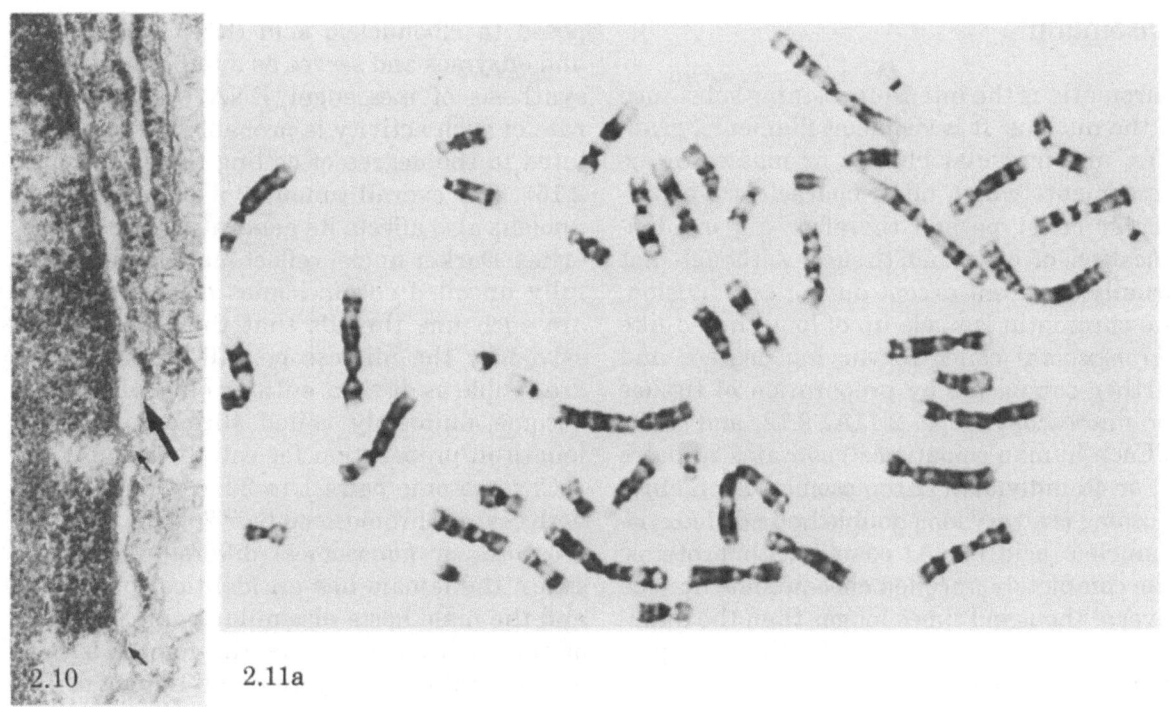

2.10   2.11a

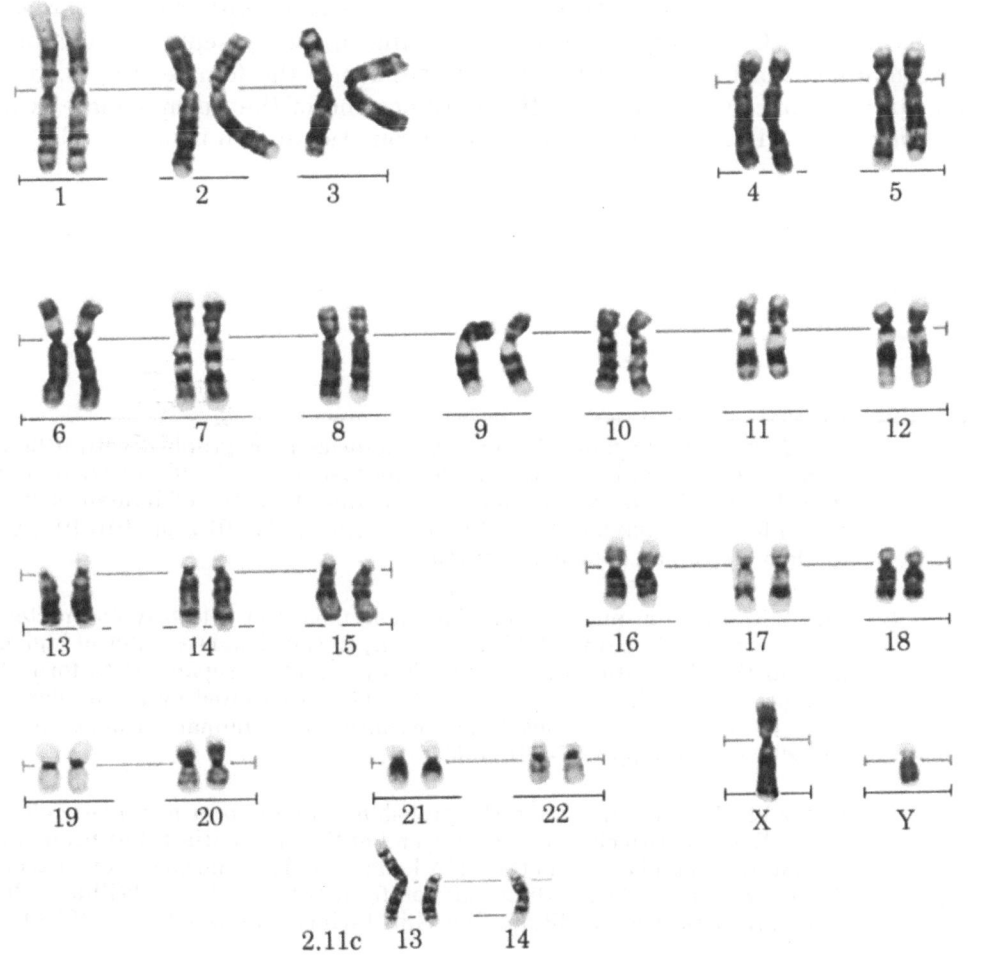

2.11b   2.11c

Chromatin

Chromatin is the intensely staining substance of the nucleus. It is visible as filaments, granules, and irregular clumps or masses in arrangements which often characterize a particular cell type and therefore aid in identification of cells and tissues. Although not usually apparent except during cell division, the chromatin is made up of long thread-like *chromosomes* coiled to varying degrees and further compacted by preparation of tissues for microscopy (Figs. 2.11A, 2.12, and 2.13).

Each human somatic cell contains 23 pairs of, or 46 individual chromosomes. Each chromosome is a very long double helix of deoxyribonucleic acid (DNA) coated with proteins. The completely uncoiled chromosome may be several thousand times longer than the diameter of the nucleus (Fig. 2.15). Different portions of the same chromosome may be coiled to varying degrees. The most tightly coiled regions of a chromosome are termed *heterochromatin* and are seen as darkly stained masses in the nucleus. Genetic information in heterochromatin is not being transcribed. The uncoiled portions of chromosomes constitute the *euchromatin*. Euchromatin is exposed to ribonucleic acid (RNA) precursors and enzymes and serves as a template for the synthesis of messenger RNA (mRNA). The rate of such activity is probably inversely related to the degree of coiling (Figs. 2.14 and 2.15). The overall amount of coiling in the nucleus also affects its general staining properties. Darker nuclei reflect more coiling. The fully uncoiled chromosomes of euchromatin are such fine threads that they are not resolved by the microscope. All chromosomes are visible as distinct entities only when they become uniformly coiled throughout their length in preparation for cell division.

Chromosome pairs 1 to 22 are identical in both sexes. Chromosome pair 23 (the *sex chromosomes* or gonosomes) differs in the two sexes; the female has an identical pair (XX) and the male has a dissimilar pair (XY). One of the X-chromosomes in the female is heterochromatic, that is, remains tightly coiled even when the cell is not dividing, unlike other chromosomes. It is visible with the light microscope as the *Barr body* or *sex chromatin* adhering to the nuclear envelope of cells in the tissues of the female (Fig. 2.16). The X-chromosome of the normal male is uncoiled (euchromatic) and thus not visible.

Fig. 2.12. Partially coiled *human chromosomes* photographed with a light microscope. The lower orders of coiling are not visible. ×3340. (Courtesy of Y. Ohnuki, from Ohnuki Y. Demonstration of the spiral structure of human chromosomes. Reprinted by permission from *Nature*, Vol 208, No 5013, pp. 916–917. Copyright © 1965 Macmillan Journals Limited.)

Fig. 2.13. Electron micrograph of a whole mount of a tightly contracted human *chromosome 1*. The chromatids are partially uncoiled and resemble at higher magnification the chromatids in Fig. 2.12. They would be separated to form daughter chromosomes by the mitotic process. ×25,000. (Reprinted by permission from DuPraw EJ. Evidence for a folded fibre organization in human chromosomes. *Nature*, Vol 209, No 5023, pp. 577–581, 1966.)

Fig. 2.14. Diagram indicating the probable *structure of a metaphase chromosome*. A and B are its two chromatids. One end of the chromatid B has been "dissected" to show the coils of coils and the DNA helix wound around the octomeres of protein. (Redrawn and modified with permission from Warwick R and Williams PL. Gray's Anatomy, 35th British edition, Churchill Livingstone, Edinburgh, 1973.)

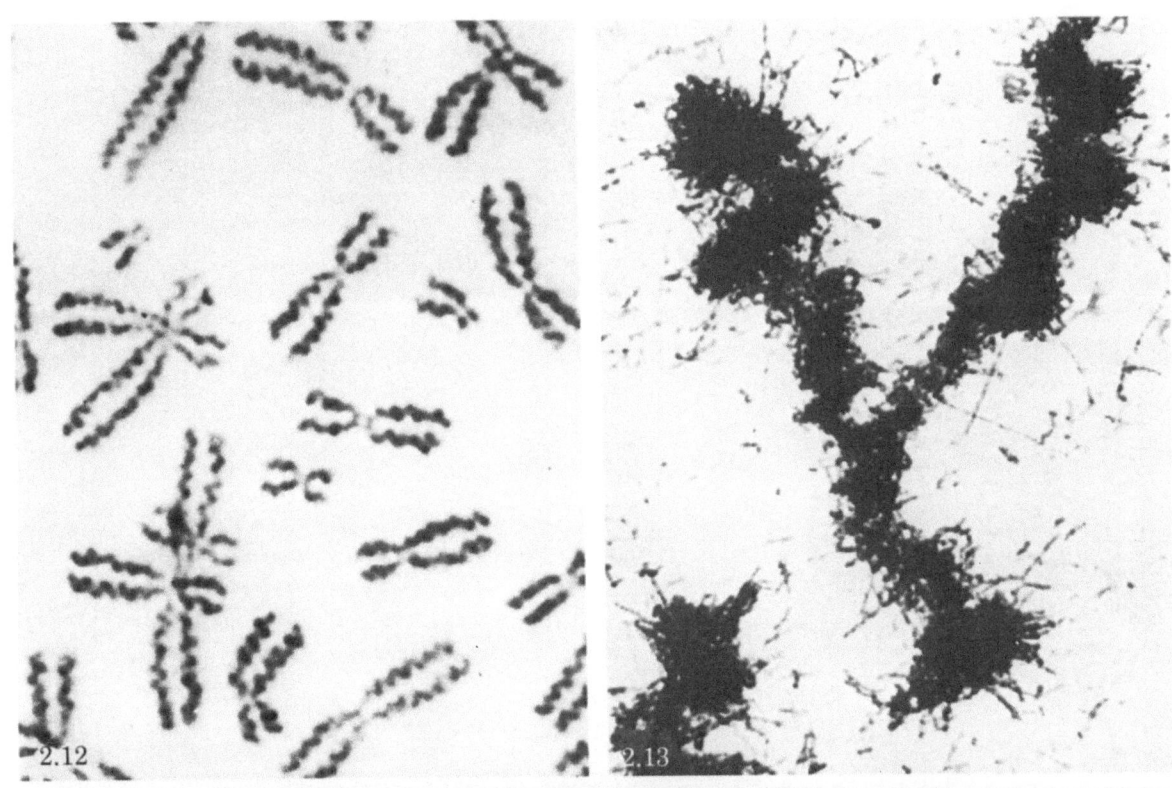

2.12

2.13

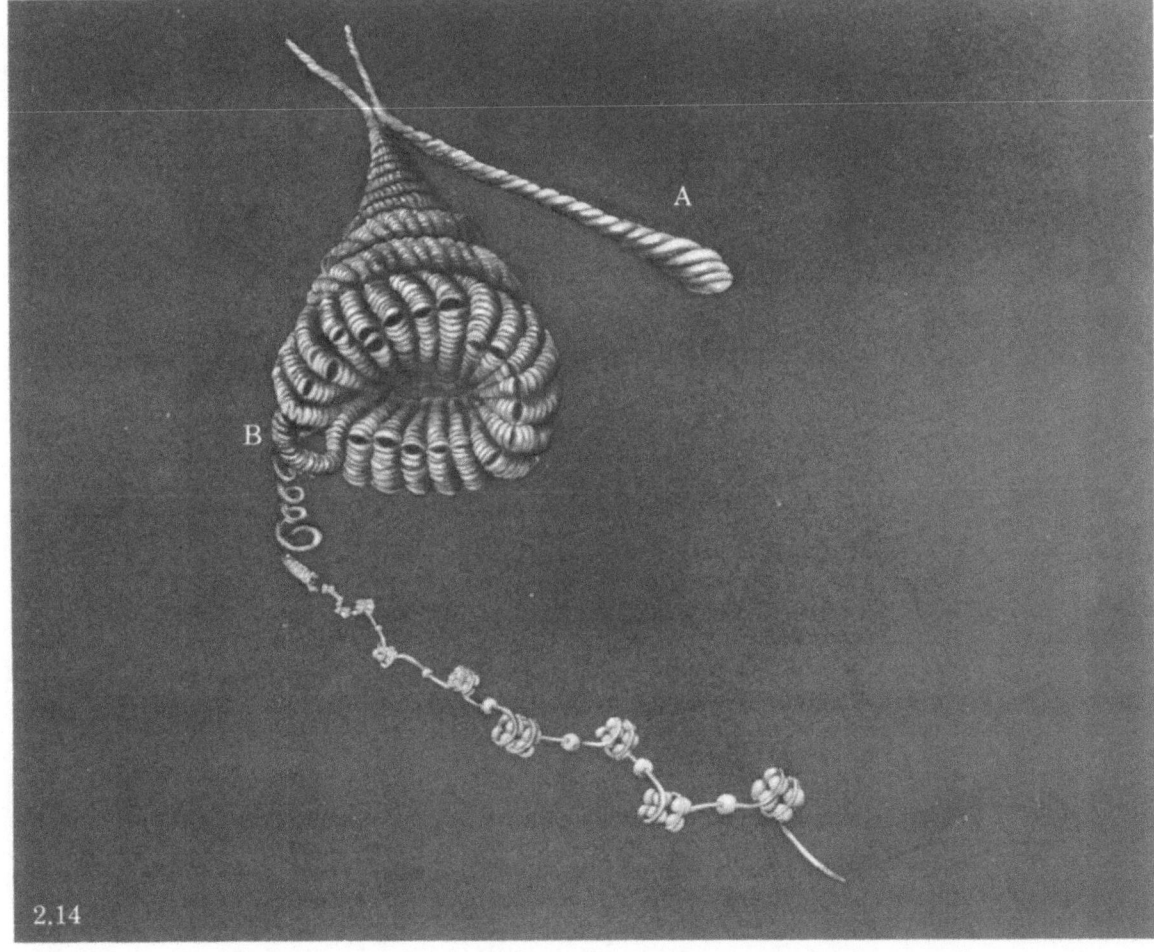

A

B

2.14

Fig. 2.15. A human *chromosome* spread out on a film after removal of the protein. ×14,000. (Reproduced with permission from Paulson JR and Laemmli UK. The structure of histone-depleted metaphase chromosomes. Cell, 12:817–828, 1977. Copyright © by The MIT Press.)

Fig. 2.16. *Sex chromatin* (Barr body) (arrows). In the epithelial cell (**A**) this is a dense granule inside the nuclear envelope; in the neutrophil (**B**), although still within the envelope, it appears as a satellite attached by a stalk to the exterior of the nucleus. (Modified with permission from Fig. 3.26 in Junqueira LC, Carneiro J, and Contopoulos A: Basic Histology. Los Altos; Lange Medical Publications, 1977.)

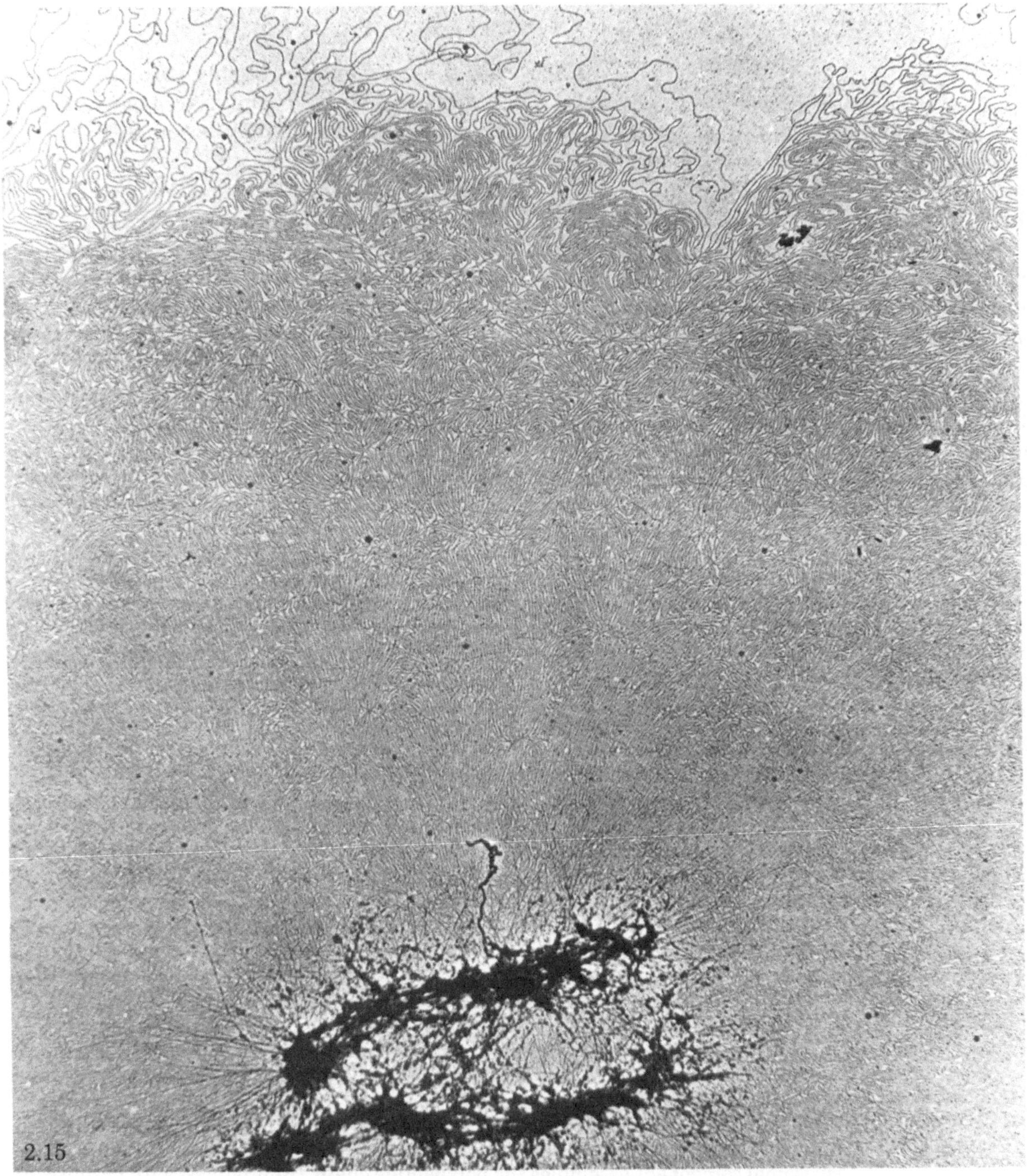

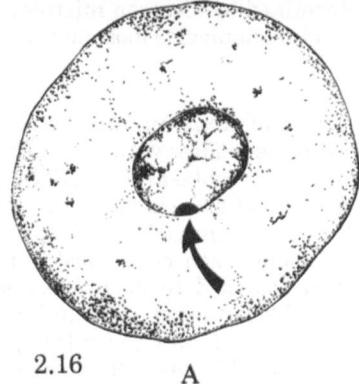

2.15

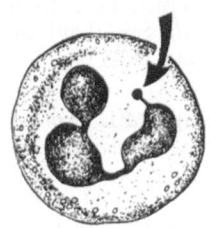

2.16   A   B

Nucleolus

The nucleolus (Figs. 2.17 through 2.19) is a densely staining, sharply outlined intranuclear body 1 μm or more in diameter and variable in form and position. It is visible in many cells with the light microscope (Fig. 2.18). With the electron microscope, the RNA which represents its chief constituent is seen in two forms: 5–8 nm filaments and 15 nm granules, both of which are probably stages in the formation of ribosomes. Also present is some nucleolus-associated chromatin that probably represents portions of chromosomes involved in synthesis of ribosomal RNA (Fig. 2.19).

Nucleoli are larger and/or more numerous in cells actively synthesizing protein either for their own differentiation and growth, as in embryonic and malignant cells, or for export as in actively secreting gland cells. They may be absent, or at least reduced in size, in cells engaged in little synthetic activity (e.g., muscle cells). They are apparently responsible for the production of the two ribosomal subunits. Nucleoli move into contact with the nuclear envelope and pass the subunits

into the cytoplasm, probably through the nuclear pores. Only in the cytoplasm are the subunits assembled into ribosomes.

Cytoplasm

Cytoplasm consists of all cellular components occupying the region between the nuclear envelope and the plasmalemma. Although there is great variation in the nucleocytoplasmic ratio, the cytoplasm generally is three to five times greater in volume than the nucleus. It contains ground substance (not to be confused with extracellular ground substance; see Chapter 4), organelles, and inclusions.

Ground Substance

The ground substance (also known as matrix, cytosol, hyaloplasm, or cell sap) is a very complex aqueous solution of proteins, amino acids, carbohydrates, minerals, gases, and other soluble substances. It has colloidal properties that lend the capacity for important sol-gel

Fig. 2.17. *Nucleolus* and *ribosomes* (rectangle), as shown in Fig. 2.1.

Fig. 2.18. *Nucleoli* (arrows) as seen with the light microscope. Sometimes it is difficult to distinguish these from masses of heterochromatin, as, for example, in the nucleus indicated by the long arrow. ×1000.

Fig. 2.19. Electron micrograph of a *nucleolus.* ×20,000. (Courtesy of R. Brooks.)

Fig. 2.20. Model of a *ribosome.* The area of contact of the two subunits is where the tRNA brings the amino acids into contact with the mRNA and where the ribosomal component assembles the polypeptide chain. (Reproduced with permission from Lake J. Ribosome structure determined by electron microscopy of *Escherichia coli.* Small subunits, large subunits and monomeric ribosomes. J Mol Biol 105:131–159, 1976.)

Fig. 2.21. *Protein synthesis.* Three forms of RNA manufactured by nuclear DNA are involved. (1) rRNA from the nucleolus associates with protein to form ribosomes, which are assembled and function in the cytoplasm. (2) mRNA in the form of a tape or ribbon is threaded through a series of several ribosomes to produce a functional group, the polysome. The mRNA carries the code for the eventual polypeptide product and passes through each ribosome. Each code word is matched with the appropriate amino acid, which is then attached to its predecessor to add a new link to the chain being produced. (3) tRNA carries specific amino acids to the ribosomes, where they are added in sequence to other amino acids to produce a polypeptide chain. (After Fig. 1.18A in Warwick R, Williams PL: Gray's Anatomy, thirty-fifth British edition. Edinburgh: Churchill Livingstone, 1973.)

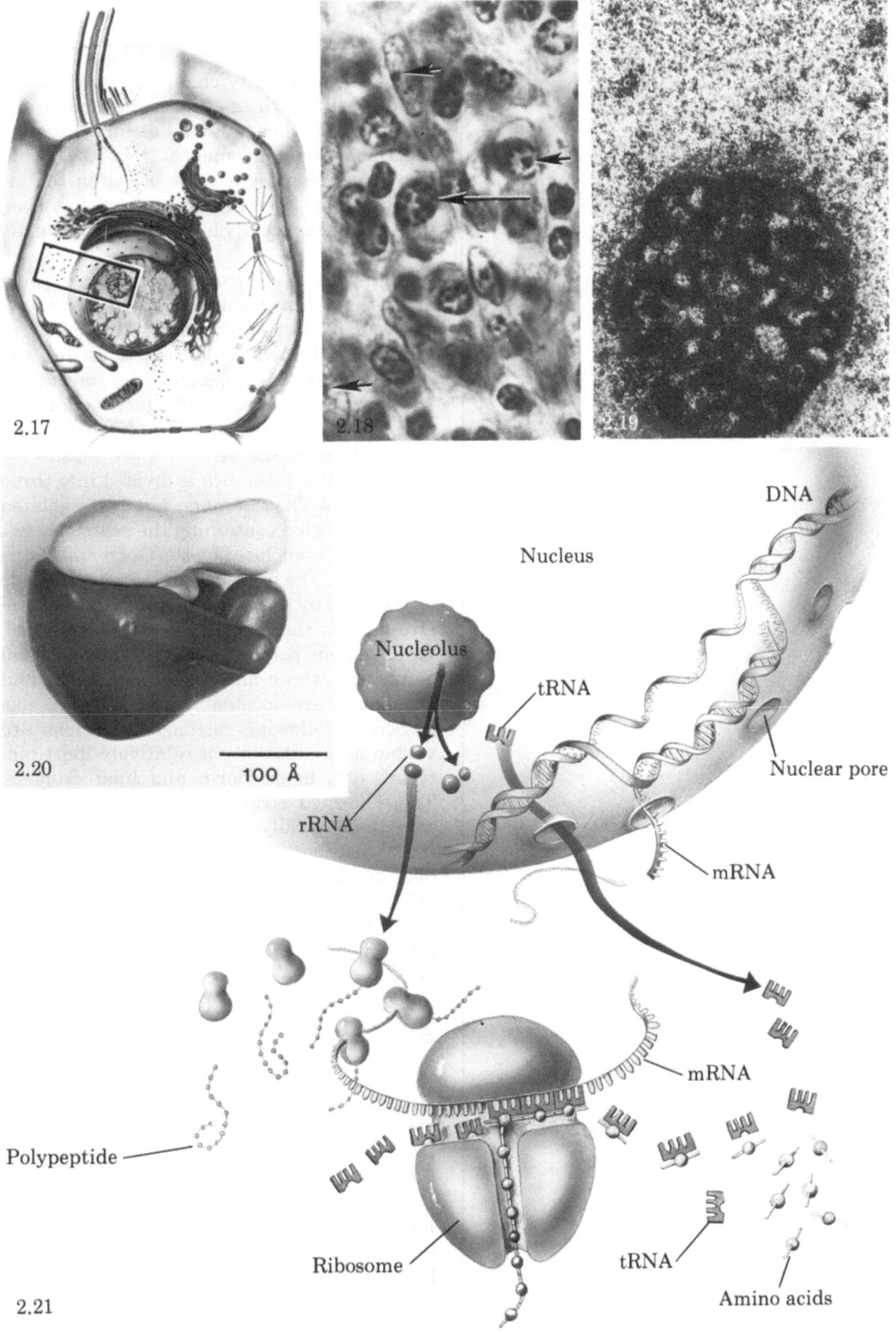

2.17

2.18

2.19

2.20

100 Å

DNA

Nucleus

Nucleolus

tRNA

Nuclear pore

rRNA

mRNA

Polypeptide

mRNA

Ribosome

tRNA

Amino acids

2.21

transformations that change cytoplasmic viscosity. Such viscosity changes permit fundamental cell activities such as movement and changes in cell form as well as internal organizational rearrangements. It is likely that the sol-gel changes may be based on the behavior of the protein actin, which has been found in unexpectedly large amounts in many cells.

High-voltage electron microscopy shows a dense three-dimensional latticework of microtrabeculae of 3–5 nm diameter. Ribosomes are located at the trabecular junctions and the trabecular system appears to be continuous with actin fibrils. Aqueous solutions and suspensions occupy and are moved about in the intertrabecular spaces.

The ground substance is divided into three major zones. The *cell center* is a firmly gelated spherical region containing the *centrioles* (*see below*) and is enclosed by the Golgi apparatus (*see below*). The nucleus is often pushed aside or indented by this structure. The most extensive zone is the *endoplasm,* a generally solvated region peripheral to the nucleus and cell center where most of the *organelles* and *inclusions* are located. Organelles are discussed in following sections. Inclusions are visible accumulations of relatively inert material, e.g., hemosiderin and lipid droplets. These formed structures are moved about, sometimes rapidly, in the cytoplasmic streaming that occurs in this zone. The zone just deep to the plasmalemma is relatively, and often completely, free of organelles and inclusions. It is termed the *ectoplasm* and is commonly gelated, but in motile cells it is capable of very rapid sol-gel transformation.

Organelles

Organelles are permanent structures with characteristic morphology that carry out specific functions in cellular metabolism.

NONMEMBRANOUS ORGANELLES are various types of naked granules, filaments, and tubules suspended in the ground substance that are not enclosed by membrane, nor is a membrane part of their structure.

Ribosomes are complex cytoplasmic particles that synthesize proteins. Individually their small size places them below the limit of resolution of the light microscope, but aggregates can be recognized because their polyanionic nature makes them strongly basophilic. Cytoplasmic basophilia is proportional to the population of ribosomes. In human cells, as in those of other organisms, each ribosome is made up of two different-sized subunits, the smaller being composed of a single RNA molecule with about 30 different small proteins. The larger contains two or possibly three RNA molecules and about 40 different proteins. Some electron microscopic observations on ribosomes treated with antibodies to their various protein components seem to be providing a morphologic model of these structures (Fig. 2.20).

Ribosomes occur as individual granules or in spiral configurations, *polyribosomes,* of several granules arranged along a thread of messenger RNA (mRNA). Single ribosomes are inactive; as polyribosomes they synthesize protein. Free polyribosomes in the cytoplasm release their polypeptide products into the ground substance, where they are assembled into structural and functional proteins for use by the cell. Polyribosomes also become attached to the outer surface of the membranous walls of endoplasmic reticulum. In this arrangement polypeptide products are segregated from the rest of the cell by injection into the cisterns where further processing occurs (Fig. 2.21). Such segregated products are usually specific cell secretions for export or are potentially dangerous proteases to be packaged in the *lysosomes (see later).*

Microfilaments. In cells other than muscle there are two classes of microfilaments in the cytoplasm, one 5 nm and one approximately 10 nm in diameter. (Figs. 2.22 and 2.23). The microfilaments measuring 5 nm are composed of actin and have been found in all human cell types that have been examined to date. They extend into microvilli on the surface of the cell, form a meshwork of variable density (the terminal web) near the apex of epithelial cells, and form a contractile ring or belt around the cell during the process of division.

In addition, they appear to be related to motility because they are involved in the formation of ruffles or folds in the surface, the invagination of portions of the plasmalemma, and cell contraction.

The microfilaments of the 10 nm class, also known as tonofilaments or tonofibrils, constitute a population probably including several special types, each related to a specific function. They do not appear to be related to motility. They often loop in and out of the cytoplasmic side of desmosomes in great numbers. Groups may extend across a cell, thus constituting a skeleton. In cells of keratinized stratified squamous epithelium, they are composed of keratin and eventually fill the cells.

Myosin is also present in many cells in the form of short segments rather than as the long filaments that characterize striated muscle. It is associated with the 5 nm class of filaments in areas where cell contraction occurs. It probably acts in this process much the same way as it does in muscle (see Chapter 6).

Microtubules. Many of the microtubular components (Figs. 2.22 through 2.27) of cells appear related to the particular cell shape. Their elongation by the assembly of subunits results in the development of the characteristic form of a cell during its differentiation, for example, the development of the long cell processes of neurons. Cell elongation does not occur if the assemblage of tubules is experimentally prevented. It has been proposed that microtubules are involved in intracellular transport along the interface between the tubule surface and the surrounding cytoplasm. Particles and organelles close to the tubules move parallel to their long axes. Microtubules are composed of approximately globular subunits known as tubulin arranged in coiled or helical stacks that produce cylinders with exactly 13 subunits per turn. Tubules do not branch. They are particularly well developed in centrioles, cilia, basal bodies, and the mitotic spindles. Antimitotic drugs that bind tubulin, such as colchicine and vinblastine, bring about dispersal of subunits and disappearance of the tubules. After the removal of the drug the tubules reassemble.

Fig. 2.22. *Microfilaments* and *microtubules* (rectangle), as shown in Fig. 2.1.

Fig. 2.23. *Microfilaments* (arrows) in the cytoplasm of a stratified squamous epithelial cell. ×28,000. (Courtesy of M. Webb.)

Fig. 2.24. *Microtubules* are the only visible structures in these three cells. In this type of preparation they are seen as fluorescent threads against a dark background. Approximately ×900. (Reproduced with permission from Osborn M and Weber K. The display of microtubules in transformed cells. Cell, 12:561–577, 1977.)

Fig. 2.25. Drawing of molecules of *tubulin* in spiral arrangement, forming a microtubule. Approximately ×1,100,000. (Redrawn with permission from Fig. 9.5C in DuPraw EJ. Cell and Molecular Biology. Academic Press, 1968.)

Fig. 2.26. Longitudinal section of *microtubules*. ×40,000. (Courtesy of M. Webb.)

Fig. 2.27. Cross sections of *microtubules*. ×247,000. (From the work of V. Mizuhira, reproduced with permission from Junqueira LC, Carneiro J, and Contopoulos A. Basic Histology, 2nd edit., 1977. Lange Medical Publications, Los Altos, California.)

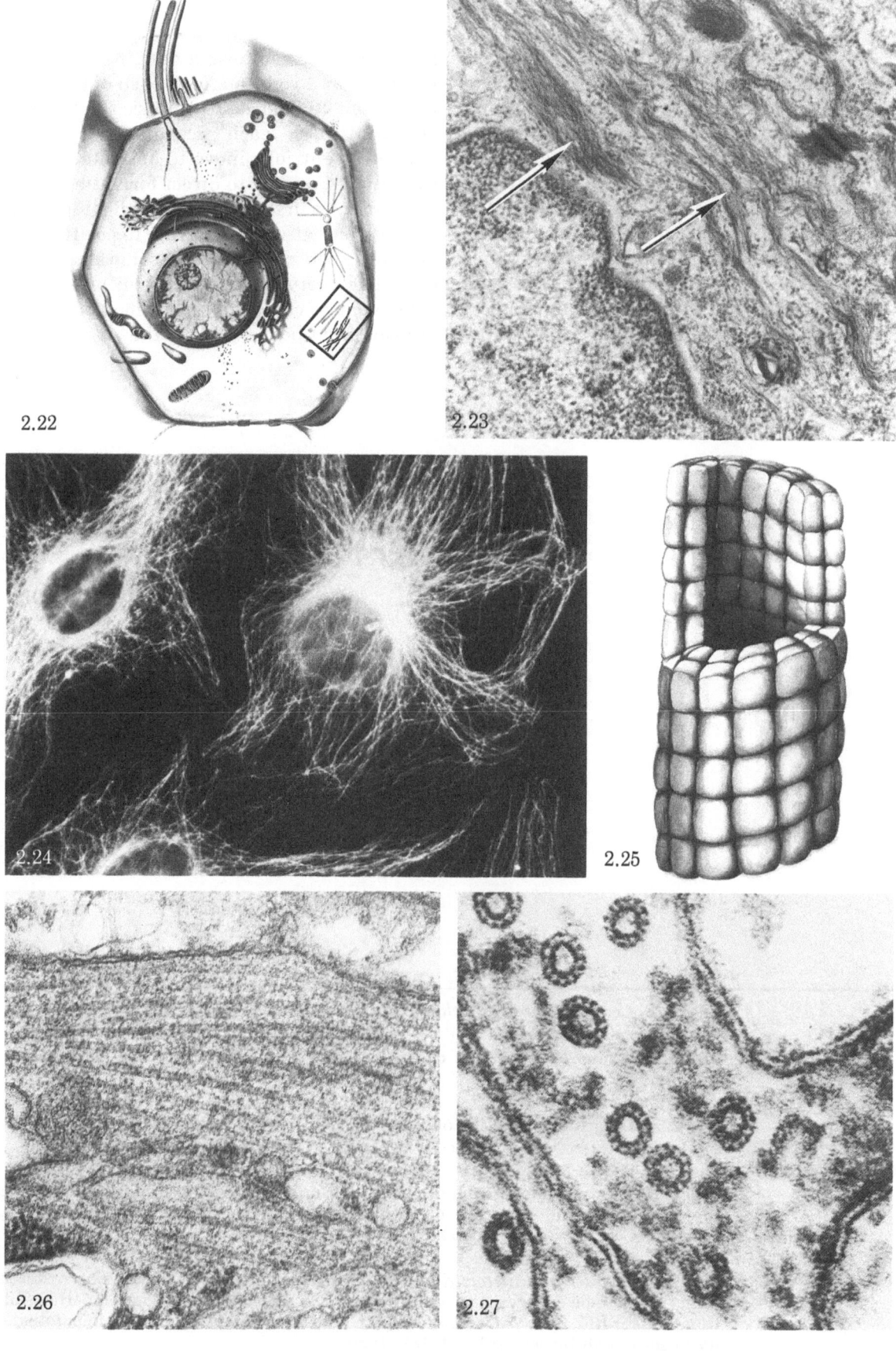

2.22

2.23

2.24

2.25

2.26

2.27

Centrioles (Figs. 2.28 through 2.30) are visible with the light microscope as tiny rods and are shown with the electron microscope to be cylindrical structures with nine fins or plates in their walls. The fins are arranged like those of a turbine and each is composed of three longitudinally fused microtubules. The inner tubule of each fin is overlapped by the outer tubule of its neighbor. Amorphous dense masses, termed satellites, are located near one end of the centriole and may be unassembled precursors or subunits for the formation of new centrioles. Most cells have one pair, but before mitosis a daughter centriole is formed at a right angle to each of the existing parent centrioles. At mitosis the two parent centrioles, each accompanied by its daughter centriole, move to opposite poles of the cell and appear to direct formation of the microtubules in the mitotic spindle (Fig. 2.60).

Centrioles also may migrate to positions beneath the cell membrane, become slightly altered in structural detail, and initiate the development of cilia. These modified centrioles are the basal bodies of the cilia.

Fig. 2.28. *Centrioles* and *mitochondria* (rectangles), as shown in Fig. 2.1.

Fig. 2.29. Transverse sections of two *centrioles*. ×67,000. (Courtesy of R. G. W. Anderson.)

Fig. 2.30. Longitudinal section of a *centriole*. ×67,000. (Courtesy of R. G. W. Anderson.)

Fig. 2.31. Electron micrograph of portions of *mitochondria* in a plasma cell. Note the unit membrane structure of both inner and outer layers of the organelle. ×73,000. (Courtesy of M. Webb.)

Fig. 2.32. *Swollen and distorted mitochondrion* in hepatocyte. This lesion resulted from the common analgesic, acetaminophen. ×12,400. (Reproduced with permission from Walker RM, Racz WJ, and McElligott TF. Acetaminophen-induced hepatotoxicity in mice. Lab Invest 42(2):181–189, 1980.)

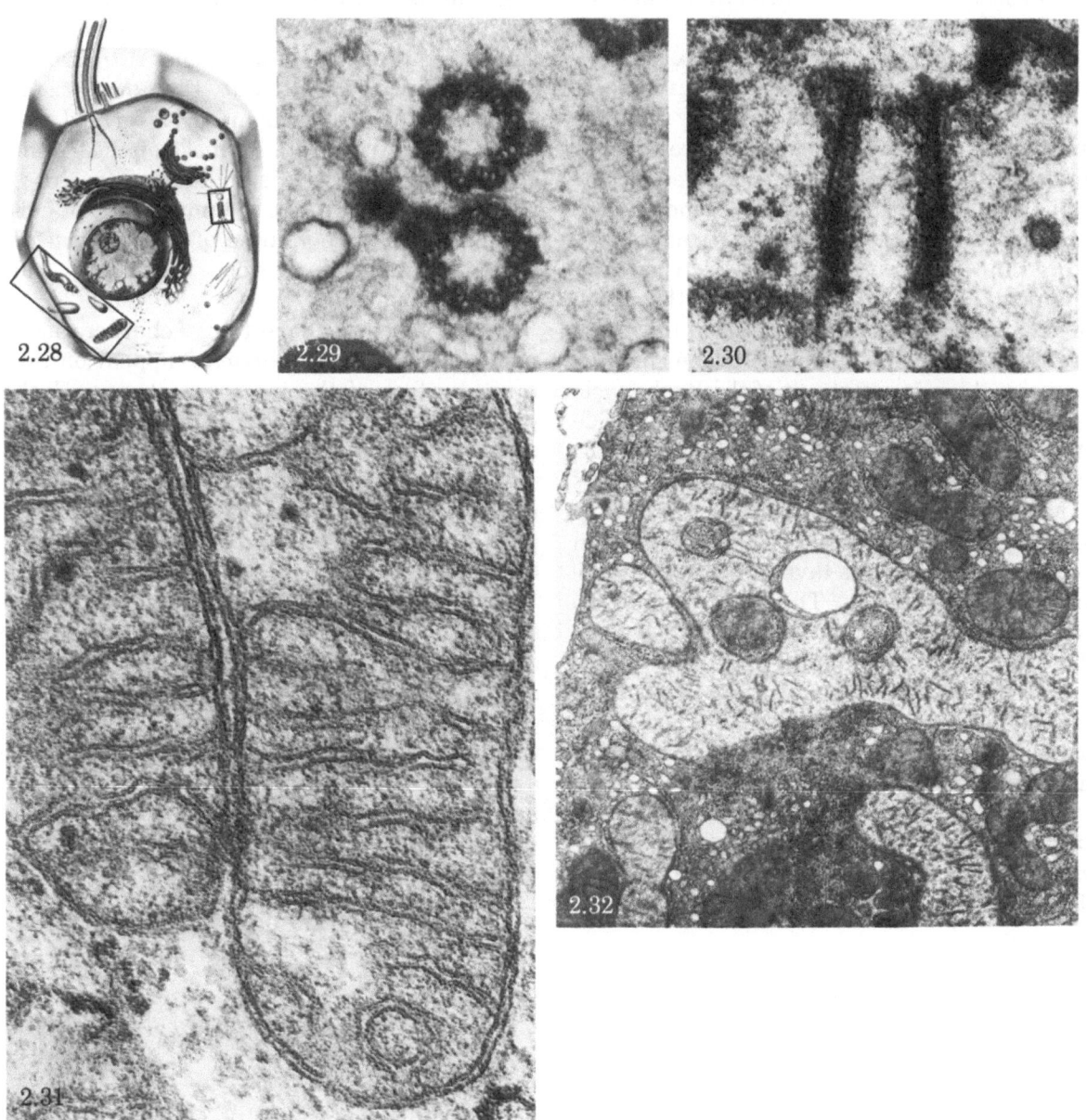

MEMBRANOUS ORGANELLES are either enclosed by, or composed of, membranes.

Mitochondria.   All animals are heterotrophic, that is, they cannot utilize the sun's energy directly, but must take in reducing substances and oxidize them. The free energy released upon oxidation is conserved by the cell through the formation of adenosine triphosphate (ATP). The energy effectively stored in ATP is available for electrical, mechanical, or chemical work through the action of various ATPases that are present in a number of locations within the cell. The complex sequential enzyme systems of the Krebs cycle and of oxidative phosphorylation that provide ATP are all located in mitochondria (Figs. 2.28, 2.31 through 2.33).

Mitochondria are spherical, sausage-shaped, or filamentous bodies occurring in considerable numbers (averaging 1000–1500) in all eukaryotic cells. They measure 0.1–0.5 nm in diameter and up to 10 nm in length. They may be randomly distributed in the cytoplasm or localized where work is being done, for example, apically in ciliated cells or basally in electrolyte transporting cells. Their average life span is about 10 days.

The electron microscope demonstrates two unit membranes; the inner has folds (*cristae mitochondriales*) projecting into the interior. The mitochondria of steroid-producing cells (e.g., adrenocortical cells) possess tubular projections of the inner membrane instead of the usual flat shelf-like folds. The *intra*cristal spaces appear clear, but the *inter*cristal spaces contain granular material termed *matrix*. The matrix contains most of the Krebs cycle enzymes and occasional dense dark bodies that may represent accumulations of calcium. The relative volume of the two cristal spaces changes in various functional and pathologic states.

Under certain conditions characteristic particles (*elementary particles*) appear on the inner surface of the inner membrane. Each particle has the form of a small granule attached to a basal thickening by a slender stalk. It is possible, but not proved, that they represent the enzymes of the electron transport system known to reside in this membrane.

Mitochondria-specific DNA and RNA are synthesized within the mitochondrion. Mitochondria also synthesize their own protein, and may self-replicate. Membrane-bound respiratory enzymes are present. These features, as well as a circular DNA structure, are also characteristic of bacteria; hence it has been suggested that mitochondria may represent descendants of an ancestral symbiotic prokaryote.

Fig. 2.33. *Structural and functional features of a mitochondrion.* The inset enlargement indicates the location of cellular respiratory enzymes.

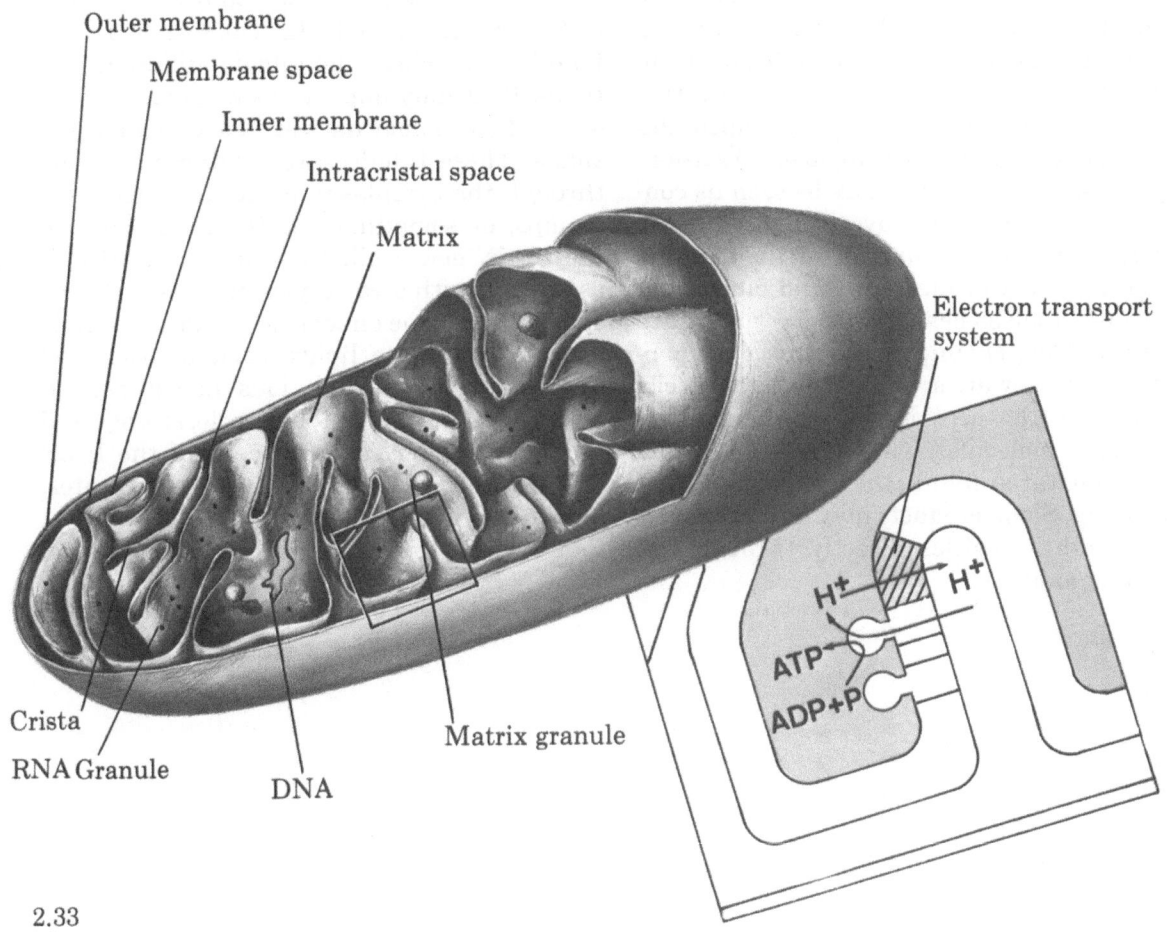

Outer membrane

Membrane space

Inner membrane

Intracristal space

Matrix

Electron transport system

H+   H+

ATP

ADP+P

Crista

RNA Granule

DNA

Matrix granule

2.33

Rough (granular) endoplasmic reticulum (RER) (Figs. 2.34 and 2.35) consists of flattened sacs (cisterns) of the unit membrane commonly occurring in stacked array in localized areas, but sometimes irregularly shaped and widely distributed in the cytoplasm. Occasionally the wall of a cistern may be seen as continuous with the outer layers of the nuclear envelope. The outer surfaces of the cisterns are studded with coiled rows and clusters of ribosomes (polysomes) that, by a procedure not yet completely understood, inject the peptide chains they are synthesizing into the cisterns. Here the peptides may be assembled into larger molecules, which then pass to the Golgi apparatus for further processing and packaging. Some products may be secreted by way of other vesicles directly through the plasmalemma.

Smooth endoplasmic reticulum (SER) (Figs. 2.36 through 2.38) lacks ribosomes and is found in varying amounts in different cell types. It usually appears as a complex mesh of tubules of somewhat variable diameter and shape. These tubules are scattered sparsely through the cytoplasm, or occur in localized clumps, or sometimes, as in Leydig cells of the testis, nearly fill the entire cell. SER is associated with a variety of functions: steroid synthesis in some endocrine organs; assembly of fatty acids into lipids; accumulation and distribution of calcium ions in contraction and relaxation of striated muscle; storage and breakdown of glycogen in cells of the liver; and detoxification, notably of barbiturates, also in the liver.

Fig. 2.34. *Rough endoplasmic reticulum (RER)* in a plasma cell. The arrows indicate cisterns, in which are sequestered the polypeptides assembled by the ribosomes. ×28,000. (Courtesy of M. Webb.)

Fig. 2.35. *Forms of the RER.* The ribosomes are mostly arranged in chains as polysomes (polyribosomes).

Fig. 2.36. *Smooth (S) and rough (R) ER* (rectangle), as seen in Fig. 2.1.

Fig. 2.37. *Smooth endoplasmic reticulum* (SER) in a section of interstitial cell of the testis, a steroid-producing cell. ×27,000. (Courtesy of J. Thliveris.)

Fig. 2.38. Drawing of the usual three-dimensional configuration of *SER* with interlaced and interconnected tubular channels.

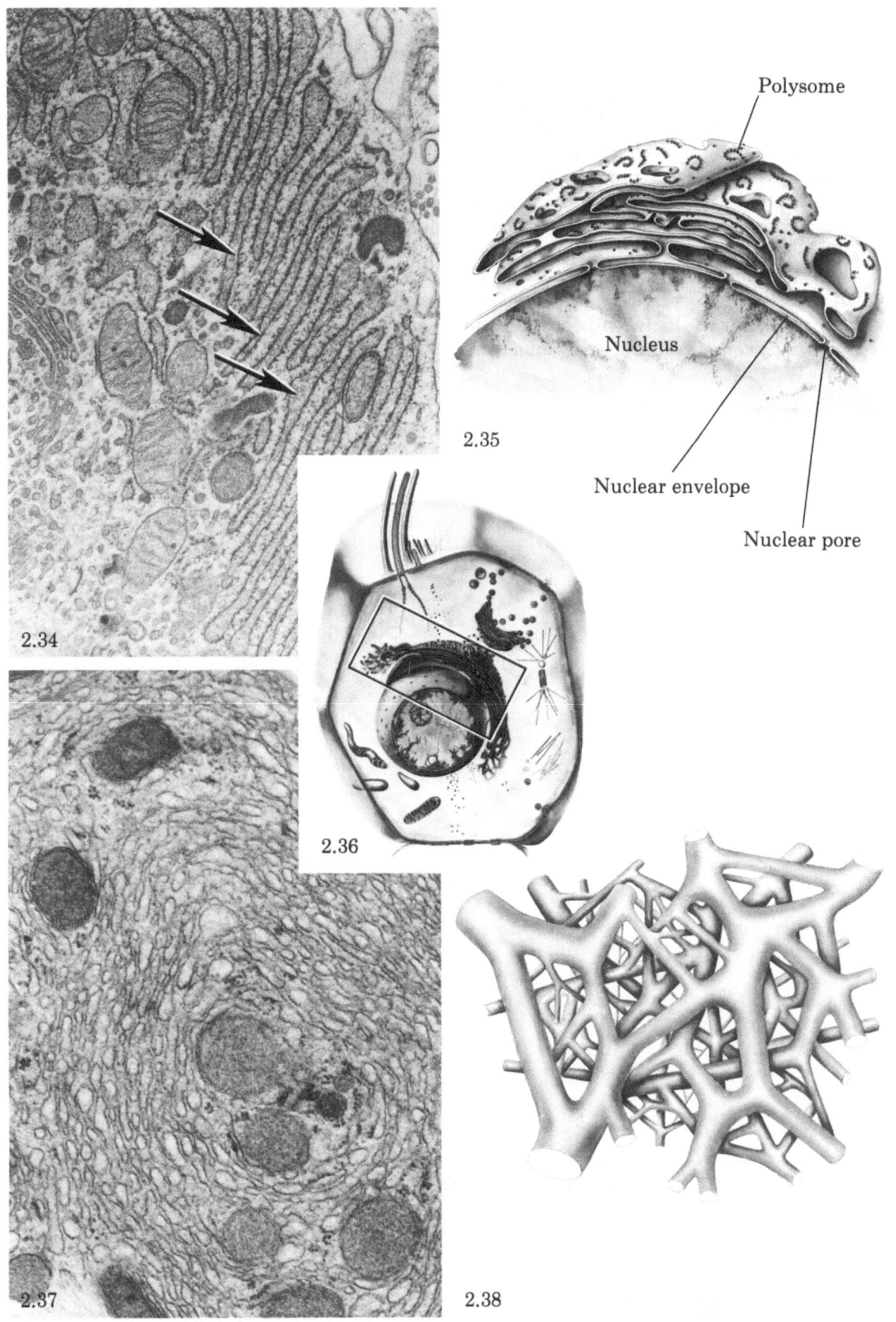

Polysome

Nucleus

Nuclear envelope

Nuclear pore

2.35

2.34

2.36

2.37

2.38

The Golgi apparatus (Figs. 2.39 through 2.41) is a complex of flat membranous sacs and round vesicles. It is visible with the light microscope. It is most highly developed in the cells of glands that secrete proteins (e.g., pancreas, pituitary). Its size is proportional to the rate of secretory activity of the cell. In highly polarized cells, such as those of most glands and of the intestinal epithelium, it is located between the nucleus and the surface from which secretion is to be released. Cells such as those of the liver, which synthesize several products, may contain a number of Golgi complexes. With the electron microscope each complex is seen as an array of flattened concave sacs stacked like saucers. Numerous small vesicles are located along the rims of the sacs and on the convex surface of the stack. Larger vesicles and vacuoles, often containing secretions, are close to the concave surface of the stack. The convex surface is referred to as the forming face and the concave surface the maturing face of the Golgi apparatus. The cisterns are connected by slender tubes or channels.

Fig. 2.39. *Golgi apparatus* (rectangle), as shown in Fig. 2.1.

Fig. 2.40. Electron micrograph showing a section of a *Golgi apparatus.* Approximately ×40,000. (Courtesy of R. S. Decker.)

Fig. 2.41. Drawing of a *Golgi apparatus* indicating its three-dimensional organization.

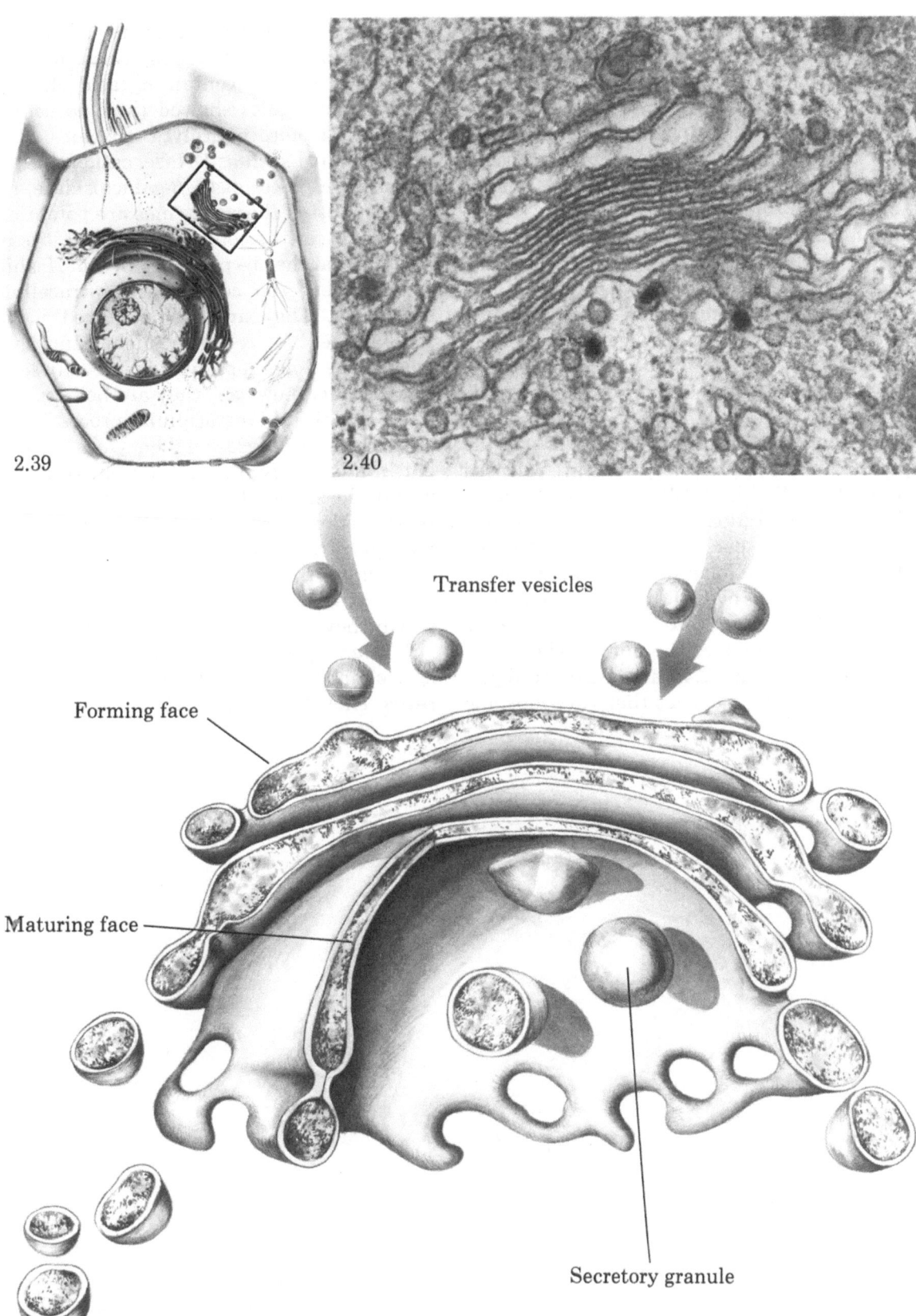

2.39

2.40

Transfer vesicles

Forming face

Maturing face

Secretory granule

As we have seen, polypeptides that have been synthesized by ribosomes and injected into the cisterns of the rough ER are moved to the forming face of the Golgi apparatus by the small, smooth transfer vesicles. Presumably the Golgi apparatus completes the secretion product by binding polypeptide chains together. In some cells that secrete glycoprotein hormones, such as those of the pituitary gland, the carbohydrate portion of the final product is added to the protein in the Golgi apparatus. The product is then concentrated and packaged at the maturing face in the form of storage granules that move toward the apex of the cell. In the secretion process, a granule fuses with the inner surface of the plasma membrane, the membrane breaks down at the point of fusion, and the contents are released from the cell (Fig. 2.42). The membrane of the empty secretion vacuole appears to become a mosaic patch in the plasmalemma. If the product is a lipoprotein, the lipid component is provided by SER, the protein component by RER, and the Golgi combines these substances to produce the final product.

Lysosomes (Figs. 2.43 and 2.44) are digestive vesicles and vacuoles that vary morphologically depending on the nature of the material being digested. Originally lysosomes were defined as vesicles containing acid phosphatase. Later studies showed them to contain at least 12 more hydrolytic enzymes active at an acid pH such as DNase, cathepsins, collagenase, α-glucosidase, β-galactosidase, and others. Most of these enzymes are potentially dangerous for the cell to handle and it is important that they be packaged in some fashion to keep them from contact with intracellular structures. They are manufactured in the RER and sequestered in the membranous vesicles of the Golgi apparatus just as any secretory product; however, they are not exported but rather used in intracellular processes. Not all of the known lysosomal enzymes are present in any one lysosome; different lysosomes within the same cell have different functions. In a complex cell such as the hepatocyte there may be several subclasses of lysosomes, depending on the enzyme or group of enzymes they contain and the different functions which they perform.

Primary lysosomes are the original packages of enzymes derived from the Golgi apparatus. They fuse with vacuoles containing the

Fig. 2.42. *Secretion.* Precursors, processes, and organelles involved in the production of a glycoprotein by a secretory cell.

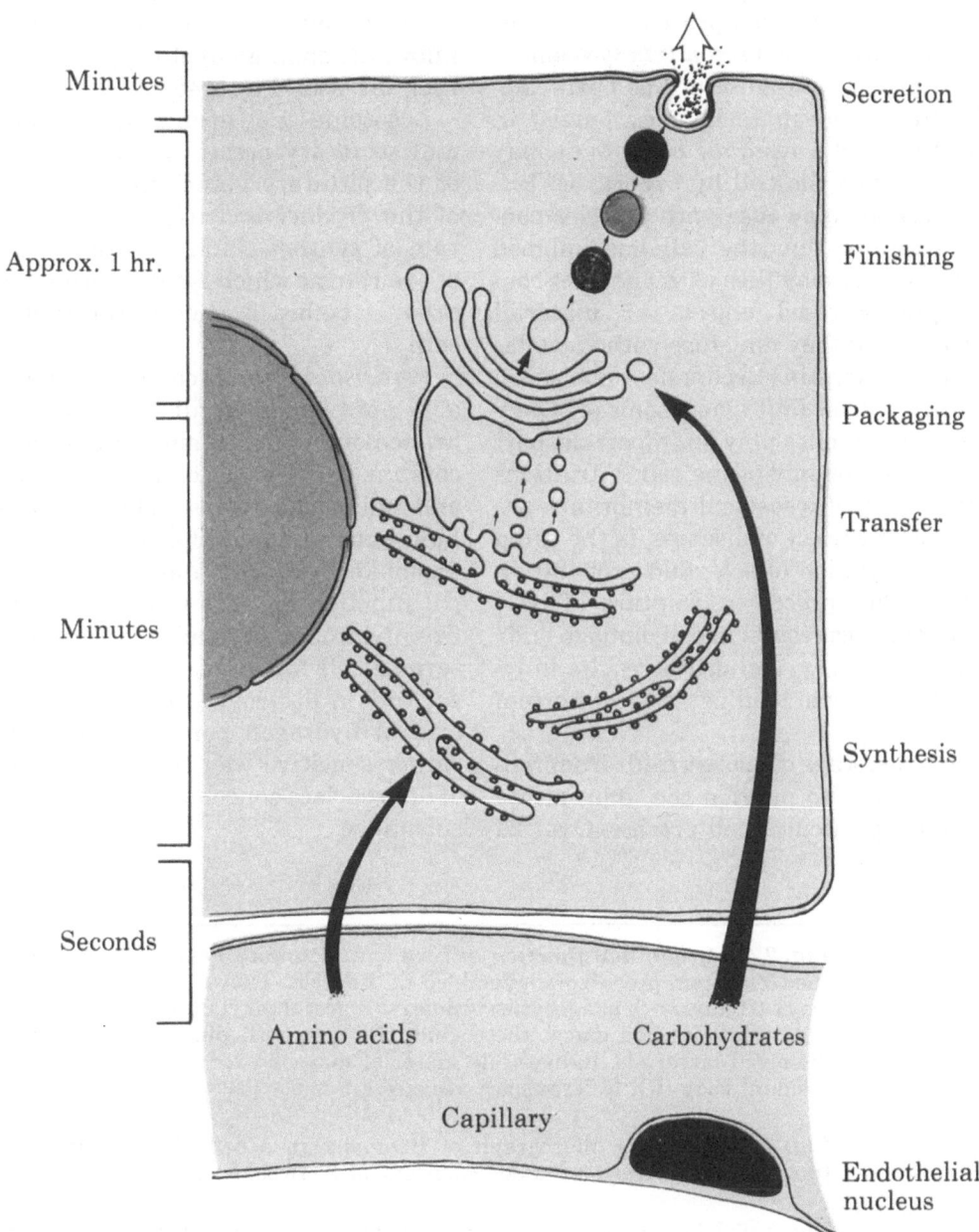

Minutes — Secretion

Approx. 1 hr. — Finishing

Packaging

Transfer

Minutes — Synthesis

Seconds

Amino acids   Carbohydrates

Capillary

Endothelial nucleus

2.42

structures or substances that are to be digested. After fusion, and presumably after the beginning of the digestion process, the resulting packages are termed *secondary* lysosomes. After the process of digestion has been completed, indigestible material may persist in a vacuole termed a *residual body,* or it may be excreted from the cell by exocytosis. Primary lysosomes may fuse with vesicles containing solutions that the cell has imbibed (pinosomes), they may fuse with vacuoles containing phagocytosed objects or material (phagosomes), or they may fuse with vacuoles enclosing degenerating organelles such as aging mitochondria (autophagosomes). Obviously these organelles play an important part in the overall economy of the cell. Variations in permeability of lysosomal membranes are important in a variety of diseases, in the aging process, in radiation effects, and probably in numerous other processes. Rupture of lysosomal membranes results in cell damage and/ or death. Conversely, cell death results in lysosomal breakdown leading to postmortem autolysis.

Lysosomal storage diseases result from failure of lysosomes to provide the appropriate enzyme for a particular cell process. Over 25 different conditions have been identified, each associated with a specific enzyme deficiency. Representative of this group is a condition known as sphingomyelin lipidosis (Niemann-Pick disease) (Fig. 2.45).

Lysosomes may even be involved in the normal secretory process of cells such as those of the pituitary gland. Here the net release of the product is a function not only of the rate of synthesis and of exocytosis, but also of the rate at which lysosomes degrade excess product before it can be released from the cell.

Peroxisomes occur commonly, but are probably not present in all cells. They are membrane-bound vesicles similar to lysosomes, but contain peroxidase, catalase, urate oxidase, and amino acid oxidase. They are particularly numerous in macrophages and in the parenchymal cells of liver and kidney. Their principal function appears to be release of oxygen from hydrogen peroxide. This is necessary in several cell functions and is particularly important in destroying bacteria. Peroxisomes control hydrogen peroxide metabolism in a rather sensitive way so as to assure the cell of appropriate concentrations of this powerful substance.

Fig. 2.43. *Origin and function of lysosomes.* Primary lysosomes (**A**) are formed by the Golgi from precursors assembled in the RER. They have three functional pathways: (**B**) fuse with phagocytic vacuoles to digest their contents; (**C**) engulf degenerating organelles and digest these, and; (**D**) fuse with pinocytotic vesicles to digest dissolved materials. Indigestible material may be exocytosed (**E**) or retained as a residual body (**F**). G, Transport vesicles.

Fig. 2.44. Electron micrograph of *lysosomes* in a cell of a proximal convoluted tubule of the kidney. ×24,300. (Courtesy of R. Brooks.)

Fig. 2.45. Niemann-Pick disease is caused by a deficiency of the enzyme sphingomyelinase which is responsible for cleaving the lipid sphingomyelin, a ubiquitous component of membranes. The lipid progressively accumulates in secondary lysosomes, especially of macrophages. The condition is incurable and progressive. It affects various organs, especially those of the lymphoid system. Involvement of the spleen may cause enlargement to ten times normal size. Cells of the central nervous system may also be involved. **a:** Photograph of bone marrow from a patient with *sphingomyelin lipidosis* (Niemann-Pick disease) shows the enlarged, foamy cytoplasm of several macrophages (arrows). At routine check-up, physical examination of an otherwise normal-appearing infant revealed an enlarged liver. In the course of investigation for this a biopsy of bone marrow established the correct diagnosis. The child later developed severe enlargement of liver and spleen and became troubled by pulmonary infections at the age of three. ×560. **b:** Electron microscopy confirms that vacuoles are engorged *secondary lysosomes,* containing membranous components. ×5050. (Courtesy of R. Brooks.)

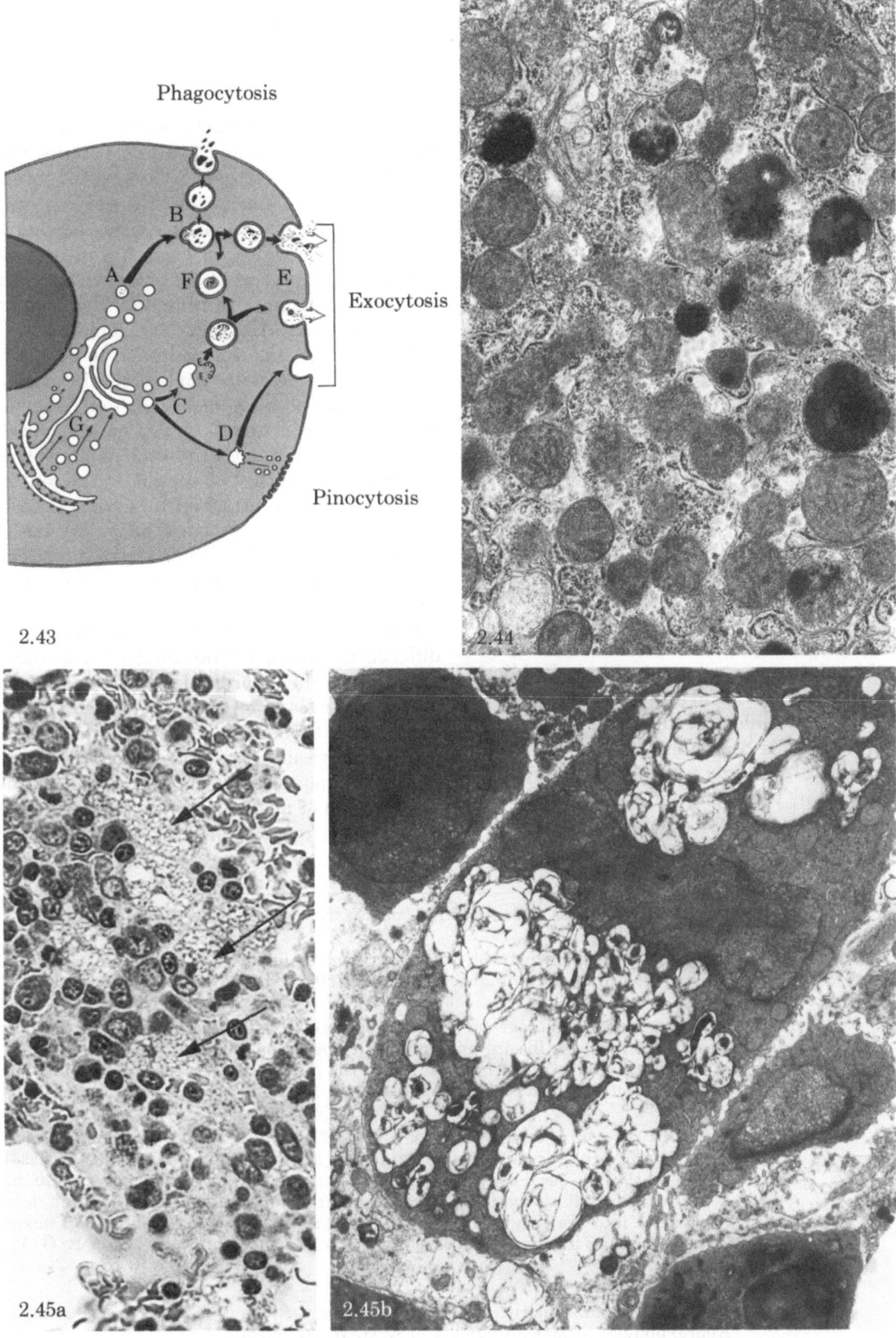

Phagocytosis

Exocytosis

Pinocytosis

2.43

2.44

2.45a

2.45b

44   The Cell

Specializations of the Cell Surface

In addition to specializations at the molecular level which are present in the glycocalyx, highly organized, microscopically visible structural modifications associated with special functions are present on the surfaces of many cells.

Microvilli

Microvilli (Figs. 2.46 through 2.48) are nonmotile finger-like projections from the cell surface. They may vary in number from a few widely scattered structures, as in hepatocytes, to as many as 2000 on the apical surface of an intestinal cell where they may be so crowded as to be visible with the light microscope in the form of a distinct surface layer. Before development of the electron microscope this layer was referred to as a striated or brush border. Such masses of microvilli vastly increased the surface area of the cell and contain enzymes associated with hydrolytic and active transport mechanisms. Microfilaments often extend into microvilli. In some parts of the male reproductive system, some epithelial cells bear numerous very long microvilli termed *stereocilia* which probably function in the secretion and absorption of material involved in maturation of stored spermatozoa.

Cilia

Cilia (Figs. 2.46, 2.48 through 2.50) are motile projections from cell surfaces. They are about twice the diameter and five to ten times the length of microvilli, and of far greater internal complexity. A cell may bear only one cilium, or in some special instances as many as 250. In the center of each cilium lie two microtubules and at its periphery, beneath the plasmalemma, are nine additional pairs of microtubules. All extend the length of the cilium. The nine peripheral pairs in each cilium are aligned with triplets in the corresponding basal body (see *centriole,* above). There are no central tubules in the basal body—only the nine peripheral triplets. The proximal ends of the two tubules in the center of the cilium are attached to a central core at the distal end of the basal body. The basal bodies of some cells have long striated rootlets extending from their proximal ends deep into the cytoplasm.

Ciliary motion is thought to be caused by differential sliding of the tubules along their neighbors. The coordination of movement among the cilia of adjacent cells is such that the beat is sequential rather than synchronous. This results in a wave of motion that effectively moves liquid or particulate material lying on or near the surface of the ciliated tissue. The free end of each cilium has an

Fig. 2.46. *Microvilli* and *cilia* with *basal body* (rectangle), as shown in Fig. 2.1.

Fig. 2.47. Electron micrograph of the apical end of intestinal epithelial cells showing *microvilli* cut in longitudinal sections. ×22,750. (Courtesy of M. Webb.)

Fig. 2.48. Electron micrograph of cross-sections of *microvilli, cilia,* and *basal bodies.* Note the differences in size and complexity between the cilia (large arrows) and microvilli (small arrows). The inset shows the plane of the section. Approximately ×31,000. (Courtesy of R. G. W. Anderson.)

Fig. 2.49. *Structural organization* of a *cilium* and its *basal body.* Note that each pair of peripheral microtubules in the cilium is replaced by a triplet in the basal body; also that the basal body has a slight spiral, and that its triplets are continuous below with the ciliary rootlet. The central pair of microtubules in the cilium does not extend into the basal body. This is the basic pattern. Many cilia, depending on cell function, have a more complex structure. (Based on the work of R. G. W. Anderson.)

Fig. 2.50. Electron micrograph of longitudinal sections of *cilia* from the oviduct. Approximately ×60,000. (Courtesy of R. G. W. Anderson.)

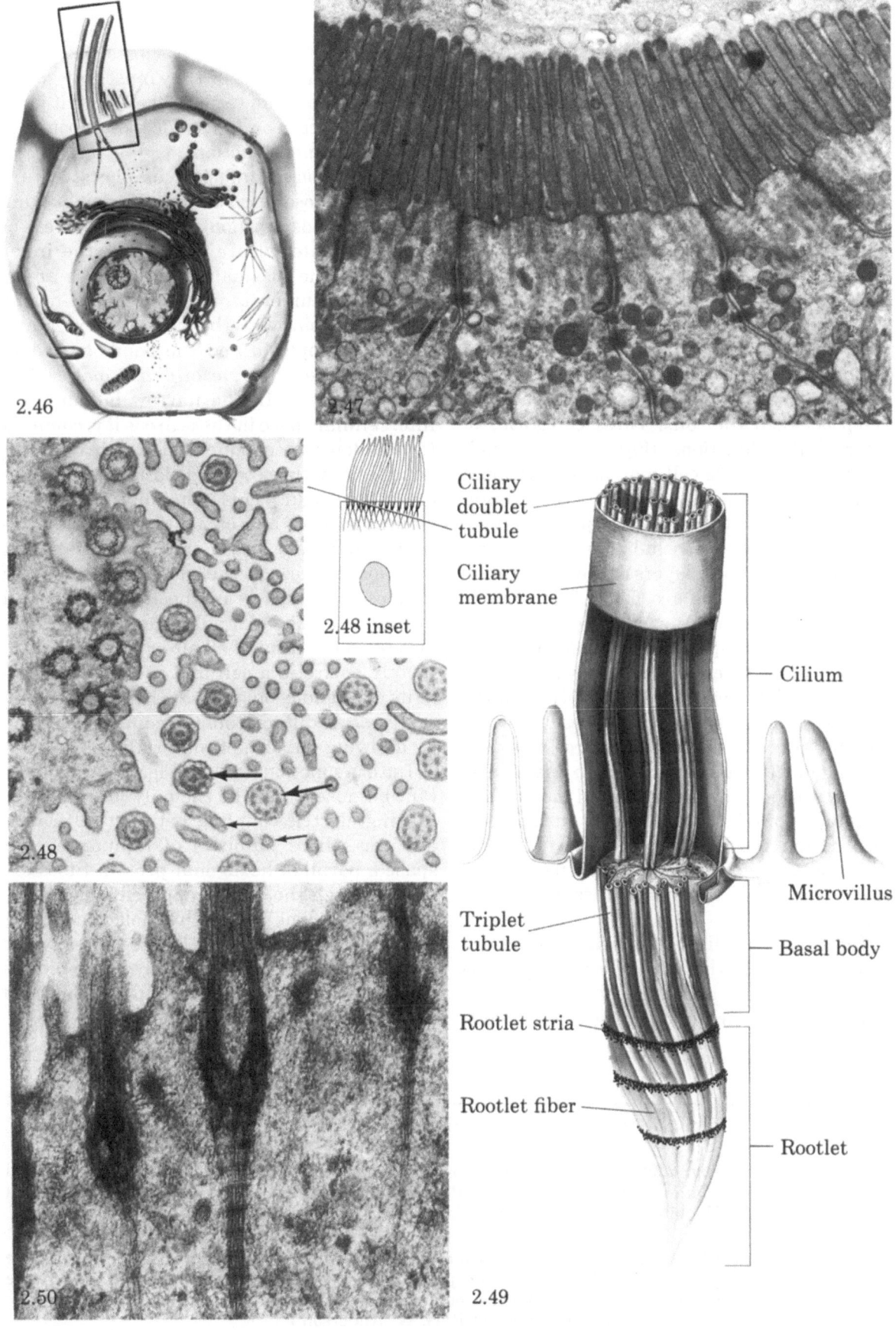

2.46

2.47

2.48 inset

2.48

2.50

Ciliary
doublet
tubule

Ciliary
membrane

Cilium

Microvillus

Triplet
tubule

Basal body

Rootlet stria

Rootlet fiber

Rootlet

2.49

especially dense tuft or crown of glycocalyx. In ciliated cells of the oviduct, this apical tuft is electrically charged and thus, in a sense, can grasp the surface of the egg in its passage toward the uterus and effectively move this large object along its course. It is not yet known whether all cilia possess this property.

Intercellular Junctions

Many cell types maintain more or less permanent contacts with others of their own kind. At these points of contact associations of varying degrees of complexity and intimacy develop between the cells. Three categories of intercellular junctions (Figs. 2.51 through 2.55) exist. A single cell may have junctional structures of a single type or may have representatives of all three types of junction.

THE TIGHT JUNCTION (occluding junction) is an area where the outer layers of the plasmalemmas of the two cells are fused. The area of fusion is indicated by a single dark line in electron micrographs. The distance between the two inner layers of the involved plasmalemmas is less than the sum of the widths of the two membranes. This suggests that the membranes actually fuse. The area of an occluding junction is composed of an anastomosing network of ridges in each cell membrane. The apices of the set of ridges on one cell surface match precisely those of the neighbor cell, and the plasmalemmas are fused along the ridges where the membranes are in contact.

Tight (i.e. occluding) junctions occur in two forms (Fig. 2.52). The *Zonula occludens* forms a belt encircling each cell, attaching it to all of its neighbors and making the layer of cells

into an effective barrier. If substances are to pass such a layer of cells they must go through the cell bodies. The second form of tight junction, the *macula occludens,* is like a spot-weld and offers no obstruction.

THE ADHERING JUNCTION is a complex structure involving close association of neighboring plasmalemmas without fusion. Masses of granular material are located on the inner surface of the plasmalemma in these areas. There are numerous microfilaments in the form of hairpins with the free edges extending into the cytoplasm and the bends buried in the attachment plaque of dense material of the *desmosome.* In the narrow but uniform intercellular space in these areas it is common to find dense or opaque material believed to be protein with associated sialic acid and glycosaminoglycan. This combination of substances may act as a cementing material. Adhering junctions occur in two forms. Most common of these is the *macula adherens* or *desmosome* which is in the form of a small button or plaque. An adhering junction may also be in the form of a belt or zone that completely encircles a cell and attaches it to all of its contiguous neighbors. This is the *zonula adherens.* It differs from the zonula occludens by allowing passage of materials.

THE GAP JUNCTION (NEXUS) (Fig. 2.53) is important because it may be the only junction permitting electric coupling between cells. It is an area where numbers of minute, evenly spaced, parallel, hexagonal protein tubes extend through the closely apposed plasmalemmas and provide direct channels connecting the cytoplasm of the cells. These tubes permit the passage of ions and probably larger biologically important molecules of up to about 2000 daltons.

Fig. 2.51. *Junctional complex* (rectangle), as shown in Fig. 2.1.

Fig. 2.52. The two *forms of intercellular junctions, macula* (or button, left) and *zonula* (or belt, right). (From Poirier J and Ribadeau Dumas J, Review of Medical Histology, p. 23, Fig. 11, WB Saunders, Philadelphia, 1977.)

Fig. 2.53. *Gap junction,* shown by scanning electron microscopy of a freeze-fracture preparation. The area of the junction is just inside the dashed line. The tissue was frozen, then split. We are looking at the surface of one of the fragments. Approximately ×33,000. (Courtesy of R. G. W. Anderson.)

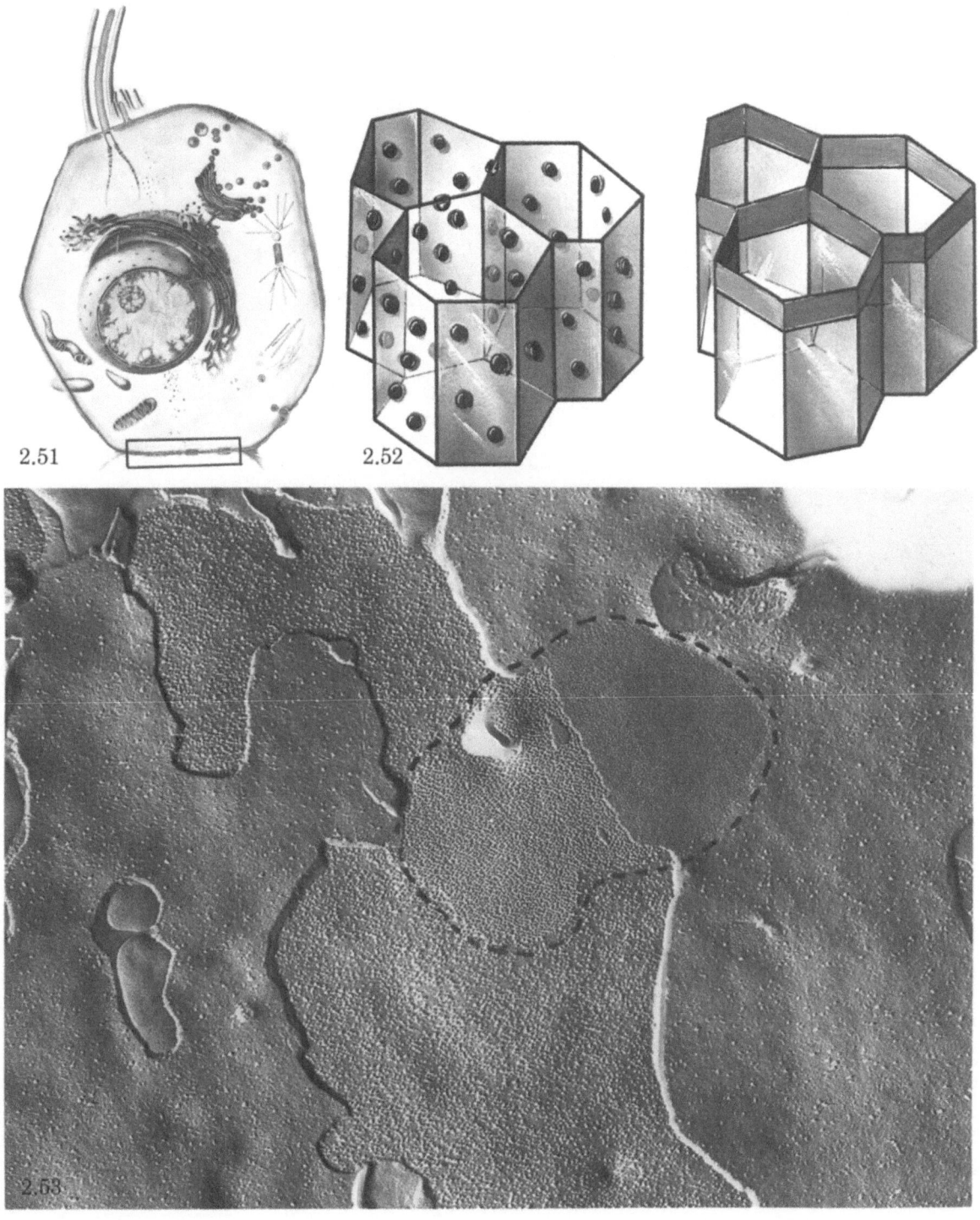

2.51

2.52

2.53

Fig. 2.54. Electron micrograph of *junctional complexes* (bracket) between apical ends of adjacent epithelial cells. ×22,750. (Courtesy of M. Webb.)

Fig. 2.55. The fine structure of a *junctional complex.*

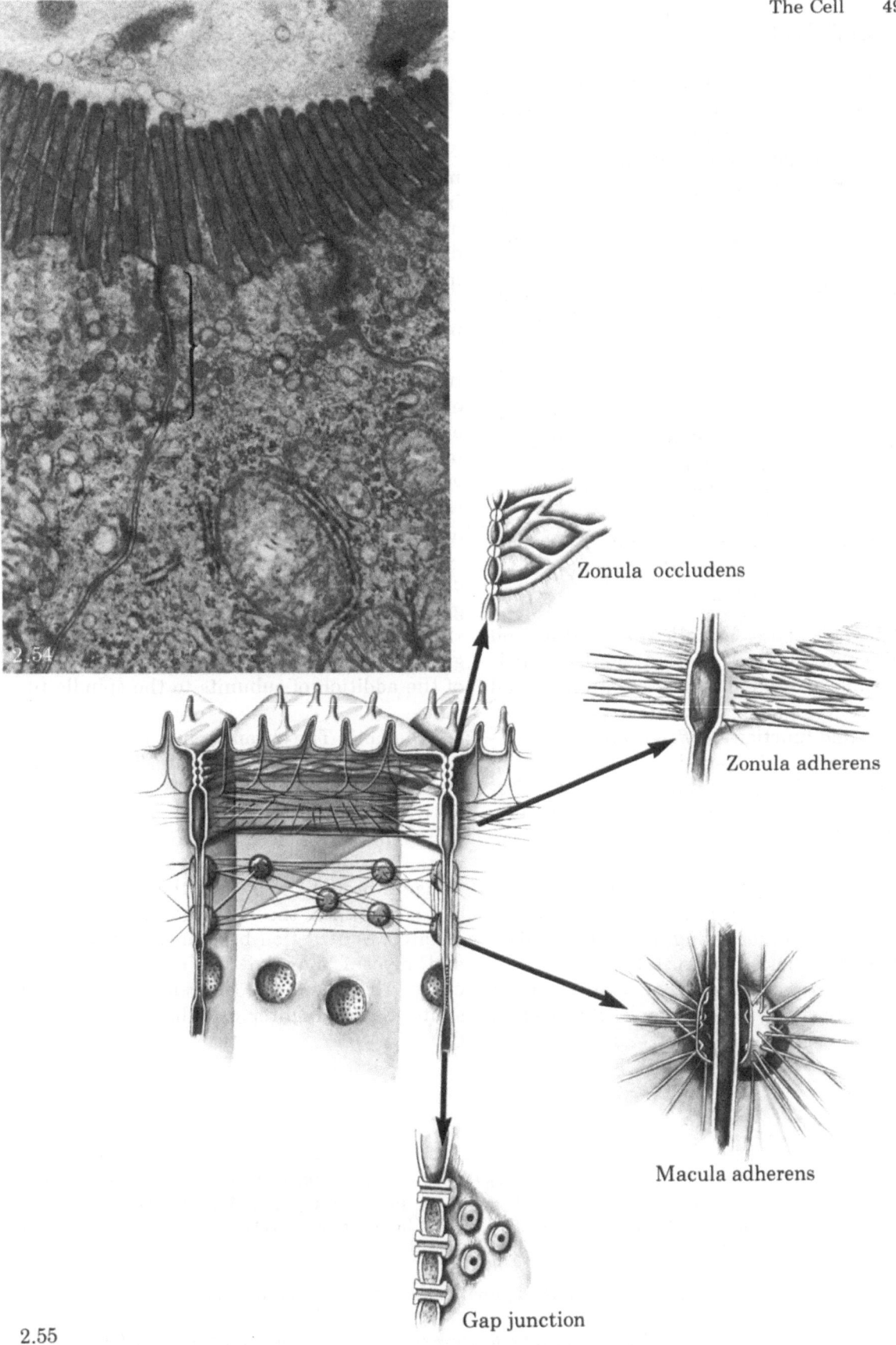

Zonula occludens

Zonula adherens

Macula adherens

Gap junction

2.54

2.55

The Cell Cycle

Not all cells are capable of mitosis. The more highly differentiated (e.g., nerve) cells are *end cells* and as such are unable to divide. Once lost they cannot be replaced. In contrast, the precursors of circulating blood cells and the simpler types of epithelium and connective tissue cells can reproduce seemingly infinitely. Most cell types lie between these two extremes. Many of the less differentiated cells are able to increase their rate of reproduction in response to stress. This is part of the reaction of regeneration after injury and it has many forms.

The period between two mitotic separations of daughter cells constitutes the cell cycle (Figs. 2.56 through 2.60). It has four basic stages. Variation in length of the cycle is largely due to differences in only one of these stages, G_1. However, in some pathologic states, such as psoriasis, the duration of all stages may be altered.

1. G_1. G_1 is the stage following mitosis and is marked by lack of DNA synthesis. It is a time of protein synthesis, growth, and the development of characteristic structure and function—*differentiation*. The remainder of this stage is spent in carrying out the cell's particular function. For human hepatocytes in tissue culture it is about 10 hours long. For end cells this stage terminates with cell death.
2. S. The second stage is that of DNA synthesis, during which the chromosomes are replicated. No other changes are appreciable. This stage lasts for 8 or 9 hours.
3. G_2. This is an interval of little apparent special activity. It is a time of preparation for mitosis and requires 1–2 hours.
4. M (mitosis). In this stage the cell components are physically separated. It requires about 1 hour and consists of four phases.

Prophase. Individual extended euchromatic chromosomes become visible with the light microscope through a process of intensive coiling and recoiling—and therefore shortening and thickening. The centrioles replicate and daughter pairs move to opposite poles of the nucleus. The nucleolus vanishes and the nuclear envelope disappears at the end of this phase.

Metaphase. The protein subunits of microtubules gather in the nuclear region, apparently together with actin and myosin. They are then assembled into discrete microtubules, some of which connect the centromeres with the centrioles. Others extend between centriole pairs. The chromosomes become aligned at the equatorial plate.

Anaphase. The centromeres divide and the chromatids, now separate chromosomes, migrate to the poles. Actin and myosin may assist in this latter process. Some further elongation of the spindle may occur as a result of the addition of subunits to the spindle tubules.

Telophase. The chromosomes now uncoil to return to the euchromatic state. Two new nuclear envelopes are formed from fragments of RER around each mass of chromatin. *Karyokinesis,* nuclear division, is now complete. The division of the cytoplasm, *cytokinesis,* is brought about by the formation of a groove called the cleavage furrow at the equator. Contraction brought about by actin and myosin may be the mechanism that causes this furrow to deepen until the cell splits. Each daughter cell then enters stage G_1.

Fig. 2.56. *The cell cycle.* Phase G_1 is variable in different cell types and in different functional and pathological conditions. Phases S, G_2, and M are relatively constant in all cell types at about 8, 3, and 1 hours, respectively. The width of the band represents the amount of DNA present.

Fig. 2.57. *Normal mitotic figures* in a section of embryonic neural tube. ×560.

Fig. 2.58. *Abnormal mitotic figures* (arrows) in a malignant tumor. ×560.

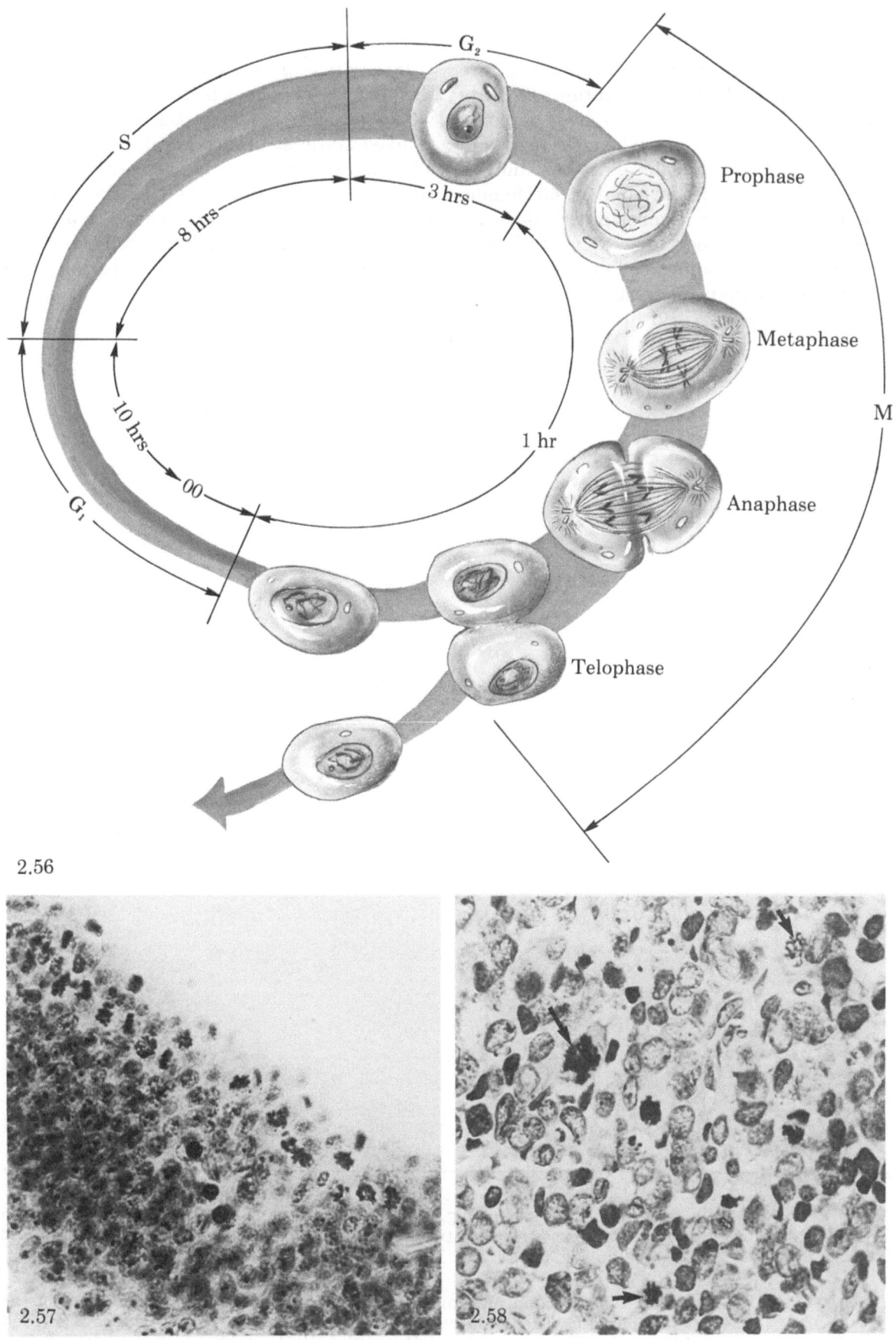

G₂

S

8 hrs

3 hrs

Prophase

Metaphase

1 hr

M

10 hrs

00

Anaphase

G₁

Telophase

2.56

2.57

2.58

Meiosis. The *gametes* (sperm and egg) are special cells, each of which contains 23 chromosomes, half the usual number (haploid). Thus after fertilization, when the egg and sperm nuclei fuse, the cells of the new individual will have the diploid number, 46. Reduction in chromosome number during development of sperm or egg is accomplished by a sequence of two modified cell divisions. These two divisions together constitute meiosis. This process will be described further in Chapter 18.

Integration of activity. We have presented the structure of the cell in a descriptive, and we hope functional, way. But the impression of fixed static structure is falsely simplistic. The picture fails to include the dynamic features of living cells as well as the complex integration of their diverse parts. To appreciate these one should see living cells in action; time-lapse cinematography is especially useful in this regard.

Fig. 2.59. *DNA replication.* In the lower drawing, strands of the double helix (left) are diagrammed as separating. The bases thus exposed are then matched with complementary bases forming two new helices (right). (From DuPraw EJ. Cell and Molecular Biology, p. 559, Fig. 18.11B, Academic Press, New York, 1968.)

Fig. 2.60. Reproduction and migration of the *centrioles* and the structure of the *mitotic apparatus.* (Redrawn with permission from Fig. 19.1 in DuPraw EJ. Cell and Molecular Biology. Academic Press, New York, 1968.)

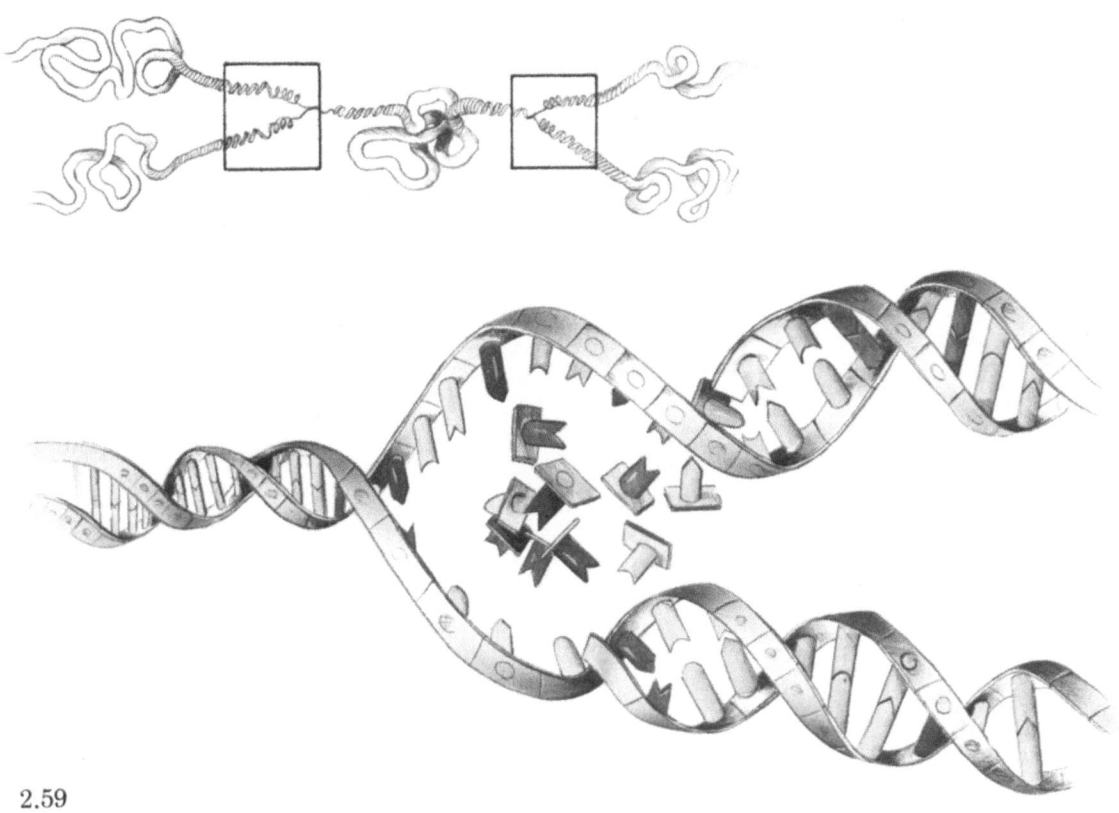

2.59

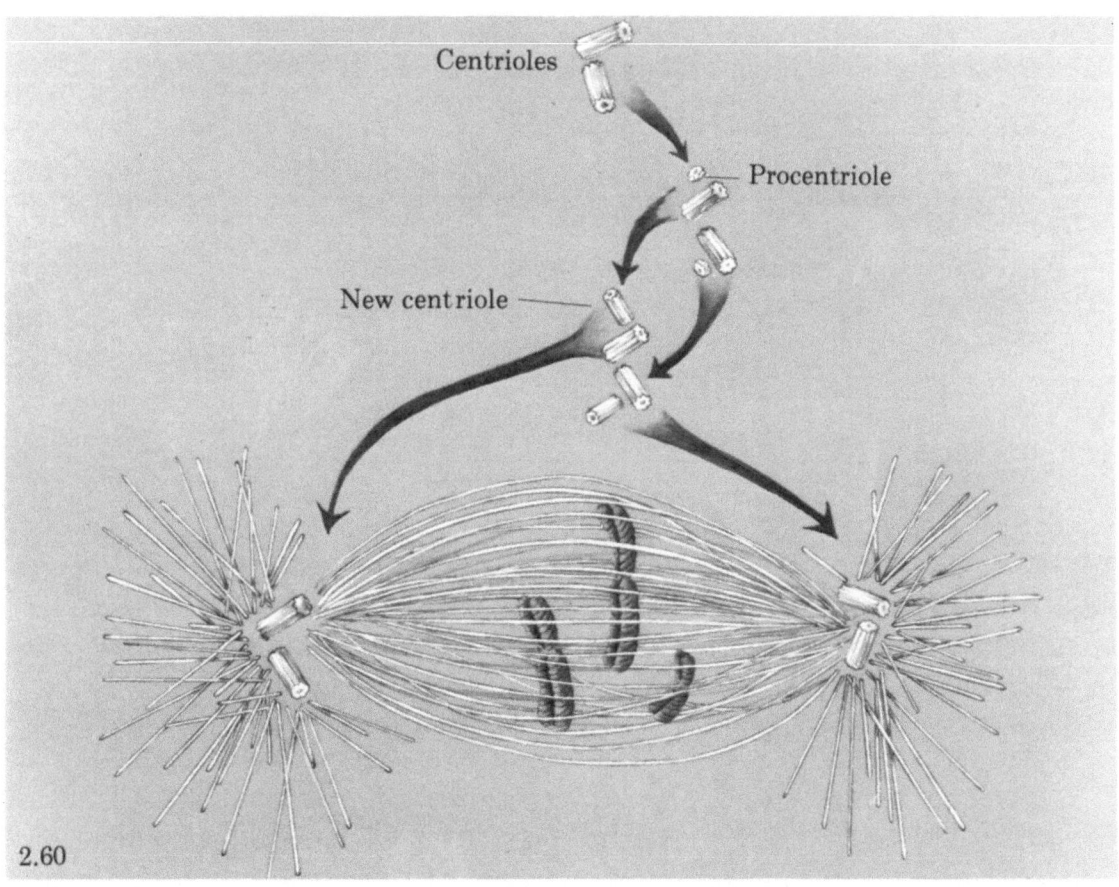

2.60

3 Epithelium

General Characteristics

Epithelial tissue covers surfaces (e.g., skin), lines cavities (e.g., stomach). The individual cells are extremely cohesive. They are also firmly attached to a basement membrane that separates them from the tissue beneath. There is little if any external matrix (intercellular substance) and no fibrous material between the cells. Because they are located at interfaces between entirely different environments, epithelial cells tend to be strikingly polarized. A basal end is firmly attached to a basement membrane that separates them from the tissue beneath and to the connective tissue support; an apical end faces the lumen or free surface. This polarization preserves the internal milieu of the body and prevents entropy by establishing and maintaining the necessary concentration gradients across epithelial membranes. As will be seen, epithelium may demonstrate considerable specialization related to function. In organs such as the intestines, epithelium may have surface modifications related to secretion and absorption. In other areas it may be thick and tough for protective purposes.

Epithelia are usually classified according to two criteria (Fig. 3.1): (1) The number of layers of cells: simple (one layer), stratified (more than one layer), pseudostratified (apparently, but not actually, more than one layer); and (2) The form of the individual cells: squamous, cuboidal, or columnar.

Most epithelia are avascular, i.e., contain no blood vessels. Epithelium derives nutrition from vessels across various intervening membranes. Its superficial position allows shedding and replacement of cells in an orderly and regular fashion by division of remaining cells. There is a continuing cycle of cell division, maturation, death, and replacement in the less differentiated types of epithelium. The more differentiated varieties are more permanent and, if lost, may be replaced only with less specialized cells if at all. For example, gastric chief cells are less likely to be replaced after loss than are mucus-secreting cells of gastric pits in the condition of chronic gastritis.

The basement membrane consists of two layers, the basal lamina and the reticular lamina. The former is applied to the deep surface of the epithelium, and varies from 50 to 75 nm in thickness; thus it is not ordinarily visible with the electron microscope. The reticular lamina lies deep to the basal lamina, is variable but much thicker, and may be clearly seen with the light microscope.

With the electron microscope, the basal lamina is seen to consist of delicate fibrils in a fine granular matrix. This lamina is produced by the epithelial cells; it contains collagen and proteoglycans. The reticular lamina consists of reticular fibers (see Chapter 4) in a dense amorphous matrix of glycosaminoglycans and proteins. This lamina may be made clearly visible either by impregnating its fibers with silver or by staining the matrix with the PAS reaction.

The term basement membrane was introduced long before the advent of the electron microscope to name the structure visible with the light microscope. Thus the terms basal lamina and basement membrane are not interchangeable in spite of current looseness in their usage. Basal lamina and reticular lamina vary independently in different physiologic and pathologic states and should be understood to be subdivisions of the basement membrane.

Types of Epithelium

Simple Epithelia

SIMPLE SQUAMOUS (Figs. 3.1 through 3.3) is the simplest type of epithelium. It consists of a single layer of flattened cells adhering to a supporting surface and facing a liquid, or at least moist, environment. Each cell is shorter in the apicobasal than in the side-to-side dimension. In some instances the individual cells may be so extremely flattened and broadened that, except for the nuclei, which are horizontal and elliptical in this form, they are almost invisible in histologic sections.

This is a very useful and widespread epithelium; it lines all blood vessels (where it is referred to as endothelium). The linings of capillaries constitute a huge surface area and the simple squamous epithelium in these is adapted for exchange of gases, nutrients, metabolic products, and wastes. It is not just a filter but is also involved in several forms of active transport.

Simple squamous epithelium also lines the serous body cavities (where it is called mesothelium). It is the only tissue thin enough for effective transport of respiratory gases, and therefore it lines the alveolar spaces of the lungs. It also constitutes a portion of the nephron in the kidney. The delicate, thin, mesothelial surfaces are easily destroyed by many processes (infections, surgical manipulation, etc.) and may then be replaced by connective tissue that forms adhesions often extensive enough to obliterate spaces as large as the abdominal cavity and cause intermittent or irreversible bowel obstruction. When endothelial surfaces of blood vessels are damaged, thrombosis (precipitation of various components of blood) is likely to result.

Fig. 3.1. *Basic epithelial types.* Note that on the cut surface of all types some cells appear to lack nuclei. The reason for this is revealed in each example shown, one nucleus not having been exposed by the knife. In a histologic section, which is a thin transparent slice, not all cells may be seen to contain nuclei. Cell size, nuclear size, and thickness of the section all affect this result.

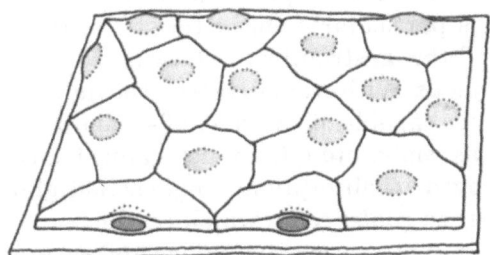

Simple Squamous

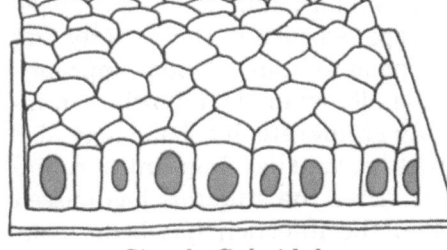

Simple Cuboidal

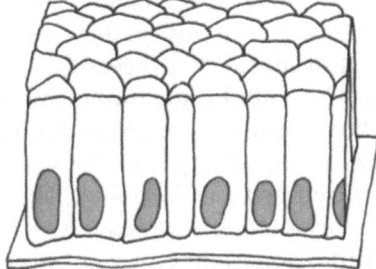

Simple Columnar

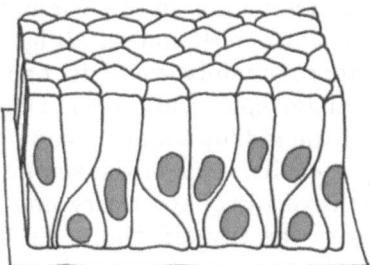

Pseudostratified

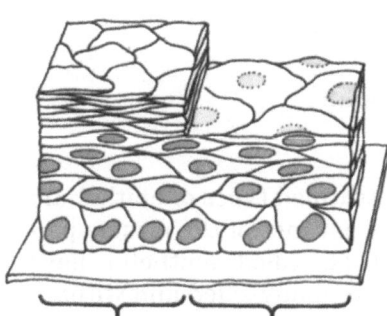

Keratinized   nonkeratinized
stratified squamous

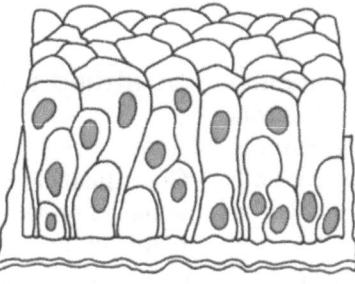

Transitional

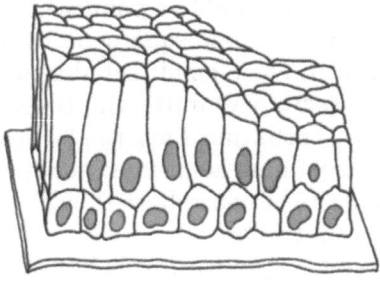

Stratified columnar cuboidal

3.1

For our initial practical understanding, simple squamous epithelium is a basic, unspecialized cell type. As such it may rapidly and markedly respond to injury. Under appropriate stimulation, for example, following an infection, it may proliferate. Its shape may also change from its normal flat shape into a round or a tall cell. After the stimulus has passed (that is, when the infection has been overcome), if a cavity still remains, this again acquires a lining similar to the original.

SIMPLE CUBOIDAL epithelial cells (Figs. 3.1 and 3.4) are approximately equal in height and width and have spherical nuclei. They make up most of the kidney tubules, many glandular secretory cells, some of the smaller gland ducts, the covering of the ovary and the parenchyma of the thyroid gland. As with almost all cells, one must remember that the external form at any given time may be related to functional status and to spatial relationships with other cells. In some glands, the accumulation of secretion in the lumen may distend the gland to a point where the epithelium may become squamous rather than cuboidal. In some small tubules and glandular acini (secretory units), the several secretory cuboidal cells may have the form of pyramids, or at least have somewhat narrow apical ends facing the lumen, where they are crowded between neighbors.

SIMPLE COLUMNAR epithelial cells (Figs. 3.1 and 3.5) are relatively tall with nuclei that vary in shape from spherical to elliptical. This type is particularly characteristic of the lining of the gastrointestinal tract below the esophagus. Within small bowel, the individual cells are capable of a variety of specializations such as: elaborate microvillous apical surface employed in absorption; single-celled glands known as *goblet cells*, which produce a large droplet of mucus occupying most of the apical cytoplasm; protein-synthesizing systems for the production of serous enzyme solutions; and endocrine-synthesizing systems involved in the control of digestive processes.

Both simple cuboidal and simple columnar epithelium have wide ranges of functional activity and both may or may not be very specialized. As discussed in Chapter 2, the various cellular organelles, surface structures, and intercellular junctions carry out different specific actions. The level of each activity is likely to be reflected by the relative prominence of the particular structure responsible.

Stratified Epithelia

Classification of stratified types of epithelium is based on the appearance of the most superficial cells. Most stratified epithelia have deeper cells that are many-sided and without a specific form.

Fig. 3.2. *Simple squamous epithelium of the peritoneum seen from above.* Photo is taken from a tissue spread, not a cut section. The mesothelial cells on the surface appear like a pavement. ×680.

Fig. 3.3. *Simple squamous epithelium of the peritoneum seen in section.* The epithelium is a very thin layer (arrows) on the surface. In many sections of peritoneum the nuclei are scarce and the layer may appear nonexistent by this method. ×400.

Fig. 3.4. *Simple cuboidal epithelium of the kidney.* This shows tubules (epithelium-lined tubes) composed of two different cell types, both simple cuboidal. The plane of the section has cut some tubules only tangentially and the lumen is not apparent in all. ×400.

Fig. 3.5. *Simple columnar epithelium.* It is not so readily apparent in all areas of the photo whether this epithelium is simple, stratified or pseudostratified (see below). Cutting of any simple epithelium in any plane other than perpendicular to its surface will appear to add both height and stratification. ×400.

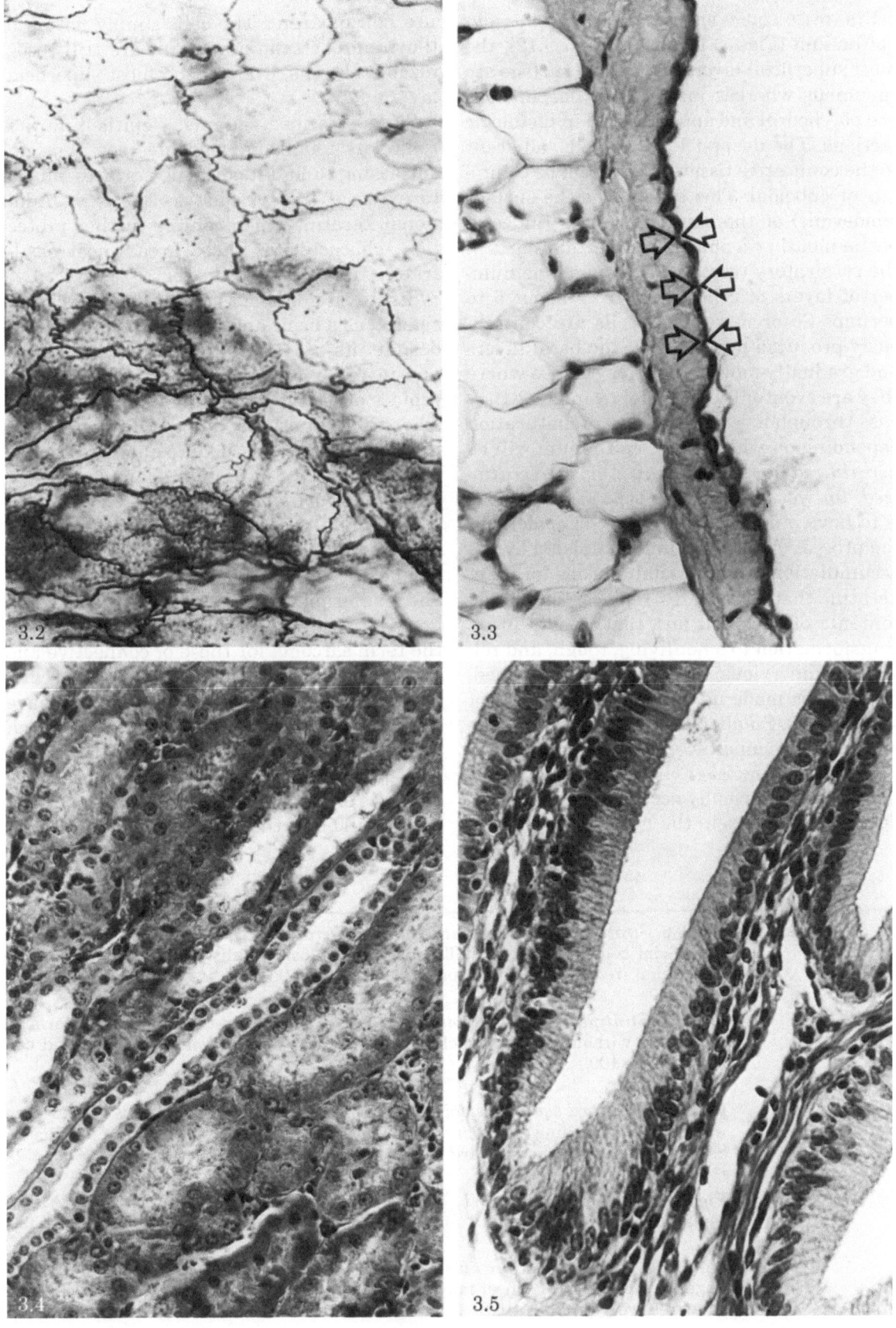

STRATIFIED SQUAMOUS. In *stratified squamous* epithelium (Figs. 3.1, 3.6, through 3.12), the most superficial layers on the free surface are squamous whereas most of the deeper cells are polyhedral and appear round in histologic sections. The deepest layer of cells, adjacent to the connective tissue, may in fact be columnar or cuboidal. This type forms the surface (epidermis) of the skin, the lining (mucosa) of the mouth, esophagus and certain parts of the respiratory tract and the anus. The number of layers of cells varies from about 5 to perhaps 25 or more. New cells are continuously produced by mitosis in the basal layers and gradually move to the free surface where they are eventually lost. As they migrate they pass through a series of stages of maturation depending on whether the epithelium will be *keratinized* for dry surfaces, or *nonkeratinized,* for wet areas. If this type of epithelium is to have a dry surface, as in the epidermis, the process of maturation is completed by the accumulation of a special fibrous protein, keratin, that eventually replaces all of the contents of each cell and that results in its transformation to a nonliving, tough, and relatively impervious plate that is finally shed. Dandruff is made up of the larger clumps of these plates. Smaller masses are not noticeable without a microscope. If the epithelium is faced with a moist environment, keratinization does not normally occur, and the sharply demarcated stages in the maturation process are not apparent. The cells simply flatten as they approach the lumen but are still recognizable as cells, even in the most superficial layers.

Since stratified squamous epithelium is a relatively tough and durable coat, it is not surprising to find it covering surfaces subject to external injury, such as the skin. Additional keratin, which confers further protection, characterizes those areas most easily traumatized (soles of the feet).

Stratified squamous epithelium may be considered as a basic and perhaps primitive type despite its relatively complex appearance, and in response to chronic irritation it may replace other types of epithelium in locations where it is not usually found. The transformation of one type of tissue into another is called *metaplasia.* This particular example is called *squamous metaplasia* (Fig. 3.9).

Of all the epithelial types stratified squamous is the most likely to undergo malignant neoplastic change (uncontrolled proliferation and extension, i.e., cancer. The term carcinoma is used for epithelial malignancies and the term sarcoma for those of connective and some other tissues. Cancer includes both categories). In this state the involved cells have certain recognizable characteristics by which the diagnosis is made. These include variations in nuclear size and shape, and excessive amounts of chromatin. Metaplasia and malignancy will be further discussed in Chapter 20.

Fig. 3.6. *Stratified squamous epithelium, nonkeratinized, from the vagina.* The more superficial cells are flattened. The basal layer continually replenishes this tissue as the mature cells are shed from the surface. ×100.

Fig. 3.7. *Stratified squamous epithelium, keratinized from the skin.* The superficial layers are without nuclei (anucleate) and consist only of heavily keratinized cell remnants. ×100.

Fig. 3.8. *Stratified squamous epithelium, smear from the vagina.* This preparation was made by touching the slide to the epithelial surface to pick up the loose cells. Several rod-shaped bacteria are also visible. Papanicolaou technique. ×480.

Fig. 3.9. *Squamous metaplasia of cervix of uterus.* Squamous epithelium (**A**) has replaced some of the normal columnar epithelium (**B**) of the cervical glands. ×320.

Fig. 3.10. *Variations of stratified squamous epithelium.* Often all of the following stages in the genesis of cancer may be found in one specimen: **a:** normal. **b:** hyperplastic (excessively proliferating). **c:** malignant noninvasive. **d:** malignant invasive.

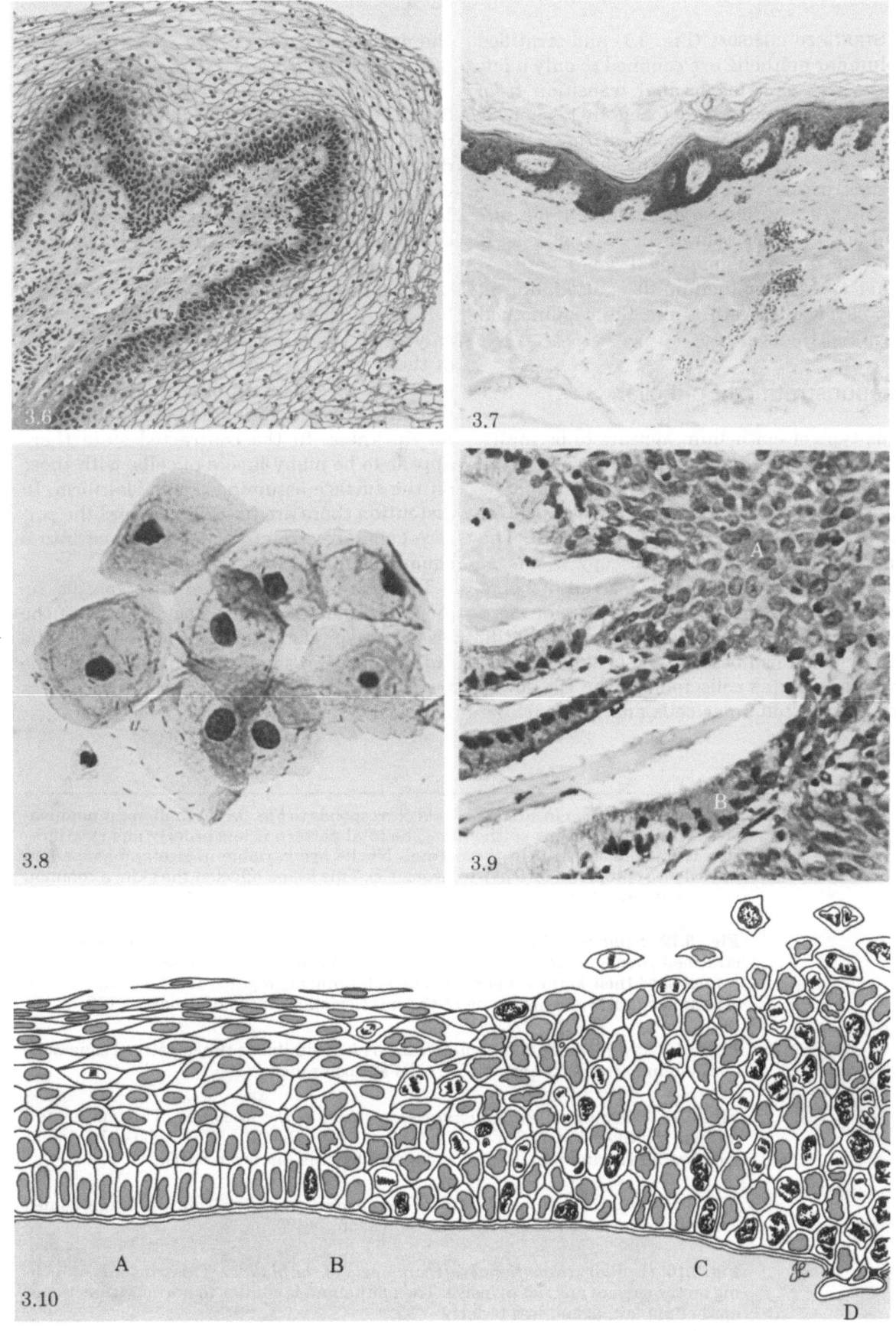

3.6

3.7

3.8

3.9

3.10

STRATIFIED CUBOIDAL (Fig. 3.1) and stratified columnar epithelia are confined to only a few sites. The zones of gradual transition from one type of epithelium to another, such as in the anal canal, may possess these types. They are also present in the ducts of sweat glands, breast, and some other glands.

STRATIFIED COLUMNAR epithelium (Figs. 3.1 and 3.13) lines the larger ducts of glands. It may be found in junctional zones between other types of epithelium. It is also found in the cavernous urethra and the conjunctival fornix of the eye.

Pseudostratified Epithelia

This type of epithelium appears to be multi-layered. However, all cells are attached to the basement membrane, although this cannot be appreciated without electron microscopy. Not all of the cells reach the free surface. The impression from light microscopy is one of such crowding that nuclei, instead of being in a single row, are squeezed into two or more levels, giving the false impression of stratification. The term basal cell is usually applied to those shorter cells found near the lower ends of the columnar cells and not reaching the surface. There are two important types of pseudostratified epithelium.

PSEUDOSTRATIFIED COLUMNAR EPITHELIUM (Figs. 3.1 and 3.14) occurs in some of large glandular ducts and in the male urethra. Ciliated pseudostratified epithelium is characteristic of the conducting portions of the respiratory system. In the tracheobronchial tree enteroendocrine cells may be present in the basal layer, and there are numerous goblet cells.

TRANSITIONAL EPITHELIUM (Figs. 3.1, 3.15, and 3.16) lines the urinary tract from the renal calyces to the distal end of the urethra. All of these structures are capable of significant reduction or expansion of their internal surface area and the lining adjusts by changing its thickness. In the contracted state there appear to be many layers of cells, with those on the surface assuming a cuboidal form. In distention there are fewer layers and the surface cells are stretched and flattened into a squamous form.

Two examples of epithelia in specific regions that do not fit these categories are the visceral layer of glomerular epithelium in the kidney and the seminiferous tubules of the testes. These will be described in Chapters 15 and 18, respectively.

Fig. 3.11. *Carcinoma in situ.* This field corresponds to Fig. 3.10C, malignant noninvasive stratified squamous epithelium. The total pattern is less orderly and stratification is less precise than in the normal. Nuclei are variable in size and shape and have dense chromatin (are hyperchromatic). This lesion affected the skin, a common site of cancer. ×100.

Fig. 3.12. *Squamous "pearls" in a lung cancer.* These are groups of malignant stratified squamous cells that have invaded the underlying tissue and therefore cannot shed their keratinized cells. The enlarging aggregates develop series of concentric laminations. This is one of the most common types of cancer. ×100.

Fig. 3.13. *Stratified columnar epithelium.* This is similar to thin stratified squamous epithelium except that the surface cells are columnar. ×560.

Fig. 3.14. *Pseudostratified columnar epithelium of the bronchus.* This epithelium appears stratified, but appropriate techniques show that all cells reach the basement membrane. The luminal surface is covered by cilia (arrows). ×400.

Fig. 3.15. *Transitional epithelium of the urinary bladder.* Note the large domed cells at the surface, which are often binucleate. ×400.

Fig. 3.16. *Papillary transitional cell carcinoma of the bladder.* This cancer is branching on the surface and not invasive. The epithelium is similar to normal transitional epithelium but, again, less orderly. ×85.

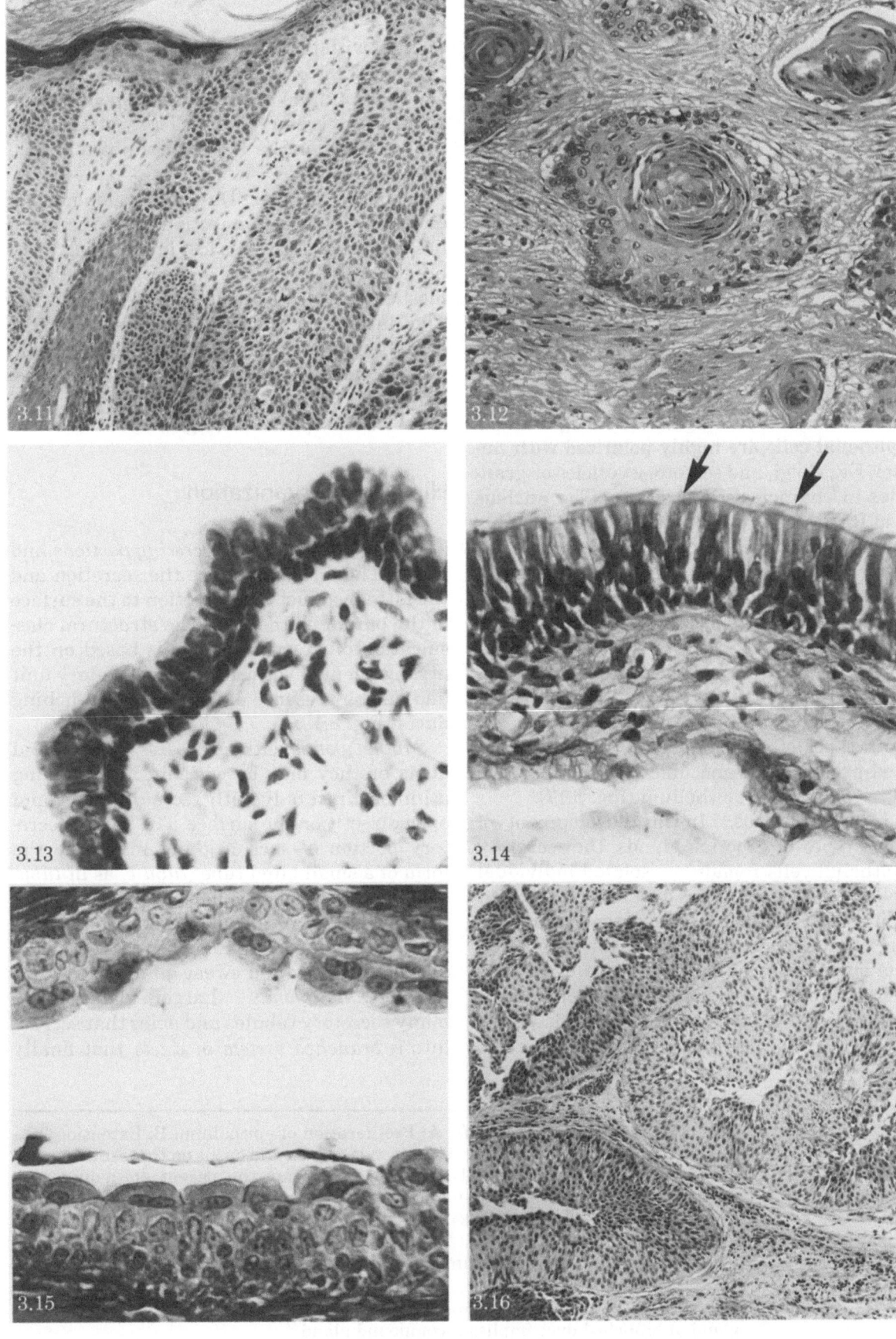

Glands

Introduction

Glands are groups of epithelial cells that synthesize and secrete specific products. *Exocrine glands* secrete fluids through ducts into lumens. *Endocrine glands* are ductless and release their secretions into the circulation. Precursors of the secretory product are absorbed by endocytosis, the product is synthesized in the RER, usually stored for various lengths of time in cytoplasmic vesicles derived from the Golgi apparatus, and finally extruded from the cell by exocytosis. Most glandular epithelial cells are highly polarized with nuclei, ER, Golgi, and secretory vesicles or granules in characteristic positions. The nucleus and RER are located basally. The Golgi apparatus is ordinarily located just apical (that is, toward the secreting surface) with respect to the nucleus. The secretory storage vesicles or granules are generally apical in position.

Development

Both types of glands develop from the localized proliferation and differentiation of cells of an embryonic epithelium (Fig. 3.17).

EXOCRINE GLANDS. In the development of some types of exocrine glands, the secretory epithelial cells remain as isolated individual cells or scattered groups of cells in the parent epithelium (Fig. 3.18). Their secretion is simply emptied into the general lumen or onto the surface of the epithelium. In other exocrine glands, the glandular epithelial mass is deeply buried in the connective tissue beneath the originating sheet and retains a connection with the parent epithelium. This connecting stalk of cells hollows out to become the *duct* and the cell mass hollows out to become the secretory units (*acini* or *tubules*). The sweat gland is an example of a simple tubular gland.

ENDOCRINE GLANDS. During development of endocrine glands, connection with the original epithelial surface is lost and the cell mass breaks up into clusters and cords of cells enmeshed in a network of capillaries (Fig. 3.17). The lumens are actually obliterated in most of the endocrine glands, and, strictly speaking, the term epithelium no longer applies. However, we may persist in this usage because of the epithelial origin.

Histologic Organization

EXOCRINE GLANDS have *secreting portions* and *ducts*. The former produce the secretion and the latter conduct this secretion to the surface of the parent epithelium. The structural classification of exocrine glands is based on the arrangement of the cells in the secretory unit and on the presence or absence of branching ducts (Fig. 3.19).

Simple glands either possess unbranched ducts or they may be without ducts, having a lumen lined only with secretory cells, and open directly on the surface. The hollow secretory portion of such a gland may take the form of a small blind tube (*tubule,* as in *tubular glands*) or of a spherical *acinus* (as in *acinar glands*), or a combination (as in *tubuloacinar glands*). Tubules may be very long, as in the kidney and sweat glands.

Compound glands. Larger glands have many secretory tubules and acini that secrete into a *branched system of ducts* that finally

---

Fig. 3.17. *Development of glands.* **A:** Proliferation of epithelium. **B:** Extension into the underlying connective tissue. **C:** Lumen is formed and opens on the free surface—an exocrine gland. **D:** The cell mass separates from the parent epithelium—an endocrine gland. **E:** Lumens are not formed (as in most endocrine glands). **F:** Lumens are formed but without openings to the surface (as in the thyroid).

Fig. 3.18. A *unicellular gland* in simple columnar epithelium.

Fig. 3.19. *Types of exocrine glands.* A single unbranched duct implies a simple gland; a branched duct implies a compound gland.

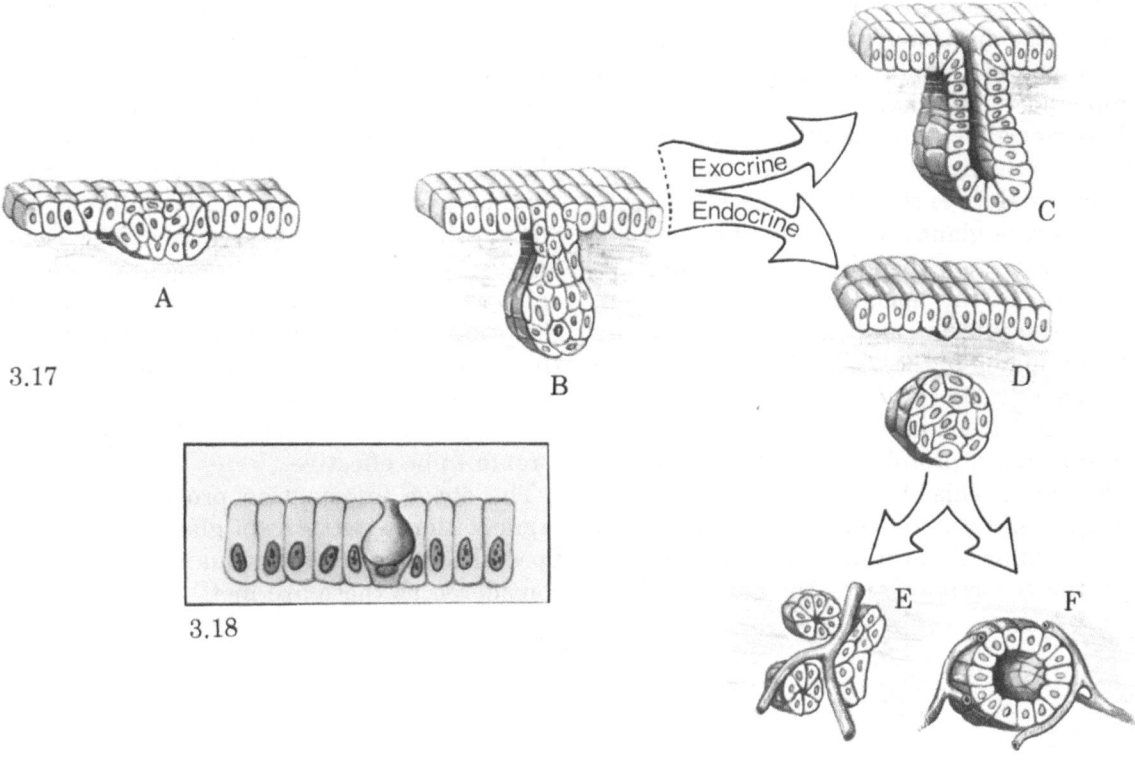

3.17

3.18

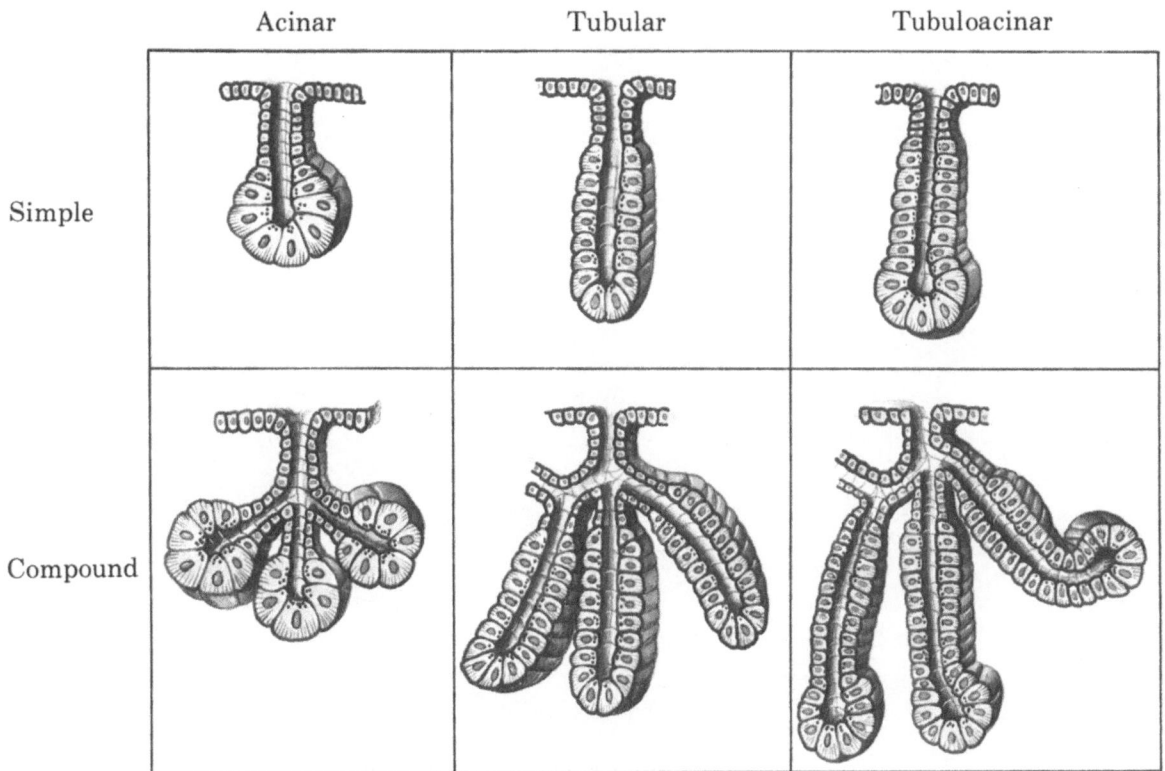

3.19

empty their secretion by a single common duct. These are compound glands. They may be compound tubular, compound acinar, or compound tubulocinar.

Exocrine glands are sometimes additionally characterized by the manner in which the secretory product is shed by the secreting cell. In *merocrine* glands, which are the most numerous, secretory vacuoles fuse with the plasmalemma of the apical surface of the cell, open to the exterior, and empty their contents into the lumen of the gland (for example, the pancreas). In *apocrine* glands, the secretory product is pushed into a bulge in the cell surface forming a protuberance into the lumen of the gland. This bleb is then pinched off as a droplet of secretion enclosed in a coat of plasmalemma (for example, breast). In a third type, the *holocrine* glands, the entire cell becomes distended with accumulated secretion, dies and is shed in its entirety into the lumen (for example, sebaceous gland).

ENDOCRINE GLANDS exhibit two patterns of organization. Most of them are composed of clumps and cords of secretory cells in close contact with a rich network of capillaries into which their secretion is passed. In some glands, the cells are arranged in hollow spheres, *follicles*, in the lumens of which their secretion is stored (for example, thyroid). In this instance the follicle is not an exit route but a temporary storage chamber. The secretion product must be passed into the blood stream to be effective.

The above information provides the basic organizational patterns of glands in general. Special features of individual glands will be considered as these are met.

4 Connective Tissue

The basic function of connective tissue is to bind together and compartmentalize other tissues and organs. It underlies epithelial sheets and their outgrowths or ingrowths, and in these positions it is important in controlling the passage of fluids and of infections across membranes. It also provides pathways into organs for vessels and nerves and fills potential spaces between adjacent structures. In addition, as will be seen in the next chapter, it forms rigid supporting columns, blocks, and plates of bone and cartilage for the body as a whole. In contrast to epithelium, the cells of connective tissue are widely separated by varying quantities of intercellular material.

Connective tissue occurs in a wide variety of forms as will be seen, but these all consist of cells and extracellular fibers embedded in an amorphous ground substance. This semi-fluid intercellular material (the ground substance) allows transport of cells, small particles, and oxygen and carbon dioxide in solution. Thus connective tissue also functions as a transport medium. One common feature of all connective tissue, no matter how highly modified, is the presence of the characteristic protein, collagen, in the form of fibers.

The precursor of all types of connective tissue is the mesenchyme of the embryo, a simple, primitive connective tissue composed of cells and ground substance but lacking fibers. Being multipotent, mesenchymal cells may differentiate into any connective tissue cell type as well as into many other cell types (e.g., muscle, endothelium).

An important characteristic of connective tissue is its ability to provide for structural, but not always functional, repair of the organism after many types of injury. One can easily see this in a surgical incision (Fig. 4.20). The surgeon removes the skin sutures only a few days after the operation because connective tissue, as scar, binds the wound edges together. As we have indicated, epithelium is also involved in repair, but it acts only to reestablish an intact surface barrier against our environment. Scar tissue is a prominent—often the major—component of healed myocardial infarcts, cirrhosis of the liver, some types of cancer, and many chronic inflammatory processes.

Scars originate mainly from fibroblasts and their extracellular products. Fibroblasts, like the simpler epithelial types, can proliferate manyfold to form thick layers over large surfaces. Connective tissue in its various forms is a normal and ubiquitous component of all organ systems except the central nervous system. The response to widespread repeated injury, as in the processes listed above, may gradually transform a soft and fragile normal organ into a firm and heavy mass which yet retains some indication of its original shape. It will be recognized that scarring, though it is often necessary for the continuing life of the organism or for the function of the part, may prove excessive and cause problems of its own.

The inflammatory response, the basic reaction of the body to injury, takes place in connective tissue and involves all of its structural elements. A variety of changes in structure and function, many of them striking, are possible. As will become apparent, with respect to many defense mechanisms, "this is where the action is."

Basic Components

The Cells

FIBROBLASTS are the primary and predominant cells of connective tissue. They are large, somewhat flattened, spindle-shaped cells. Long, branching extensions of their cytoplasm can be seen in tissue spreads where the entire cell is visible. This feature is not apparent in most histologic sections. Their nuclei are the largest of any connective tissue cells and are oval, with finely granulated chromatin and one or two obvious nucleoli. These nuclei may appear to be naked, since the cytoplasm is barely visible in most preparations. These cells are responsible for the production of fibers and of the glycoprotein components of the ground substance (Fig. 4.1).

One of the neoplasms (tumors) that may be found in many sites of the body, but especially the skin, is the fibroma (Fig. 4.2). This is usually an innocent accumulation of fibroblasts, forming a small palpable nodule beneath the skin surface.

MACROPHAGES are the second most prominent cell, at least in loose connective tissue. They are phagocytic cells with more variable appearance, less regular outline, and shorter, blunter processes (pseudopodia) than the fibroblasts. The nuclei are smaller and more darkly stained because of the coarse chromatin. The nucleoli are not noticeable.

There are both transient and permanent populations of macrophages. The transients are derived from immigration of monocytes from the blood. Once monocytes enter a tissue they are called macrophages. The permanent inhabitants, called histiocytes or fixed macrophages, have two possible origins. Some may be derived from differentiating mesenchymal cells; others may be immigrant monocytes.

The cells of both populations are strongly phagocytic (Fig. 4.3). Their cytoplasm contains numerous lysosomes and residual bodies as well as vacuoles and vesicles.

Although the most obvious function of macrophages is (1) phagocytosis and scavenging of particulate materials, they also have other important functions in body defenses. They (2) take up and process antigens. This processing somehow changes the antigen so that the lymphocytes are more responsive to them. They may (3) bind antibodies to receptors in their membranes, and armed with these weapons, hunt down the antigens for which the particular antibodies are specific (Fig. 4.4). (4) Apparently they are attracted by factors known as lymphokines, which are products of T-lymphocytes (see Chapter 10). Lymphokines call macrophages to areas where they are needed, and proceed to activate them. Such activated macrophages are highly phagocytic. Macrophages also secrete several important substances; among these are collagenase (an enzyme that hydrolyzes collagen), some components of the complement system, and an important antiviral agent known as interferon, among others.

Macrophages in inflammatory processes often become fixed in the tissue and produce collagen, contributing to the formation of scars. Thus macrophages in this situation may become fibroblasts. Fusion of macrophages occurs in certain types of chronic inflammation, sometimes forming multinucleated giant cells (Fig. 4.4).

For further discussion of cellular activities in the immune response see Chapter 10.

ADIPOCYTES are also called fat cells and are among the permanent residents of connective tissue, particularly the loose variety. They are special, differentiated cells somewhat resembling fibroblasts, but they have the capability of storing fat. When fat is available from the diet, it first appears in the adipocyte as cytoplasmic droplets that later coalesce into a single large fat-filled vacuole (Fig. 4.5). When the fat is used up, the cells return to a less distended condition, often coming to resemble fibroblasts. Adipocytes with single large droplets are referred to as unilocular adipocytes and are basically energy-storing cells. Multilocular adipocytes are found in the fetus and the newborn. Their lipid is present in the form of many small droplets which gives the cells a foamy appearance. Their function appears to be heat production, a process thought to be controlled by the action of norepinephrine (see Chapter 17).

The deposit and removal of lipids in adipocytes appear to be controlled by neuroendocrine secretions as well as by the dietary status of the organism. The mechanisms by which adipocytes respond to environmental changes to release or store fat are poorly understood. In addition to being a source of energy, adipose tissue (i.e., collections predominantly of adipocytes; *see below*) serves as a thermal insulator and as a physical shock absorber. Adipocytes have been shown to have receptors for several hormones such as adrenal corticotrophic hormone (ACTH), thyroxin, and glucagon.

MAST CELLS (Fig. 4.6) most frequently occur along the course of small blood vessels. They have relatively small nuclei that are often obscured by the great numbers of coarse basophilic granules occupying the cytoplasm. They are often termed tissue basophils, although they probably are not related to the basophils of the blood. Their cytoplasmic granules apparently contain histamine and heparin. Histamine dilates blood vessels and increases endothelial permeability. Heparin, an anticoagulant, has several complex functions. Both substances are important chemical mediators of the inflammatory process.

LEUKOCYTES. Representatives from all the various categories of leukocytes, white cells, of the blood are common in the connective tissues. These originate from the lymphoid system and bone marrow and will be considered in more detail elsewhere. They may come and go from the blood depending on the needs of the tissues. For example, neutrophils (Fig. 4.7) may accumulate rapidly in great numbers in acute inflammation.

PLASMA CELLS (Fig. 4.8) may also be found in the loose connective tissue, particularly in that underlying the epithelium of the digestive and respiratory tracts. They are especially plentiful in regions of chronic inflammation. They are important in the production of antibodies. The large amount of rough endoplasmic reticulum, which often practically fills the entire cytoplasm, is necessary for the production of these complex large protein molecules and gives the cell its characteristic intense basophilia. Plasma cells are derived from the differentiation of B-lymphocytes that have migrated into the connective tissue from the circulation, and have responded to the presence of antigens by developing the ability to produce antibodies to these antigens. The plasma cell is an end cell, so highly specialized that it probably cannot be altered into other cell types, and survives for a period of about 2 weeks.

MELANOCYTES are melanin-forming cells that may be found in the connective tissue, particularly that of the skin, the pia mater, and the choroid coat of the eye. They may sometimes be confused with macrophages that have ingested hemosiderin or some other pigment.

OTHER CELLS. In any sample of connective tissue, the observer finds some cells that defy

Fig. 4.1. *Fibroblasts*. Elongated cytoplasm, oval nuclei, and distinct nucleoli. ×1000.

Fig. 4.2. *Fibroma* (arrows) of skin. This common abnormality is a local cellular aggregation resulting from simple, benign proliferation of fibroblasts. ×30.

Fig. 4.3. *Macrophages* in thoracic lymph nodes. **a:** These cells contain many black granules of carbon inhaled and transported from lung. ×1000. **b:** Sketch of **a** with identification of macrophages.

Fig. 4.4. *Foreign-body reaction* to suture. **a:** Teflon fibers in cross-section. Collagen has been laid down around these, and there are several unclassifiable connective tissue cells and a large multinucleated giant cell, characteristic of reaction to foreign bodies. ×250. **b:** Sketch of **a.**

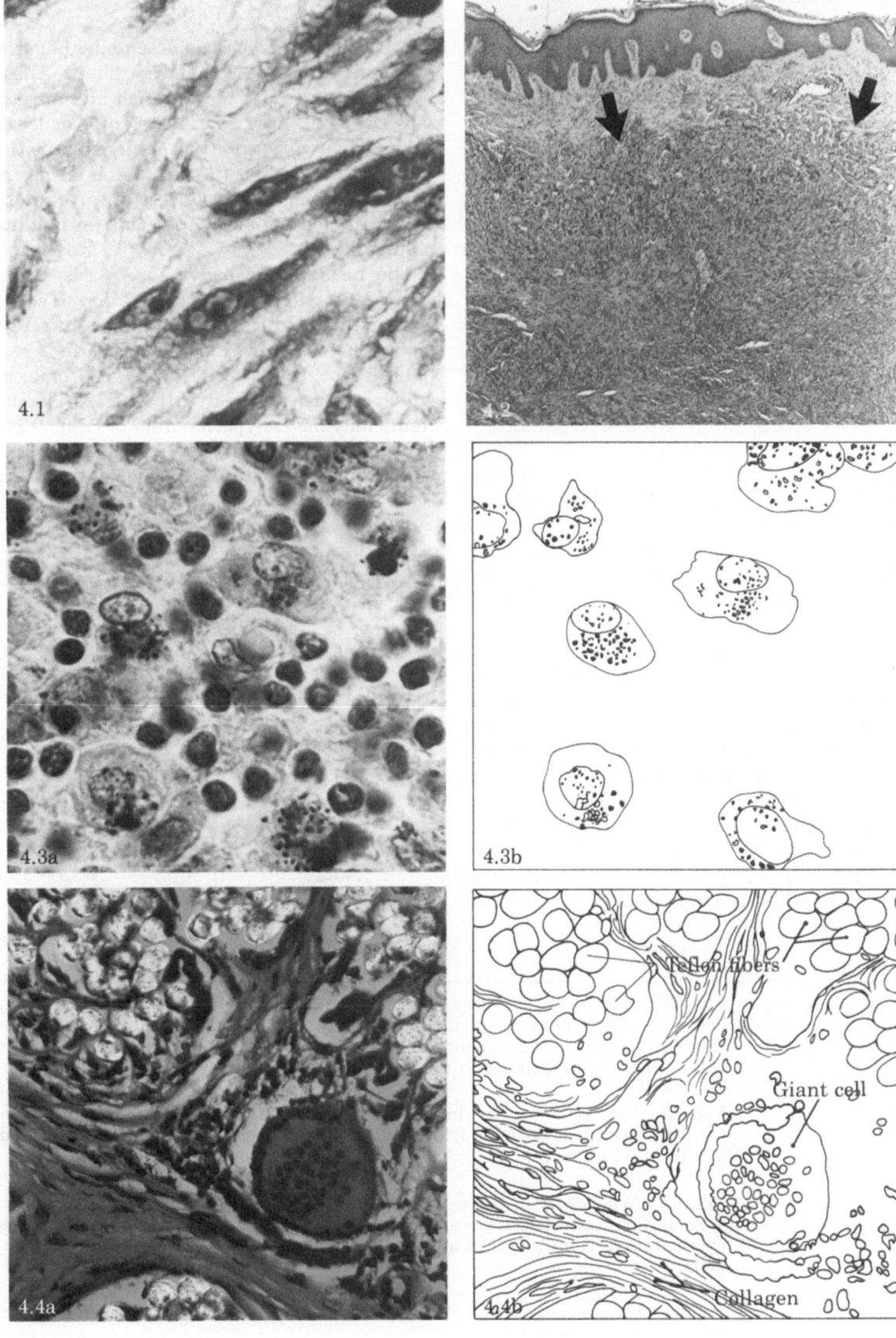

4.1

4.2

4.3a

4.3b

4.4a

Teflon fibers

Giant cell

Collagen

4.4b

certain identification. Therefore, the student should not feel compelled to classify every cell he sees. Some unclassifiable cells may be so because they are undifferentiated and either capable of, or actively in the process of, transition from one type to another. The fibroblast may be the precursor of some of these. It can actively multiply and assume a less mature form, which implies that it may be able to differentiate into other cell types. Under certain circumstances the fibroblast may produce myofilaments which are generally regarded as a specific feature of muscle.

The Fibers

The adult connective tissues contain two chemically different kinds of fibers, collagenous and elastic.

COLLAGENOUS FIBERS.   The fibroblasts produce collagen in a complex series of steps ranging from the assembly of the amino acids to the formation of the characteristic triple helix and its secretion into the surrounding matrix as tropocollagen (Fig. 4.9). The fibers are formed outside of the cell by a process which aligns the tropocollagen molecules end-to-end and side-to-side in a fashion such that, with the electron microscope, fully assembled fibers are seen to have uniform transverse striations at 64-nm intervals (Figs. 4.10 and 4.11). Fibrils 100 nm or less in diameter are of variable length and do not branch. The larger bundles seen with the light microscope

in sections are made up of assemblies of great numbers of these elementary fibers. These bundles or fascicles may branch and anastomose as small groups of fibers enter or leave them. They vary greatly in thickness in the different connective tissues. These strong fibers are arranged in a variety of ways in different tissues and are responsible for holding us together.

The form that a body possesses is essentially a function of the organization of collagen, without which we would be shapeless blobs. There are several varieties of an inherited disease, the Ehlers-Danlos syndrome, in which collagen is defective (Fig. 4.12). The patients may have: hypermobility of joints; easy bruising; poor wound healing; hyperelastic, thin, velvety, fragile skin; congenital heart

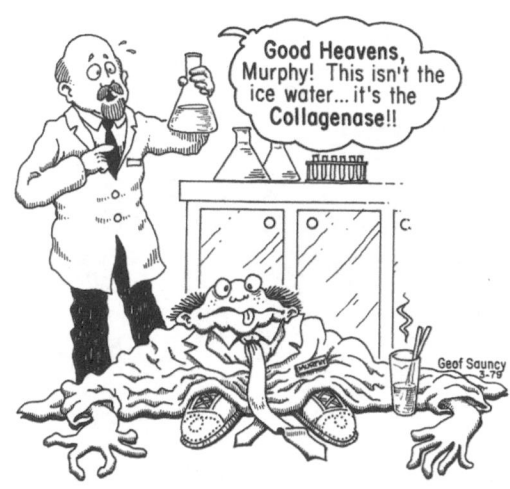

Fig. 4.5. *Adipocytes.* The stored lipid has been extracted in processing of the tissue, leaving a large empty space in each cell. The signet-ring appearance is due to the peripheral displacement of the nucleus by the fat droplet. Often a nucleus will not have been included in the plane of section. ×400.

Fig. 4.6. *Mast cells* (arrows) in subcutaneous tissue. The section is stained with toluidine blue to demonstrate cytoplasmic granules. Fragility of the cells is indicated by the evident disruption of two of the four cells shown. ×400.

Fig. 4.7. *Neutrophils* in the serosa of the appendix. **a:** A single small aggregate such as this has no determinable significance, but large numbers of these cells characterize certain bacterial infections. ×1000. **b:** Sketch of **a** to identify neutrophils.

Fig. 4.8. *Plasma cells.* **a:** "Clock-face" nuclei and, in ideal examples, paranuclear pallor. ×1000. **b:** Sketch of **a.**

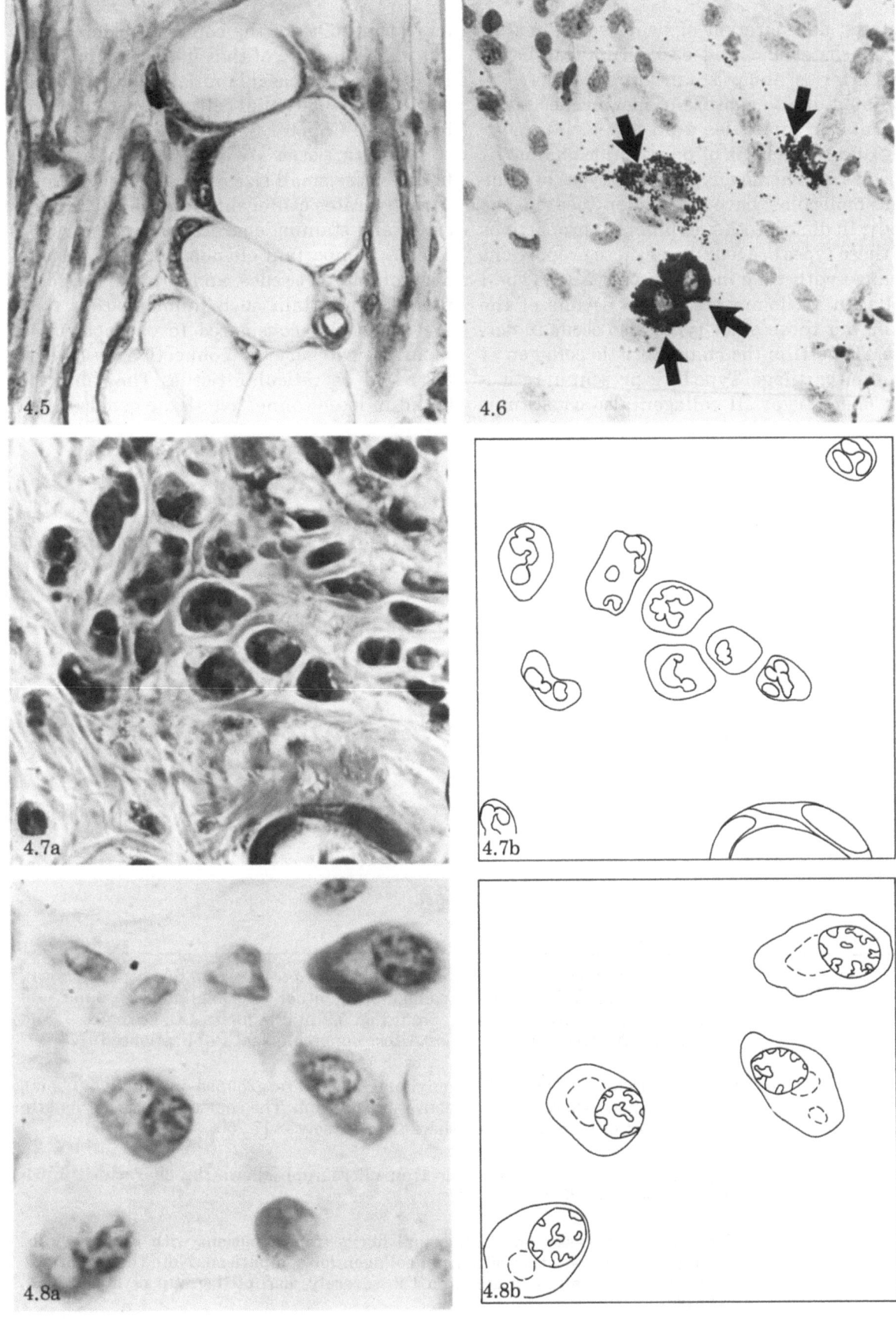

4.5

4.6

4.7a

4.7b

4.8a

4.8b

defects; degeneration of heart valves; excessively distensible and easily ruptured bowel and arteries; and pregnancy prematurely terminated due to rupture of membranes.

Collagen molecules are rods, each consisting of a triple helix of polypeptide chains. At least seven chemically different types of collagen molecules have been identified in the body. In different tissues different proportions of these types are found and these proportions change with time in the same tissue. Type I collagen predominates in the dermis of the skin, but three other types also occur in dermis. Type II is the characteristic collagen of hyaline cartilage. Type III is present in reticular fibers. Type III collagen also constitutes more than 60% of the collagen in fetal skin but less than 20% of that in adult skin. Type IV is present in basal laminae and is probably produced by epithelial cells rather than fibroblasts (see Chapter 3).

RETICULAR FIBERS are very fine collagenous fibers whose small size and coat of additional carbohydrates confer different physical properties and staining characteristics (Fig. 4.13). They are important elements of internal support of many tissues and organs; in some places they attain such numbers that they are sometimes considered to characterize a separate category of connective tissue referred to as reticular tissue. They may be found in loose connective tissue generally, in

Fig. 4.9. *Formation of collagen and ground substance.* Two pathways are shown, one through the RER and Golgi (collagen), the other via Golgi alone (ground substance). (Modified with permission from Fig. 5.9 in Junqueira LC, Carneiro J, and Contopoulos A: Basic Histology. Los Altos: Lange Medical Publications, 1977.)

Fig. 4.10. *Collagen fibers.* The individual fibrils are grouped in bundles (fibers), four of which are shown in this electron micrograph. The central fiber is cut lengthwise for most of its course, the others transversely. ×17,750.

Fig. 4.11. *Collagen fibril.* This electron micrograph shows the characteristic 64-nm periodicity. ×133,000.

Fig. 4.12. a: Cross-section of abnormal fibrils from a patient with Ehlers-Danlos syndrome. **b:** Cross-section of normal collagen for comparison. Note the larger size of fibrils, the variation in size and the severely disrupted group of fibrils in **a.** ×114,000.

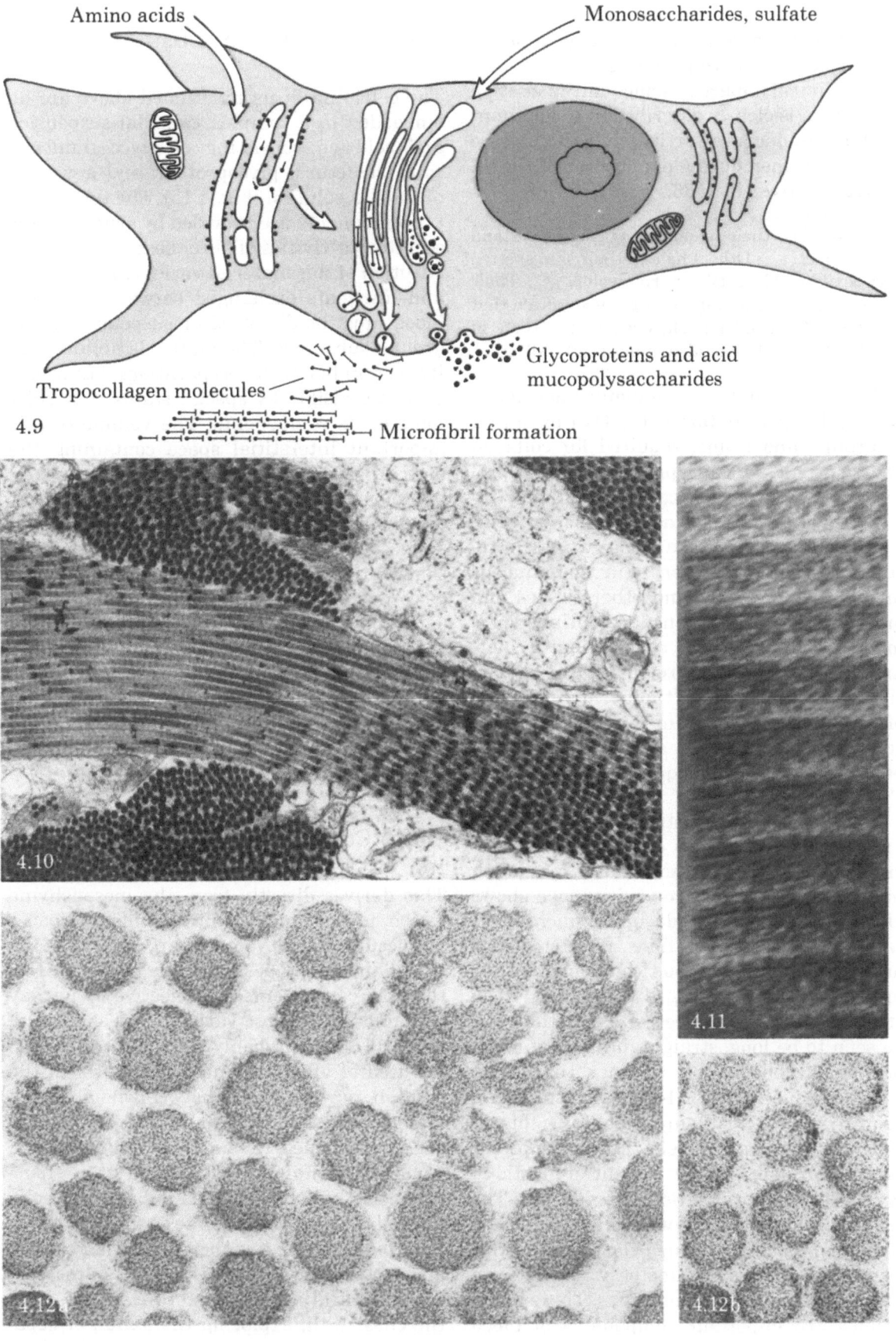

Amino acids

Monosaccharides, sulfate

Tropocollagen molecules

4.9

Glycoproteins and acid mucopolysaccharides

Microfibril formation

4.10

4.11

4.12a

4.12b

bone marrow, and in the parenchyma of the liver, spleen, and lymph nodes.

The clinical impact of inadequate formation of collagen is clearly described in the account of scurvy by Jacques Cartier when this disease affected his men during exploration of the St. Lawrence River in 1536:

"Some did lose their strength and could not stand on their feet. . . . Others had all their skin spotted with spots of blood of a purple color. . . . Their mouths became stinking, their gums so rotten that all of the flesh did fall off, even to the roots of the teeth, which did also almost all fall out."

Scurvy results from the dietary deficiency of ascorbic acid (vitamin C). Hydroxylation of proline and lysine, required for collagen fiber construction, fails, probably because protocollagen hydroxylase cannot function without the vitamin to act as a reducing agent. The weakened structure of blood vessels results in hemorrhages in skin and mucous membranes, muscles, and other tissues and organs. Bones are weakened by continued normal absorption without replacement by new matrix. All structures requiring the formation of new collagen in the normal turnover of this substance are damaged. Scurvy is not commonly encountered at the present time because the need for adequate dietary vitamin C is generally known.

ELASTIC FIBERS are constructed of a glycoprotein material known as elastin, which is secreted by fibroblasts or, sometimes, by smooth muscle cells. The electron microscope shows elastic fibers to be made up of microfibrils without transverse striations, associated with an additional amorphous component. They are truly elastic and, if examined in a stretched piece of connective tissue, they will be seen to be long, straight, branching fibers ordinarily considerably thinner than most collagen bundles (Fig. 4.14). Special stains are required to render them visible for light microscopy. The varying elasticity of different tissues is related to the content of elastic fibers in the connective tissue component. The ligamentum nuchae may contain so much as to be appropriately termed elastic connective tissue. Elastin occurs not only in the form of fibers but also as membranes. These membranes are important components of blood vessels.

The Matrix (ground substance)

The cells and fibers mentioned above are all embedded in a complex colloidal suspension and solution consisting of glycosaminoglycans, structural glycoprotein, and a variety of salts in solution (Fig. 4.15). The fundamental components are provided by synthetic and secretory activities of fibroblasts. But the constitution of this material varies since all gases and nutrients exchanged between cells and blood must be dissolved or suspended in the ground substance. The matrix is not ordinarily seen in histologic preparations, but it may be made visible by special stains that color some of its components. The volume of this important interstitial space containing the matrix varies in different physiologic and pathologic states and control of the amount of fluid in it is a necessary homeostatic mechanism. The total interstitial space is so large that clinically significant weight change can be produced by the accumulation of fluid (edema), as in heart failure. Also localized swelling is extremely common. Mosquito bites, bee stings, bruises, "pink eye," and stuffy nose are a few familiar examples.

Types of Adult Connective Tissues

Loose Connective Tissue

This derives directly from the mesenchyme which, in early embryonic life, fills the spaces not occupied by developing organs (Fig. 4.16). All of the cell types and fibers described as the basic components of connective tissue may be found in the loose variety (Figs. 4.14, 4.15, and 4.17). It is probably the most widely distributed of all the connective tissues. In the adult it may be found between neighboring organs, under the skin, and in serous and mucous membranes. In the dissecting room, the demonstration and separation of gross structures and of fascial planes is largely accomplished by splitting the loose connective tissue that binds them together. The macroscopic appearance of the tissue is best appreciated when separating the pectoralis major from the chest wall, exploring the axilla, or separating some of the other large muscles from one another. When this is done the loose connective tissue is seen to resemble a spider's web or strands of wet cotton. In the latter analogy the cotton fibers represent the connective tissue fibers, the moisture represents ground substance, and the interstices are occupied by the cells, which of course would be visible only with a microscope. Loose connective tissue supplies the stroma, or general embedding substance, for most parenchymatous organs. It provides adhesion between parts and organs, but at the same time it allows considerable mobility. It supports the skin and other membranes, attaching them to deeper structures. It binds muscle together. It underlies the simple squamous epithelium of serous membranes and the epithelium of mucous membranes.

Because of its looseness, this tissue tends to form planes of dissection, not only for the anatomist in the dissecting room, but also for blood or other fluids or gases that may find their way into the tissues. The subcutaneous periorbital hematoma (black eye) is one example. For another, air may pass from a ruptured bronchus into the interstitial, loose, peribronchial connective tissue, and dissect along the septa in the lung. If the amount of air is sufficient, it may extend into the mediastinum between the thoracic muscles and into the subcutaneous tissue of the chest to be visible on a standard chest X-ray film.

Dense Connective Tissue

The predominant feature of this type of connective tissue is its fiber content. In some examples, such as tendon or ligament, there may be very little space for ground substance and cells. Tendon, for instance, is almost pure collagen, with space for only a few fibroblasts squeezed between the massive fiber bundles.

DENSE IRREGULAR CONNECTIVE TISSUE. In this category the connective tissue fibers are more or less randomly oriented and composed of large bundles with little room for other components. A good example of this type is the dermis of the skin (Fig. 4.18). This is the layer which, after tanning, becomes leather. Scars are composed largely of dense irregular connective tissue.

Dense irregular connective tissue is usually not regarded as elastic, but there are many instances (e.g., scars of skin and normal aging skin) of stretching with time. The stretchability may be a function of the particular types of collagen present.

DENSE REGULAR CONNECTIVE TISSUE. This type is best exemplified in tendons (Fig. 4.19), aponeuroses and ligaments, where dense aggregates of collagenous fibers are oriented predominantly in one direction in response to mechanical needs. Tendons for instance, must resist very strong pull. Collagen, with its lack of elasticity and its great tensile strength, is the material of choice for this purpose. This form of collagen does not stretch.

Adipose Tissue

This tissue forms a subcutaneous layer (Fig. 4.20) and sizeable depots in the mesenteries, greater omentum, and breast, as well as many smaller collections throughout the body. It is bright yellow in gross appearance because of its high lipid content and its relatively sparse blood supply. Microscopically it is composed of packed adipocytes with a delicate stroma of connective tissue fibers arranged in a more or less lobular pattern. Scattered blood vessels and other connective tissue cell types are seen.

Upon depletion of intracellular lipid, the cells come to resemble fibroblasts and the overall tissue comes to resemble loose connective tissue. As with the fibroblast, the potentiality of the adipocyte is unclear. Is the difference in appearance between loose connective tissue and adipose tissue only a matter of nutrition? We do not know.

Connective tissue regenerates easily, sometimes excessively. The new tissue is of the dense irregular variety. First think of this regeneration as in a healing wound of the skin (Fig. 4.20). A complex series of processes—including entry of inflammatory cells and proliferation of fibroblasts and capillaries—is involved. Then consider that injury and resulting scar formation, called fibrosis, may often occur in internal tissues. This sequence is involved in many of the diseases mentioned at the beginning of this chapter, conditions that are usually chronic and often progressive.

Fig. 4.13. *Reticular fibers* in liver. These provide a delicate pervading framework in which liver cells and blood vessels are arranged. The stain is specific for reticulum. Cell details are indistinct. ×400.

Fig. 4.14. *Collagenous and elastic fibers* in connective tissue. This is not a section but a spread out piece of subcutaneous tissue stained by aldehyde fuchsin to demonstrate the thin, branching elastic fibers. Collagen fibers here are broad and faintly stained. ×400.

Fig. 4.15. *Loose connective tissue.* This shows three distinct cell types: a neutrophil (upper left); a typical branched fibroblast (center); and a mast cell (lower right). Also note two fiber types: large, irregular collagenous and thin, straight, branched elastic. These are suspended in a homogenous fluid matrix occupying the interstitial space.

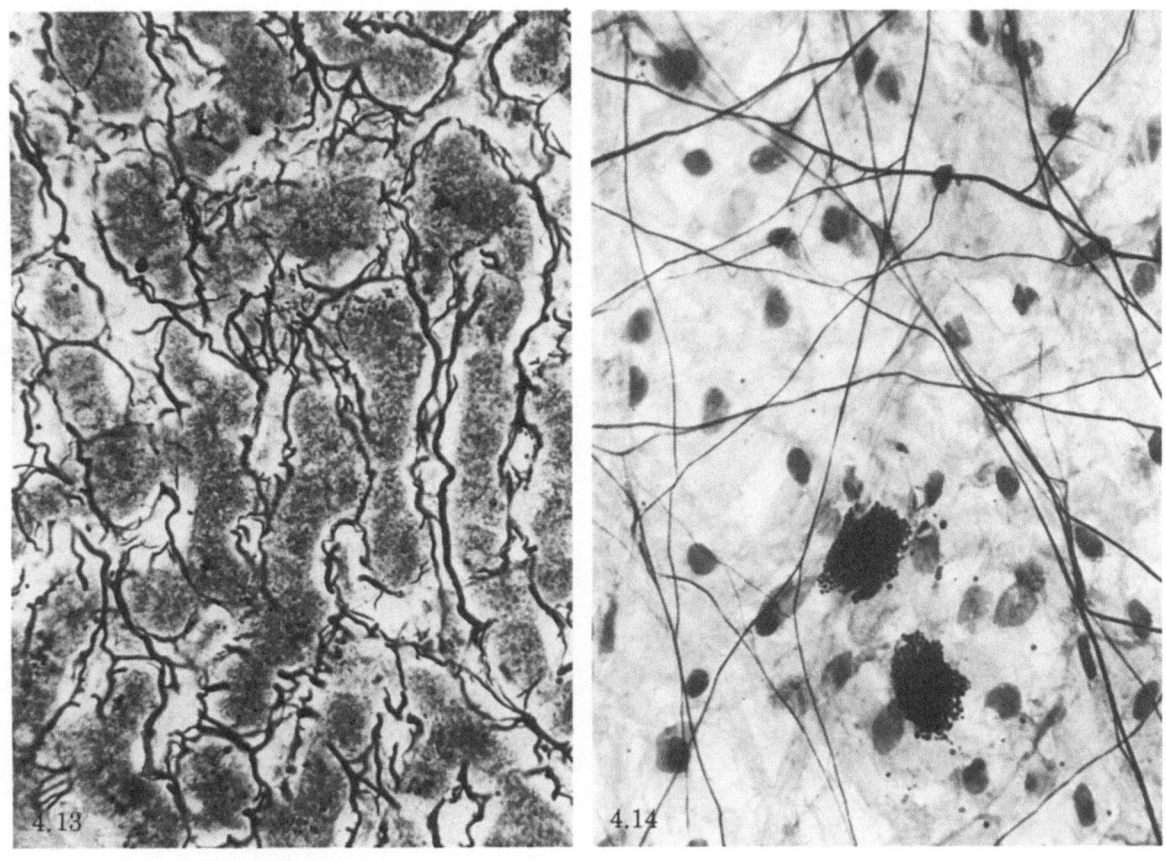

4.13

4.14

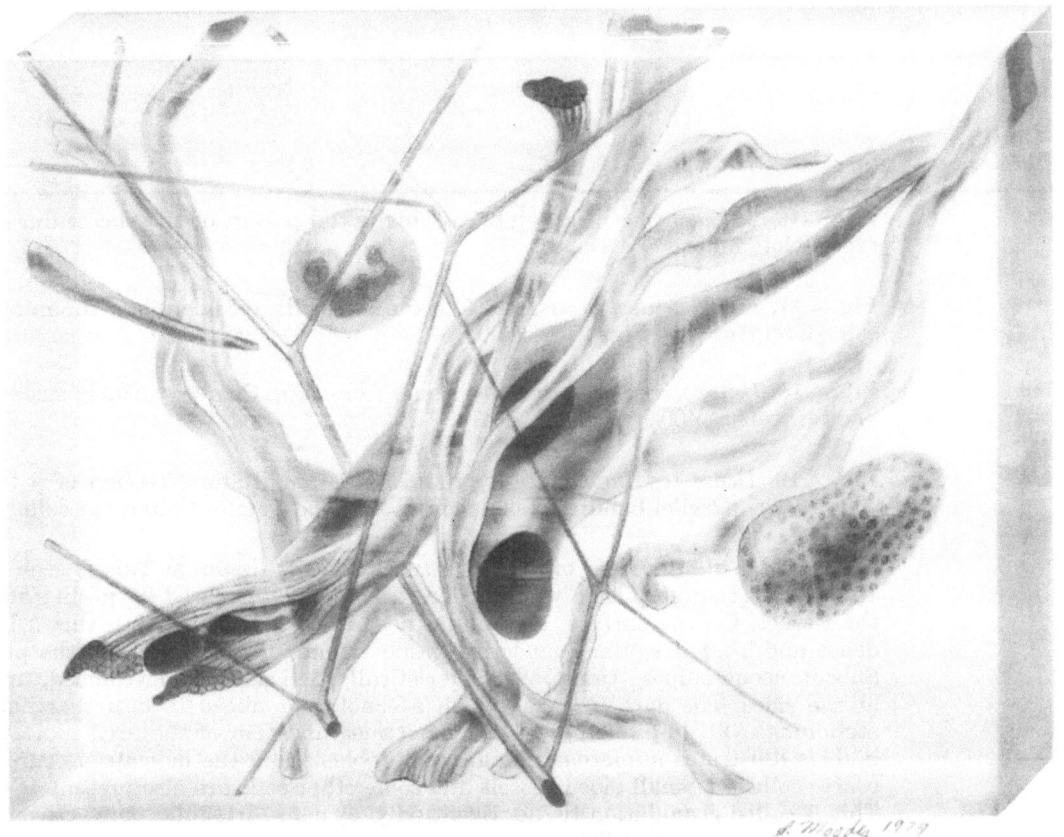

4.15

Fig. 4.16. *Mesenchyme* in an embryo. This is the parent of the succeeding tissue types. Note mitosis. ×400.

Fig. 4.17. *Loose connective tissue.* Note the fine collagen fibers and the numerous cells. Compare with Fig. 4.19. ×400.

Fig. 4.18. *Dense irregular connective tissue* from skin. Coarse, variably sized fibers and few cells. ×400.

Fig. 4.19. *Dense regular connective tissue.* This longitudinal section of a tendon shows large parallel bundles of collagen fibers appearing to flatten the cells. ×400.

Fig. 4.20. *Healing wound* of skin and subcutaneous tissue. **a:** This is seen about 10 days after surgery. The wound edges are completely fused by proliferation of the tissues. On the surface, epithelium does its part, but beneath this a line of dense and loose irregular connective tissue extends to the bottom of the picture. Subcutaneous adipose tissue, characteristically delicately honeycombed, appears at the sides. The dark streaks, which are not reproduced in b, are artifacts of sectioning. ×21. **b:** Sketch of **a. c:** Higher magnification of the area indicated in **b.** This illustrates numerous immature fibroblasts and the delicate precursors of coarse collagen. Small blood vessels and some other cells are also present as usual. This is called granulation tissue. Eventually, as dense irregular connective tissue, it will become a scar. ×250.

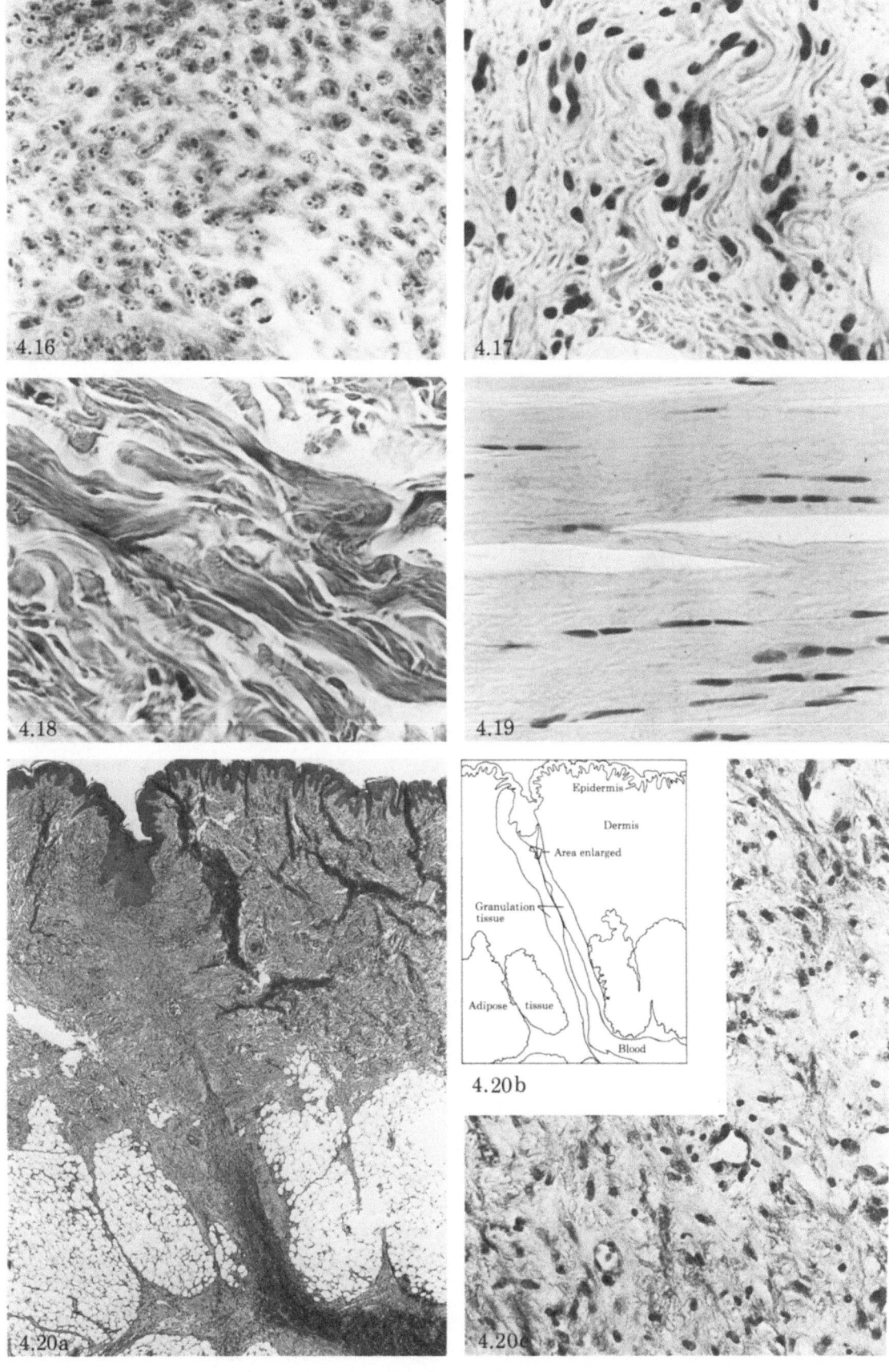

4.16

4.17

4.18

4.19

4.20a

Epidermis

Dermis

Area enlarged

Granulation
tissue

Adipose   tissue

Blood

4.20b

4.20c

5 Cartilage and Bone

Cartilage

Cartilage has a solid and comparatively firm consistency, although it is not as rigid as bone. In adult humans it functions most importantly as a shock absorber in joints and prevents collapse of some tubular structures such as the airway. It also serves in the fetus as the model upon which many of the long bones are later built, and it allows rapid growth of these structures as they mature.

Unlike almost all other tissues, cartilage is avascular (without blood vessels).

At the interface between cartilage and surrounding tissue lies a layer of dense connective tissue called *perichondrium*. The portion of the perichondrium nearest the cartilage contains undifferentiated fibroblast-like cells, the *chondroblasts*, which can develop into cartilage cells, *chondrocytes*.

Types of Cartilage

HYALIN CARTILAGE is the most abundant and the most rigid of the three types. It has approximately the consistency of a rubber eraser. It covers the ends of long bones, providing them with smooth sliding surfaces for joints. It forms tracheal rings, bronchial plates, anterior ends of ribs, the framework of the larynx, and the walls of the anterior portion of the nose. The chondrocytes have single round central nuclei and a small amount of light-staining cytoplasm. They lie in small spaces, *lacunae*, surrounded by an abundant matrix secreted by the cells (Fig. 5.1). The matrix is rich in glycosaminoglycan and contains fine collagenous fibrils visible only by electron microscopy.

FIBROCARTILAGE is softer and more pliable than hyalin cartilage. It contains a much greater amount of collagen and this is visible with the light microscope (Fig. 5.2). Fibrocartilage composes intervertebral discs, the pubic symphysis, menisci of the knee, and some tendon insertions.

ELASTIC CARTILAGE is even more pliable than fibrocartilage. It gives both form and flexibility to the pinna of the external ear and the epiglottis. The matrix contains a meshwork of interlacing elastic fibers in addition to collagen (Fig. 5.3).

The distribution of cartilage types is illustrated in Fig. 5.4.

Growth of Cartilage

Cartilage grows in two patterns (Fig. 5.5). The first, and more important, is *appositional growth* and refers to the formation of new cartilage at the surface of the perichondrium by chondroblasts. The second is *interstitial growth,* the expansion of the mass of cartilage by mitotic division of chondroblasts and the formation of matrix internally.

Nutrition and Degeneration of Cartilage

Because cartilage contains no vascular or lymphatic channels nutrients are supplied entirely by diffusion and imbibition. Cartilage is therefore vulnerable to degeneration. Its bluish-white translucency diminishes with age and it becomes opaque and yellowish. Calcification follows and eventually renders the tissue hard and relatively brittle.

Bone

Bone is a type of connective tissue made especially rigid by crystals of inorganic salts in the ground substance. The dense rigid structure is well known and easily identified both grossly and microscopically. It is supplied with nerves and blood vessels. The long, stress-bearing beams or columns are arranged and supported with architectural precision (Fig. 5.6). Consider the physical tension placed on bone by strenuous work or exercise; it is said to reach as high as 800 pounds.

Bone is a living cellular tissue that not only grows in the young and in conditions of healing, but also metabolizes and undergoes continuous remodeling throughout life. It is especially influenced by growth hormone, parathormone, calcitonin, vitamin D, and steroid hormones as well as by basic nutrition and factors affecting calcium and phosphate metabolism.

Types and Structure of Bone

Whereas cartilage is solid and not interrupted by the presence of blood vessels, the structure of bone appears more finely engineered. It has a dense outer *cortex* of compact bone and an internal *marrow* containing adipose tissue

---

Fig. 5.1. *Hyalin cartilage.* Cartilage is avascular. ×150.

Fig. 5.2. *Fibrocartilage.* The collagen fibers give pliability and strength. ×150.

Fig. 5.3. *Elastic cartilage.* Contains thin straight fibers visible only with an elastic tissue stain. ×400.

Fig. 5.4. *Distribution of cartilage types.* (Based on Fig. 27 in Poirier J, Ribadeau-Dumas JL: Review of Medical Histology. Philadelphia; W B Saunders, 1977.)

Fig. 5.5. A: *Interstitial growth* is growth of all parts throughout, like the development of an apple. **B:** *Appositional growth* is the addition of layers to the surface, as of a coral reef. Stippled area represents new cartilage formed by the overlying perichondrium (solid line).

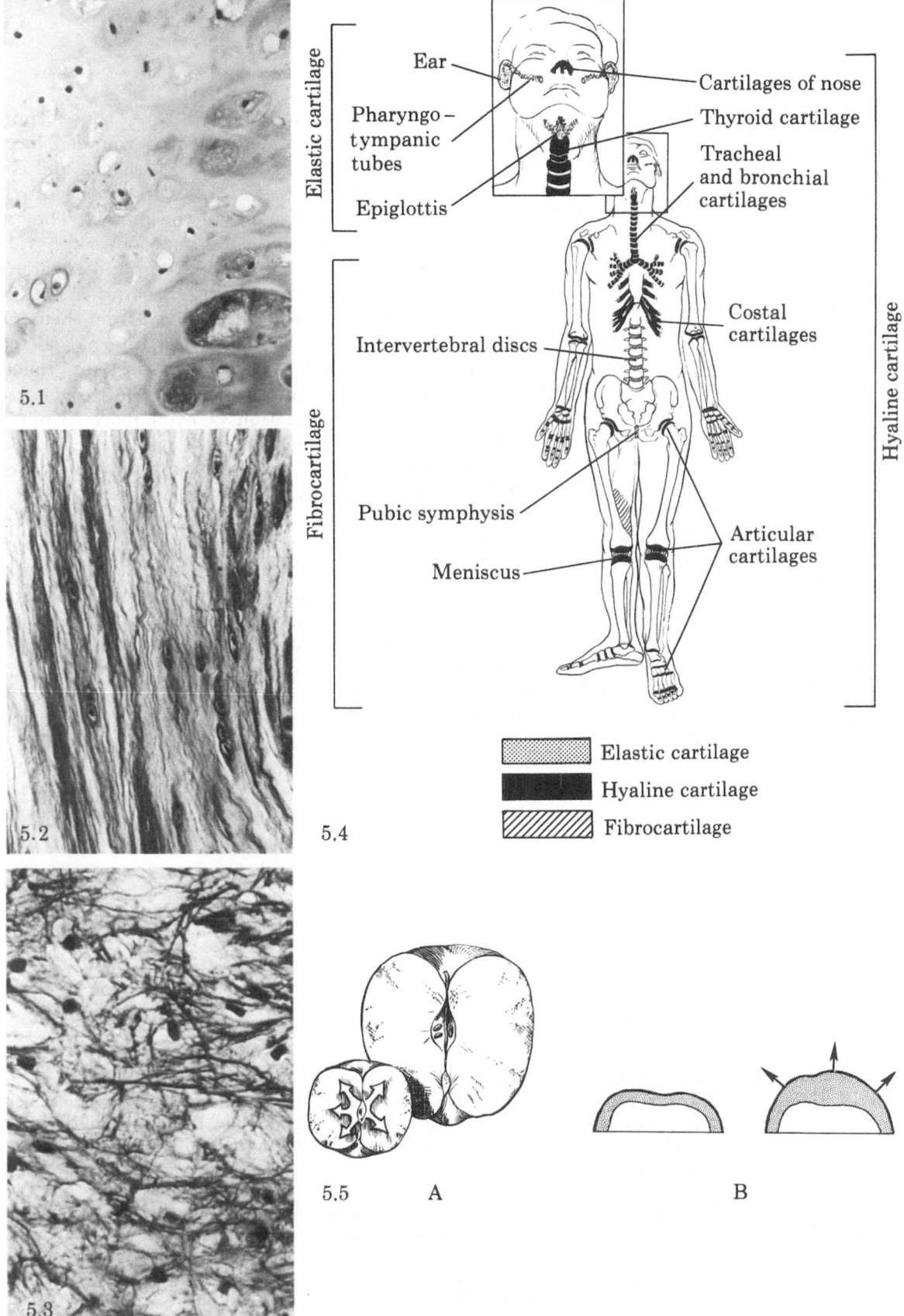

5.1

5.2

5.3

Elastic cartilage

Fibrocartilage

Hyaline cartilage

Ear

Pharyngo-
tympanic
tubes

Epiglottis

Cartilages of nose

Thyroid cartilage

Tracheal
and bronchial
cartilages

Intervertebral discs

Costal
cartilages

Pubic symphysis

Meniscus

Articular
cartilages

5.4

Elastic cartilage

Hyaline cartilage

Fibrocartilage

5.5   A   B

and blood-forming cells. The *medullary* or *marrow cavity* is crossed by columns called *trabeculae* of bone. The interior bone is appropriately called spongy bone (*see below*).

All bones are composed of lamellae (layers); the fibers of each lamella run parallel to each other, but different lamellae are arranged for maximum support by having different directions. This is similar to the arrangement of plies of an automobile tire (Fig. 5.7).

COMPACT BONE is formed mainly of *osteons* or *haversian* systems. An osteon is a column of 4–20 cylindrical lamellae concentrically arranged about the *haversian canal*. An haversian canal contains vessels and nerves and connects with other canals and with the medullary cavity. Transverse canals (Volkmann's canals) connect neighboring haversian canals and penetrate from the periosteal surface. Filling the gaps between osteons are less regular interstitial lamellae. Additional circumferential lamellae formed by the periosteum cover the entire exterior of all bones. Others lie on the interior (medullary cavities) of the diaphyses of long bones.

Lamellae and osteons are not visible in most histologic preparations of bone because the process of decalcification blurs the lines that define them (Fig. 5.8).

SPONGY (CANCELLOUS) BONE is a loose meshwork of bone trabeculae containing spaces for marrow and connective tissue. In the smaller trabeculae osteons and lamellae are less obvious.

Components

CELLS

Osteoblasts (Fig. 5.9) are bone-forming cells. They are medium-sized, rounded, or cuboidal with cytoplasmic extensions and contain numerous organelles to synthesize the organic constituents of the matrix. They secrete glycoproteins and mucopolysaccharides that form the uncalcified ground substance of bone called *osteoid. Osteocytes* and *osteoclasts* (*see below*) are derived from them. Osteoblasts are found on the internal surface and externally under the periosteum, reflecting active bone formation. The existence of another population of even more primitive bone cells was established not long ago. (See discussion of progenitor cells in Chapter 10 for general consideration of this subject.)

Osteocytes. These cells are osteoblasts that have become surrounded with matrix and lie within *lacunae* (Fig. 5.9). From each of the lacunar spaces several delicate cytoplasmic extensions branch and extend into small channels known as *canaliculi* (Fig. 5.10). The function of osteocytes is to maintain appropriate concentrations and arrangements of various molecules that compose the matrix. If blood supply to a portion of bone is cut off, the osteocytes die and the entire bony substance supported by them is resorbed and eventually replaced by new osteoblasts and new matrix.

Fig. 5.6. *The architecture of bone.* Delicate trabeculae and compact cortical bone supply maximum strength with least bulk, as suggested by this section of the upper end of a femur. Notice the different ratio of amounts of compact to spongy bone in the shaft versus the end of the bone.

Fig. 5.7. *Lamellar bone.* A dried undecalcified specimen showing osteons in cross section with their central Haversian canals. ×85.

Fig. 5.8. *Bone of a newborn infant.* This shows cement lines (arrows) separating lamellae. In older subjects the decalcification, which is usually the first step in processing calcified tissues for sectioning, renders these lines less distinct. ×90.

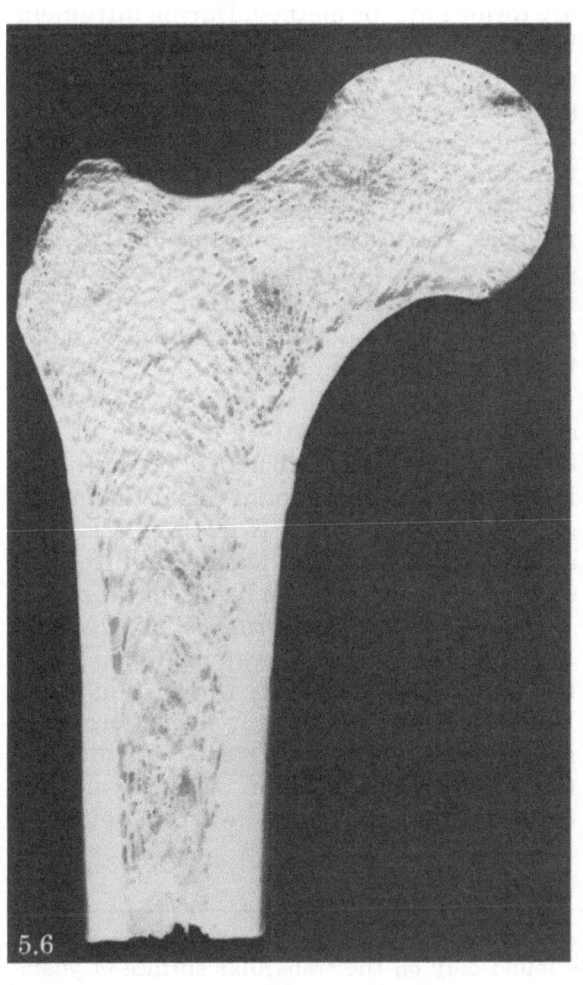

5.6

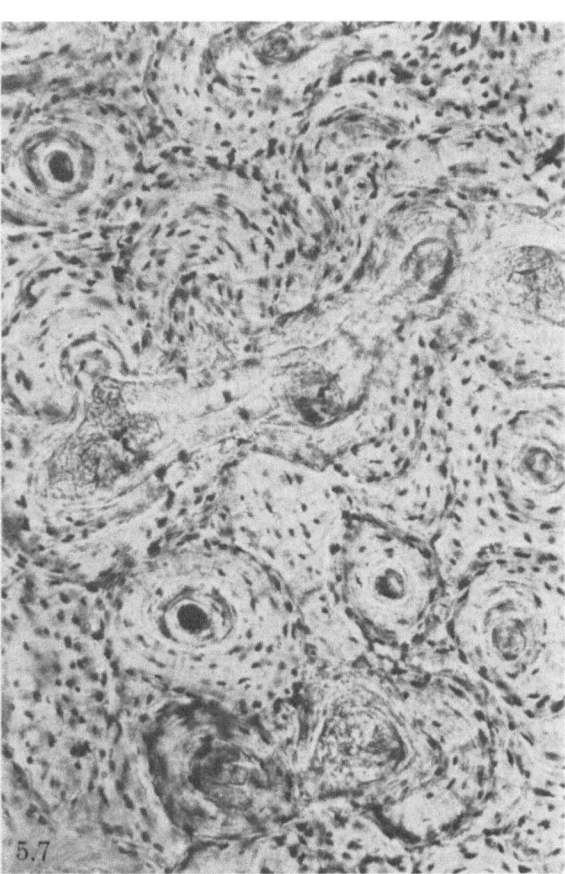

5.7

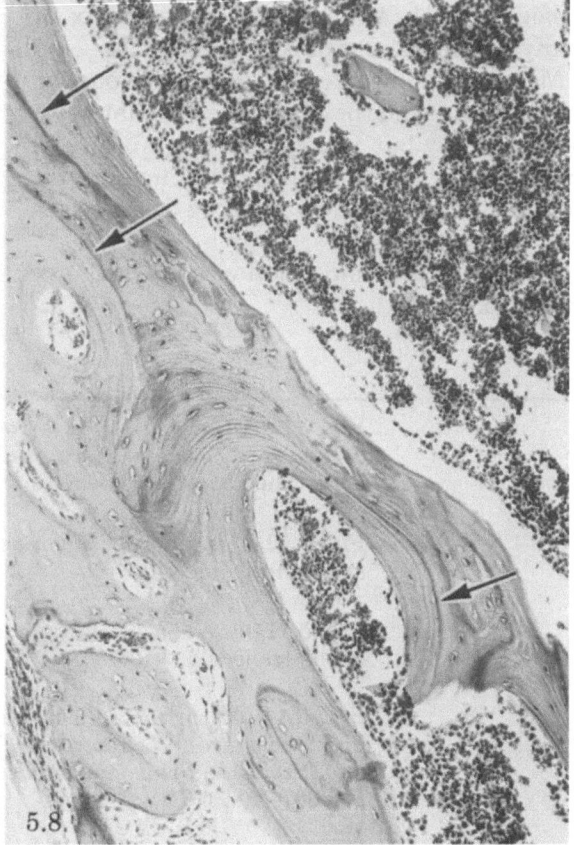

5.8

Osteoclasts occur only on the inner and outer surfaces of bone in portions that are being resorbed (Figs. 5.11 and 5.12). They are large, up to 50 μm in diameter, and have 6–25 nuclei. At the interface of the cell with the matrix a brush border of microvilli seems to carry out the erosion, supported by cytoplasmic vesicles, vacuoles, and lysosomes.

MATRIX is the extracellular substance of bone. It is similar to other forms of connective tissue in its base of collagen fibers, but differs by having them arranged in highly ordered lamellae, reinforced with mineral. The characteristic hardness of bone comes from hydroxyapatite, a crystalline form of calcium phosphate. The body carefully regulates the amounts of calcium and phosphate in the blood and interstitial tissues and uses the mineralized matrix as a storehouse either to extract or deposit these ions under various physiologic and pathologic conditions. This accounts for the variable density of bone in different stages of nutrition and in disease. The collagen base confers some flexibility.

PERIOSTEUM is a specialized dense connective tissue covering the bone. It contains osteoblasts as well as fibroblasts and collagen. It is bound firmly to the underlying matrix by many small fibers (Sharpey's fibers).

MARROW occupies the central spongy portion of bone and may be either yellow (fatty) or red (cellular) but is commonly a mixture of both. The cells are erythrocytic, myelocytic, and megakaryocytic, and will be described in Chapter 9.

The general organization of bone is shown in Fig. 5.13.

Formation and Reformation of Bone

FORMATION (OSSIFICATION). The first event in bone formation is the deposition of immature uncalcified matrix called osteoid. From this point we distinguish two different processes of development of bone structure:

Intramembranous ossification (Fig. 5.14) occurs within connective tissue and not by the replacement of cartilage. Most cranial bones are formed by this method. During intramembranous ossification a group of mesenchymal cells, presumably osteoblasts but not distinguishable as such until this point, begins to produce osteoid at a nidus called an ossification center. Ossification extends progressively into surrounding tissue, lamellar bone soon replaces the osteoid, and maturation and growth are accomplished by remodeling (see later). Neighboring ossification centers in a given bone expand and later fuse to produce the final form of the bone.

Intramembranous ossification is also responsible for the growth in diameter of long bones. In this instance bone is laid down first in the form of a short collar about the middle of the diaphysis (shaft). Growth results from addition of bone to the outside, and from resorption of bone from the inside, of the collar.

Endochondral (intracartilaginous) ossification. In this process a cartilaginous model is replaced by bone from within (Fig. 5.15). Long bones of the extremities are formed in this manner. The process starts with differentiation of cartilage from mesenchyme and ends only after puberty with cessation of

---

Fig. 5.9. *Osteoblasts* (thick arrows) *and osteocytes* (thin arrows). Osteoblasts show a variety of forms and are easily found only on the trabecular surface of young bone. They become osteocytes when entrapped in bone. ×560.

Fig. 5.10. The same specimen as in Fig. 5.7 at high magnification showing *lacunae* and *canaliculi*. ×400.

Fig. 5.11. *Osteoclast.* A large multinucleated cell in a typical recess on the surface of the trabecula. ×1000.

Fig. 5.12. *Osteoclast* seen by scanning electron microscopy. Extensive branching projections are in contact with bone surface to the right. ×1280. (From Jones SJ and Boyde A. Some morphological observations on osteoclasts. Cell Tissue Res 185:387–397, 1977.)

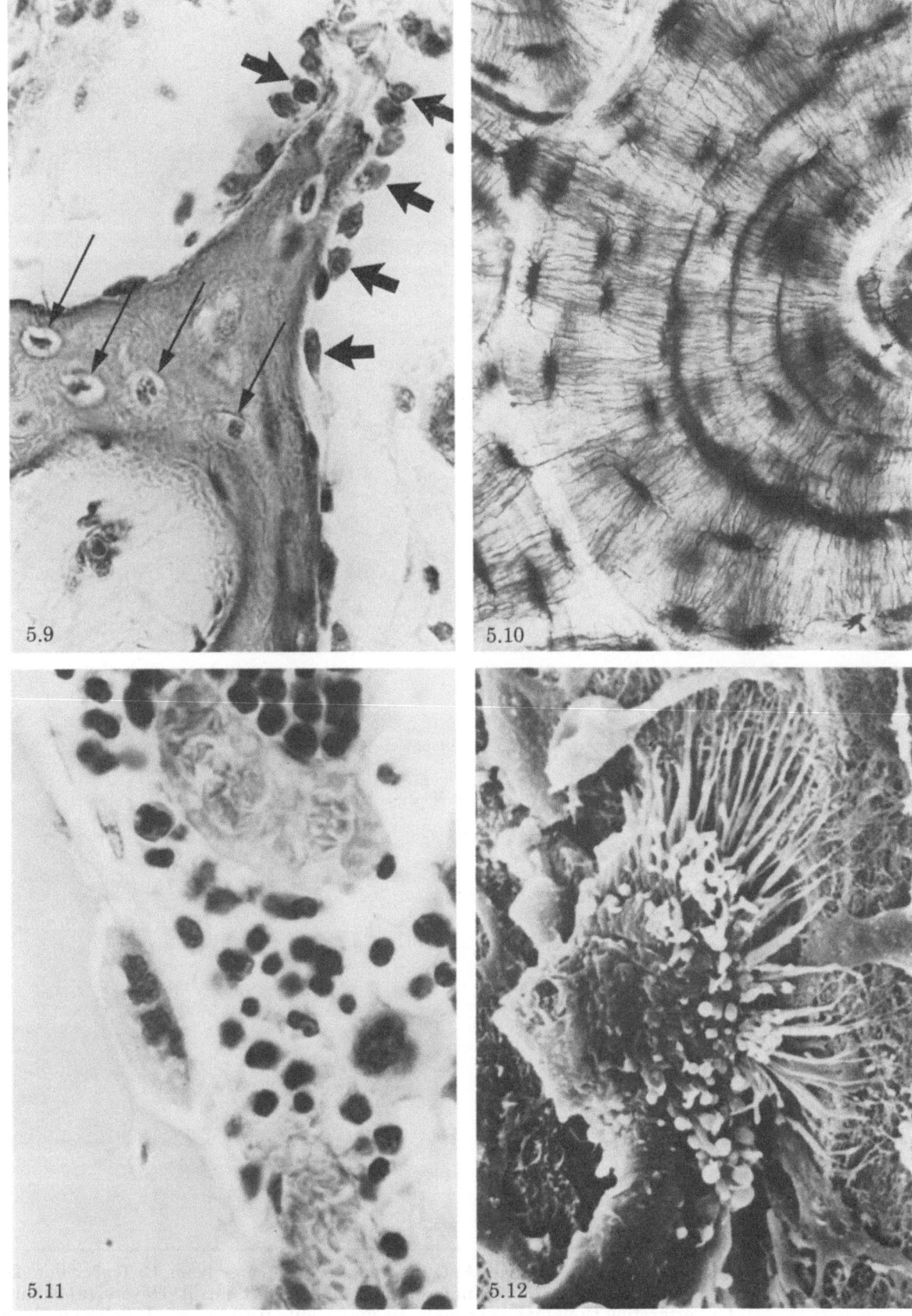

5.9

5.10

5.11

5.12

Fig. 5.13. *Structure of bone.* **A:** Compact bone. **B:** Spongy bone. **C:** Trabeculae. **D:** Interstitial lamellae. **E:** Circumferential lamellae. **F:** Central (Haversian) canals. **G:** Perforating (Volkmann's) canals. **H:** Periosteum (two layers). **I:** Collagen fibers binding periosteum to matrix (Sharpey's fibers). **J:** Osteon. **K:** Blood vessels.

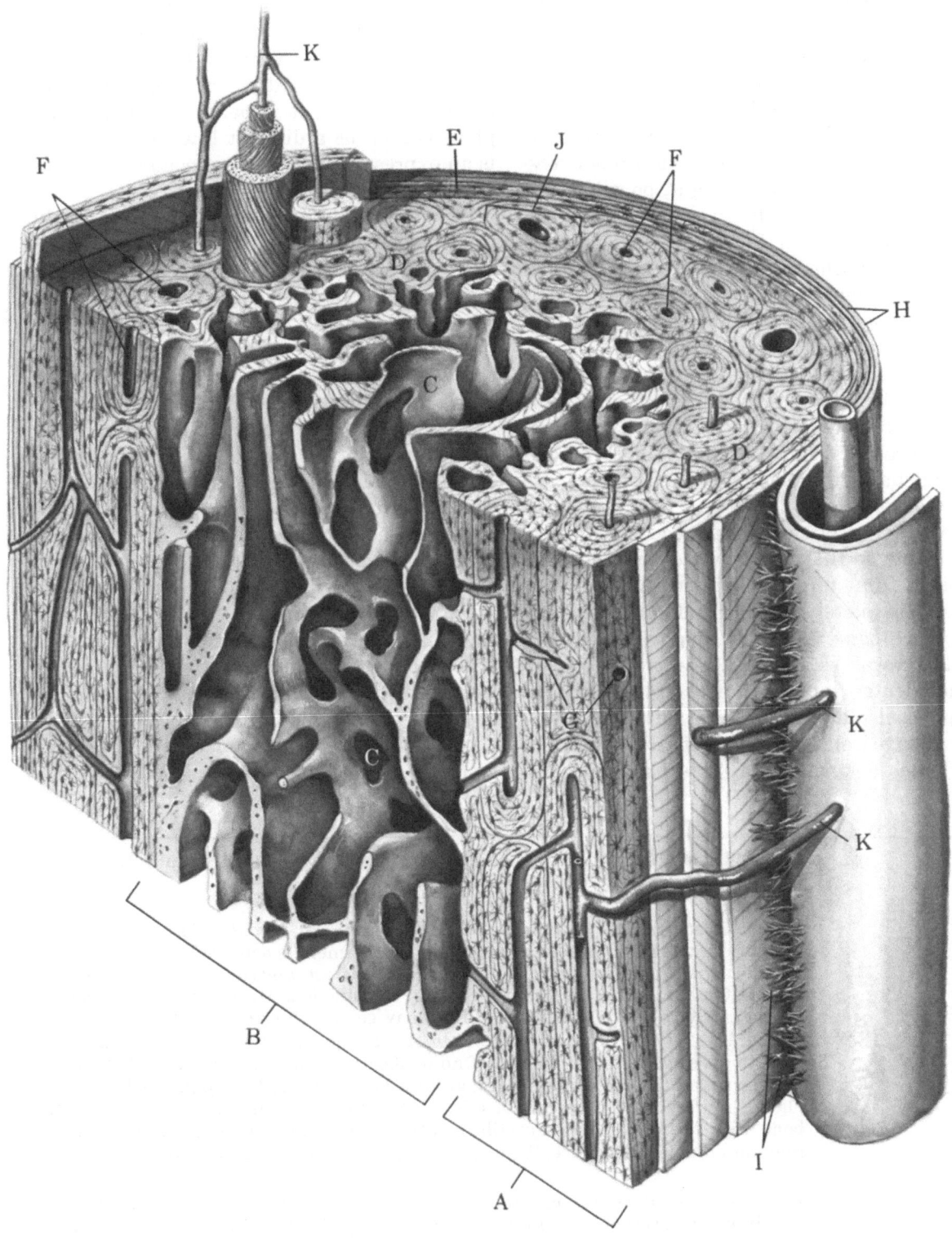

5.13

growth. In fairly rapid programmed sequence the cartilage *grows, calcifies, degenerates,* is *vascularized,* and then *resorbed.* This last is accompanied by the appearance of *primitive cells* that occupy the lacunae left by the degenerated cartilage and differentiate into osteoblasts that begin to lay down osteoid. The process takes place in straight, parallel, and evenly spaced columns extending from the center of ossification (Fig. 5.16). This sequence is so tightly scheduled that the new uncalcified bone is laid down on the columns of calcified cartilage (Fig. 5.17) that are left after the partial resorption. Each column then is gradually transformed from cartilage to bone. The delicate bony columns then undergo progressive remodeling into Haversian systems.

Ossification begins in the middle of the young shaft—the diaphysis—and spreads evenly toward the two ends—the epiphyses. The orderly series of changes progresses through the tissue so that the appearance of the advancing front remains the same until it has passed completely through and replaced cartilage with bone. After the diaphyseal growth center is well established, a secondary ossification center appears in each epiphysis. The epiphyseal plate, or growth plate, is a layer of cartilage isolated between these two enlarging areas of ossification. This plate appears to persist in most bones for the entire growth period while the bone is becoming severalfold larger and longer. Actually the cartilage is continually proliferating at approximately the same rate as it is being destroyed. The plate is seen as a distinct line by X-ray and is an expression of active endochondral ossification and growth.

RESORPTION. Living bone, being constantly involved in the exchange of ions with blood, is continually remodeling itself. Although more obvious in the young, remodeling continues throughout life. Osteoclasts are the most important agents of *resorption,* but osteocytes may also perform this function in lesser degree. Parathyroid hormone is the chief stimulus of osteoclast activity. Excessive production of this hormone, as by a tumor of parathyroid tissue, may cause severe depletion of bone calcium and produce the condition known as osteomalacia. Calcitonin, secreted by parafollicular cells of the thyroid, opposes the action of parathormone on bone.

GROWTH of bone involves an increase in either diameter or length. Growth in diameter of long bones, like growth of the axial skeleton, results from resorption and intramembranous ossification with remodeling. The addition of new matrix on the outside of a bone is produced by appositional growth

---

Fig. 5.14. *Intramembranous ossification,* the formation of bone in connective tissue without a previous cartilage model. ×150.

Fig. 5.15. *Steps in the development of a long bone.* **A:** A mass of hyalin cartilage with the first form of the bone. Subsequent enlargement is achieved by both interstitial and appositional growth of this uncalcified cartilage, and continues until maturation. **B:** Ossification occurs in a collar about the middle of the shaft. **C:** Calcification of the cartilage of the shaft inside the bony collar. **D:** Cartilage grows, calcifies, degenerates, and is replaced by bone in strict sequence. Vessels are required for bone to develop. **e:** The formation of an ossification center in the head of the bone has narrowed the remaining cartilage to a single layer, the epiphyseal (growth) plate. Proliferation of this cartilage is responsible for the increasing length of the bone. Growth stops when the cartilage of the plate is entirely resorbed. **F:** Cartilage remains on the joint surface; the epiphyseal plate has closed and growth has ceased.

Fig. 5.16. *Zones in endochondral ossification.* Some of the primary bony trabeculae are absorbed and others are enlarged in remodeling. **A:** Resting cartilage. **B:** Proliferating cartilage. **C:** Hypertrophied cartilage. **D:** Calcified cartilage. **E:** Ossification. ×130.

Fig. 5.17. Higher magnification of Fig. 5.16 to show relationship of calcified *cartilage* to *ossification.* **A:** Hypertrophied chondrocytes. **B:** Degenerating chondrocytes. **C:** Calcified cartilage matrix. **D:** The start of ossification. ×200.

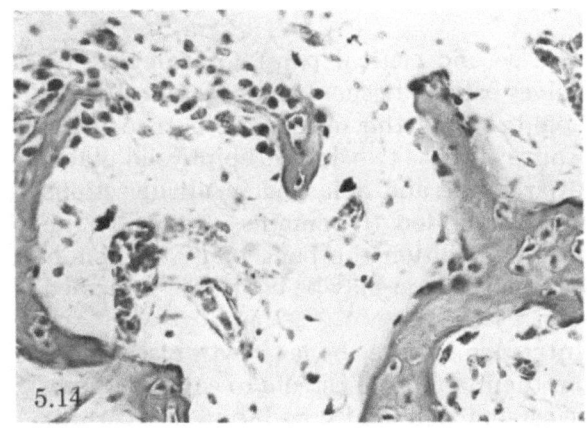

5.14

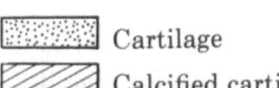
Cartilage
Calcified cartilage
Bone

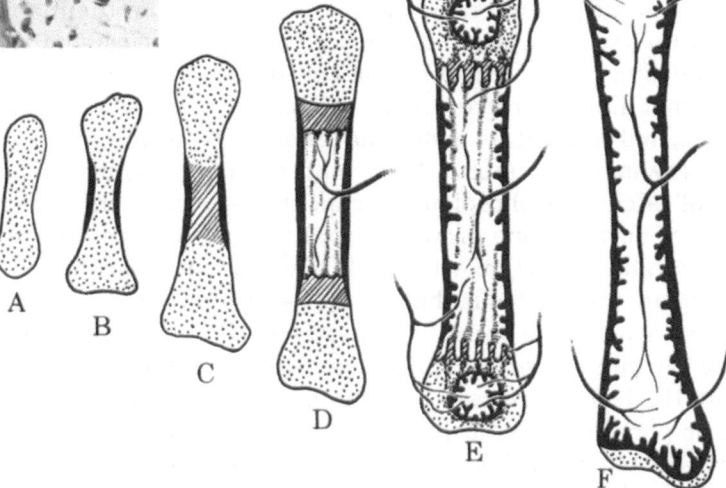

A   B   C   D   E   F

5.15

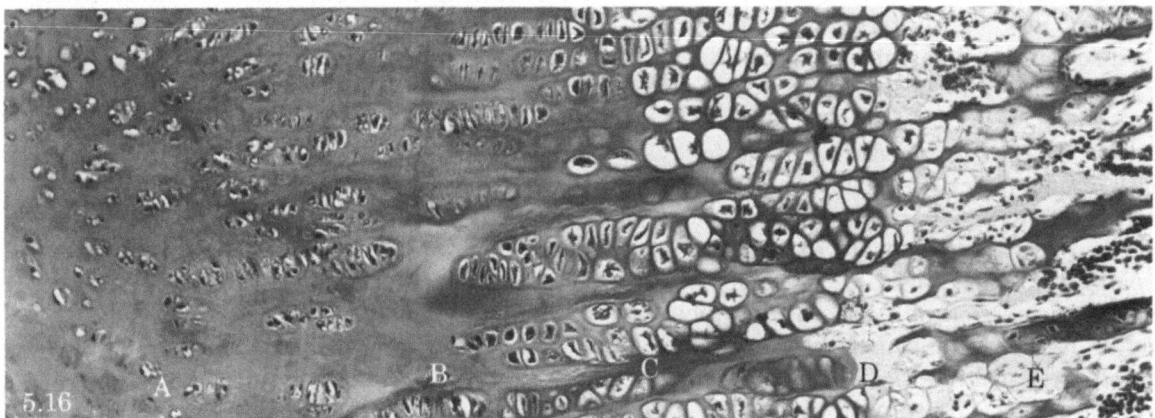

5.16   A   B   C   D   E

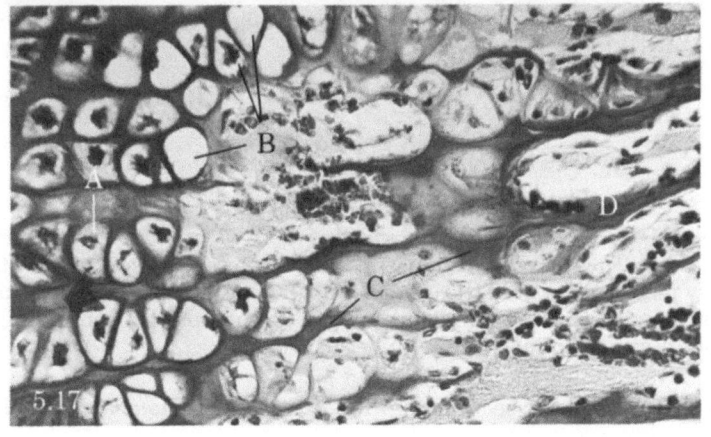

5.17   A   B   C   D

of the periosteum. Growth in length of long bones occurs entirely by endochondral ossification, especially on the diaphyseal side of the epiphyseal plate. The plate "closes" as the last layers of cartilage and osteoid are replaced by mature bone and as the epiphyses and diaphysis fuse. After the epiphyseal plate disappears longitudinal growth of bones ceases.

REMODELING involves the formation of new osteons and the gradual relocation of old ones by coordinated resorption and deposition of lamellae (Figs. 5.18 and 5.19). It continues throughout life, is proportionate to changes in stress, and responds to endocrine influence.

RICKETS AND OSTEOMALACIA. Abnormal serum levels of calcium or phosphate disrupt the sequence of normal bone growth. Usually this is attributable to lack of vitamin D which is provided in certain foods, but which is also produced within the human organism with the aid of sunlight. Certain renal diseases may deplete the body of excessive amounts of calcium or phosphate; critically low levels may occur. In children the clinical condition caused by calcium deficiency is known as *rickets*. Since the bone matrix does not calcify, bone growth and formation are affected. These abnormalities best seen by X-ray (Fig. 5.20).

Calcification is a necessary step in two phases of endochondral ossification. If the intercellular matrix of cartilage does not calcify the cells will not degenerate as regularly or as readily as they normally do. This interrupts the succession of steps and produces a broad uneven layer of uncalcified or partially calcified cartilage that may become only irregularly resorbed and replaced by bone.

The second critical point for calcification involves osteoid tissue. Lack of mineral deposition prevents the formation of true bone. Because of these two defects epiphysial plates are irregular and enlarged in all directions but the bone length remains practically the same. In addition the bone ends are abnormally pliable and may be bent; this is termed bowing.

Intramembranous bone growth also suffers from the inability of osteoid to calcify. Excessive osteoid is produced and therefore certain characteristic distortions of membranous bones occur, such as parietal bossing of the skull.

Mature bone is less susceptible to all of these influences but as it is a living tissue it requires normal maintenance. Therefore if the serum concentration of calcium or phosphate is severely depressed for a long time the adult may suffer a variety of the same condition; this is then called osteomalacia.

OSTEOPOROSIS occurs when a reduction of the bone mass has progressed to the point where it is deemed abnormal. It is a common disorder resulting not from a lack of mineralization, as in osteomalacia, but apparently from a more basic defect that allows osteoclastic activity to exceed osteoblastic activity. The decision as to this diagnosis is obviously arbitrary and depends on several factors. The significance of this condition lies mainly in the fractures which may result from it. For example fracture of the neck of the femur is rather common, serious, and life-threatening among the elderly; it usually occurs following a fall on the hip. Similar falls seldom cause such fractures in young or middle-aged persons (Fig. 5.21).

Fig. 5.18. *The remodeling process.* **A:** Completed osteon, made of laminae successively placed one within the other. **B:** Beginning excavation. **C:** Advanced excavation. This is eccentric due to unequal rates of absorption. **D:** Rebuilding by again successively placing laminae one within the other.

Fig. 5.19. Histologic section showing *osteons in various stages.* ×100.

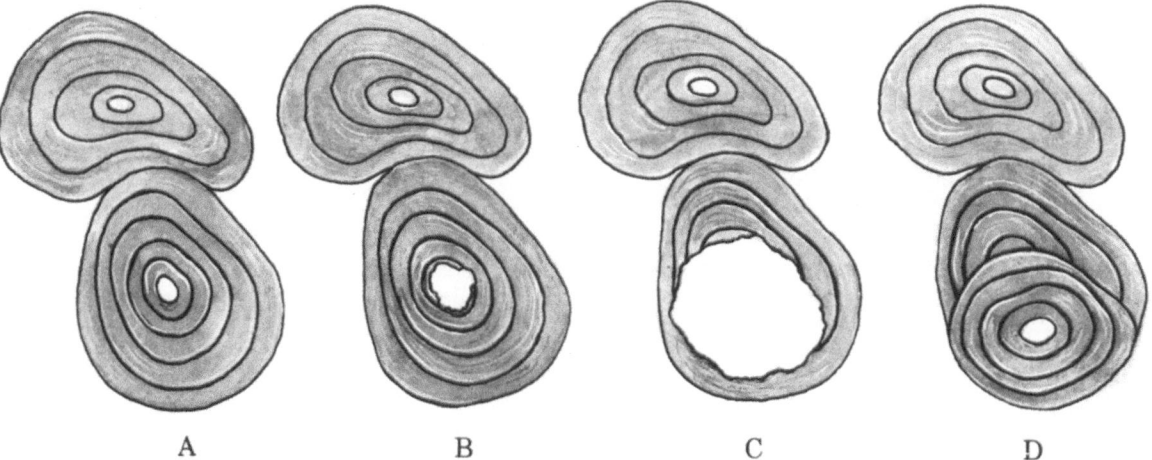

A   B   C   D

5.18

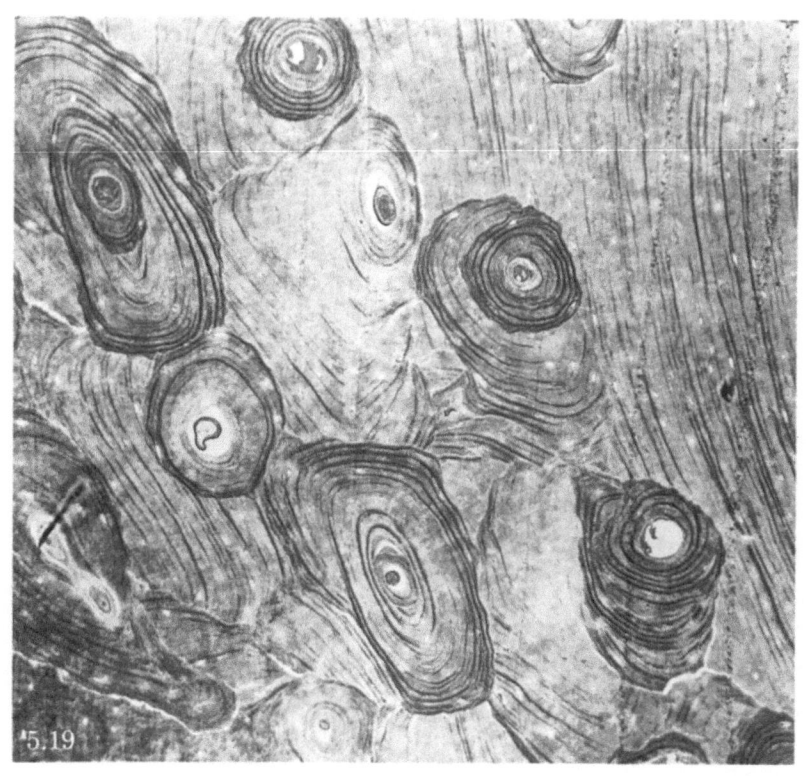

5.19

Fig. 5.20. X-rays of developing bones of the knee joint in two children. (Courtesy of Dept. of Diagnostic Radiology, Oregon Health Sciences University.) **a:** *Normal* 4-year-old. The smooth surfaced radiolucent epiphyseal line (between the short arrows) represents residual cartilage, the radiopaque layer, calcification (between the long arrows). **b:** A 2-year-old with dietary *rickets*. The epiphyseal discs are thick and rough-surfaced. The zones of calcification are indistinct.

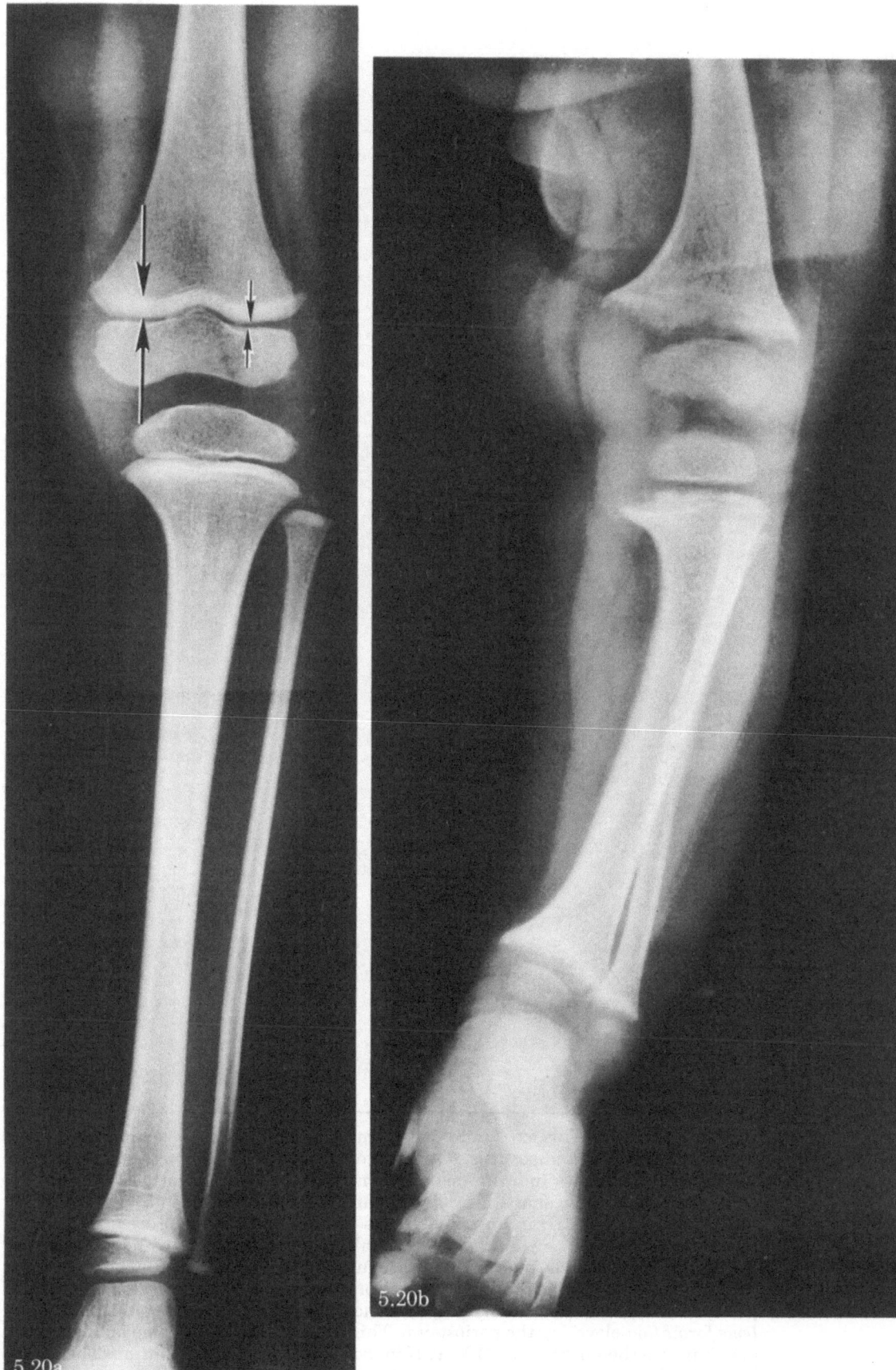

5.20a

5.20b

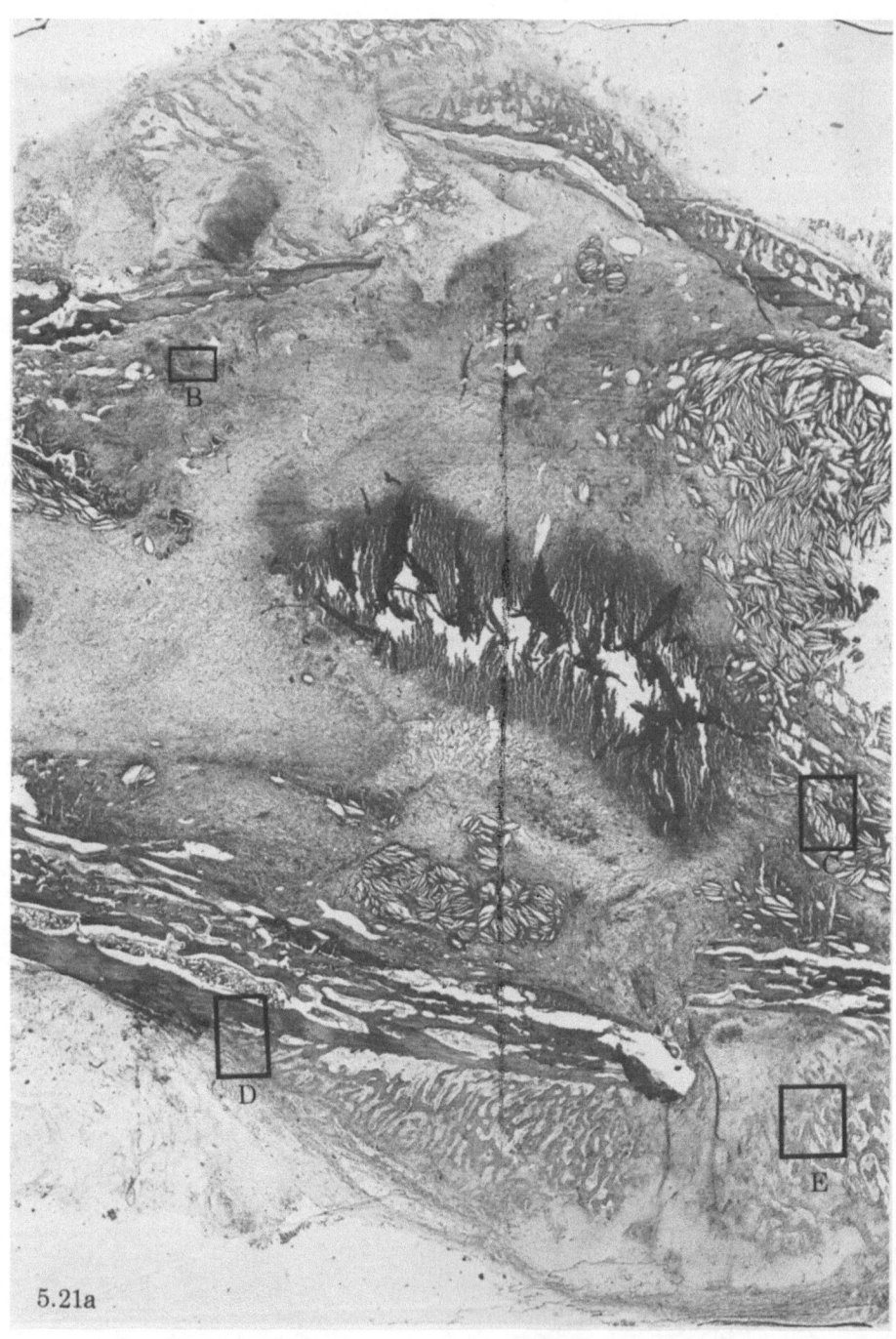

5.21a

Fig. 5.21. *Fracture.* This extraordinarily complex healing process demonstrates the capacity of bone for homeostasis. (Courtesy of S. Jacobson.) **a:** Longitudinal section of fracture. Rectangles indicate fields shown in higher magnifications. Sections of fresh blood clot often shatter, producing artefacts like the one in the center of the picture. ×7.5. **b:** *Granulation tissue* is part of the repair process as in any healing wound. ×160. **c:** *Cholesterol.* Actually this compound has been dissolved in the tissue processing and the pointed, fusiform, empty spaces in more or less parallel bundles now give the only evidence of its presence. This substance commonly precipitates in sites of unresorbed hemorrhage. ×100. **d:** *New* (intramembranous) *bone formation* elevating the periosteum. This will be followed by remodelling which may improve the alignment. ×100. **e:** New *bone and cartilage formation.* The cartilage will disappear as healing progresses. ×100.

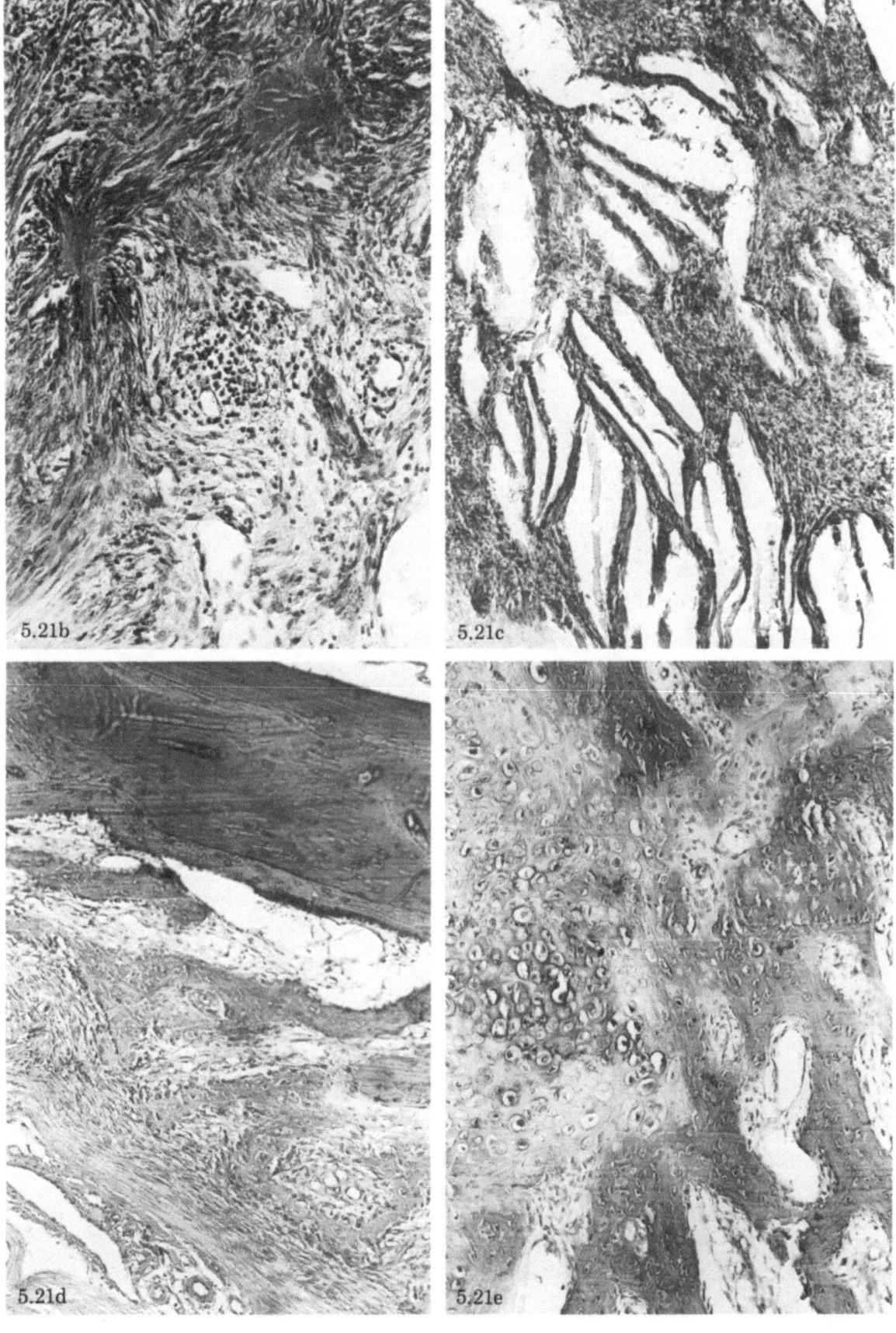

5.21b

5.21c

5.21d

5.21e

6 Muscle

Muscle tissue consists of elongated cells or multinucleated fibers specialized for contraction. To accomplish this function each cell or fiber contains the proteins actin and myosin, which undergo alterations resulting in contraction.

Types of Muscle

On the basis of microscopic morphology and function muscle is classified into three types. *Smooth muscle* is made up of elongated spindle-shaped cells somewhat resembling fibroblasts which do not show cross-striations. The contraction of these cells is not under voluntary control. *Skeletal muscle* is made up of elongated, cylindrical, multinucleated fibers that show transverse striations as a result of the alignment of contractile filaments. This type constitutes the voluntarily controlled musculature of the body. *Cardiac muscle,* also showing striations, is made up of individual cells firmly attached at points of end-to-end contact by *intercalated discs,* which are unique to cardiac muscle. Cardiac muscle contraction is involuntary and rhythmic.

Smooth Muscle

Smooth muscle (Figs. 6.1 through 6.6) cells are usually arranged in layers in the walls of hollow organs of the digestive tract, blood vessels, and the respiratory and genitourinary systems. They also occur as scattered individuals or small groups or irregular bundles in the stroma of some organs including skin. In a longitudinal section of smooth muscle (Fig. 6.1) the tapering elongated nature of the cells may be observed as well as the elongated, central nuclei which often assume the shape and proportions of a cigar. The cells are bound together by a meshwork of reticular fibers (Fig. 6.2) embedded within and lying upon an extracellular coating equivalent to the basal laminae of epithelia. In general the cells are separated but in certain special areas they are in contact with each other. At these locations the facing cell membranes are joined by gap junctions which apparently permit spread of the contraction stimulus from one cell to another.

Smooth muscle is not under voluntary control but maintains function without our having to think about it. It is innervated by autonomic nerves but not every cell has its own innervation. The contraction stimulus, once started, is passed directly from cell to cell. Movements tend to be slow and rhythmic, and to pass through the muscle as a wave rather than to involve the muscle as a whole. Such contractions make possible the function of smooth muscle in peristalsis.

Fig. 6.1. Two views (**a** and **b**) of *smooth muscle* cells of gut cut longitudinally. Both are normal. ×560.

Fig. 6.2. *Smooth muscle* (gut). Note the variation in appearance of the cross sections depending on the level at which the cells are cut. Stained for reticulum. ×560.

Fig. 6.3. A single *smooth muscle fiber* cut at different levels to explain variations seen in Fig. 6.2.

Fig. 6.4. *Hypertrophy* of smooth muscle in a pregnant uterus—an adaptation to functional needs within the range of normal histology. Note that this and Fig. 6.5 are taken at the same magnification. ×125.

Fig. 6.5. *Atrophy* of smooth muscle in a uterus after the child-bearing age. Normal? ×125.

Fig. 6.6. *Tumors* (leiomyomas, two) of smooth muscle. These are in the wall (myometrium) of the uterus, where they occur in about 50% of adult women. The appearance at this magnification is typical. ×21.

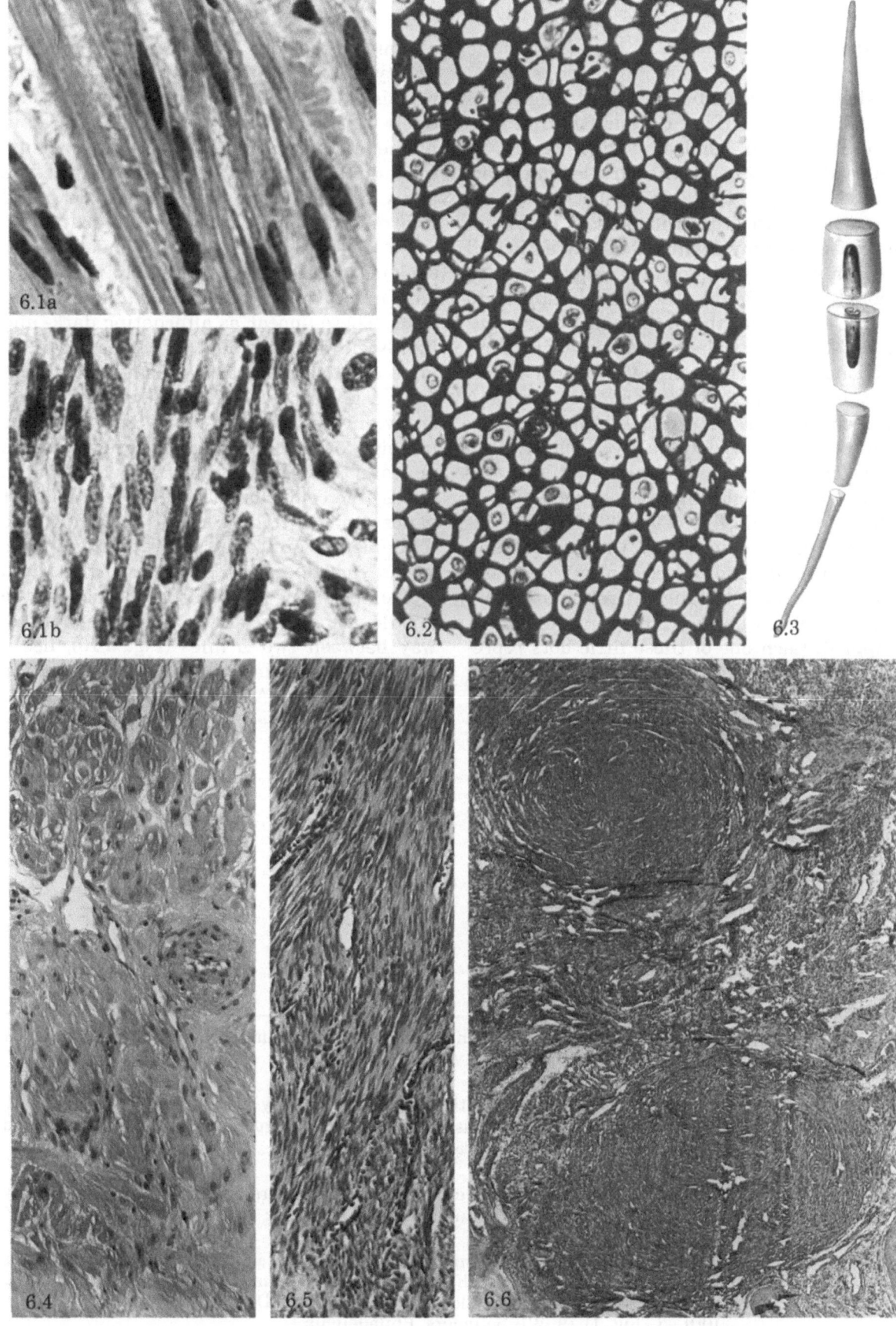

6.1a

6.1b

6.2

6.3

6.4

6.5

6.6

Skeletal Muscle

A skeletal muscle fiber is a very long cylindrical syncytium (Figs. 6.7 and 6.8) that may contain several hundred nuclei located at intervals just beneath the sarcolemma (plasmalemma of a muscle fiber). The cytoplasm is packed with great numbers of longitudinally oriented myofilaments of both actin and myosin precisely aligned in parallel array. Although at first glance there would appear to be little space for them, the usual organelles are present, particularly great numbers of mitochondria, which provide the energy necessary for contraction. The endoplasmic, here termed sarcoplasmic, reticulum is elaborate. There is also considerable glycogen.

In cross-sections of skeletal muscle observed with a light microscope, each fiber is limited by a thin line (Fig. 6.9). This line includes three components: the sarcolemma (Fig. 6.12), an external coat of glycoprotein, and a delicate "stocking" of reticular fibers. The cytoplasm appears finely granulated or stippled. Each one of these little dots represents a cross-section of a *myofibril*. Within each myofibril, but visible only with the electron microscope, are hundreds of *myofilaments* of actin and of myosin. Those of myosin

are much thicker. The arrangement of the two types in cross section is such that each myosin filament is surrounded by six precisely placed actin filaments, and each actin filament is equidistant from three myosin filaments (Figs. 6.10 and 6.11). Between the two types are connecting bridges that break and reform during contraction and relaxation.

THE SARCOMERE. In longitudinal sections, skeletal muscle fibers are seen to possess evenly and regularly spaced transverse striations. These appear as alternating dark- and light-staining bands (Fig. 6.7). The cross banding is due to the exact alignment of the myofibrils; a given component of one fibril is precisely aligned with the equivalent structures in neighboring fibrils. Thus a series of bands appears to stretch across the entire fiber. Across the center of each of the largest light bands is a very fine dark line, the *Z line*. The fundamental unit of structure of the fiber is the *sarcomere* and is defined as that portion of the fiber lying between two Z lines. In the middle of each sarcomere, and therefore midway between two Z lines (Fig. 6.10), lies a broad, darkly staining band, the *A band*. On each side of the A band is a lightly stained band representing half of the entire lightly stained band (the *I band*).

Fig. 6.7. *Skeletal muscle.* Longitudinal section stained to show the striations. A (dark) and I (light) bands are visible. ×400.

Fig. 6.8. *Skeletal muscle.* With the more commonly used stains, such as H & E, striations may be faint or invisible. Hence other morphologic criteria must be used in recognizing the tissue. ×125.

Fig. 6.9. *Skeletal muscle* in cross-section. The fibers are bound into bundles by connective tissue. **A:** Epimysium. **B:** Perimysium. **C:** Endomysium. ×40.

Fig. 6.10. The structural *organization of striated muscle.* The two rectangular insets depict the fine structure of the two types of filaments. (Modified from a drawing by Sylvia Colard Keene in Bloom W and Fawcett DW. A Textbook of Histology, 10th ed., Fig. 11.19, WB Saunders, Philadelphia.)

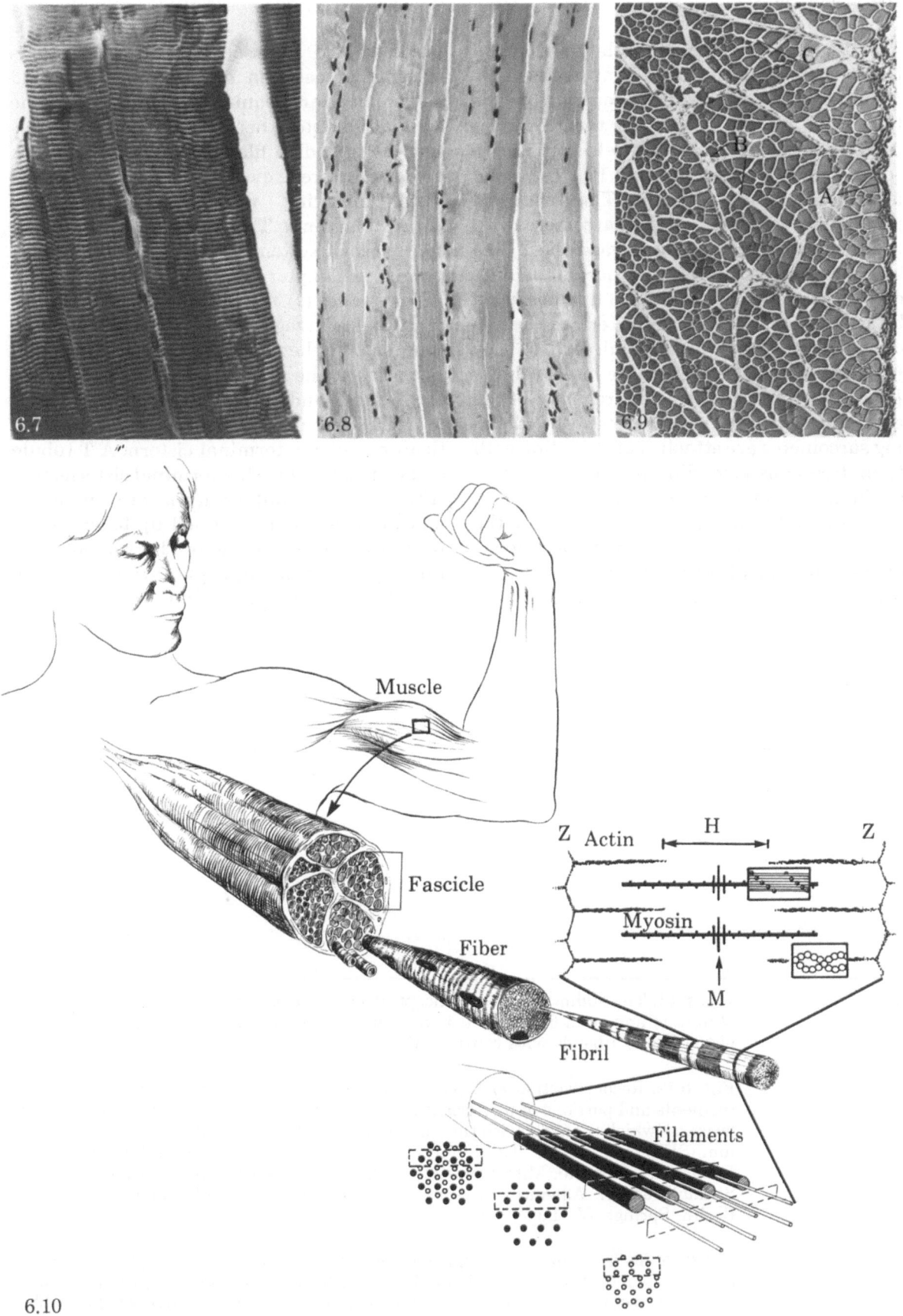

6.7

6.8

6.9

C
B
A

Muscle

Fascicle

Fiber

Fibril

Z Actin   H   Z

Myosin

M

Filaments

6.10

Although changes in the relative width of these bands have long been known to be associated with varying states of contraction, the true basis for the bands and their changes can be appreciated only at the electron microscopic level. As shown in Fig. 6.10, the A band is formed by myosin filaments. These are lined up across the center of the sarcomere with their free ends projecting toward the Z line but not reaching it. Precisely across the middle of the sarcomere is a faint line produced by swellings at what might be termed the median ends of the myosin molecules where they join with each other. This line bisects the *H band* which lies between the free ends of the actin filaments. The actin filaments of adjoining sarcomeres are attached at the Z line with their free ends extending toward the center of the sarcomere. The free ends of the actin filaments interdigitate with or overlap the free ends of the myosin filaments, the amount of overlap being directly related to the degree of contraction of the sarcomere. Dephosphory-lation of ATP is associated with alterations in bonding between myosin and actin, and calcium ions are required for this process. The current accepted theory of muscular contraction is the sliding filament theory of Huxley, although there is evidence of another mechanism involving molecular reorientation within filaments. This process is initiated by the nervous system through the motor end-plate (see Chapter 7).

TRANSVERSE (T) TUBULES (Figs. 6.12 and 6.13) are tubular invaginations of the sarcolemma that encircle the myofibrils of each sarcomere. Each lies at the level of the junction between the A and I bands. On each side of and parallel to each T tubule is a sac of sarcoplasmic reticulum called a terminal cistern. A T tubule and its two neighboring terminal cisterns constitute a triad. Mitochondria are numerous and most of them are lined up between the myofibrils. The cisterns of the sarcoplasmic reticulum contain large quantities of calcium ions that are necessary to initiate contraction.

Fig. 6.11. The sliding filament concept of *muscle contraction*. The area of overlap of myosin and actin filaments is indicated by stippling. Note the decrease in width of the H and I bands with contraction.

Fig. 6.12. Reconstruction of a portion of a *skeletal muscle fiber*. Six myofibrillar segments and portions of four triads are included. Each triad consists of a T tubule (arrows), which connects with the sarcolemma, and a cistern of sarcoplasmic reticulum (SER) on each side. The tubules and cisterns are intimately related but their lumens are separate. Mitochondria are shown between neighboring triads. (After Schmalbruch H: Advances in Anatomy, Embryology and Cell Biology, 43: No. 1, Berlin, Springer-Verlag, 1970.)

Fig. 6.13. *Skeletal muscle* shown in a transmission electron micrograph of a longitudinal section. Portions of four T-tubules (arrowheads); Z lines (Z). Myosin filaments, having been cut obliquely, appear as short segments (arrows). (Courtesy of M. Webb.) ×28,000.

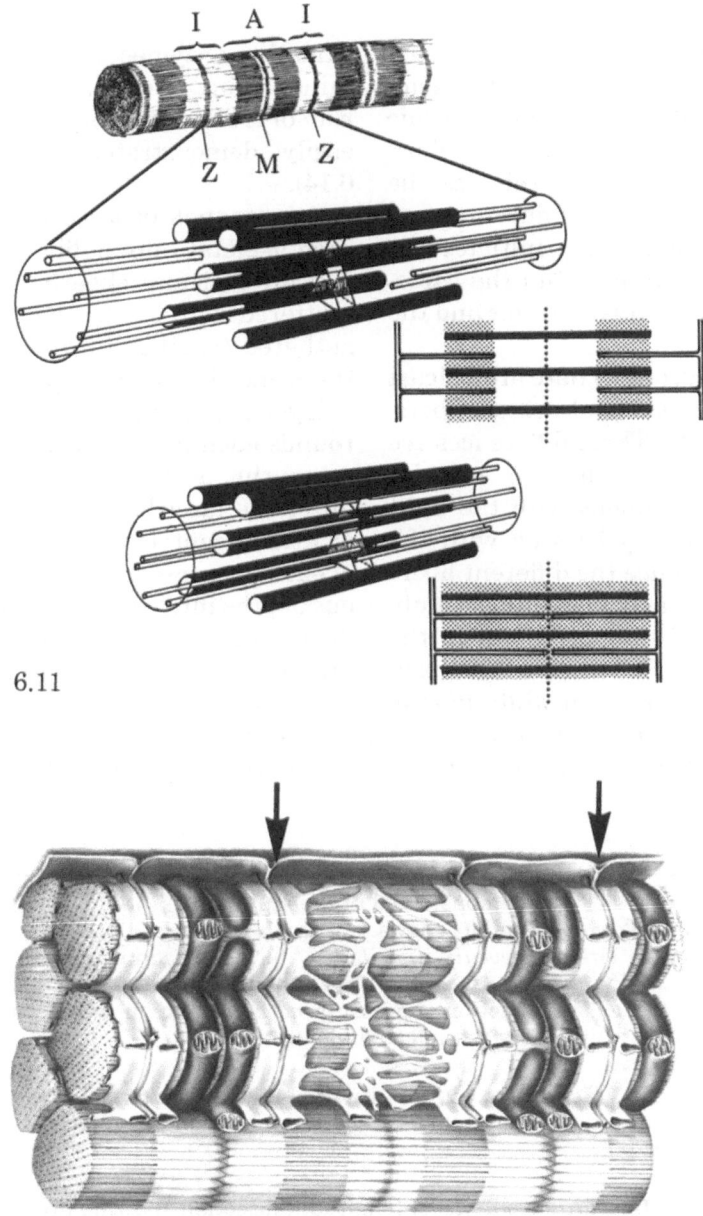

I A I

Z M Z

6.11

6.12

6.13

Depolarization originating in the motor end-plate (see Chapter 7) passes along the membranes of the T tubules to the sarcoplasmic reticulum in the region of the triad. Depolarization of the triad membranes releases the calcium from the cisterns and induces muscular contraction. Repolarization initiates the reaccumulation of calcium within the sarcoplasmic reticulum. ATP then reforms and the muscle relaxes.

TYPES OF SKELETAL MUSCLE. There are at least two different types of skeletal muscle fibers, red (or dark) and white. These differences are not easily recognized in human muscles grossly or in fixed specimens with the light microscope, but they may be seen with the electron microscope. Since the different fibers react somewhat differently to certain stimuli, the patterns produced may be useful in the study of some diseases. Red muscle cells react and contract more slowly than white muscle cells. They also contain more myoglobin and more mitochondria; hence they are richer in oxidative enzymes and capable of more sustained effort. The white fibers show a higher rate of ATPase activity. These differences are easily demonstrated histochemically (Fig. 6.14).

ORGANIZATION OF MUSCLES. As stated above, each skeletal muscle fiber is enclosed by the delicate reticular sheath of endomysium and scattered fibroblasts. Numerous fibers are gathered together into fascicles coated with the somewhat more prominent perimysium. A layer of similar loose connective tissue surrounds each muscle as seen in the dissecting room; this is the epimysium, which encloses all of the fascicles of a muscle. At the place of attachment to a tendon the sarcolemma of each fiber has several invaginations of various depths into which the ends of the collagen fibers insert. Amazingly, this junction has greater tensile strength than either the muscle or the tendon.

CONTROL. There are more than 500 separate pairs of muscles of the human body, and

Fig. 6.14. ATPase demonstrated in skeletal muscle. ×85. (Courtesy of A. D'Agostino.) **a:** The *normal* reaction shows two types of fibers. Both types are approximately *equal* in size and *evenly distributed*. **b:** The reaction here is typical of *systemic disease*, in which the *red* (darkly stained) fibers are *more affected* and therefore *smaller*. **c:** This reaction represents *nerve injury*, in which some of *both* the red and the white fibers are affected about *equally*.

Fig. 6.15. *Cardiac muscle*, longitudinal section. The separation of fibers by interstitial connective tissue makes their branching more apparent. Compare with Fig. 6.16. ×200.

Fig. 6.16. *Cardiac muscle*. A longitudinal section showing branching fibers, intercalated discs, and blunt-ended, centrally located nuclei. One rarely finds all these features in a single microscopic field. Nuclei of endothelial cells and connective tissue cells are also present. ×250.

Fig. 6.17. *Cardiac muscle*, cross-section. Nuclei are usually central in location, but this is not apparent in every cell. ×320.

Fig. 6.18. Myocardial *succinate dehydrogenase* reactions. ×740. **a:** Normal; note the longitudinal and cross striations. **b:** Hypoxia; striations are not visible although the reaction is just as strong as in the normal specimen. This change correlates with weak contraction of the muscle and with heart failure. H & E stains of serial sections from the same tissue blocks show histologically normal myocardium. In other words, the histochemical reaction reflects abnormal function in spite of normal histology.

Fig. 6.19. *Acute Myocardial infarction*. Both normal (left) and necrotic myocardium are visible. The necrotic tissue has hazy and poorly defined or absent nuclei. However, the fibers still appear well preserved. ×250.

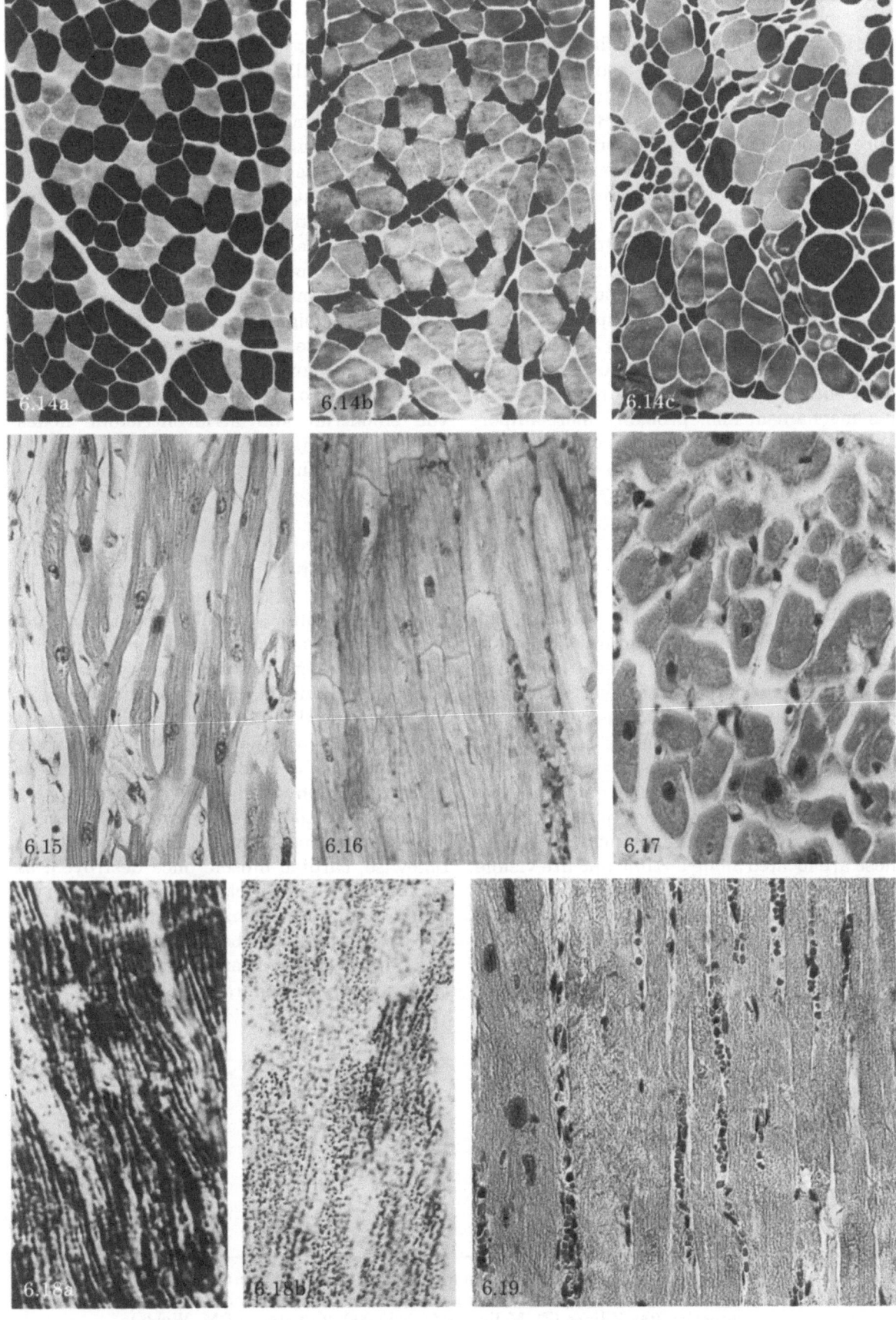

each has its own innervation. Thus each muscle can be separately and voluntarily controlled, although most people are not able to master this feat without a lot of practice. More important, we have the ability to control movement of all parts of our bodies without having to think about which muscle is doing the work.

Each muscle fiber is innervated by a single nerve fiber originating in the central nervous system; one nerve fiber may supply several muscle fibers. Because of the speed of transmission of impulses in nerves (see Chapter 7), a muscle that may consist of many separate fibers can contract as a unit. Details of this mechanism and, probably more importantly, of just how the necessary refinements of timing and strength of contraction work, are only partly understood.

Cardiac Muscle

Cardiac muscle (Figs. 6.15 through 6.19) has the same basic organization of myofibrils and myofilaments as skeletal muscle and thus shows similar striations. However, each fiber is a single cell with one nucleus centrally located among the myofibrils (Figs. 6.15 through 6.17). Each cylindrical cell is attached to its neighbors at each end by a complex junctional system of desmosomes, zonulae adherentes and tight junctions. All of these are located along a Z line and are visible with the light microscope as dark transverse lines called *intercalated discs* (Fig. 6.20). Many of the cells branch and connect with other branched neighbors to give a woven or interlaced appearance in longitudinal section.

Nuclei are of a characteristic form; that is, short and usually blunt, sometimes square at their ends.

The T system of cardiac muscle cells is irregular and variable. It differs from that of skeletal muscle in that each T tubule encircles the fibril at the level of the Z line, rather than at the junction of A and I bands, as in skeletal muscle, and lies between cisterns of adjacent sarcomeres.

All cardiac muscle cells can and do conduct impulses to neighboring myocytes. However, some specialized muscle fibers are required for the necessarily more rapid distribution of this impulse to the entire myocardium from the sinoatrial and atrioventricular nodes. This, the cardiac conduction system, will be described in Chapter 8.

Regeneration of Muscle

Unlike epthelium, connective tissue, and bone, striated muscle (both skeletal and cardiac) has no regenerative capacity. This lack is associated with a high level of differentiation. In general, highly differentiated tissues are less able to regenerate. Skeletal muscle can be induced to regain much of its lost mass after the atrophy of disease or disuse but this is accomplished by enlargement—hypertrophy—rather than by multiplication of fibers. Likewise, cardiac muscle once destroyed, as for example by infarction (Fig. 6.19), can be replaced only by a connective tissue scar but not by regenerated fibers. Smooth muscle is less highly differentiated than the striated types and can regenerate more readily.

Fig. 6.20. Transmission electron micrograph through an *intercalated disc* of *cardiac muscle*. In addition to myofilaments and mitochondria, note desmosomes (D), gap junction (G), Z lines (Z), M lines (M). ×20,000. (Courtesy of M. Webb.)

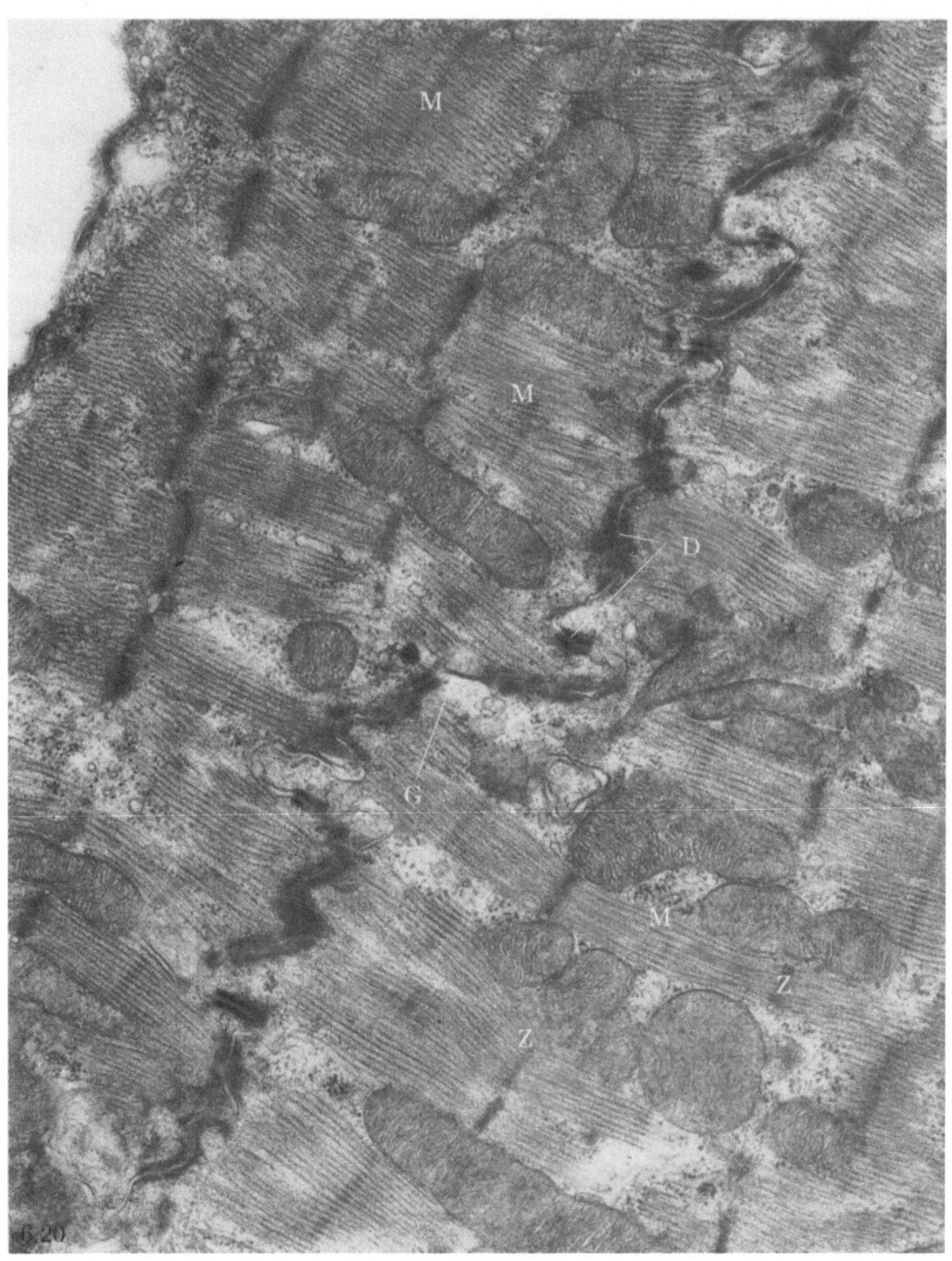

7 Nervous Tissue

The gross and microscopic anatomy of the nervous system is so complex and special that it deserves an entire course and a considerably larger text than can be accommodated in this volume. Nervous tissue is distributed throughout the brain and spinal cord and its extensions, like those of the vascular system, appear in every other organ and tissue.

Organization of the Nervous System

The nervous system is composed of nerve cells or *neurons* and supporting cells, *glia*. Anatomically it is divided into the central nervous system (CNS) and the peripheral nervous system (PNS).

Central Nervous System

The CNS consists of the brain and spinal cord and lies within the cranial cavity and the vertebral canal (Fig. 7.1). The CNS comprises the integrative centers for communication, coordination, thought, and emotion and has an estimated 10^{14} functional interneuronal connections. Internally the CNS lacks the collagen, elastin, and ground substance that impart resilience and pliability to the rest of the body. Glial cells and their processes take the place of these components. The bony case surrounding the CNS is vitally important for its physical protection and support.

Peripheral Nervous System

The PNS is composed of nerves, ganglia, and end-organs. Most neuronal bodies reside in the CNS; thus nerves are essentially cables of long neuronal processes carrying impulses between the CNS and the end-organs. The nerves branch as they extend into all tissues. The PNS is the means of rapid (0.5–100.0 m/sec) transfer of stimuli between the CNS and the functioning and feeling periphery.

The most striking feature of the nervous system is its many fibers, which group, course, regroup, and branch in the nerves like cables of wires. The lines of communication must remain intact, even though they are extremely numerous and the wiring accordingly complex. Peripheral nerve trunks and branches contain fibers that are bound together and encased in connective tissue sheaths.

CRANIAL AND SPINAL NERVES. Cranial and spinal nerves include both motor and sensory fibers. The motor fibers originate from cell bodies within the CNS and carry impulses to skeletal muscles or to ganglia of the autonomic nervous system (see below). The sensory fibers conduct information to the CNS from sensory nerve endings throughout the body. The cell bodies of the sensory neurons are located in the cranial and spinal ganglia (Fig. 7.1; also see later).

AUTONOMIC NERVOUS SYSTEM. This division of the peripheral nervous system is connected with the CNS through some of the cranial and spinal nerves. The autonomic nervous system is the means by which we unconsciously regulate: the degree of dilation of, and thus the rate of flow in, all blood vessels; peristalsis of the gut; some endocrine and exocrine secretions; and numerous other bodily functions.

Fig. 7.1. *General features of the nervous system.* **A:** Overview of central nervous system. The connections with the peripheral nervous system, by way of cranial and spinal nerve roots, are shown. **B:** Cut surface of the brain shows white matter with folded covering of gray. Two nerve fibers are indicated bringing information into the cerebral cortex from lower levels. **C:** Transverse section of spinal cord. Here the gray matter is centrally located in a butterfly-shaped area, and the white matter, composed of ascending and descending tracts, is peripherally located. **D:** Area boxed in **A**. Spinal cord in situ. The cord and spinal nerve roots are shown in relation to meninges, vertebral column, and sympathetic trunk. **E:** Cross-section of spinal nerve. Three fascicles are shown; there may be several or only one, depending on the diameter of the nerve.

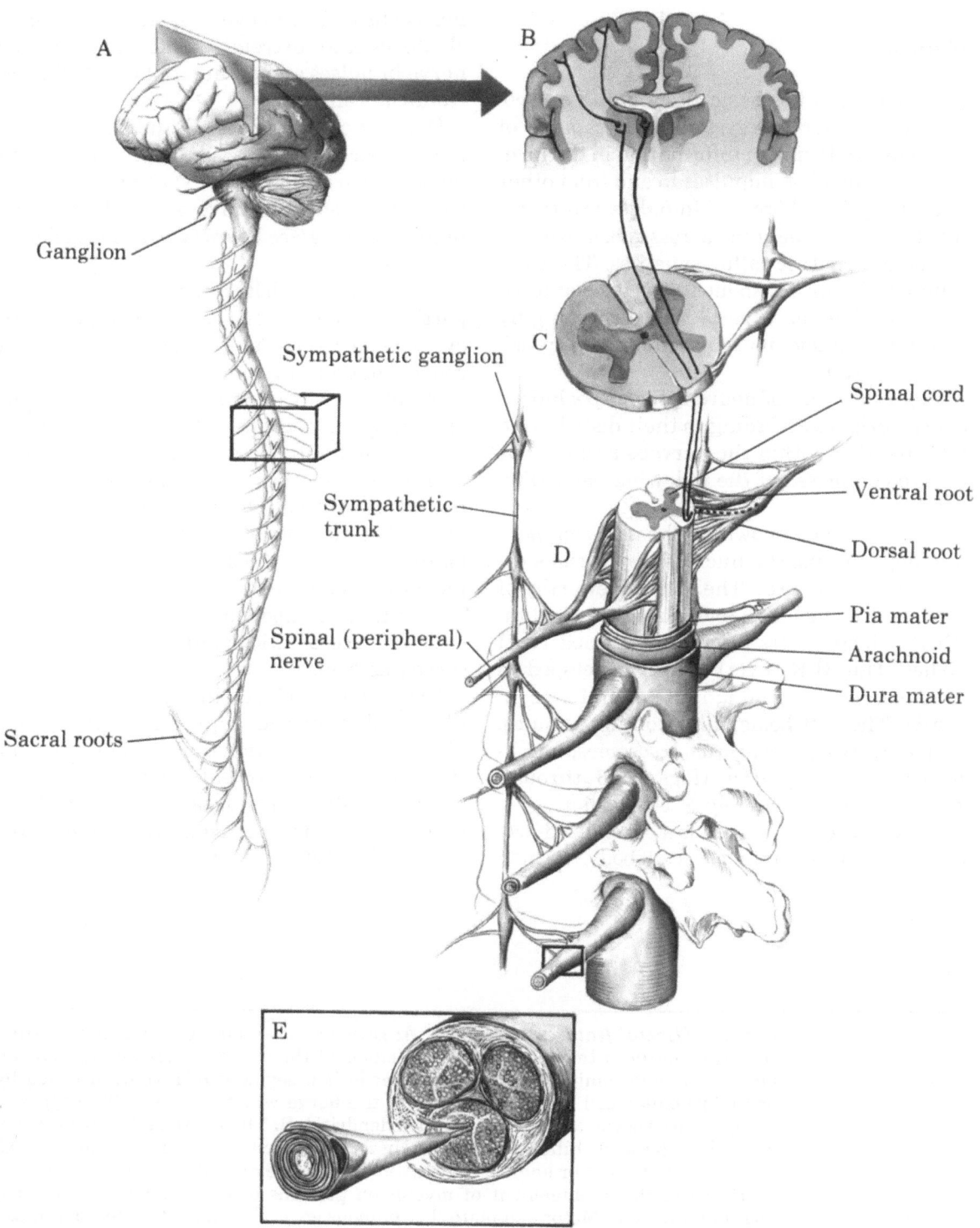

Ganglion

Sympathetic ganglion

Sympathetic trunk

Spinal (peripheral) nerve

Sacral roots

Spinal cord

Ventral root

Dorsal root

Pia mater

Arachnoid

Dura mater

A

B

C

D

E

7.1

Cells

Neurons

The neuron is the basic functioning component of the nervous system. It is capable of receiving and sending information in the form of electrochemical impulses to and from other neurons and end-organs. Impulses are transmitted between neurons across specialized areas of cell contact called synapses. The total number of neurons, about 10^{10}, is fixed at birth and, as might be expected in such a highly specialized tissue, no replacements are possible thereafter.

Different types of neurons have specialized characteristics according to their distribution and function within the nervous system, but all are comprised of the following parts (Fig. 7.2):

THE CELL BODY, known as the *soma* or *peri-karyon*, contains the nucleus and various cytoplasmic structures. The most noteworthy of the latter is the rough endoplasmic reticulum (RER) which occurs in clumps, termed Nissl bodies. The RER is very highly developed in neurons, reflecting a high rate of protein synthesis. The cell bodies also contain tubules, filaments, Golgi apparatus, lysosomes, and lipofuscin. *Gray matter* (Figs. 7.23 through 7.25) is composed largely of cell bodies.

A SINGLE AXON. An axon is a specialized process originating from the cell body. It may be very long. The axons of spinal anterior horn cells extend to even the most distal muscle fibers of an extremity. The axon conducts nerve impulses and products of the RER away from the cell body.

ONE OR MORE DENDRITES. Dendrites are long, fine, branching processes that conduct impulses toward the cell body; some are as long as axons. Dendrites have along their course many synapses (see below) with axons of other neurons.

Axons and dendrites in fascicles with supporting fibrous astrocytes and oligodendrocytes (*see below*) form the *white matter* of the central nervous system.

SYNAPSES are the points of functional contact between neurons. These are characterized as cholinergic, catecholaminergic, serotoninergic, or other, reflecting the chemical neurotransmitter released at the end of the axon. The neurotransmitter acts at the adjoining surface of the dendrite, only to be immediately destroyed and partially reabsorbed. In addition to axodendritic synapses, axoaxonic and axosomatic synapses have been observed as well.

Examination of cells in sections of nervous tissue fails to give an appreciation of the complexity and proportions of a single neuron. If the cell body were enlarged to the size of a tennis ball, its dendritic tree would fill a living room and the axon would equal the length of a football field.

Fig. 7.2. *General features of neurons.* **A:** Drawing of an entire motor neuron from the gray matter of the spinal cord. The stems of the dendrites are shown, but not all of their fine ramifications. The internode is a segment of myelin provided by one neurilemma cell and that portion of the nerve which it covers. Two types of synapses are shown, axosomatic, and axodendritic. **B:** The nerve cell body or soma. Note that the axon hillock is free of Nissl bodies and most other organelles. **C:** The terminal bouton or endfoot of an axon. This is the axonal portion of a synapse. **D:** Detail of the arrangement of myelin on portions of two internodes and at a node of Ranvier. **E:** Motor end-plate. The bulbous ends of the axon fit into a depressed area of the sarcolemma whose floor has numerous folds extending into the muscle fiber. Nuclei, mitochondria, and other organelles are usually more numerous here than in other portions of the muscle fiber. **F:** Photomicrograph of a *multipolar neuron* and neighboring nerve *fibers.* ×400. **G:** Electron micrograph of a section through a *synapse.* ×21,000. (Courtesy of A Peters with permission from Fig. 5.5 in Peters A., Palay S and Webster H: The Fine Structure of the Nervous System. Philadelphia, W B Saunders, 1976.)

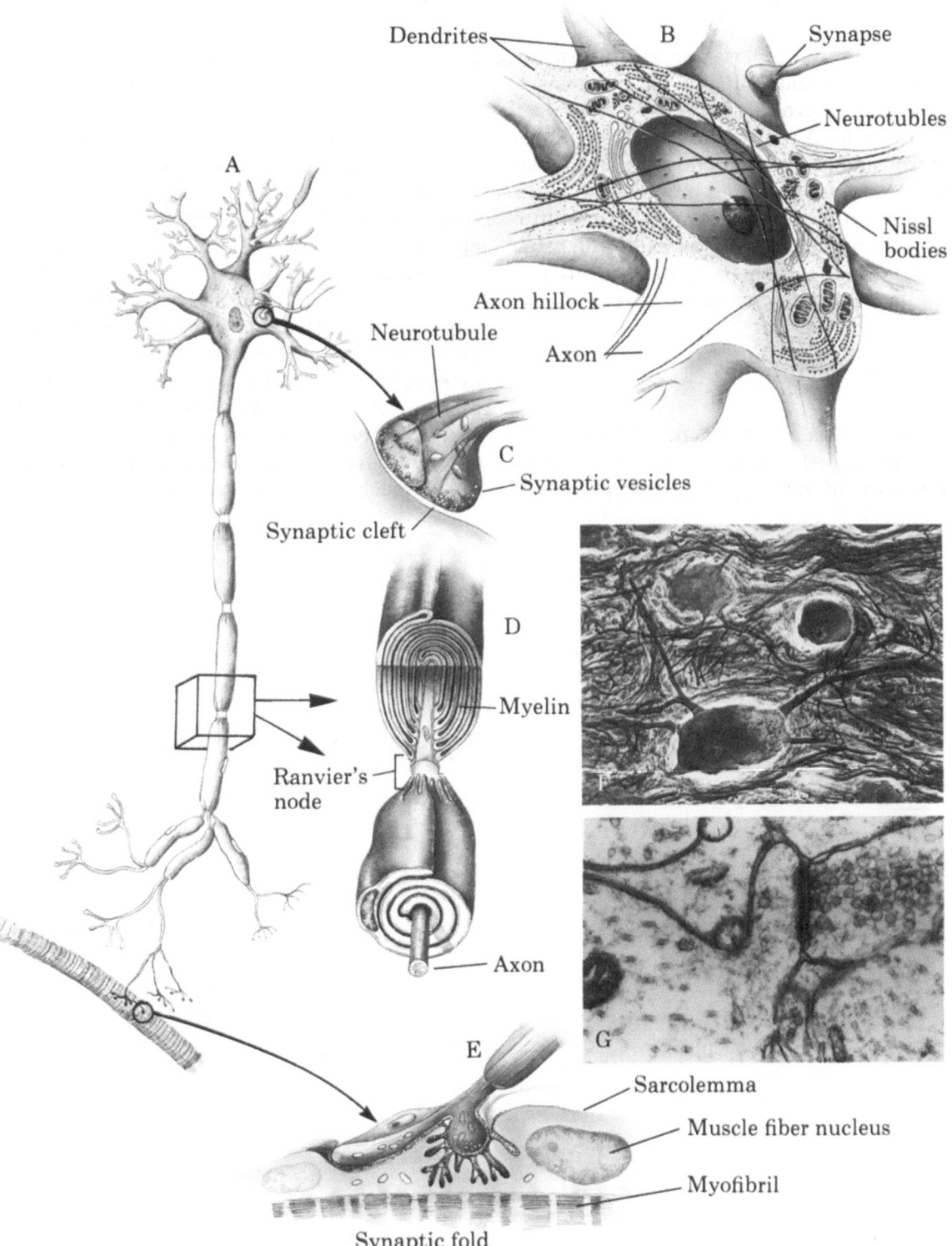

Dendrites

B

Synapse

Neurotubles

Nissl
bodies

Axon hillock

Axon

A

Neurotubule

C

Synaptic vesicles

Synaptic cleft

D

Myelin

Ranvier's
node

Axon

F

G

E

Sarcolemma

Muscle fiber nucleus

Myofibril

Synaptic fold

7.2

Neurons may be classified as multipolar, bipolar, and pseudounipolar on the basis of the number of processes attached to the cell body (Fig. 7.3). A multipolar cell (Fig. 7.2) has numerous dendrites and one axon. A bipolar cell has one dendrite and one axon. A pseudounipolar cell has a single process that bifurcates, one branch serving as axon, the other as dendrite. In all these types the cell processes may have few or many branches.

Glial Cells (Neuroglia)

Glial cells (Figs. 7.4 through 7.9) have processes that intertwine with those of the nerve cells and are of three types. All except microg-lia are ectodermal in origin. All are found only in the central nervous system.

ASTROCYTES (Fig. 7.5) give neurons both structural and nutritional support. They also serve to insulate synaptic receptor surfaces, thereby preventing diffusion of the neurotransmitter. Protoplasmic astrocytes lie chiefly in the gray matter and have large nuclei, abundant cytoplasm, and rounded or thick processes. Fibrous astrocytes tend to occupy white matter and have longer, thinner processes. A characteristic feature of astrocytes is their expanded pedicles or "end-feet" at the ends of their processes. These attach to the outer surfaces of blood vessels or to the deep surface of the pia mater, a meningeal layer which coats the exterior of the CNS.

Fig. 7.3. *Three basic types of neurons:* bipolar, multipolar, and pseudounipolar (from left to right).

Fig. 7.4. *Types of neuroglia.* **A:** Protoplasmic astrocyte. **B:** Fibrous astrocyte. This type is especially numerous just beneath the pia mater on which its feet often terminate. **C:** Microglia. The phagocytes of the CNS accumulate at sites of infection and other damage. **D:** Oligodendrocyte provides the myelin wrappings of nerve fibers in the CNS.

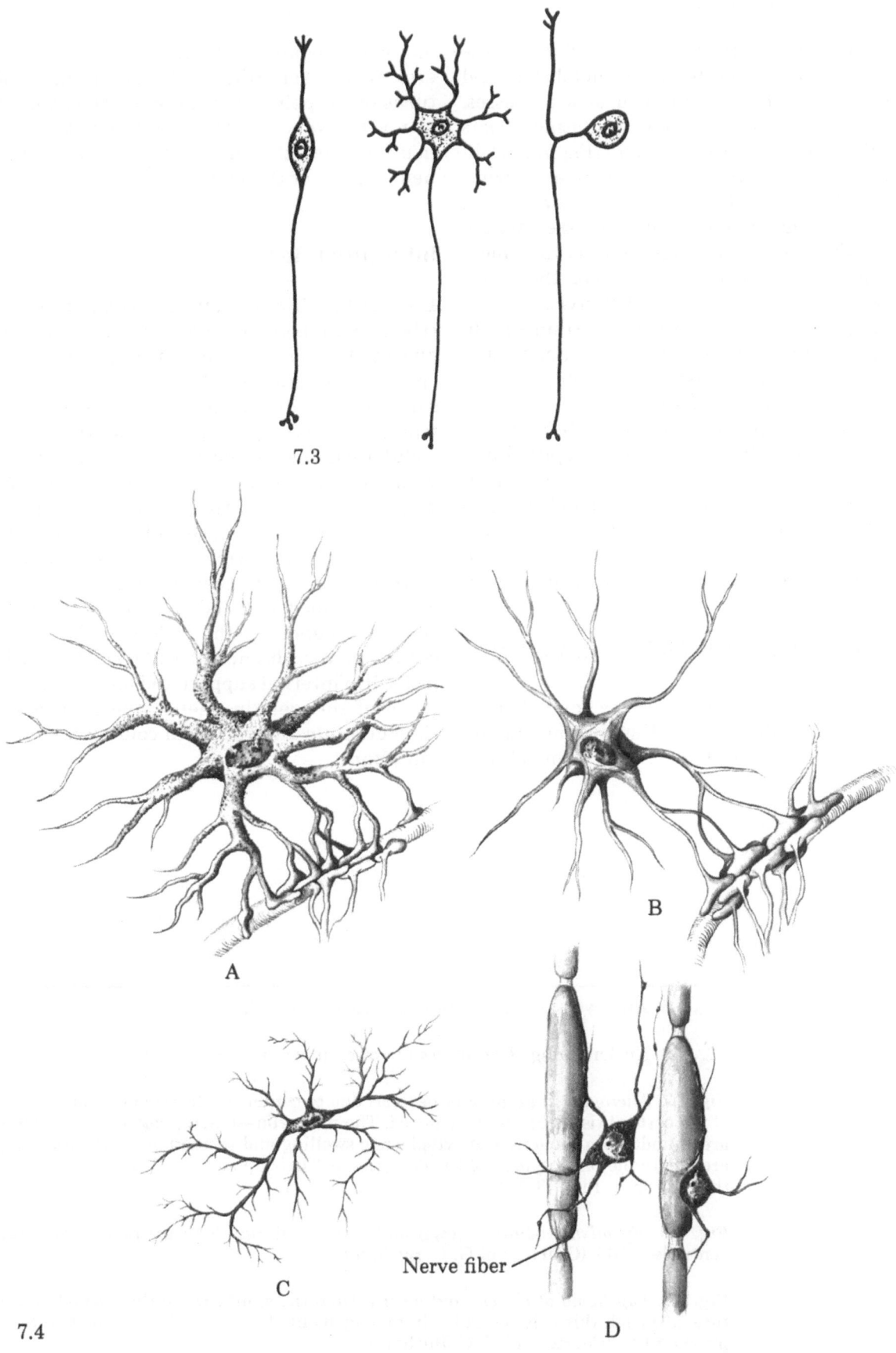

7.3

7.4

Nerve fiber

A

B

C

D

OLIGODENDROCYTES (Figs. 7.6 and 7.10) produce extensive sheets of cell membrane and roll them tightly around neuronal processes, constituting multilayered, insulating sheets of lipoprotein known as myelin (Fig. 7.11). Oligodendrocytes are smaller than astrocytes; they have smaller nuclei and fewer, less branched, and more slender processes. Where the sheaths of two oligodendrocytes meet along the course of a nerve fiber there is a short gap called the node of Ranvier.

MICROGLIA (Fig. 7.7) are of uncertain significance, but probably serve as macrophages and repair cells for the CNS. Their embryonic origin is probably mesodermal.

EPENDYMOCYTES (Figs. 7.8 and 7.9) make up a simple cuboidal or columnar epithelium. They line the ventricular cavities of the brain and the central canal of the spinal cord, as well as cover the choroid plexuses (see below). Most ependymocytes are ciliated and probably assist in the circulation of spinal fluid.

Neurilemmal Cells (Schwann Cells)

In the PNS, Schwann cells are equivalent to the oligodendrocytes and supply myelin by the same process (Fig. 7.10). The myelin is an insulating and supporting coat for peripheral nerve fibers (Fig. 7.11). The number of turns of wrapping, and therefore the amount of myelin, vary greatly in different types of neurons. Neurilemmal cells arise from the neural crest of the embryo (Fig. 7.12).

Interstitial Space

Because the CNS has a unique structural matrix, lacking both collagen and glycosaminoglycans, the passage of fluid through it merits special consideration. The basic process is the same as elsewhere: Nutrient-containing filtrate of capillary blood passes into the extracellular (that is, interstitial) space; metabolic wastes are removed by flowing in the opposite direction. Because of the high density of glial cells and neuronal (nerve cell) processes this space is normally visible only by electron microscopy, but may be seen by light microscopy when expanded, as by edema. The interstitial space surrounds all the cells and their processes. In the absence of collagen, the CNS lacks firm internal support and has the consistency of soft gelatin. Hence the protective, rigid cranium and vertebral column are very important.

Fig. 7.5. *Astrocytes* and *fibers*. Gold chloride stain. ×225.

Fig. 7.6. Nuclei of *oligodendrocytes* (arrows) in cerebral cortex. ×560.

Fig. 7.7. *Microglia* in an area of necrosis due to cerebral infarction (stroke). Much of the cortical tissue has been removed. The microglia—macrophages of the CNS— are abundant on the left. The cytoplasmic swelling and retraction of cell processes are due to the phagocytosis of the dead tissue. Their appearance has changed from that shown in Fig. 7.3. ×250.

Fig. 7.8. *Ependyma* (short arrows) and *choroid plexus* (long arrows) in cerebral ventricle. ×100. (Courtesy of G. C. Buchan.)

Fig. 7.9. *Papilloma of the choroid plexus*. Note the similarity to the normal structure, although this is less regular in arrangement. This is a relatively benign neoplasm. ×100. (Courtesy of G. C. Buchan.)

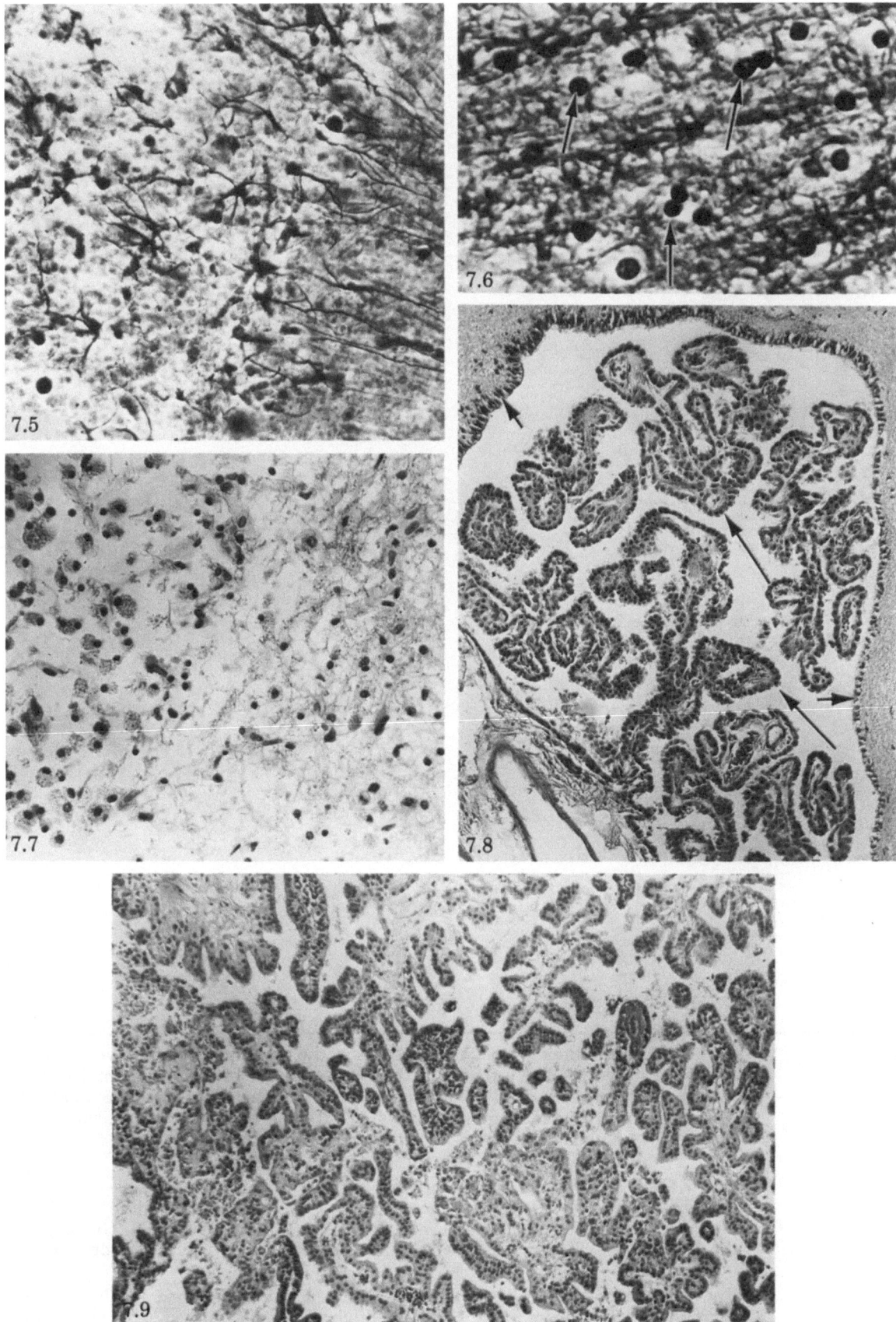

Fig. 7.10. *Myelination.* **A:** Sequential steps in the development of a myelin sheath around a nerve fiber by growth of the plasmalemma of a neurilemmal cell. **B:** Five nerve fibers embedded at different depths in grooves in a neurilemmal cell. The single layer of neurilemma is invisible with the light microscope; thus these are termed unmyelinated fibers.

Fig. 7.11. A *cross-section* of a *nerve fiber* with its myelin sheath as seen with the electron microscope. The process shown in Fig. 7.10A has produced numerous fused layers of neurilemmal cell membrane. ×39,000. (From J. Alvarado, Histology of the Human Eye, Hogan MJ, Alvarado JA, and Weddell JE. WB Saunders, 1971.)

Fig. 7.12. Cross-sections of *nerve fibers.* ×250. **a:** The unstained myelin sheaths surround the dark fibers. H&E. **b:** Fibers. Silver stain. **c:** Myelin sheaths are stained darkly. Osmium tetroxide.

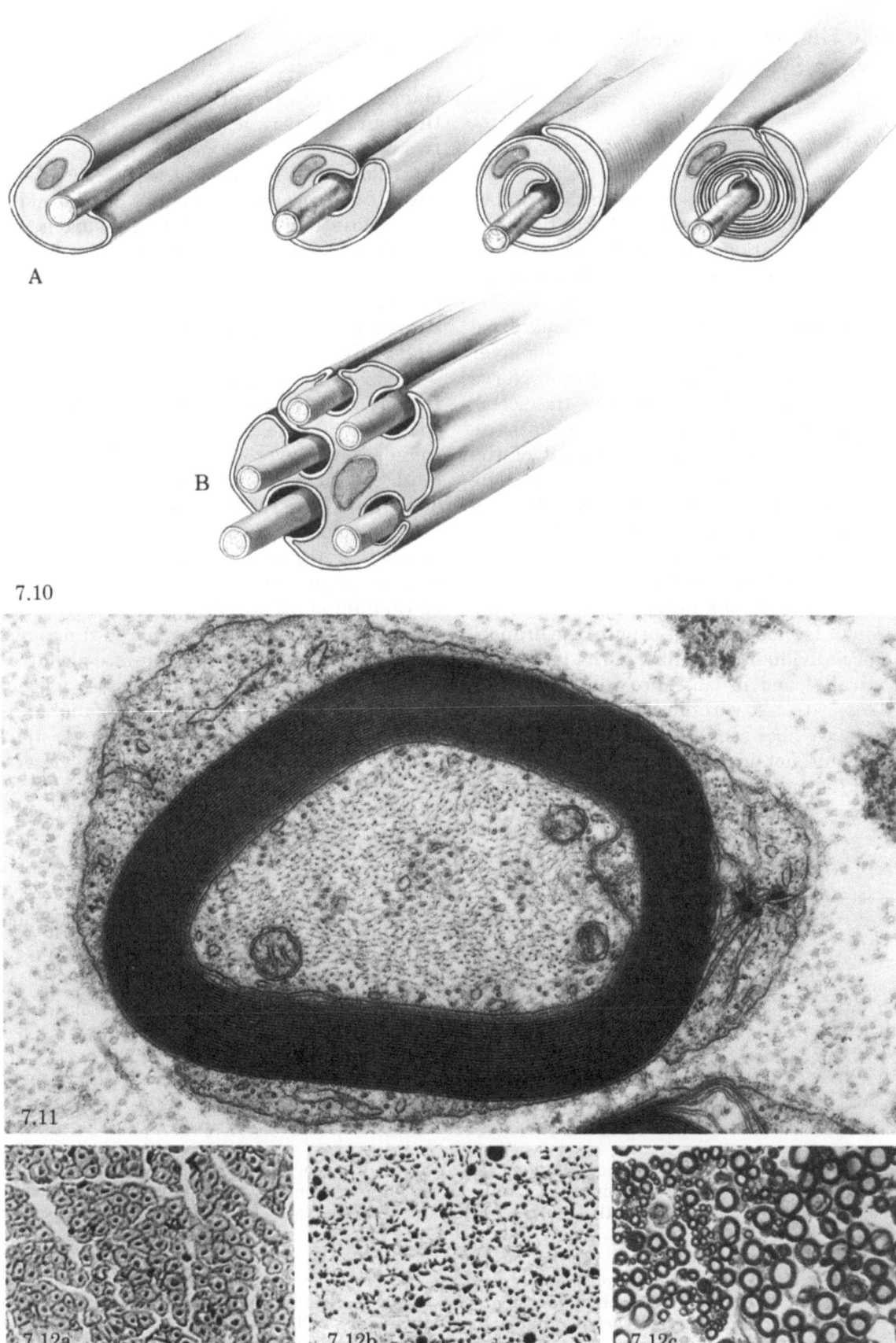

7.10

7.11

7.12a   7.12b   7.12c

Basic Histology of the Peripheral Nervous System

Nerves

Nerves vary in size depending on the number of fibers (axons and dendrites) and their degree of myelination. Cross-sections vary in diameter from a few micrometers to about 1.5 cm (Fig. 7.13).

Each nerve fiber is surrounded, and separated from its neighbors, by a tenuous layer of connective tissue, the *endoneurium*. Nerve fibers are grouped into bundles (fascicles), each with an obvious connective tissue sheath, the *perineurium*. Finally all of the bundles constituting a nerve are bound together by a coat of connective tissue, the *epineurium*. The parallel with muscle in arrangement, sheathing, and nomenclature is obvious (Figs. 7.14 and 7.15).

The branching of a nerve implies the separation of fascicles but not usually the branching of individual nerve fibers. The latter run in parallel and in close proximity but they are separate, like wires in a cable. Terminally, each nerve fiber connects to one of the following: an autonomic ganglion; a motor end-plate (Figs. 7.2 and 7.19); one of several types of sensory receptors.

Ganglia

Ganglia are clusters of nerve-cell bodies along the course of peripheral nerves. They are of two types.

CRANIAL and SPINAL GANGLIA (Fig. 7.16) are entirely sensory and are located on the nerve roots close to the CNS. Their neurons are pseudounipolar; one of the two heavily myelinated branches extends distally to a sense organ, and the other enters the CNS and transmits impulses that have originated peripherally.

Cranial and spinal ganglia are characterized by closely packed spherical cell bodies with central nuclei. Each cell body is surrounded by a layer of satellite cells of neural crest origin and by a layer of capsule cells of connective tissue origin.

AUTONOMIC GANGLIA (Fig. 7.17) are composed of motor neurons whose axons carry impulses distally to smooth muscle and/or glandular epithelium in *all of the organs*. Clearly, autonomic ganglia may have profound functional effects that are not under voluntary control.

Autonomic ganglia are located in various positions. Some, the sympathetic ganglia, lie along the paired sympathetic trunks or more distally on the nerves that supply the viscera. Others, the parasympathetic ganglia, are on or near the organs they innervate. The nu-

---

Fig. 7.13. A *peripheral nerve* in cross-section showing epineurium (E), perineurium (P), and endoneurium (arrows). ×100.

Fig. 7.14. *Small nerve* in cross-section. Neurilemmal cells appear to be aligned across the nerve, rather than along it. This is commonly seen, due to the shrinkage and distortion of the tissue. ×150.

Fig. 7.15. *Neurilemmoma.* This is a benign tumor of neurilemmal cells. Many of the cells are arranged in parallel bundles, simulating the appearance seen in Fig. 7.14. ×125.

Fig. 7.16. *Spinal ganglion.* **a:** Collection of sensory neurons and nerve fibers. ×35. **b:** The pseudounipolar nature of the neurons is not ordinarily apparent in such a section. Note the central nuclei and the layer of satellite cells. Methylene blue stain. ×250.

Fig. 7.17. *Autonomic ganglion.* **a:** The arrangement of these cells is less regular than in the spinal ganglion. ×35. **b:** These cells are multipolar and appear more ragged and variable than the spinal ganglion cells. Also satellite cells are so close to the neurons as to appear in some cases to be within them. ×200.

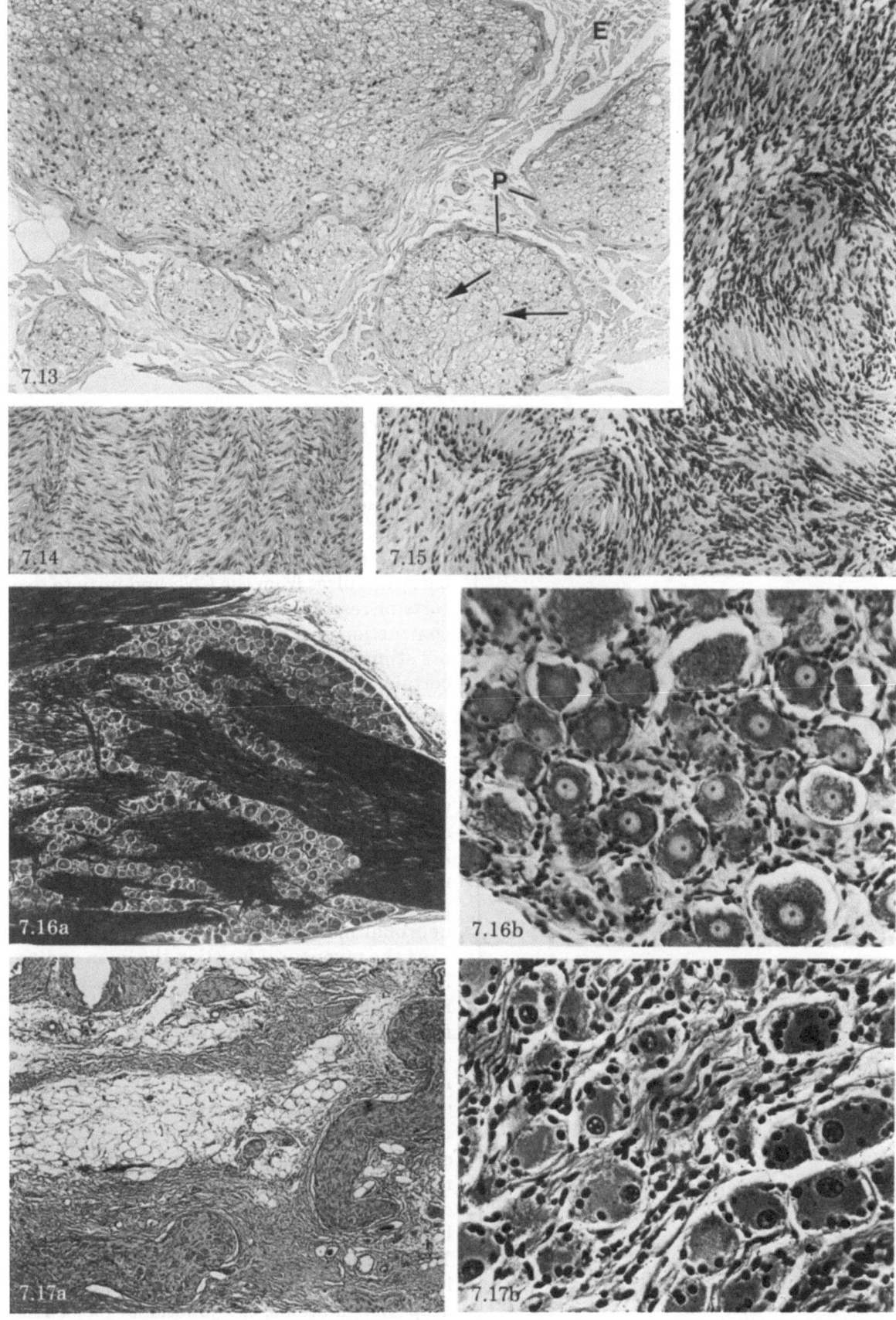

7.13

7.14

7.15

P

E

7.16a

7.16b

7.17a

7.17b

merous dendrites of autonomic neurons receive impulses from preganglionic neurons, whose cell bodies are located within the CNS.

The ganglion cells are multipolar neurons, each with several dendrites and a single axon. Because of the presence of numerous processes, these cells appear irregular or ragged in histologic sections. Their satellite cells are located between the cell processes and sometimes falsely appear to be within the neuronal cytoplasm. The neurons have eccentric nuclei. In most autonomic ganglia the cell bodies are more or less scattered, not closely packed as in spinal ganglia.

End Organs

End organs (Fig. 7.18) are of two major types, motor (efferent) and sensory (afferent).

MOTOR ENDINGS (Fig. 7.19) are the terminations of the axons of efferent nerves. The fibers carry impulses from the CNS and initiate two sorts of responses. Some fibers stimulate the contraction of skeletal or smooth muscle; others stimulate the secretory epithelial cells in certain glands. The best known motor ending is the *motor end-plate* or *myoneural junction* of skeletal muscle.

A single motor neuron may supply only a single muscle fiber, or it may branch many times to innervate as many as 150. In any case the nerve fiber or its branch terminates in a structure similar to a synpase. Here the neurotransmitter acetylcholine initiates depolarization of sarcolemma rather than of neuronal membrane.

At the myoneural junction the axon ending is unmyelinated. The end of the nerve fiber is dilated and has a flattened or rounded surface that fits into a shallow oval depression on the surface of the muscle fiber. This terminal dilation is covered by the cytoplasm of one or more neurilemmal cells and contains numerous mitochondria and synaptic vesicles. Between the membranes of the axon and the muscle is a narrow space, the synaptic cleft. Within the cleft are the conjoined basal laminae of the neuron and the muscle fiber. The surface area of the sarcolemma is greatly increased here by the presence of numerous deep invaginations, the junctional folds. The area immediately beneath these folds, within the muscle fiber, is free of myofilaments and contains numerous mitochondria and ribosomes, glycogen granules, and several muscle nuclei. This portion of the sarcolemma contains acetylcholine receptors, to which the acetylcholine from the synaptic vesicles binds in the process of initiating sarcolemmal depolarization. Unused acetylcholine is broken down by cholinesterase, an enzyme located within the synaptic cleft.

Patients with myasthenia gravis, a disease of intermittent or progressive muscular weakness, have circulating antibodies to the acetylcholine receptors. These antibodies prevent normal binding of the neurotransmitter.

SENSORY ENDINGS, of which there are several types, receive information from the external and internal environments and transmit it to the CNS via afferent or sensory neurons. They are transducers, each type of which converts a specific kind of stimulus (temperature, touch, light, etc.) to a wave of depolarization of the neuronal membrane. This wave passes centrally along an afferent nerve fiber. When it reaches the appropriate region of the brain the impulse is interpreted as a specific sensation.

Some sense organs are very elaborate and complex and their functions are limited to special parts of the body. These are called organs of special sense. For example, although we can feel pain from any part of the body, both internally and externally, we perceive light only with a special structure restricted to a particular location. Endings to be considered in this chapter are of general sense; the organs of special sense are considered in Chapter 19.

Naked nerve endings (Fig. 7.18) are probably the simplest sensory structures, at least morphologically, and probably also the most common. Although they may be the most useful and informative of the general sensory endings, little is known about them. The tiny terminal branches simply end in intimate association with the cells of the tissue from, or through, which stimuli are being received. The best known examples are the free nerve endings of the epidermis. They are believed to be responsible for sensations of pain and temperature. However, some, such as those around hair follicles, are probably tactile and others in different regions may have different functions.

Encapsulated nerve endings are supported by special arrangements of connective tissue and enclosed by connective tissue capsules. Three types are described here, although there are others.

Tactile corpuscles (of Meissner) (Fig. 7.20) are numerous in the skin of the palmar surfaces of the hand, especially on the digits. These are barrel-shaped structures that lie in the connective tissue papillae of the skin just beneath the epithelium (epidermis). They are composed of connective tissue within which lie nerve fiber endings in irregular, spiral, or zigzag arrangements. Slight compression or distortion of a corpuscle initiates a nerve impulse interpreted in the CNS as touch or light pressure.

Other forms of tactile corpuscles are present in the skin of the lips, portions of the genitalia and other areas that are particularly sensitive to touch and pressure.

Pacinian corpuscles (Fig. 7.21) are elliptical or long, sausage-shaped, sometimes worm-like structures. They are formed of numerous concentric layers of connective tissue separated by narrow, fluid-filled spaces. There is a thin central core within which lies a nerve fiber. A cross-section of a corpuscle viewed with the light microscope resembles a slice of onion. Some of these corpuscles are large enough to be visible with the unaided eye. They are common in the fatty loose connective tissue layer beneath the skin, but are also found elsewhere. Compression or distortion apparently initiates impulses generally interpreted as pressure, but these corpuscles are not likely to be the only source of pressure sense.

Muscle spindles (Fig. 7.22) provide information to the CNS about the state of contraction and tension in skeletal muscles and thus play a role in the reflexes involved in postural mechanisms. They are located within, or adjacent to, the fasicles of ordinary muscle and parallel to them. Structurally they are the most complex of the organs of general sense. Each spindle consists of a few thin, short, modified skeletal muscle fibers (intrafusal fibers) enclosed in a fairly dense connective tissue capsule with tapered ends. Both sensory

Fig. 7.18. *Sensory nerve endings.* **A:** Naked nerve ending. Fine branches of a nerve fiber rebranch and terminate among the cells of an epithelium. **B:** Tactile corpuscle (of Meissner). The nerve terminates in an irregular spiral arrangement within a fibrous bulb of connective tissue just beneath an epithelium, usually epidermis. **C:** Pacinian corpuscle. The nerve terminal lies in the center of a sheath composed of numerous concentric layers of connective tissue fibers and cells. **D:** Muscle spindle. A motor nerve fiber (above) gives off a branch to a large extrafusal muscle fiber and then penetrates the spindle's sheath and ends on the small intrafusal muscle fiber. A sensory nerve (below) enters the spindle and its terminal portion is coiled around the intrafusal fibers.

Fig. 7.19. Two *myoneural junctions* viewed with a scanning electron microscope. ×1010. (Courtesy of E Uehara from Fig. 11.3A in Fujita T, Tanaka K, and Tokunaga J: SEM Atlas of Cells and Tissues. New York: Igaku-Shoin, 1981

Fig. 7.20. *Tactile* (Meissner's) *corpuscle* just beneath the epidermis. Silver stain. ×185. (Courtesy of W. Montagna and N. Roman.)

Fig. 7.21. *Pacinian corpuscle.* Note the laminated, onion-like structure. ×55.

Fig. 7.22. *Muscle spindle* in cross-section. Note capsule (C) and intrafusal fibers (I). ×520.

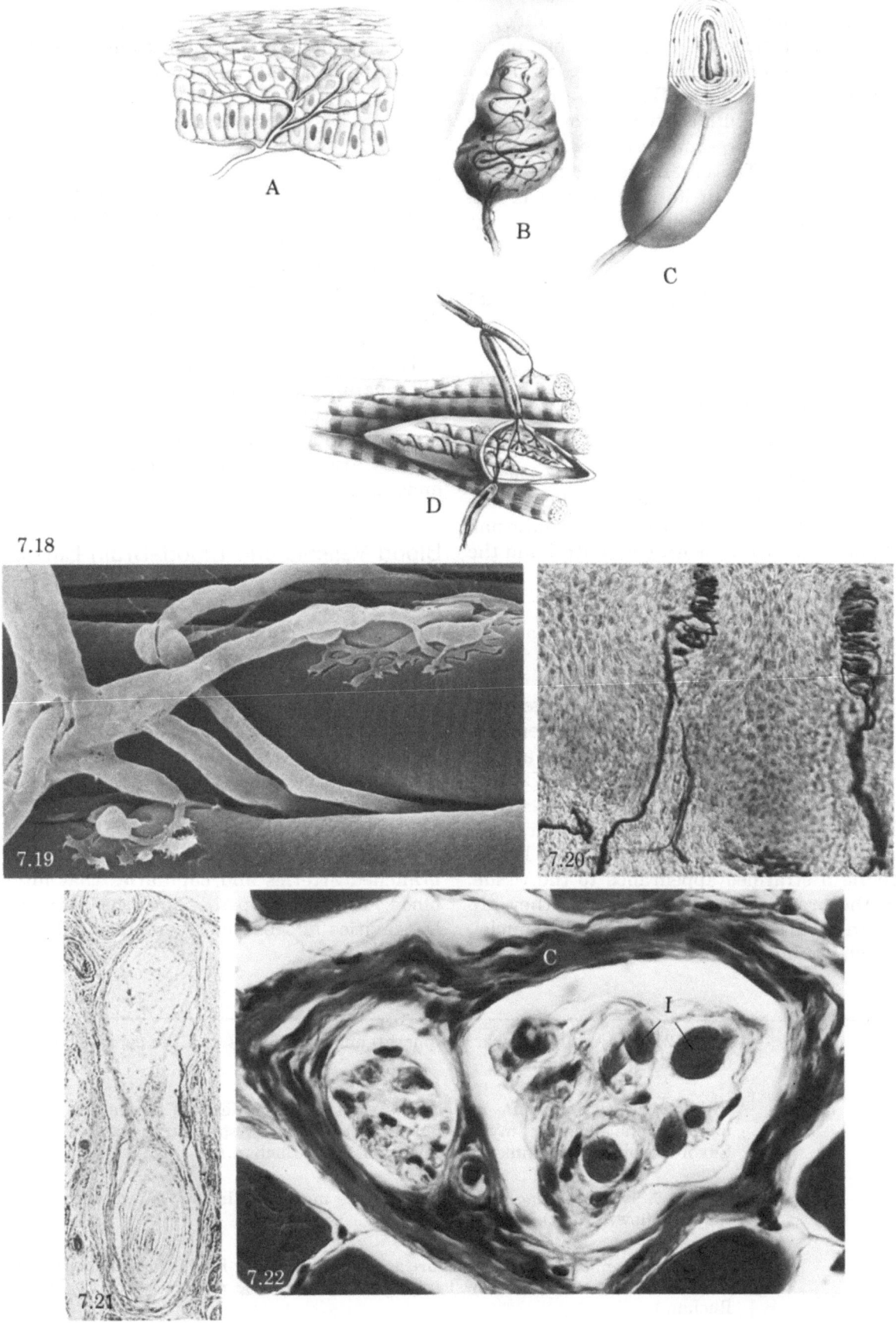

A

B

C

D

7.18

7.19

7.20

7.21

7.22

C

I

and motor nerve fibers enter the spindle. The motor fibers terminate in motor end-plates on the intrafusal fibers and thus control contraction of these fibers. Each intrafusal fiber is also wrapped with a few turns of a sensory nerve fiber that presumably senses the degree of contraction. This organ has both motor and sensory endings, but its net function is sensory and thus is described in this category.

Basic Histology of the Central Nervous System

In most parts of the CNS there is a sharply visible boundary between two different types of substance, and this distinction is apparent both grossly (as gray vs. white matter—a distinction in shading only) and microscopically (as cells vs. fiber tracts). The gray lies on the surface of the brain and the white is internal. In the spinal cord the gray is central and the white external (Figs. 7.1 and 7.23).

Gray Matter and Nuclei

The gray color is derived from the large number of neurons and the relative absence of myelin. The cells in the gray matter are arranged in precisely ordered patterns. Certain patterns are unique to specific areas of the CNS (Figs. 7.24 and 7.25). In the cerebral cortex, for example, they are arranged in layers, giving a stratified appearance to the tissue. In the brain stem and spinal cord they are arranged in columns and groups called nuclei, which are functionally as well as structurally

discrete. (Note that the term nucleus here has distinctly different meaning from its earlier definition as a cell component.)

White Matter and Tracts

White matter and tracts (Figs. 7.23 through 7.25) contain few nuclei, either of neurons or other cells; cell processes are the main component. Many of these axons and dendrites are arranged in bundles called tracts. All of them are myelinated, which accounts for the whiteness grossly.

The tracts are functional entities, not visibly separate either grossly or microscopically. They constitute groupings of fibers with similar connections and functions. A given tract usually arises from a particular nucleus and ends in a specific region.

Blood Vessels and Blood–Brain Barrier

Blood vessels pervade the entire nervous system. The endothelial cells of capillaries in the CNS possess many tight junctions. Certain substances present in the circulating blood are unable to pass into the tissue of the CNS. This has led to the concept of the blood–brain barrier. This barrier appears to be the capillary endothelium, which has properties unique to the CNS.

The *choroid plexuses* in the CNS (Fig. 7.26) are fine networks of abundantly and finely branched arteries and capillaries that filter blood. The filtrate passes into the ventricular cavities and becomes cerebrospinal fluid (CSF).

Fig. 7.23. *Gray matter* (dark, peripheral) and *white matter* of the cerebral cortex. (Courtesy of G. C. Buchan.)

Fig. 7.24. *Gray* and *white matter* in a section. The difference in shading is due mainly to the amount of myelin, which takes the darker stain, in the white matter. Luxol-fast-blue-PAS stain. ×2. (Courtesy of G. C. Buchan.)

Fig. 7.25. The *white matter* (upper left) has more myelin and fewer nuclei than the *gray* (lower right). ×85.

Fig. 7.26. *Choroid plexus* (same figure as 7.8.). Ventricular fluid is formed by passage from the blood vessels (arrows) into the ventricle (V). ×100. (Courtesy of G. C. Buchan.)

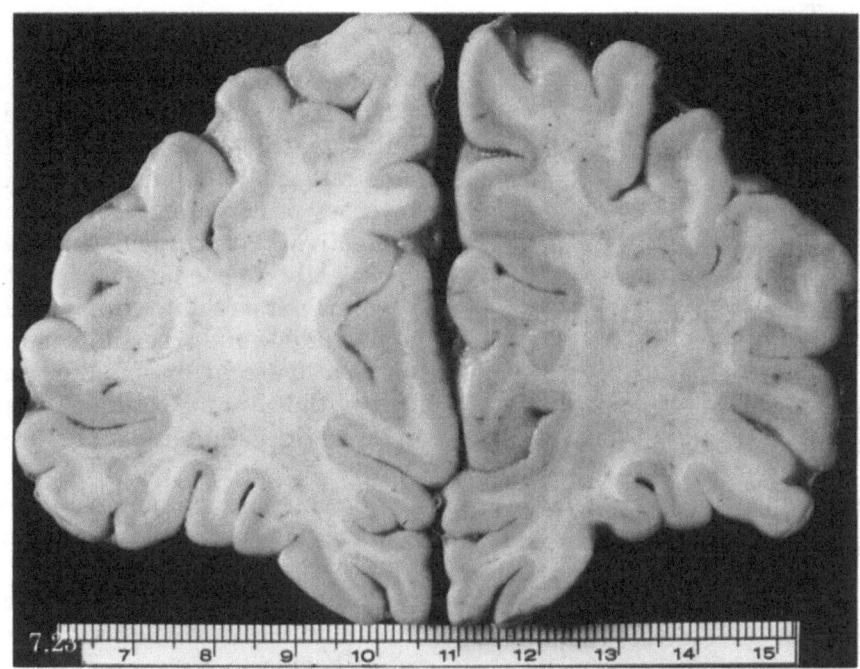

7.23

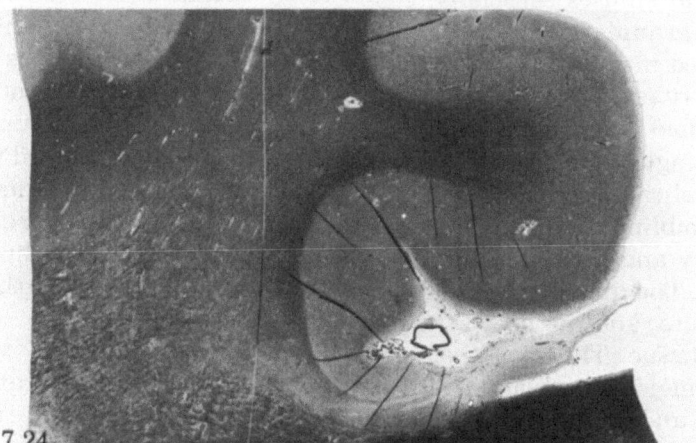

7.24

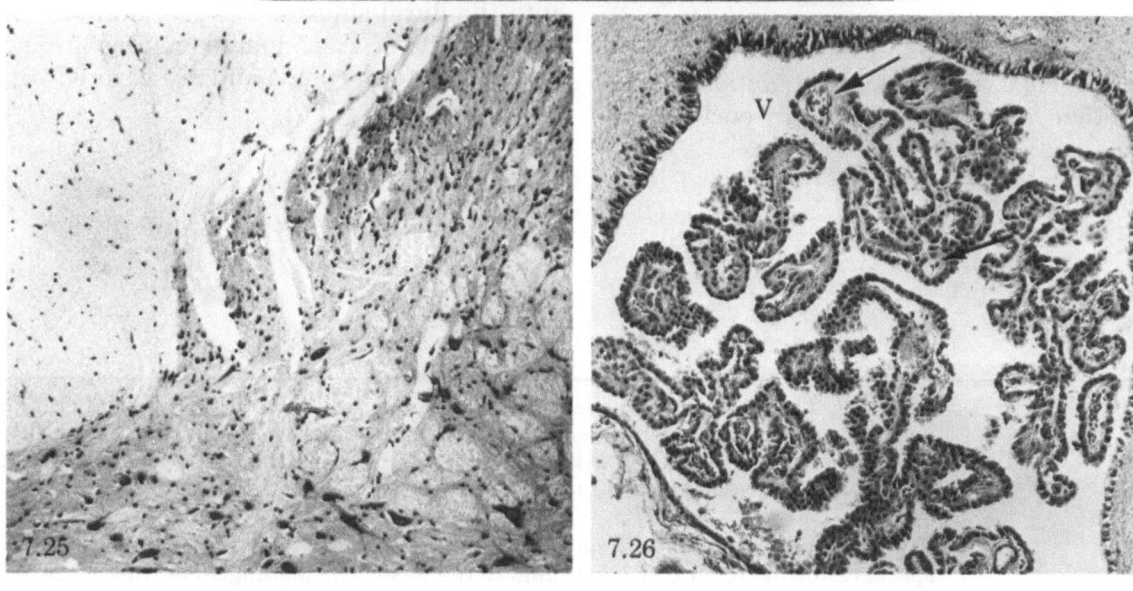

7.25

7.26

Meninges and Spaces

The brain and cord have three enveloping layers of connective tissue, the meninges (Figs. 7.27 and 7.28).

DURA MATER (pachymeninx) is the outermost layer. In the skull it is adherent to the cranium. The extradural (epidural) space external to this is of significance only rarely, as when a cranial fracture lacerates the middle meningeal artery and causes hemorrhage into the space. This may result in compression of the brain.

The spinal canal has a wide epidural space containing loose fatty tissue and many veins. In both the cranium and spinal canal the dura is tough and fibrous. It encloses several large venous sinuses. Some of these, the superior and inferior sagittal sinuses especially, contain the arachnoid granulations by which the CSF may be drained into veins.

ARACHNOID, PIA MATER, AND SUBARACHNOID SPACE. The arachnoid and the pia mater (often known as a single membrane, the pia-arachnoid) are delicate connective tissue layers grossly resembling cobwebs. Their separation is arbitrary and they may be called the leptomeninges. The arachnoid adheres to the surrounding dura, and the pia to the underlying nervous tissue. The space between them, the subarachnoid space, contains many fine fibrous strands and small veins that carry blood from the brain to the dural sinuses. These thin-walled veins are relatively easily ruptured by trauma to the head, resulting in hemorrhage. Such an accumulation of fluid or other material in the rigidly enclosed cranium need not be massive to be serious.

The subarachnoid space contains CSF. This fluid also fills the ventricles and normally amounts to 80–100 ml but may be much more in cases of cerebral atrophy. It serves as a protective physical cushion. Because it is chemically a poor buffer it must be replaced regularly. It circulates freely. The fluid serves as a valuable and accessible material for diagnosis, as one may by spinal or cisternal puncture withdraw and examine samples for cells, chemical constituents, and infectious organisms.

No lymphatic channels are present in the CNS, and the interstitial space, although similar in concept to that of other tissues, has no collagen or glycosaminoglycans, and is finer and less visible except when distended as by edema.

The SUBDURAL SPACE is only a potential space because the arachnoid is closely applied to the dura. However, in some cases of cranial trauma, veins may be ruptured as they pass through the space toward the dura, and bleed in small or large amounts. Subdural hemorrhages (Fig. 7.28) are more likely to be limited in extent than subarachnoid ones; thus the clinical presentation of the two lesions may be different.

CSF flows from the ventricular system through three small foramens into the subarachnoid space. It returns to the vascular system through the arachnoid granulations into the dural sinuses. The granulations are villous tufts of arachnoid extending through the dura into the veins and are covered with endothelium.

Fig. 7.27. *The meninges* and their relationships to brain, blood vessels, and cranial bone. The meningeal artery lies in the epidural space between the dura and periosteum. The venous sinus lies within the dura. Thin-walled, bulbous arachnoid villi project into the venous sinus and allow cerebrospinal fluid to pass into the blood.

Fig. 7.28. *Subdural hemorrhage.* The tearing of small veins crossing the subdural space, resulting from external trauma to the head. The meningeal outline conforms approximately to the line of the skull, and the brain is correspondingly deformed.

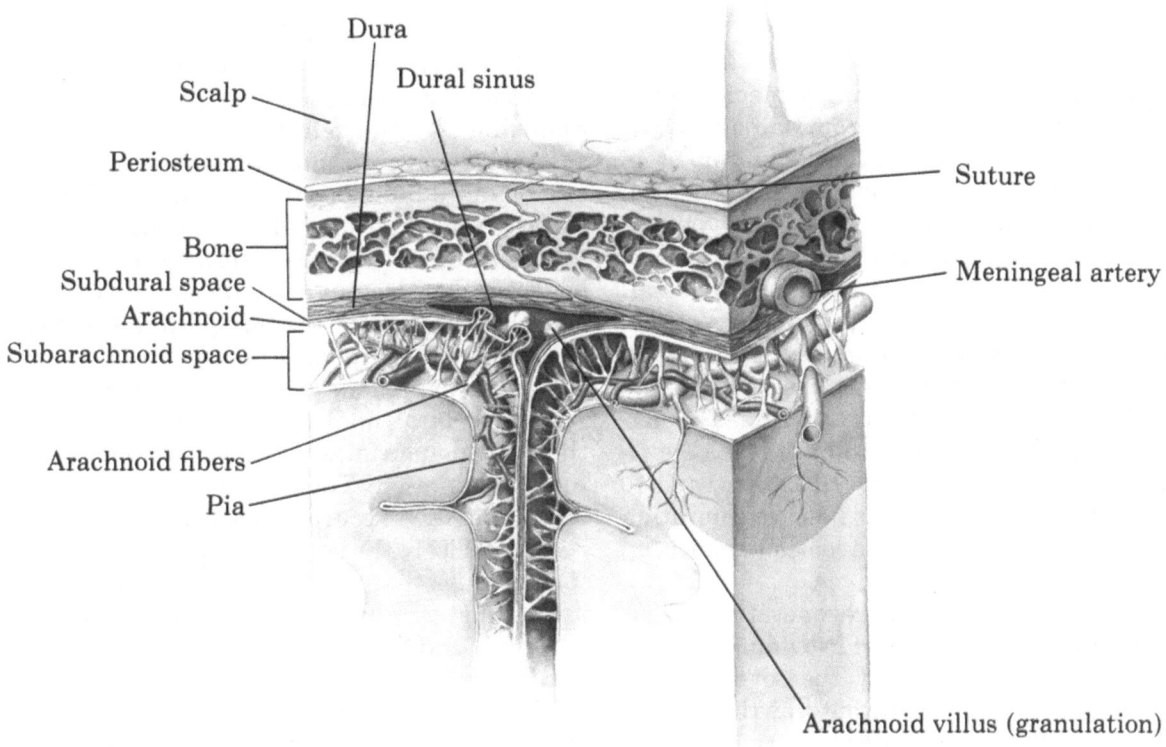

Scalp

Periosteum

Bone

Subdural space

Arachnoid

Subarachnoid space

Arachnoid fibers

Pia

Dura

Dural sinus

Suture

Meningeal artery

Arachnoid villus (granulation)

7.27

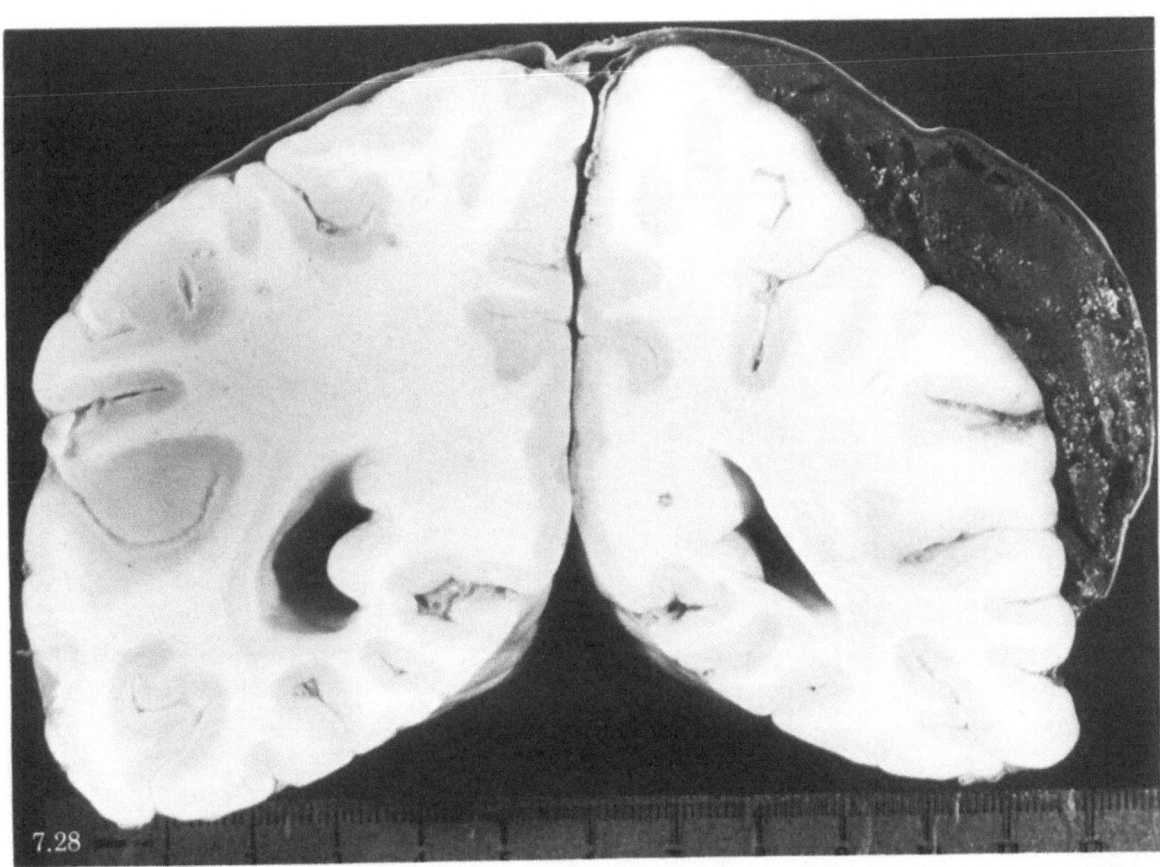
7.28

Regeneration

Some of the most devastating of medical problems are those resulting from damage to the CNS. All neurons are end cells and no stem cells are present to provide replacement if these are destroyed by disease or trauma. Even very small localized lesions in the nervous system which interrupt relatively small tracts of nerve fibers may produce severe loss of sensory and/or motor functions. Such losses are permanent, because, within the CNS, nerve fibers do not regenerate. The permanent paralysis following damage to the spinal cord, for example, is well known, and to date efforts to bring about fiber regeneration and functional recovery have been unsuccessful.

In the PNS, however, regeneration of cut nerve fibers occurs readily. Providing that the cell body is not damaged, the severed axon or dendrite is replaced by outgrowth of a new fiber from the cut end of the portion that remains attached to the cell.

When a nerve fiber is cut, chromatolysis occurs, i.e., the Nissl bodies in the cell disappear, and the nucleus moves close to the plasmalemma. As the cell recovers from the insult, it resumes its normal appearance and one or more pseudopodial sprouts develop at the cut end. The fiber distal to the cut has degenerated in a process termed Wallerian degeneration, leaving only its connective tissue sheaths intact. Providing that the two ends of a cut peripheral nerve can be surgically approximated, the regenerating fibers will grow into the distal portion and follow the old endoneurial sheaths back to their original termination. The reinnervation is only approximately accurate; that is, few fibers reach precisely the same muscle fibers or sensory endings that they supplied before the injury. Thus some bizarre distortions of sensory pattern or disturbances of motor function may occur but can be overcome by relearning. Much research effort is being directed toward stimulating similar regeneration within the CNS.

8 Cardiovascular System

Introduction

The cardiovascular system is a continuous series of tubes transporting blood (Fig. 8.1). It intimately connects the cells of the body with their sources of supply and their sites of waste disposal, thereby allowing a huge population of cells to live in a small area.

Within its volume of approximately 15 liters, the cardiovascular system carries:

1. Oxygen, most of which is in red blood cells.
2. Other food substances to tissues for their consumption. In some cases intermediate stops, such as the liver, are necessary for processing of these substances before their ultimate distribution.
3. White blood cells, platelets, antibodies, and other elements for protection against injury (the inflammatory response system).
4. Chemical integrators, some of which are hormones that stimulate or repress the functions or growth of various tissues.
5. Wastes for excretion by the respiratory, gastrointestinal, and urinary systems.

Basic Histologic Organization

The various organs that comprise the cardiovascular system are lined with a simple squamous epithelium known as endothelium. Outside of the endothelial lining are layers of connective tissue and muscle arranged in patterns characteristic of each of the structural components of this system (see Structural Components). The walls of all blood vessels are composed of the following layers (Fig. 8.2):

1. An inner layer consisting of endothelium and a supporting layer of fine connective

Fig. 8.1. *General plan of circulatory system.* All blood is pumped from the heart to the lungs (pulmonary circuit). It passes through arteries, which branch progressively and become smaller, then through capillaries where gas is exchanged. Blood returns to the heart from the pulmonary capillaries through veins that increase in size as they join. Oxygenated blood flows from the heart through branching arteries to systemic capillaries, where nutritive, secretory, and excretory products are exchanged. Blood, now deoxygenated, is returned to the heart by the veins. Within this plan are many different routes that supply the tissues and organs of the body. In three of these circuits there are two distinct capillary beds for each. These are located in kidney, hypophysis, and gastrointestinal system.

Fluid leaks from all capillary beds into the interstitial space. This fluid (lymph) returns via lymph vessels to the blood after being filtered by lymph nodes. This system of vessels begins with lymphatic capillaries. Lymph flows through merging channels to enter the largest veins.

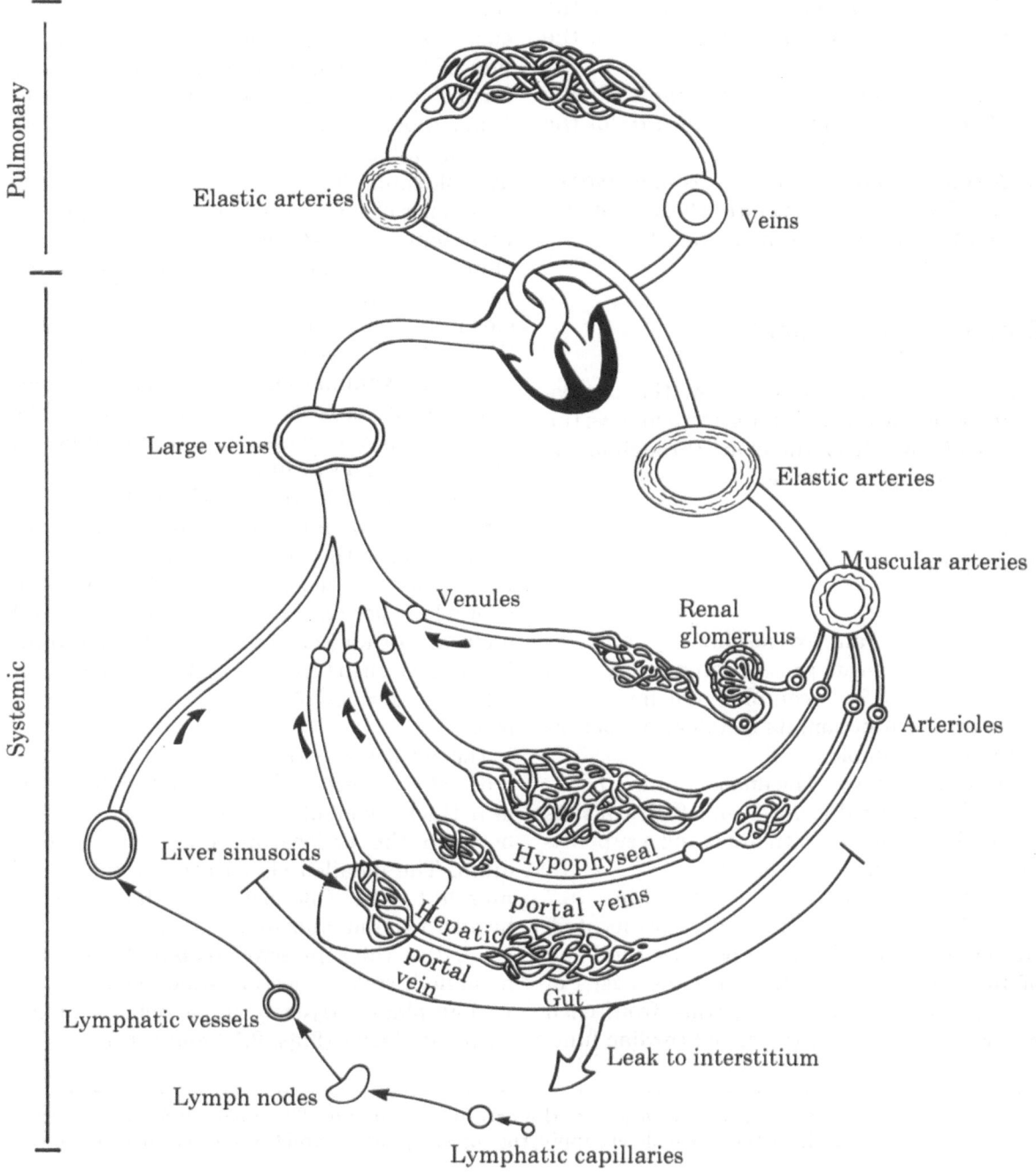

tissue. This is the *tunica intima* of the blood vessels and the *endocardium* of the heart.

2. A layer of muscle. This is the *tunica media* of the vessels and the *myocardium* of the heart.
3. An outer supporting layer of connective tissue. This is the *tunica adventitia* of vessels and the *epicardium* of the heart.

Structural Components

Our sequence of description of the components of the cardiovascular system follows the course of blood from the heart through arteries, capillaries, and veins.

The Heart

The heart is an extraordinarily efficient pump. Although its gross anatomy (Figs. 8.3 through Fig. 8.7) is complex and important to its proper function, its histologic structure is relatively simple.

THE ENDOCARDIUM. The endocardium, the inner heart layer (Figs. 8.2 and 8.4), consists of simple squamous epithelium and a supporting layer of connective tissue.

FIBROUS SKELETON AND VALVES (Figs. 8.7 through 8.11). Where the valves are located, the walls of the heart must be more rigid and of limited diameter; otherwise the cusps of the closed valves might separate from each other. It is important to normal cardiac func-

tion that, when the heart valves close, their cusps approximate each other to prevent reflux of blood. Dense connective tissue in the form of rings, *annuli fibrosi* (Fig. 8.7) provides firm support for the bases of each of the four cardiac valves. These rings constitute the cardiac skeleton. The valves between the atria and ventricles are provided with cordlike attachments termed *chordae tendineae*. The chordae arise from the free margins of the valves and attach to tips of the papillary muscles in the ventricular walls. The valve cusps (Figs. 8.8 and 8.9), although thin and delicate on gross examination, are extremely tough and durable as well as freely flexible. They contain layers of collagen and elastic fibers, covered by endocardium.

This admirable tissue called the cardiac skeleton can be injured. Following injury, as in the aftermath of rheumatic fever, scarring may gradually distort the cardiac skeleton over a long period of time (Fig. 8.10). Bacterial endocarditis may destroy a part of it, perforating a valve cusp (Fig. 8.11). These lesions usually have serious physiologic and clinical effects.

THE MYOCARDIUM (Figs. 8.2 and 8.4) is the most characteristic feature of the heart. It is a thick layer of cardiac muscle, situated between the endocardium and the epicardium. The detailed structure of this type of muscle has been described in Chapter 6. Its branching and anastomosing fibers are arranged in thick interwoven bundles so that a single histologic section shows them cut in various planes. Myocardium is richly supplied with capillaries (Figs. 8.12 and 8.13).

Fig. 8.2. The *three layers* of the *cardiovascular tube.* The heart and larger vessels all have their own blood supply, the coronary vessels and the vasa vasorum (arrows).

Fig. 8.3. *Frontal view of the heart.* Transverse plane shows orientation for Fig. 8.6.

Fig. 8.4. *Wall* of the *heart* (see Fig. 8.5 for location). Endocardium (En); myocardium (M); epicardium (Ep). ×3.8.

Fig. 8.5. *Frontal cutaway diagram of heart. Rectangle* shows area of section in Fig. 8.4. Arrows indicate the flow of blood.

Fig. 8.6. *Heart cut* in plane shown in Fig. 8.3 and *viewed from above.*

Fig. 8.7. *Cardiac fibrous skeleton* traced on Fig. 8.6.

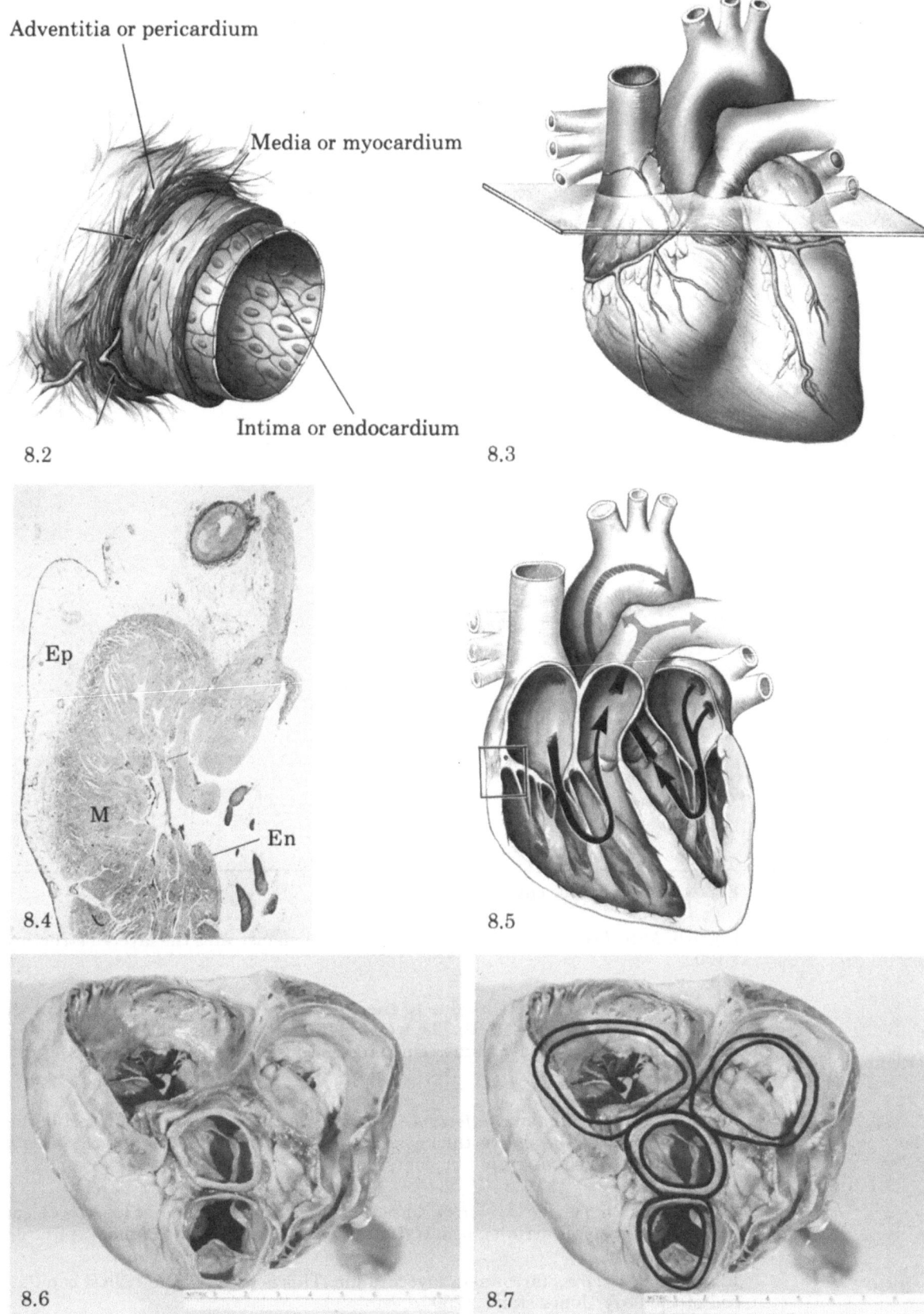

Adventitia or pericardium

Media or myocardium

Intima or endocardium

8.2

8.3

Ep

M

En

8.4

8.5

8.6

8.7

Fig. 8.8. *Aortic valve cusp* (arrow). ×12.

Fig. 8.9. *Mitral valve cusp.* The stain for elastin demonstrates the layered structure. ×100.

Fig. 8.10. A: *Valvular disease* due to rheumatic fever. Note the thickening of the valve and the annulus. ×10. **B:** The well-organized pattern of the normal valve is replaced by immature scar tissue. This process causes valvular deformity and malfunction. ×250.

Fig. 8.11. *Calcification and infection involving annulus fibrosus.* The infection has extended through the entire thickness of the heart wall and eroded the base of the mitral valve (M). Atrium (A), ventricle (V). ×2.

Fig. 8.12. *Coronary arterial system.* Closeup view of an injection cast to show epicardial branches (small arrows), penetrating branches (large arrows), and capillaries.

Fig. 8.13. *Capillaries* (arrows) in myocardium. This is possibly the richest capillary bed of the body. Jones stain. ×250.

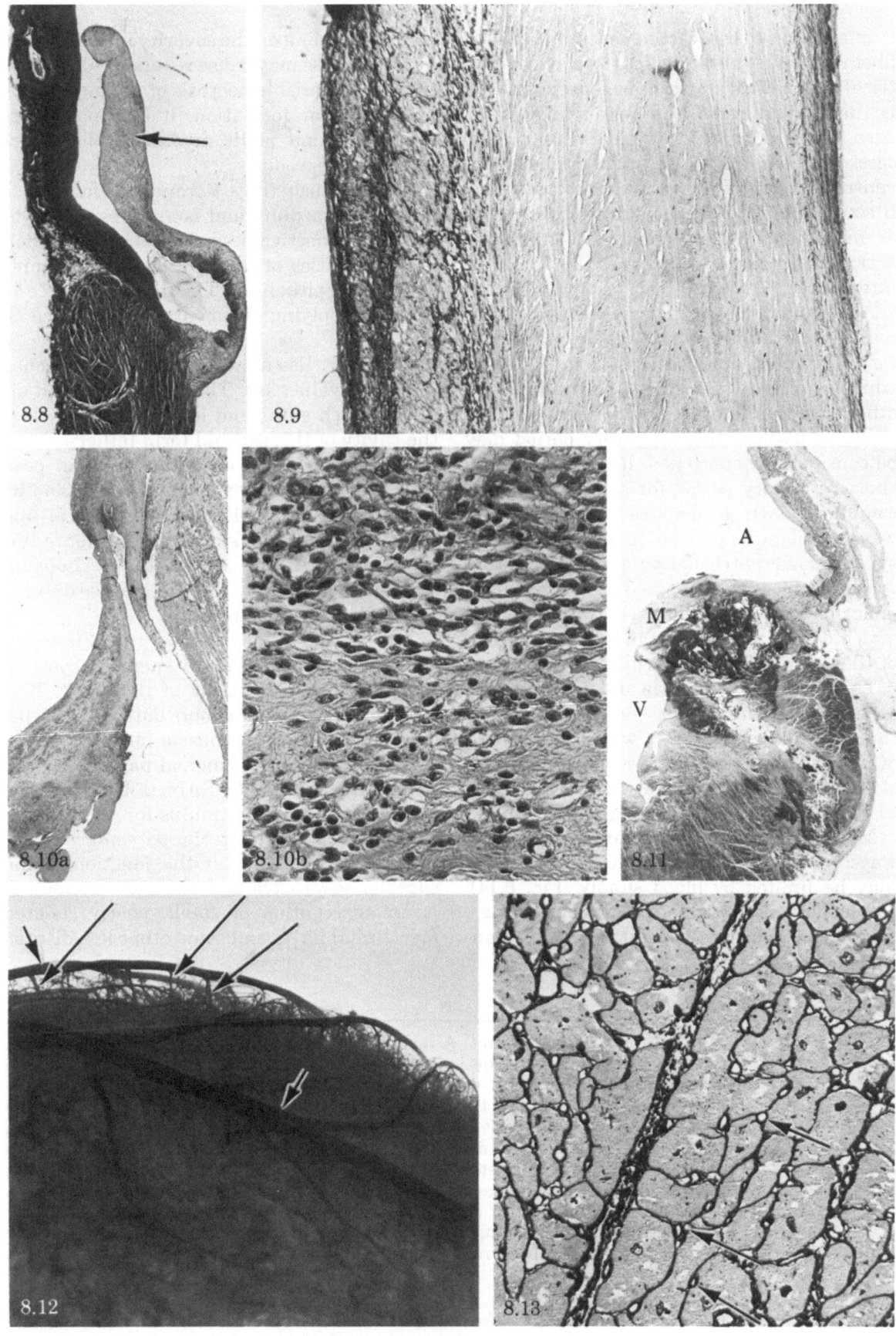

8.8

8.9

8.10a

8.10b

8.11

8.12

8.13

In addition to contracting, each myocardial fiber (cell) must also conduct the wave of electrical depolarization to the adjacent cell. It is therefore inherently a conducting tissue. Also, the direction of this wave through successive cells of the entire atrial or the entire ventricular myocardium must be controlled. If some cells should be avoided by the wave, as might happen if others ahead of them were destroyed, this orderly progression would be interrupted.

Another important biologic feature of normal myocardium is a relatively long refractory period after each contraction during which it cannot respond to, or conduct, another stimulus. However, under conditions of stress or disease, this refractory period may be considerably shortened. If the abnormally short refractory period for some fibers were combined with a detoured depolarization wave, it might be possible to prevent entirely synchronous ventricular or atrial contraction. Actually this is the supposed basis for several abnormalities of cardiac rhythm, some of which can be abruptly fatal. The best known of these is ventricular fibrillation.

The myocardium of atria and ventricles are separated by the fibrous skeleton except at the AV bundle (see later), which is a strand of myocardial fibers that passes through the skeleton. This allows the atria and ventricles to contract in appropriate sequence.

Myocardium may be injured in several ways: by reduction of available oxygen, which may be limited by blood supply (Fig. 8.14); by alcohol; and by certain therapeutic drugs. These are probably the most important dangers. Depending on the severity in the particular case, these may cause reversible degeneration or irreversible necrosis of the muscle, followed by scar formation. It is important to remember that adult myocardial fibers are unable to reproduce.

THE EPICARDIUM (Figs. 8.2 and 8.4) lies outside of the myocardium and is an irregular layer of loose connective tissue containing considerable quantities of fat covered with a simple squamous epithelium. The larger vessels and nerves supplying the heart are included in this layer.

The heart lies almost free and unattached in a thin-walled sac. The large veins and arteries which enter and leave the heart cross the cavity of this sac and form tethering connections which maintain the heart in position. The sac is the pericardial cavity and its inner and outer walls are the visceral and parietal pericardia—similar to the pleura surrounding each lung and to the peritoneum of the abdomen. The visceral pericardium is also called the epicardium.

THE CARDIAC CONDUCTION SYSTEM (Fig. 8.15) controls the regular and sequential contraction of different portions of the heart. It is not composed of nerve fibers but rather of special modified cardiac muscle fibers. This system contains three principal parts:

The sinoatrial node (SAN) (Fig. 8.16) is the site of origin of the stimulus for cardiac contraction; it is therefore the pacemaker of the heart. The SAN lies at the junction of the superior vena cava and the right atrium. It is an aggregation of small, poorly striated myocardial fibers and some other less distinc-

Fig. 8.14. *Myocardial infarct.* A man sustained a large infarct and died of heart failure 17 days later. **a:** The left ventricle is much enlarged as indicated by the position of the left anterior descending artery (arrow). The thin flabby wall is collapsed (bracket) in this postmortem specimen. **b:** Transverse section through the ventricles shows patchy discoloration, indicating infarction, for most of the left ventricular wall thickness and about 75% of its circumference. The wall is also extremely thin due to stretching. The amount of viable myocardium remaining was unable to maintain adequate blood flow to the body. Rectangle indicates area of **c. c:** Section of the full thickness of the ventricular wall shows necrosis and scarring at all levels. Rectangle indicates area of **d.** ×18. **d:** An island of recognizable and viable myocardium (arrows), is surrounded by necrotic debris and scar tissue. ×85.

Fig. 8.15. The *cardiac conduction system.*

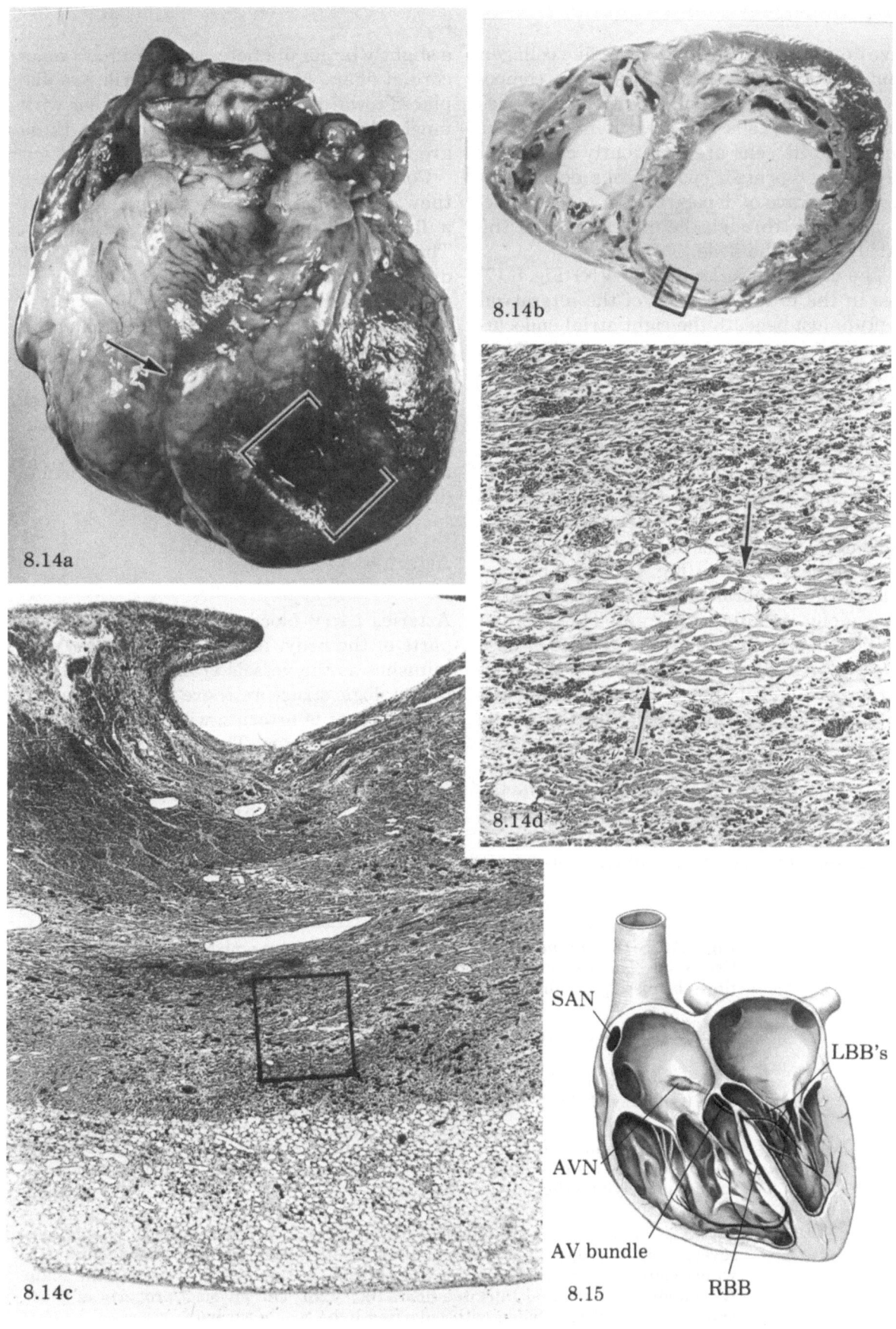

8.14a

8.14b

8.14d

8.14c

8.15

SAN

LBB's

AVN

AV bundle

RBB

tive appearing cells, all bound in fine collagen and elastic fibers. Connective tissue components of the SAN increase with age. Nerves and ganglion cells are present in and near the node. Its cells are apparently capable of regularly repeated, spontaneous depolarization. The wave of depolarization and contraction spreads through the musculature of the atrium from the node.

The *atrioventricular node* (AVN) (Fig. 8.17) lies in the inferior portion of the interatrial septum just beneath the right atrial endocardium and is similar in structure to the SAN. However, in the process of passing on the depolarization wave to the ventricle, the AVN seems to slow or delay it. This act may serve to allow more atrial emptying before ventricular contraction begins.

The *atrioventricular (AV) bundle* of His *and bundle branches.* The fibers of the AVN become more parallel anteriorly and gather to form the AV bundle (Fig. 8.18). This courses within the membranous interventricular septum along its inferior margin. This position makes the bundle vulnerable in some disease states (especially congenital defects of the interventricular septum, and bacterial endocarditis). Groups of fibers branch from the bundle and fan out beneath the entire left ventricular endocardium as left bundle branches (Fig. 8.19). The main trunk continues within the muscular interventricular septum as the right bundle branch. As seen in sections, the conduction fibers in the bundle branches have a slightly larger diameter than ordinary myocardial fibers. Most of the myofibrils are displaced toward the periphery of the fiber with much glycogen occupying the center; these are *Purkinje fibers.*

Conduction fibers are so named because they can carry a depolarization impulse at a faster rate than other myocardial cells. Therefore they form the major pathways for dissemination of the impulse to the myocardium generally. Interruption of one of these pathways thus delays the transmission of the impulse to, and the contraction of, specific segments of myocardium (Fig. 8.20). Depending on the anatomic site of obstruction, a patient may develop either left bundle branch block, right bundle branch block, partial atrioventricular block, or complete atrioventricular dissociation.

Arteries

Arteries carry blood from the heart to all parts of the body. Arterial caliber slowly diminishes as the vessels branch. On the basis of histologic structure there are three fundamental types of arteries, with gradual transitions between them. The structural features of these types relate to functional differences.

ELASTIC ARTERIES (sometimes called conducting arteries) (Fig. 8.21). This group includes the pulmonary artery with its right and left main branches, and the aorta with its eight

Fig. 8.16. *Sinoatrial node* (SAN) (arrows). The cells are embedded in dense connective tissue. The artery is a helpful landmark because conduction tissue may sometimes be distinguishable from other myocardium only with difficulty. ×18.

Fig. 8.17. *Atrioventricular node* (AVN) (arrows). ×18.

Fig. 8.18. *Atrioventricular bundle* and fibers of the *left bundle branch* (arrows). ×35. (Courtesy of W. A. Stotler.)

Fig. 8.19. *Purkinje fibers* (arrows). These are less dense than other myocardial fibers and often slightly larger. They tend to run in planes perpendicular or oblique to the underlying other myocardial fibers. ×125.

Fig. 8.20. Cardiac dysrhythmias may result from a variety of causes. In this case several electrocardiographic abnormalities resulted from an inborn metabolic error, which caused the deposition of *oxalate crystals* in, among other tissues, the main AV bundle (**a,** ×36), and Purkinje fibers (**b,** ×125). The physical property of these crystals makes them visible with polarized light, as shown here.

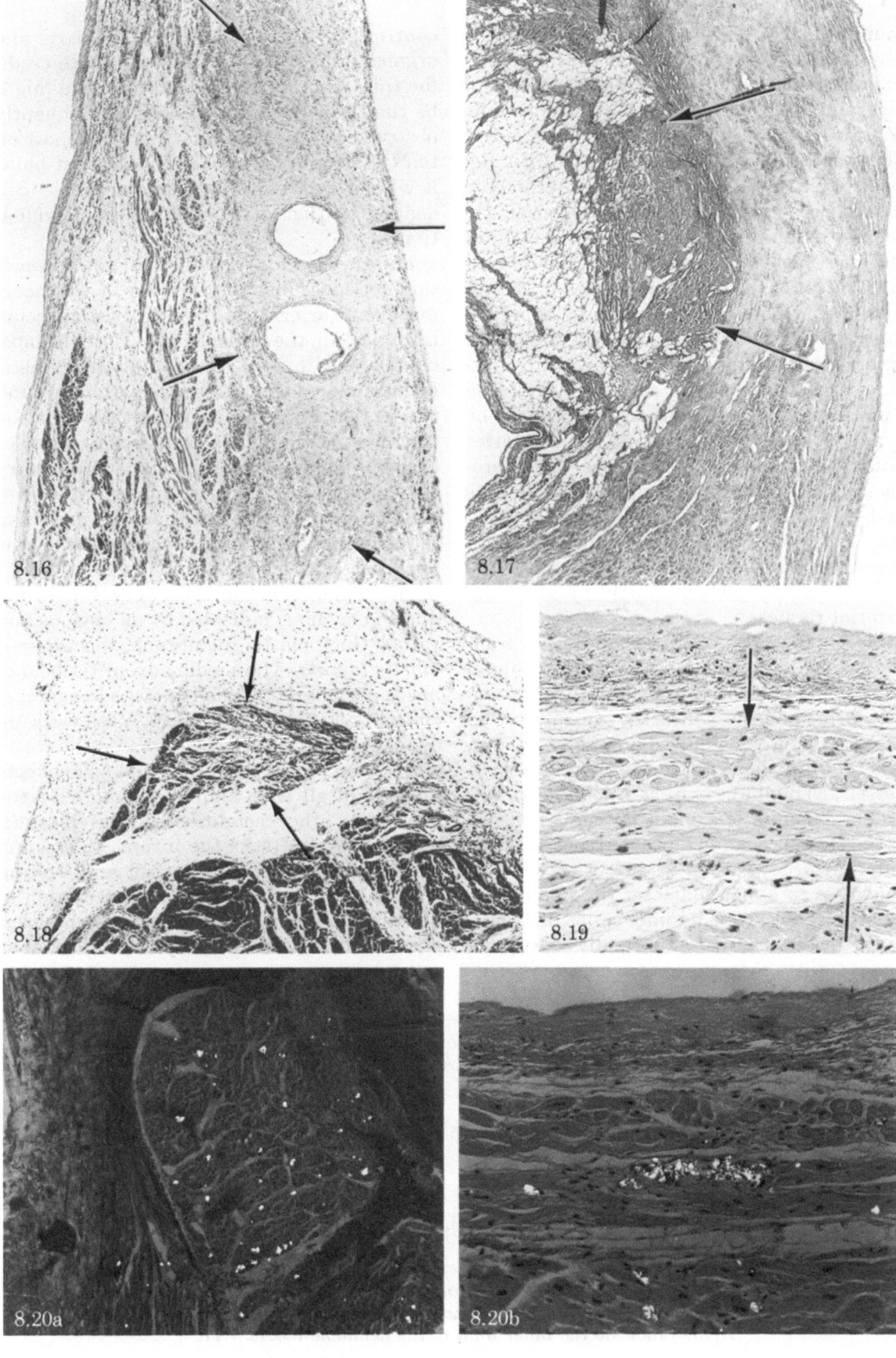

8.16

8.17

8.18

8.19

8.20a

8.20b

main branches. The aorta and pulmonary artery receive blood directly from the heart during ventricular contraction and stretch considerably each time this occurs. Their walls contain elastin in the form of circumferential fibers and fenestrated sheets (Fig. 8.21b). Between contractions the aortic and pulmonic valves close and pressure in the arterial systems is maintained by passive contraction of the stretched elastin back to its more relaxed state. Most of the elastin is located in the tunica media and is clearly seen in appropriately stained sections as numerous lines with intervening spaces occupied by smooth muscle, fibroblasts, and fine collagen fibers. The tunica intima of elastic arteries may be slightly thicker than that in other arteries and it may become quite thick in atherosclerosis. It also contains some smooth muscle cells and elastic fibers. The media, and especially the adventitia, of elastic arteries contain small blood vessels, the vasa vasorum ("vessels of vessels"), which supply blood to the arterial tissues.

MUSCULAR ARTERIES (Fig. 8.22) derive from the branching of the elastic arteries, supply the organs and extremities (e.g., liver, stomach, arm) and most directly control flow to these structures. Required flow rates vary in different functional states and therefore these vessels, as might be expected, contain considerable amounts of smooth muscle which responds to nervous and hormonal control. Muscular arteries have a higher ratio of wall thickness to lumen diameter than do elastic arteries. They are sometimes called distributing arteries because they normally exert some

control over blood flow to specific parts and organs, but arterioles are given more credit for this. Another reason for this title might be that they are the vessels most frequently obstructed by disease and therefore most often the cause of *ischemia* (insufficient blood flow) and *infarction* (ischemic necrosis—cell death due to lack of blood supply) of individual tissues.

The three tunics are most distinct in sections of muscular arteries. As in the heart and elastic arteries, the characteristic specialization lies in the tunica media. Here the muscle fibers, with a sparse population of elastic fibers, are arranged in a spiral pattern around the vessel. There is some variation in the thickness of the media of muscular arteries between different systems. The pulmonary and cerebral arteries are comparatively thin-walled, which may reflect the lower pressures in the former and the tendency for aneurysms (localized dilations) to occur in the latter.

The boundary between the very thin intima and the media is indicated by an obvious and rather thick elastic membrane, the *internal elastic lamina*. The media-adventitia boundary is also marked by a less discrete aggregation of elastic fibers and sheets. Vasa vasorum are present in the adventitia.

Arteriosclerosis (Figs. 8.23 and 8.24) affects arteries of all sizes and causes more deaths than any other condition in the Western world. It first attacks the intima, thickening it with a heterogeneous deposit and inciting thrombosis (the intravascular coagulation of blood). Second, this initial deposit progressively becomes more complex and extends

Fig. 8.21. *Aorta.* Note small arteries and vasa vasorum (arrows) in adventitia. ×85. **a:** H & E stain. **b:** Elastin stain. Adventitia (A); media (M). Intima is not identifiable in this picture.

Fig. 8.22. *Muscular artery.* ×85. **a:** H & E. Adventitia (A); media (M); intima (I). **b:** Elastin stain.

Fig. 8.23. *Arteriosclerotic* aorta. The full thickness of the media has been replaced by a nonelastic material (M), which is liable to stretch and rupture. Elastin stain. ×24.

Fig. 8.24. *Coronary artery occlusion.* Arteriosclerosis has replaced the inner portion of the media and all of the intima, setting the stage for the occlusion by thrombosis. Arrows indicate the inner limit of the definable media. ×17.

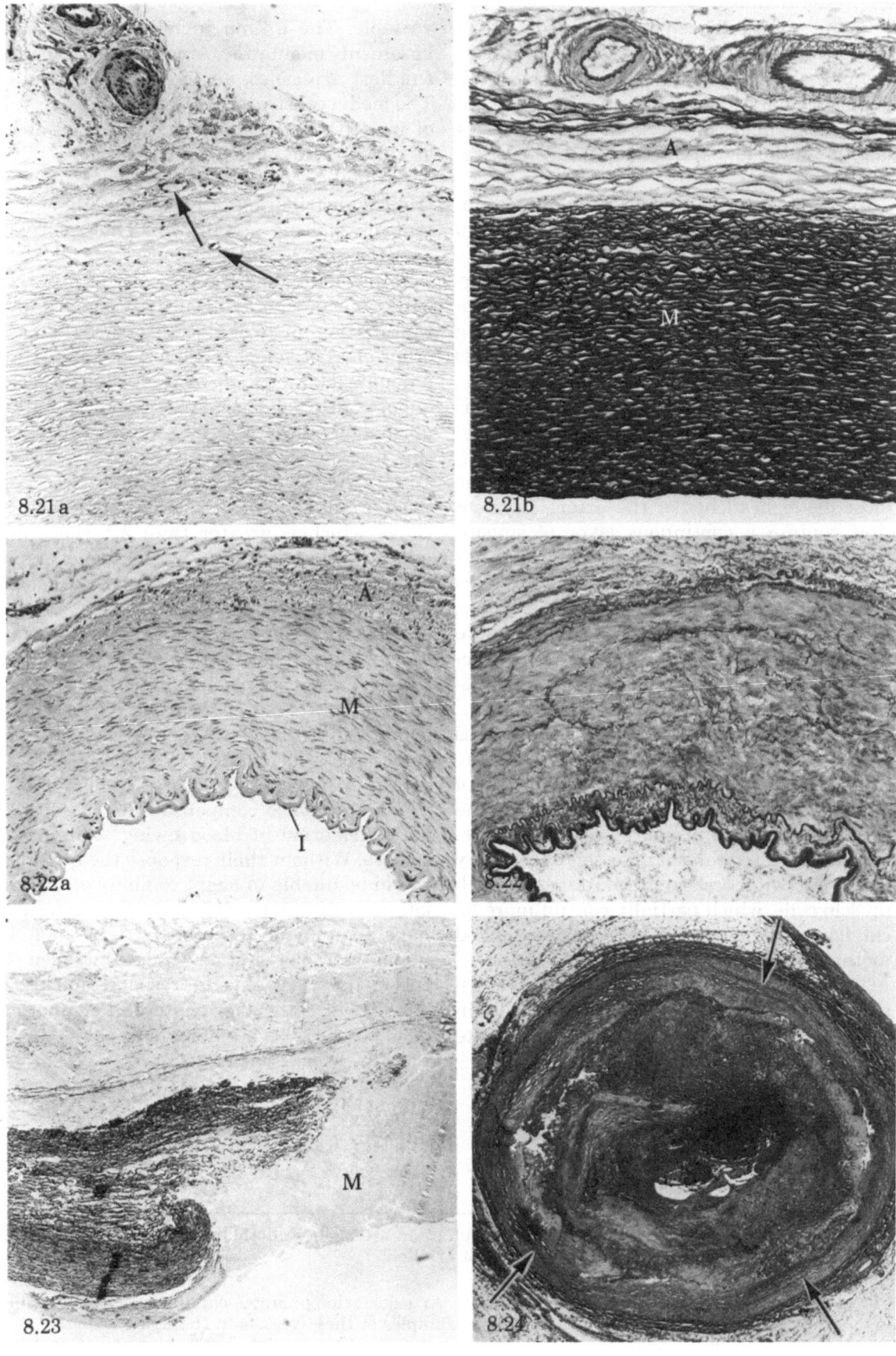

8.21a

8.21b

A

M

8.22a

A

M

I

8.22b

8.23

M

8.24

into and eventually replaces the media. With the loss of medial muscle and elastin, arteries are prone to the formation of *aneurysms* (dilated segments) and to rupture (Figs. 8.23 and 8.28). Most aneurysms occur in elastic arteries because of the low wall-to-lumen thickness ratio.

Muscular arteries are more subject to occlusion and any of these may be affected, often with serious results (Fig. 8.24). The coronary arteries are associated with the highest mortality rates. The narrowing and occlusion limits myocardial blood flow, eventually causing myocardial infarction. The arterial process may be localized, patchy, or diffuse; therefore, accurate anatomic detailing of the disease is critically important in evaluation before bypass operation.

ARTERIOLES (Figs. 8.25 through 8.28) are the most distal branches of the arterial system that contain a continuous layer of smooth muscle. They are basically muscular arteries measuring less than 0.5 mm in diameter. Morphologic definitions are not fully satisfactory; the term arteriole reflects physiology more than anatomy. Within the various tissue components of extremities and organs these vessels deliver blood into the local capillary beds. By their combined action in different areas and tissues of the body, arterioles bear the principal responsibility for the distribution of blood flow. Normally the arterioles are the site of the greatest pressure drop in the arterial side of the circulation. Vessels of capillary diameter, with occasional scattered smooth muscle cells, which partially control more local flow through capillary beds, are called metarterioles.

The thickness of an arteriolar wall in a histologic section is about the same as the diameter of its lumen, but is obviously quite variable. The intima includes endothelium, basement membrane, and, in all but the smallest arterioles, an inner elastic lamina. The media consists of one to four or five layers of smooth muscle, and the adventitia is about as thick as the media.

As implied above, arterioles basically control the distribution of blood flow under normal physiologic conditions. The relatively small size of arteriolar lumens, their high content of muscle, and the viscosity of blood, together mean that arterioles are more important in the control of blood pressure than any other class of vessels. The loss of a moderate amount (500 ml) of blood usually causes enough arteriolar constriction to maintain normal pressure (120/80 mm Hg). In *shock* this pressure is severely reduced, say to 70/10 mm Hg, in which case life is threatened. Such a reduction may be caused by a hemorrhage which is greater than arterioles and other vessels can cope with, for example, about 1500 ml. In another example, shock may result from arteriolar paralysis without the loss of any blood at all, as in the state of acute hypersensitivity (anaphylaxis).

Arterial hypertension is one of the prevalent diseases of our civilization. This is caused by excessive contractile tone in the arteriolar smooth muscle generally. Resting blood pressure may be 250/150 mm Hg or higher.

Arterioles also compensate for the loss or maldistribution of blood owing to injury or disease. Without their response the organism would be unable to adapt to many of the major, or even minor, stresses of life. Arterioles have a supply of nerve fibers from the autonomic nervous system and, controlled by these, they are able to respond quickly to changes in activity of one organ or another, or of the body as a whole.

Fig. 8.25. Electron micrograph of an arteriole. Endothelial (E) and smooth muscle (M) cells. ×7100. (Courtesy of M. Webb.)

Fig. 8.26. *Small blood vessels.* Arterioles (long arrow), capillaries (circle), venules (short arrow). Identify other examples of these vessels in the figure. ×250.

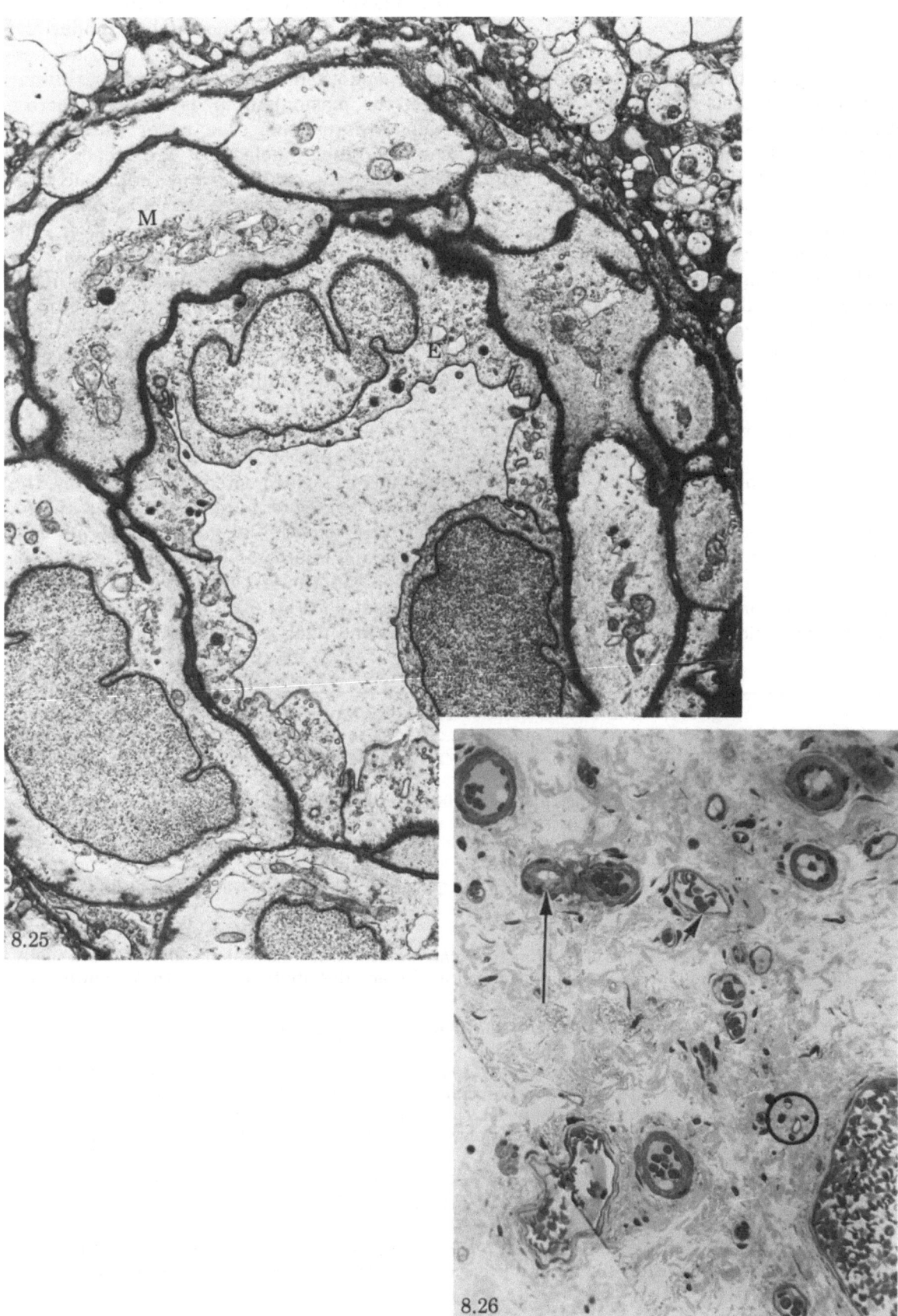

8.25

8.26

Capillaries

The capillary bed (Figs. 8.26 through 8.33) is a close mesh of innumerable branching and anastomosing vessels with a luminal diameter of 7–9 μm (Fig. 8.27). There are no blind ends because the cardiovascular system is basically a closed circuit. Movement, though most sluggish in capillaries, is still practically continuous. This allows the maximum exchange of components between blood and tissue, thus fulfilling the purpose of the system. The capillary wall consists only of endothelial cells and basal lamina, with an occasional *pericyte* applied to the outer surface. Pericytes are apparently multipotent cells which can differentiate into other cell types. They may be of importance in maintenance and repair.

On the basis of differences in endothelial cell structure, two types of capillaries are known, continuous (Figs. 8.30 and 8.31) and fenestrated (Figs. 8.30 and 8.32). Continuous capillaries have no pores and their endothelial cells commonly show great numbers of pinocytotic vesicles. In fenestrated capillaries the endothelial cells possess minute (less than 100 nm in diameter) pores that render the vessel wall more permeable. In most fenestrated endothelial cells a diaphragm, thinner than the plasmalemma, is stretched across each pore. In either case, water, solutes, and complex macromolecules are readily exchanged between blood and the tissue fluid of the interstitial spaces. Also, it is apparently not difficult for inflammatory and other cells to pass through these capillary walls by squeezing themselves between endothelial cells (diapedesis). This occurs quickly and in relatively large numbers if there is the slightest injury, but also happens to a lesser degree under normal conditions. The total surface area of capillaries available for such important interchanges is approximately 6000 m².

Another type of small vessel is sometimes classified as a third category of capillary, the so-called *sinusoidal capillary* or *sinusoid*. These are endothelial vessels of larger and less regular diameter (30–40 μm) with gaps between endothelial cells and a discontinuous basal lamina (Figs. 8.30 and 8.33). It is common to find phagocytic cells in close relation

Fig. 8.27. *Small blood vessels.* These vessels are from a retina which has been spread out on a slide and stained. Arteries (long arrow), capillaries (circle), and veins (short arrow). ×28. (Courtesy of D. Johnson.)

Fig. 8.28. *Aneurysms* (localized dilated segments) and minor abnormalities of retinal vessels from another retinal spread. Such lesions cannot be seen as clearly in the usual histologic section. ×85. (Courtesy of D. Johnson.)

Fig. 8.29. *Hemangioma* in liver. This is a collection of various-sized, thin-walled, vascular spaces. ×34.

Fig. 8.30. Types of *capillary endothelium.* In some fenestrated endothelia, especially of the kidney, pores are uniform in size and distribution, unlike those shown here.

Types of *capillary endothelium* (electron micrographs).

Fig. 8.31. *Continuous endothelium.* Transport of materials in and out of capillaries with this type of endothelium takes place in vesicles. These begin on one surface as pits which take in material, close over to form vesicles (endocytosis), move across the cell and empty their contents (exocytosis). ×22,000. (Courtesy of R. S. Connell.)

Fig. 8.32. *Fenestrated endothelium.* Arrows indicate pores. Lumen with red blood cells is to the left. ×12,750. (Courtesy of M. Webb.)

Fig. 8.33. *Discontinuous endothelium.* The long arrow is in the lumen of the vessel and indicates the inner surface. Small arrows indicate microvilli of cells outside the vessel. ×8500.

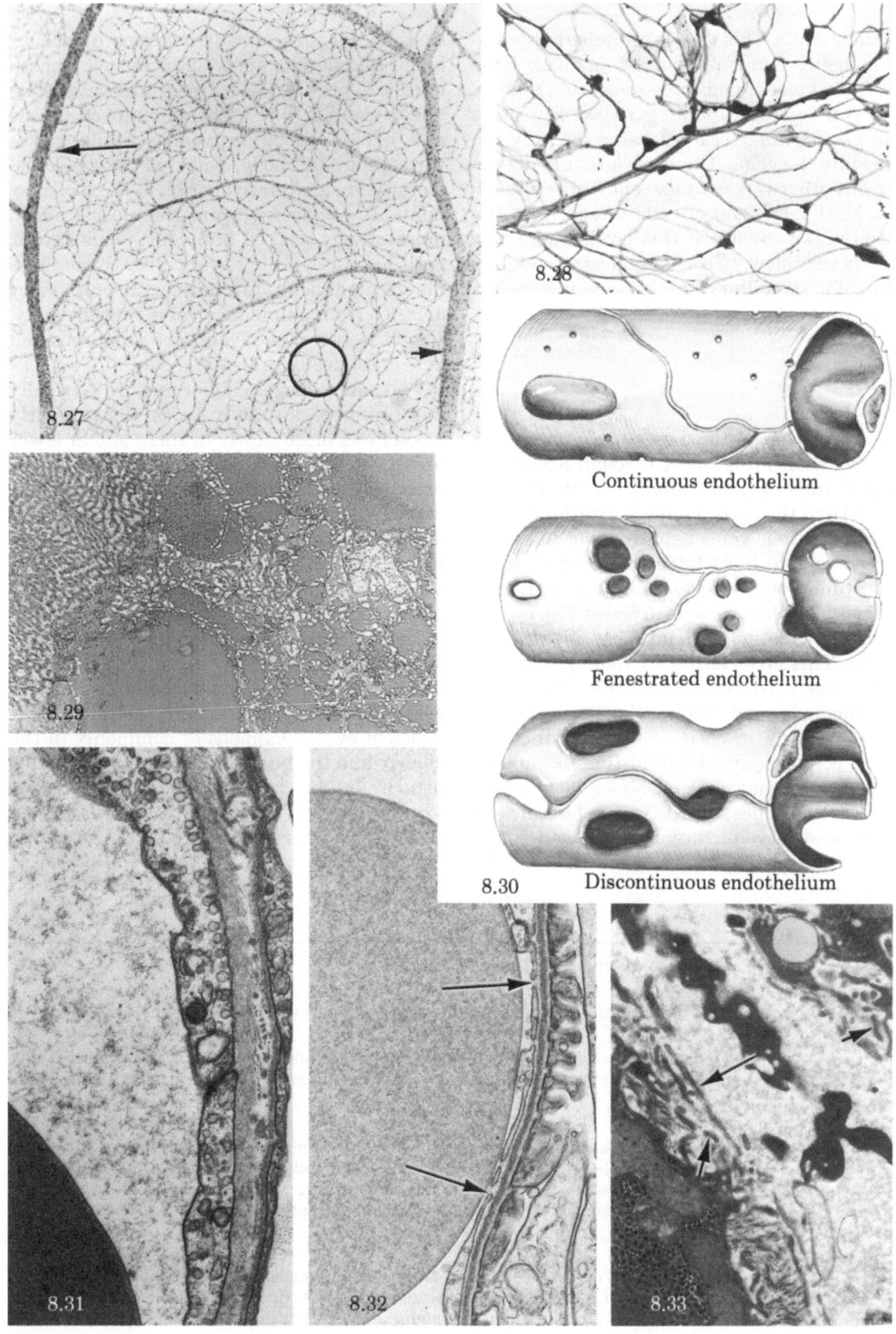

Continuous endothelium

Fenestrated endothelium

8.30 Discontinuous endothelium

to their walls. This type is of limited distribution, being found principally in liver, bone marrow, spleen, and some endocrine organs.

Distal to true capillaries, blood flows into the *postcapillary venules* before being gathered into the veins. These are larger in diameter but otherwise not different from capillaries. Most migration of cells to and from the blood vessels occurs at this level, where flow rate is very slow. In some organs the endothelium of postcapillary venules is more cuboidal than squamous.

Veins

As is apparent in the dissecting room and at surgery, veins (Figs. 8.34 through 8.38) have larger lumens and usually much thinner walls than the corresponding arteries. In histologic sections veins usually seem to be collapsed and to have folded walls (Fig. 8.34), with tunics that are generally less distinctly demarcated than those of arteries. The intima has only endothelium and a basement membrane. This layer forms, by folding, the thin semilunar valves of veins of the extremities. The media is much thinner than that of corresponding arteries (Fig. 8.35) and includes more collagen and less elastin. Its smooth muscle is arranged much more loosely and in bundles. The adventitia is the thickest layer, and in veins larger than about 5 mm

in diameter, it generally contains numerous longitudinal and spiral bundles of smooth muscle. This reaches its maximum in the venae cavae (Fig. 8.38). The amounts of muscle and elastic tissue in venous walls varies throughout the body, veins of the lower extremities being relatively rich in these components. In pulmonary veins the muscle lies in more closely packed and continuous layers, with less intervening connective tissue. This makes it difficult to distinguish pulmonary arteries from pulmonary veins histologically. The vasa vasorum of veins are numerous and penetrate deeply into the media.

Veins have larger caliber and are generally more numerous than arteries. Consequently blood flows more slowly in them and at lower pressure. With a tourniquet or with finger pressure one can temporarily halt venous flow rather easily. Venous obstruction may also occur, but often subtly and without being planned, from such ostensibly innocent practices as immobilization. In a bedridden adult, prolonged inactivity may cause stagnation of blood in veins of the lower extremities. This may lead to venous thrombosis (Figs. 8.36 and 8.37) and, later, pulmonary embolism (transport of thrombi to pulmonary arteries). This series of events happens so commonly in the elderly and the infirm, that pulmonary embolism is one of the leading causes of death. The practice of intentionally restricting patients to bed is rare now.

Fig. 8.34. *Medium-sized vein.* ×100.

Fig. 8.35. *Medium-sized vein and artery.* Note nerve between vessels. ×34.

Fig. 8.36. *Venous thrombus.* This, like most venous thrombi, is not occlusive and may not seriously impede blood flow. Clinical signs and symptoms may be minimal. ×34.

Fig. 8.37. *Thrombosis of deep leg veins.* The veins of the leg are large, and when such thrombi become detached and ride the blood stream to the lungs, they cause major problems. **a:** A portion of the calf muscles with thrombi in the vessels. **b:** A thrombus removed from a vein of the same leg. It has formed a cast of venous valves.

Fig. 8.38. *Inferior vena cava.* **a:** H & E stain of transverse section showing longitudinal bundles of smooth muscle in adventitia (A). **b:** Elastin stain of longitudinal section showing elastic fibers in media and adventitia. ×85.

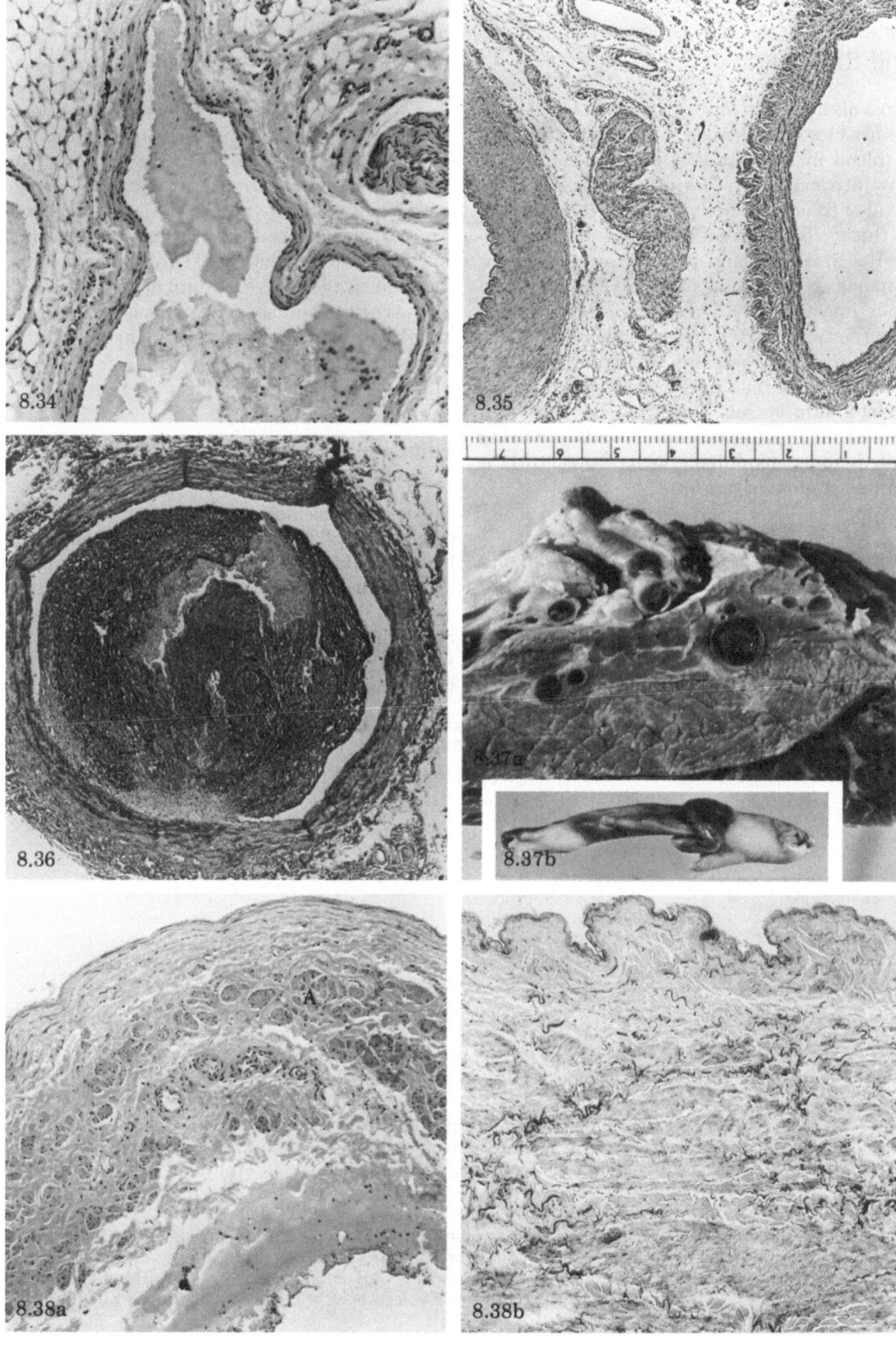

8.34

8.35

8.36

8.37a

8.37b

8.38a

8.38b

Arteriovenous Anastomoses (Figs. 8.39 and 8.40)

Most of the time a large proportion of capillaries are closed and empty, but both the amount of blood in the capillary bed and its rate of flow are extremely variable and reflect the level of functional activity of the tissue. Much of this variation, remember, is under the control of arterioles and metarterioles. Another important control is provided by arteriovenous anastomoses. These are direct connections between arterioles and venules which make possible complete bypass of capillary beds. In some areas, particularly in skin, these anastomotic vessels appear to be somewhat specialized, having very thick walls and being coiled and convoluted. Such a structure is termed a *glomus.*

Sensory Receptors

Highly specialized sensory nerve endings exist at certain sites within the arterial tree. One type, called *chemoreceptors* (Fig. 8.41), respond to changes in blood pressure, pH and oxygen and carbon dioxide levels, providing sensory input for the homeostatic mechanism. Nerve fibers from these cells pass via the autonomic nervous system to the central nervous system. There are two pairs of major chemoreceptors. The first are the carotid bodies, located at the bifurcations of the carotid arteries just outside the vessel walls. The second pair, the aortic bodies, are near the origins of the subclavian arteries. The principal *baroreceptors* (pressure receptors) are in the walls of the carotid sinuses. The sinus is an enlargement of each common carotid artery at its bifurcation.

Functional Correlations of Structure

The cardiovascular system must perform a great deal of work reliably and throughout the life of the individual. Clearly the organization of these structures is arranged to carry out this duty effectively. Only the basics are considered here (Fig. 8.42). Presentation of further detail would be beyond the scope of this book.

Fig. 8.39. *Arteriovenous anastomosis.*

Fig. 8.40. *Arteriovenous anastomosis,* skin of fingertip. Many vascular loops are cut in various planes. ×85.

Fig. 8.41. *Carotid body.* A mass of small blood vessels, among which are numerous small sensory nerve endings (chemoreceptors). Nerve endings are not visible at this low magnification. Portions of the walls of the internal and external carotid arteries are also shown. ×24.

Fig. 8.42. Graph illustrating some of the changes in *function* (above) and *structure* (below) *of blood vessels.* This is not quantitatively accurate and no scales are indicated; the relationships are important. All changes are gradual. (Modified with permission from Fig. 4.2 in Cowdry EV. Textbook of Histology, 4th edit. Philadelphia, Lea & Febiger, 1950.)

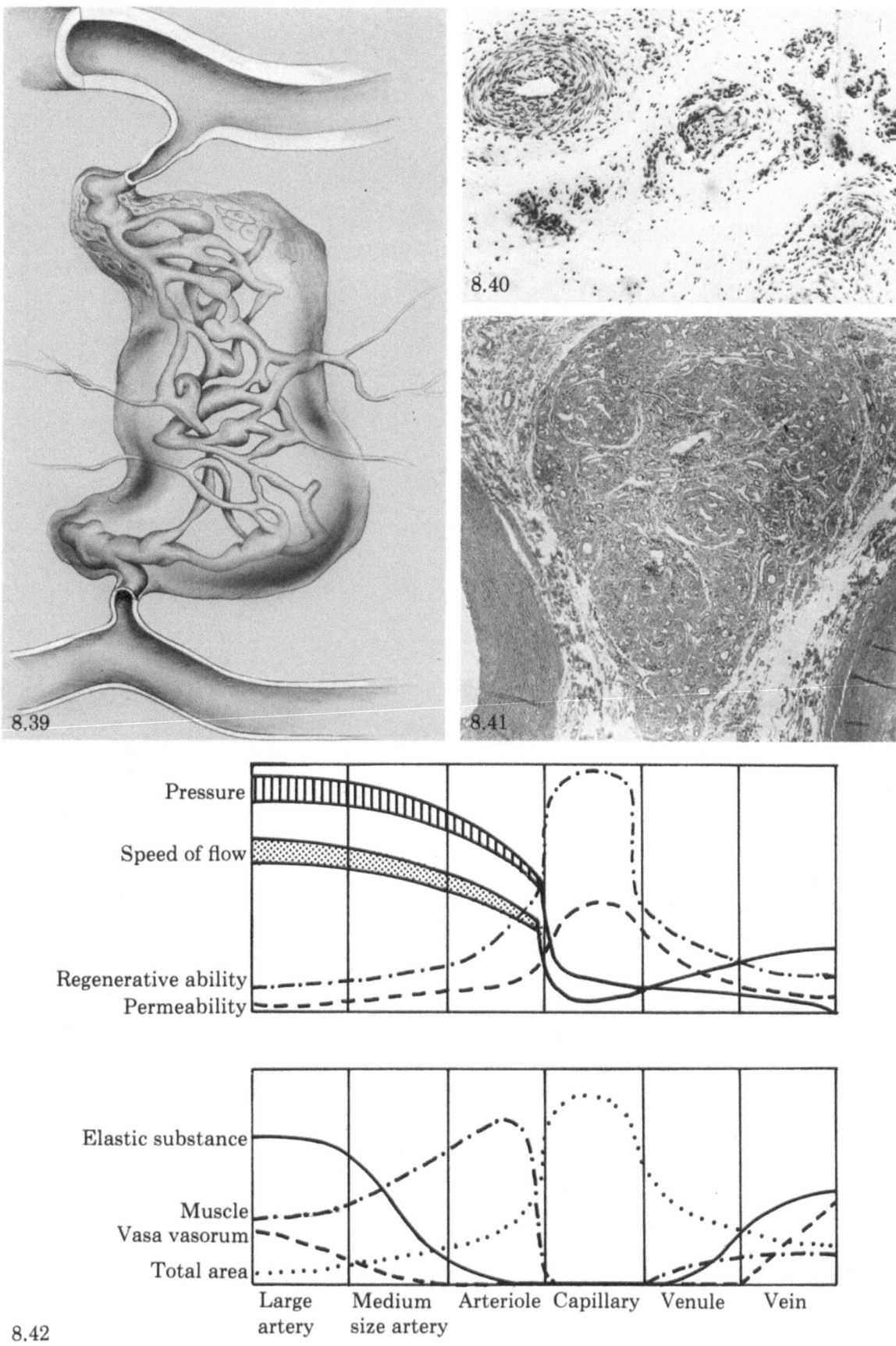

8.39

8.40

8.41

Pressure

Speed of flow

Regenerative ability
Permeability

Elastic substance

Muscle
Vasa vasorum
Total area

Large
artery   Medium   Arteriole   Capillary   Venule   Vein
          size artery

8.42

9 Blood and Bone Marrow

Blood

Blood is a liquid tissue that is pumped by the heart through the circulatory system. About 45% of the volume of blood is composed of cells; the remaining 55% is liquid plasma in which these cells are suspended. The percentage of blood volume occupied by packed cells, which is determined by centrifugation in a standardized tube, is the hematocrit. This volume varies widely in different diseases (Table 9.1, page 170).

The plasma is a complex fluid containing proteins, vitamins, lipids, hormones, and inorganic salts. The plasma proteins consist of α, β, and γ-globulins, albumin, and fibrinogen. Fibrinogen is a precursor of fibrin in the clotting process (Figs. 9.20 and 9.21). Serum is the fluid that separates from a clot; it is essentially plasma without the components of coagulation.

The cells originate from precursors in bone marrow and lymphoid tissue and the relative and absolute numbers of the different types seen in blood samples reflect the productivity of these tissues. Microscopic examination of blood samples, both for *absolute* numbers in a counting chamber and for *relative* numbers of different cell types in a fixed and stained film on a slide (called a blood smear) (Fig. 9.1), constitutes one of the most valuable diagnostic aids available to the physician. Since specific cell types are particularly responsive to different infections and other disease processes, a differential blood count can often be of material assistance in the identification of a disease (Table 9.1). Morphologic as well as numerical departures from the normal range are important in such studies. In the discussion that follows, the normal morphology as seen in blood smears, normal numerical data, and brief comments on function will be provided for each cell type. The appearances of all of these cells in smears differ from those in tissue sections (see Chapters 4 and 10).

Erythrocytes

Erythrocytes (red blood cells or RBCs) (Figs. 9.2 and 9.3) occur in the range of 4–5 million per mm^3 of blood. They are nonnucleated (anucleate) structures, very uniform in size and shape except in certain disease states (Figs. 9.3 and 9.4). They are biconcave discs averaging 7.5 μm in diameter, and this form is maintained by a ring of cytoplasmic microtubules arranged beneath the membrane at the perimeter of the cell. They contain hemoglobin, a respiratory pigment, for transport of oxygen and carbon dioxide, and the necessary enzymes to maintain this substance in an effective functional state. The glycocalyx of the cell membrane has built into it various genetically determined antigens that characterize the various blood types (A, B, O, Rh, etc.). Although they are not regarded as complete cells because of their lack of a nucleus, they do have a fairly constant functional life span of about 120 days and are removed from the blood in spleen and bone marrow. Some of the products of their breakdown (e.g., bilirubin) are excreted and others (e.g., iron) are recycled.

Young erythrocytes, freshly released from bone marrow, still contain some RNA that is synthesizing the last bit of the cell's hemoglobin. This RNA imparts a slight diffuse basophilia to the cell in stained blood smears. When the living cell is stained with cresyl violet, the RNA is precipitated as a darkly stained reticulum. Cells thus stained are reticulocytes and constitute about 1% of circulating red cells. When the marrow is called upon to increase its output, as following blood donation, this percentage increases.

Fig. 9.1. Steps in the *preparation of a blood smear.* By moving the upright glass slide to the right to contact the drop of blood and then pushing it to the left, the blood is pulled on the horizontal slide to form a thin film. The smear can then be dried, or fixed, and stained for microscopic examination.

Fig. 9.2. Smear of normal *peripheral blood* colored with Wright's stain. ×175.

Fig. 9.3. Scanning electron micrograph of *red blood cells.* The biconcave form of the round cells is clearly shown. Some cells have lost water during preparation and have undergone a shrinking process (called crenation), which gives the cells a spinous appearance. Such cells have been termed echinocytes. About ×8000. (Courtesy of M. Bessis from Fig. 10, Chapter III in Bessis M: Corpuscles, Atlas of Red Blood Cell Shapes. Berlin, Springer-Verlag, 1974.)

Fig. 9.4. Scanning electron micrograph of a red cell from a patient with *sickle-cell anemia.* In this disease red cell form varies greatly but generally tends toward an elongated crescent. About ×10,000. (Courtesy of M. Bessis from Fig. 5, Chapter V in Bessis M: Corpuscles, Atlas of Red Blood Cell Shapes. Berlin, Springer-Verlag, 1974.)

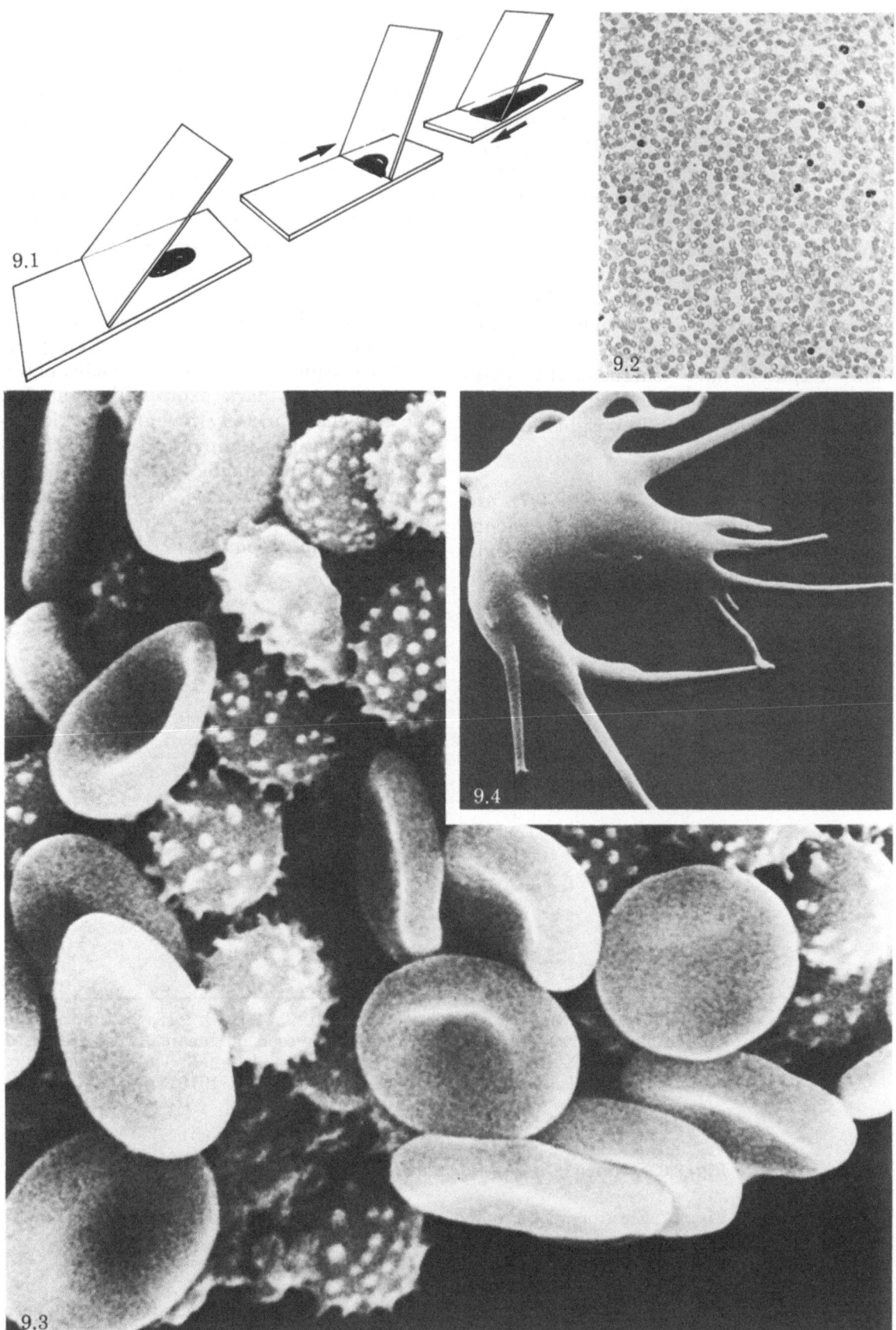

9.1

9.2

9.3

9.4

Leukocytes

Leukocytes (white blood cells or WBCs) occur as five principal types. They all arise, function, and die outside of the circulatory system in which they are transported and which constitutes a convenient source for obtaining samples. There are normally from 5000 to 10,000 WBCs per mm³ of blood. Of the five types, two, the agranulocytes, as the name implies, have no specific cytoplasmic granules; three, the granulocytes, again as the name implies, have characteristic cytoplasmic particles. The following descriptions pertain to the cells as seen in Wright's-stained smears.

AGRANULOCYTES

Lymphocytes (Fig. 9.5 through 9.7) are small cells, 6–9 μm in diameter (an occasional one may be as large as 13). The lymphocyte has a darkly staining, round or slightly indented nucleus so dense that little or no internal nuclear structure can be seen, and a narrow rim of sky-blue cytoplasm, which sometimes contains a few sharply defined but small, nonspecific, azurophilic granules. The various complex functions of these cells will be considered in Chapter 10. They characteristically accumulate in large numbers in some tissues in chronic bacterial inflammation.

Monocytes (Figs. 9.8 and 9.9) are 12–18 μm in diameter. They have a grayish-blue cytoplasm with a "ground glass" or foamy appearance, sometimes with visible vacuoles and a few very small, dark azurophilic granules. The nucleus is usually indented or kidney-shaped, sometimes lumpy, with chromatin appearing as coarse, tangled strands. Monocytes originate in bone marrow, leave the circulation, and enter the tissues. They are then referred to as *macrophages*.

The following drawings (Figs. 9.5, 9.6, 9.8, 9.10, 9.11, 9.13, 9.15, 9.17, 9.25, 9.26, 9.27) of blood and marrow cells are as they are seen in smears. These are based on paintings by D. Sturm in Diggs LW, Sturm D and Bell A: The Morphology of Human Blood Cells. North Chicago, Abbott Laboratories, 1978.)

Fig. 9.5. Drawing of a *small lymphocyte.*

Fig. 9.6. Drawing of a *large lymphocyte.*

Fig. 9.7. Electron micrograph of a *lymphocyte.* ×10,000. (Courtesy of R. S. Connell.)

Fig. 9.8. Drawing of a *monocyte.*

Fig. 9.9. Electron micrograph of a *monocyte.* In this instance the cell has been elongated in passage through a capillary in the lung. ×4100. (Courtesy of R. S. Connell.)

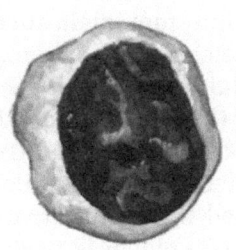

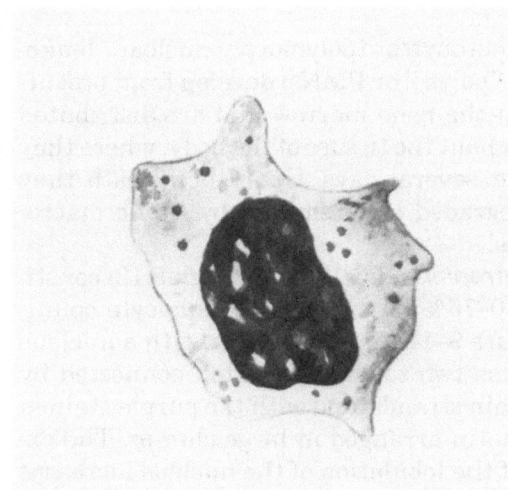

9.5

9.6

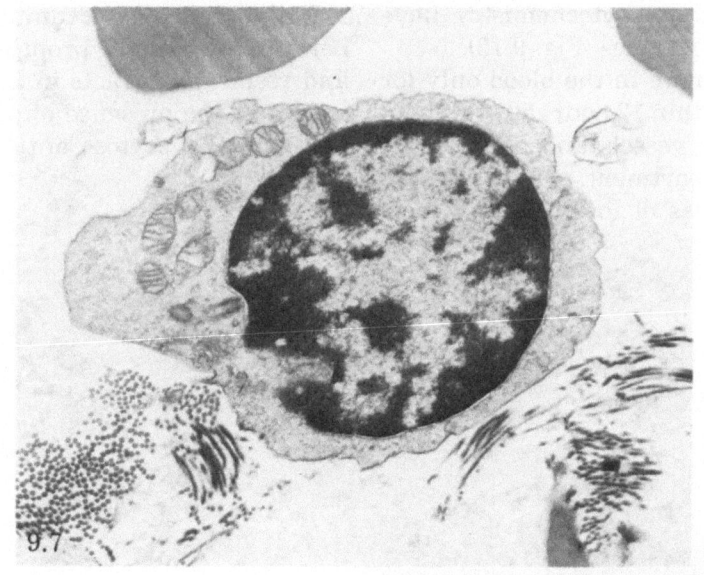

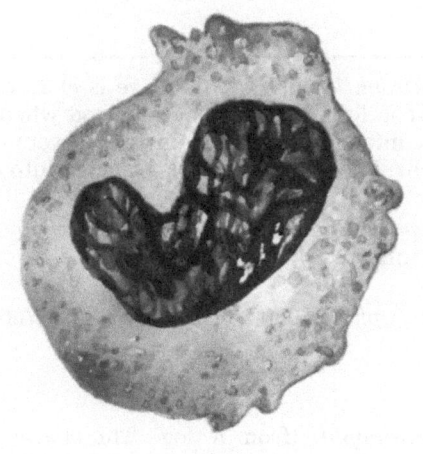

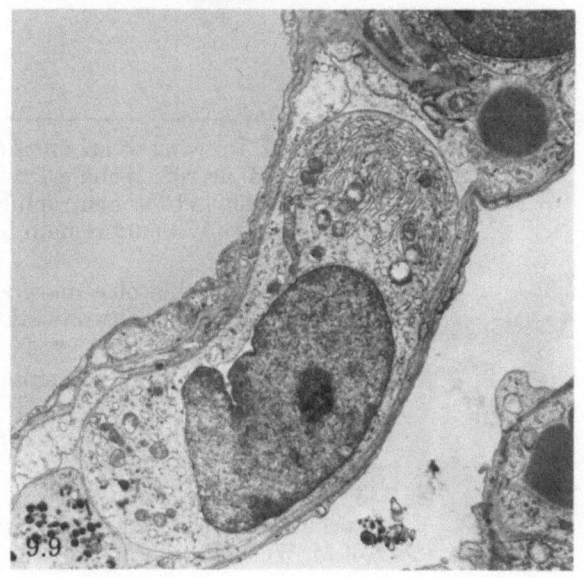

9.8

9.9

GRANULOCYTES (polymorphonuclear leukocytes, "polys," or PMNs) develop from precursors in the bone marrow and are distributed throughout the tissues of the body, where they live for several days. Upon their death they are degraded and removed by tissue macrophages.

Neutrophils (Figs. 9.10 through 9.12) constitute 40–75% of the normal leukocyte count. They are 9–14 μm in diameter with a nucleus that has two to six lobes often connected by very thin strands, and with the purple-stained chromatin arranged in large clumps. The extent of the lobulation of the nucleus increases with the age of the cell. The cytoplasm usually has a lavender hue due to the presence of fine, evenly distributed, characteristic granules which by electron cytochemistry have been found to be lysosomes (Fig. 9.12).

Neutrophils circulate in the blood only for a short time, and within 12 hours 50% of them have left the blood vessels and entered the extravascular compartment. They migrate rapidly to local areas of infection and their presence in unusual numbers, either in the blood stream or locally in tissues, indicates acute inflammation. They are phagocytic and particularly active in ingesting small, discrete, particulate materials such as bacteria. The lysosomes contain lytic enzymes utilized in the degradation of this ingested material.

Eosinophils (Figs. 9.13 and 9.14) constitute 1–6% of leukocytes and are 10–14 μm in diameter. The nucleus is usually bilobed, with the lobes connected by a thin strand or a broad isthmus. The cytoplasm is packed with large uniform-sized, orange to red, acidophilic granules that do not cover or obscure the nucleus. With the electron microscope each granule may be seen to contain a crystalline structure in its center (Fig. 9.14).

Eosinophils may accumulate in large numbers in the lamina propria of the digestive and respiratory tracts in allergies and in response to the presence of parasites. They apparently phagocytose antigen–antibody complexes.

Fig. 9.10. Drawing of an *immature neutrophil (band)*. This stage is characterized by a band- or ribbon-shaped nucleus. It is found in peripheral blood when there is extra demand for neutrophils, as in infections. In such instances young cells, which normally would remain in the marrow until mature, are rushed into action.

Fig. 9.11. Drawing of a *mature neutrophil*. This stage is characterized by a segmented nucleus with two to six lobes connected by thread-like strands.

Fig. 9.12. Electron micrograph of a *neutrophil.* ×6300. (Courtesy of M. Webb.)

Fig. 9.13. Drawing of an *eosinophil.*

Fig. 9.14. Electron micrograph of an *eosinophil* (from a dog). The characteristic specific granules contain centrally located crystalline components. ×7000. (Courtesy of M. Webb.)

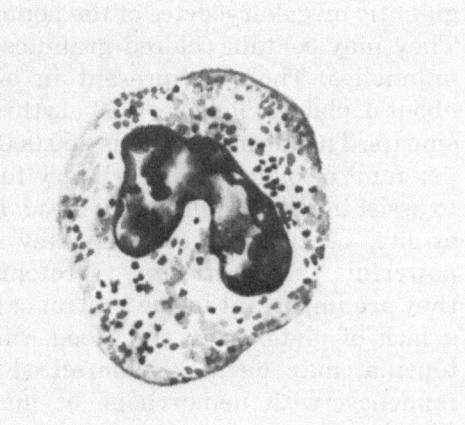

9.10

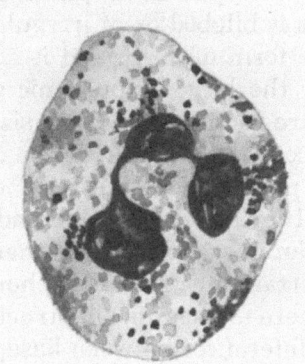

9.11

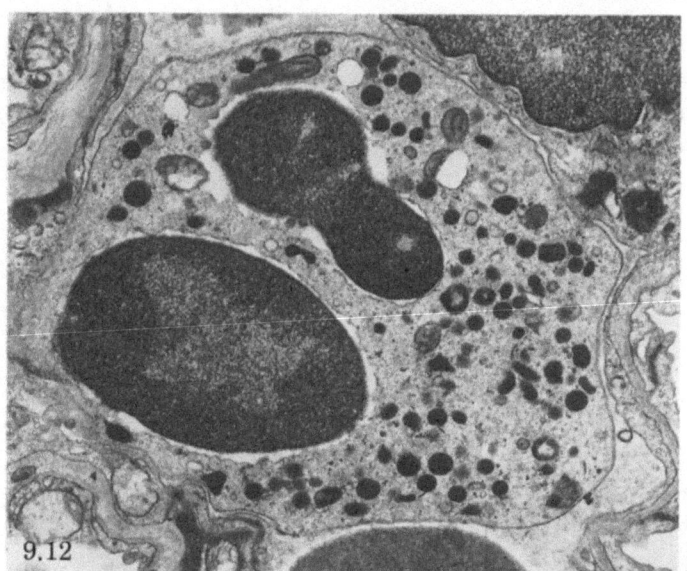

9.12

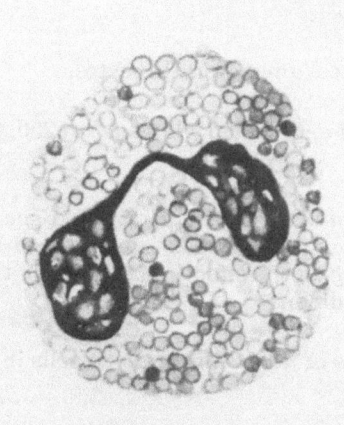

9.13

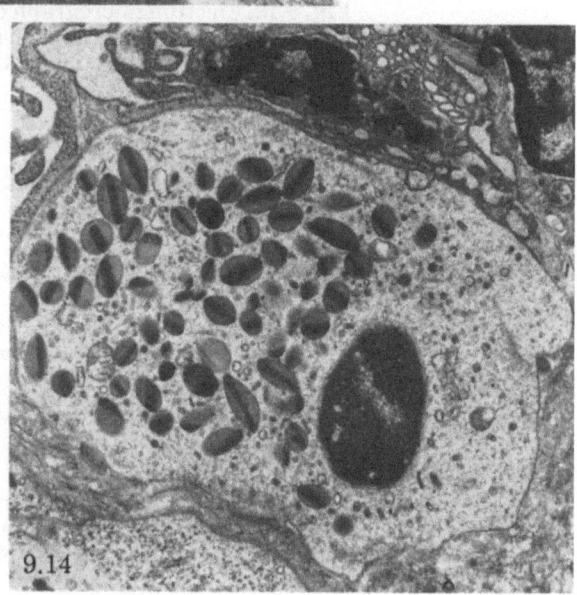

9.14

Basophils (Figs. 9.15 and 9.16) are the least common of the leukocytes, constituting 0–1% of the count. They are 10–12 μm in diameter. The nucleus is bilobed or of irregular shape, often in the form of an S, and is commonly obscured by the large cytoplasmic granules. The latter are round, variable in size, deeply basophilic, sometimes black. These cells may be slightly phagocytic. Like mast cells (see Chapter 4), they have histamine and heparin in their granules and release them in response to certain antigens and other stimuli. However, there are significant structural and functional differences between basophils and mast cells.

Platelets

Another important component of blood identifiable in smears but easily overlooked is the *platelets* (thrombocytes) (Figs. 9.17 through 9.19; 9.21). These are small (1.5–2 μm), flat-tened cytoplasmic fragments derived from the gigantic megakaryocytes of the bone marrow. They may contain colored granules and cell organelles. They are present in a ratio of about 1 platelet for every 20 erythrocytes in smears. The normal count is 250,000–500,000 per mm³ of blood. Their primary function is to assist in the coagulation of blood. However, at sites of injury to collagen they release a powerful vasoconstrictor, serotonin. Thus they are important in the control of bleeding; a lack of platelets in the blood, thrombocytopenia, may mean a generalized bleeding tendency, with hemorrhage at many sites. Platelets live for 8–12 days and are removed from the blood by the spleen and liver.

In addition to the recognizable cells described above, blood smears commonly contain occasional ruptured or otherwise damaged cells or cell fragments, some produced in the preparation of the smear. They cannot be classified by cell type.

Fig. 9.15. Drawing of a *basophil*. The dense and numerous granules often obscure the nucleus.

Fig. 9.16. Electron micrograph of a *basophil*. The specific granules are very electron-dense and, although variable in size, are generally larger than those of other granulocytes. ×7400. (Courtesy of R. S. Connell.)

Fig. 9.17. Drawing of *platelets* (thrombocytes) among erythrocytes.

Fig. 9.18. Electron micrograph of a group of aggregated *platelets*. ×6250. (Courtesy of R. S. Connell.)

Fig. 9.19. Scanning electron micrograph of the inner surface of a small artery with a loop of suture through its wall. Numerous *platelets* and several red blood cells (some of which are crenated) are resting on the endothelial lining of the vessel. ×1000. (Courtesy of P. Amstutz and B. Hindman.)

Fig. 9.20. Histologic section showing strands of *fibrin* and trapped cells in a thrombus. ×560.

Fig. 9.21. Scanning electron micrograph of part of a blood filter. A fine mesh of *fibrin* lies on the coarse fibers of the filter. *Platelets* and some erythrocytes are also present. ×450. (Courtesy of R. S. Connell.)

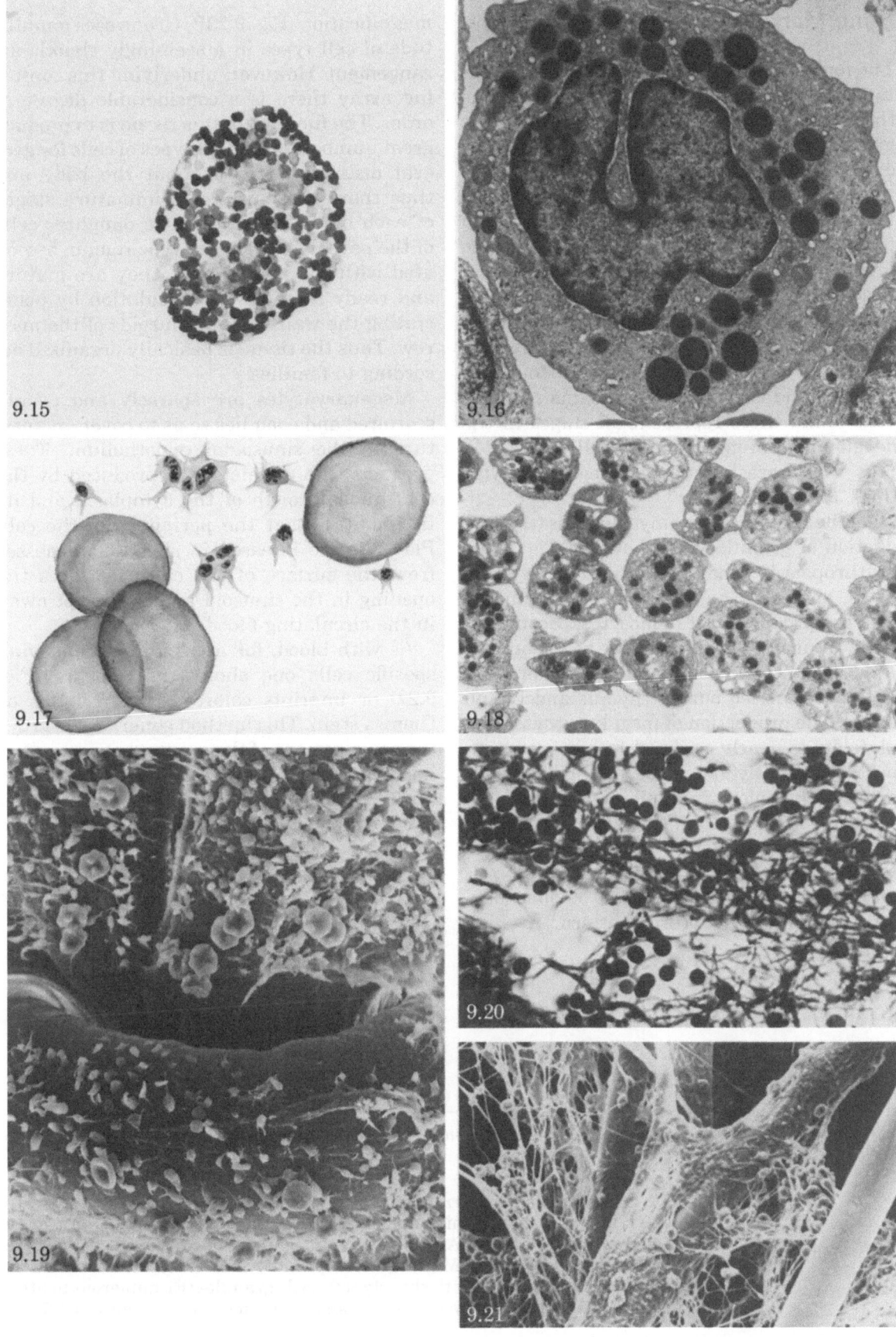

9.15

9.16

9.17

9.18

9.19

9.20

9.21

Bone Marrow

The formation of all types of blood cells begins in the mesoderm of the yolk sac during the third week of gestation. This function shifts gradually to the liver, spleen, and thymus during the third month and continues here until, or shortly after, birth. In the sixth month bone marrow and lymph nodes begin to assume this function. Normally during the first few years, bones of the extremities and head resign this duty and their marrow becomes largely or entirely fatty and yellow. The bones of the trunk (sternum, clavicles, vertebrae, ribs, and pelvis) continue to generate cells and their marrow remains red. The cells found there represent all stages in the development of mature blood cells (Fig. 9.24), plus the characteristic big megakaryocytes (Figs. 9.23, 9.27).

As the fetus matures, myelopoiesis (the production of granulocytes, shown in Fig. 9.26), erythropoiesis (the production of erythrocytes, shown in Fig. 9.25), and presumably also the production of monocytes, become entirely or nearly restricted to the bone marrow. As will be seen in Chapter 10, lymphopoiesis is largely carried out by thymus and lymph nodes. The production of megakaryocytes and platelets is nearly confined to bone marrow, but occasionally one may find megakaryocytes in the spleen in adult life.

At low magnification (Fig. 9.23A) a section of active (red) marrow appears to be a uniform cellular tissue with scattered, large fat cells and spicules of bone. There is no obvious lobulation or other structural pattern. At high magnification (Fig. 9.23B, C) one sees a multitude of cell types in a seemingly chaotic arrangement. However, underlying this confusing array there is a considerable degree of order. The function of this tissue is to produce great numbers of several types of cells for general distribution throughout the body and thus there are clusters of immature stages of each of the cell lines. The daughter cells of the parent cells of each type remain associated with the parent until they are mature and ready to enter the circulation by penetrating the walls of the sinusoids of the marrow. Thus the tissue is basically organized according to families.

Megakaryocytes are sparsely and evenly scattered and each lies so as to cover an aperture in the sinusoidal endothelium. Their products, the platelets, are produced by the continuous growth of the cytoplasm and its fragmentation at the periphery of the cell. Platelets are released in sheets and masses from the surface of the cell that faces the opening in the sinusoid and are swept away in the circulating blood.

As with blood, for accuracy in identifying specific cells one should use smears (Fig. 9.22) or imprints colored with Wright's or Giemsa stain. This method generally destroys the arrangement of the groups; however, even here related cells may remain associated (Fig. 9.22). At present in the clinical examination of bone marrow, both smears and sections are usually employed.

For the components of each of the various cell lineages in bone marrow see Figs. 9.24 through 9.26.

Fig. 9.22. Smear of *bone marrow*. Notice the clump of nucleated red cells and the cell in mitosis. ×520.

Fig. 9.23. Sections of *bone marrow*. **a:** Adipocytes and a variety of cell types are present. ×175. **b:** At slightly higher magnification the individual cells are more easily distinguished. ×250. **c:** At still higher magnification more cell details are visible. Note: megakaryocyte (M); large cell (possibly megakaryoblast) in mitosis (Mi); several eosinophilic cells with sharply refractile granules (E); numerous neutrophils including band and mature forms. Not all cells seen can be categorized. ×1000.

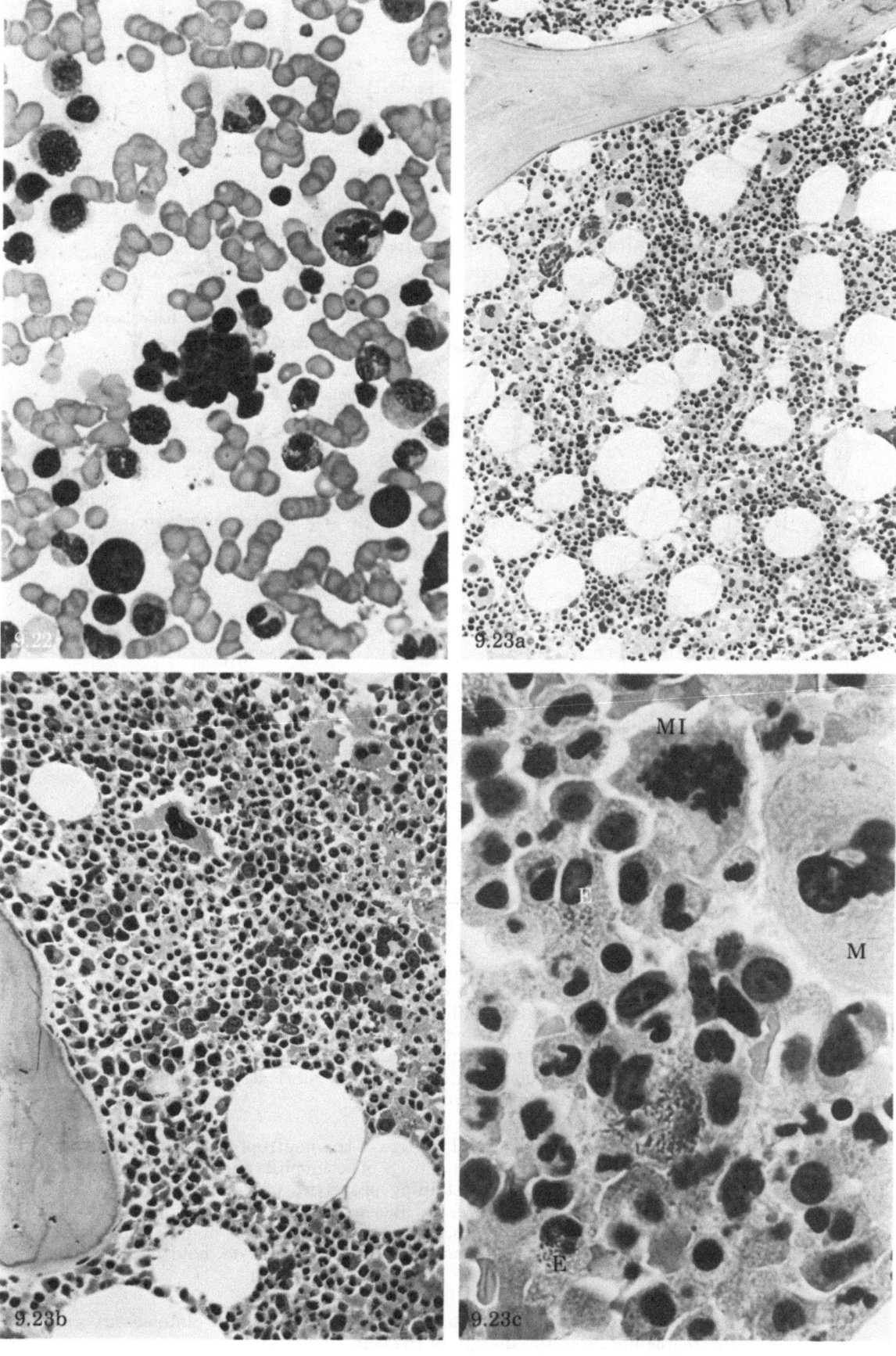

9.22

9.23a

9.23b

9.23c

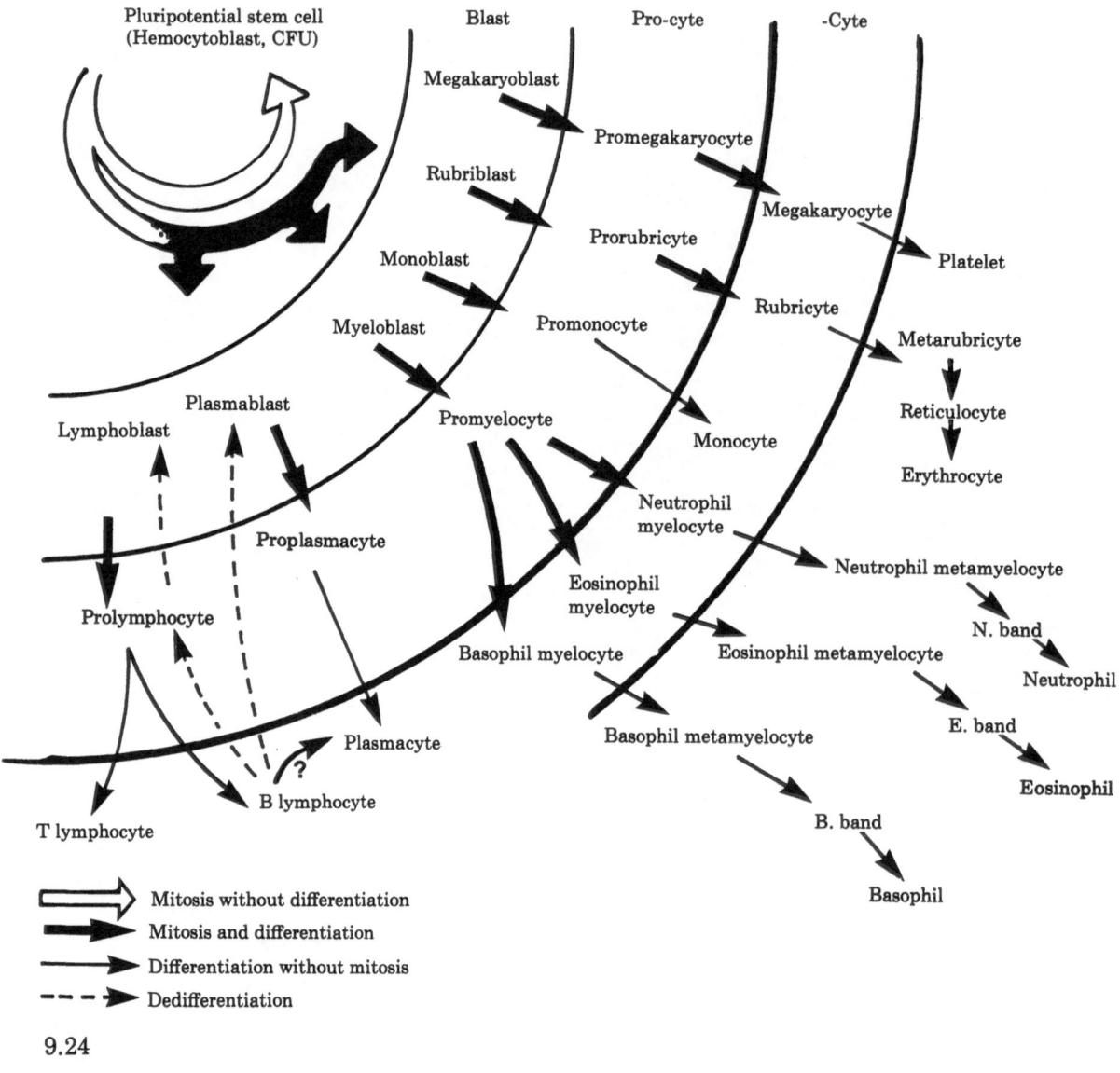

Pluripotential stem cell
(Hemocytoblast, CFU)

Blast · Pro-cyte · -Cyte

Megakaryoblast

Promegakaryocyte

Rubriblast

Megakaryocyte

Monoblast

Prorubricyte

Platelet

Myeloblast

Rubricyte

Promyelocyte

Metarubricyte

Promonocyte

Reticulocyte

Plasmablast

Monocyte

Lymphoblast

Erythrocyte

Neutrophil
myelocyte

Proplasmacyte

Neutrophil metamyelocyte

Eosinophil
myelocyte

Prolymphocyte

N. band

Basophil myelocyte

Neutrophil

Eosinophil metamyelocyte

Plasmacyte

E. band

Basophil metamyelocyte

Eosinophil

B lymphocyte

?

T lymphocyte

B. band

Basophil

⬜➔ Mitosis without differentiation
➔ Mitosis and differentiation
—➔ Differentiation without mitosis
---➔ Dedifferentiation

9.24

Fig. 9.24. Chart of *hemopoietic cell lines*.

Fig. 9.25. *Erythropoiesis.* Drawings of the red cell line to show changes that occur during differentiation. The cell diameter is markedly reduced and the cytoplasm changes from intensely basophilic to acidophilic. In the nucleus the nucleoli disappear and the chromatin pattern changes from fine threads or stippled, to coarse strands, to compact clumps, to a single dense pyknotic mass, before disappearing. From top to bottom: Rubriblast, prorubricyte, rubricyte, metarubricyte, basophilic erythrocyte (reticulocyte), erythrocyte.

Fig. 9.26. *Myelopoiesis.* The cell lineage of the neutrophil is shown as an example of myelopoiesis. The stages in the lineage of eosinophils and basophils are essentially the same except for size and staining properties of the specific granules. There are also some slight differences in nuclear morphogenesis. From top to bottom: myeloblast, promyelocyte (characterized by large numbers of dark nonspecific granules), neutrophilic myelocyte, neutrophilic metamyelocyte, neutrophilic band, neutrophilic segmented form.

Fig. 9.27. Drawing of a *megakaryocyte.* Great numbers of platelets are produced by fragmentation of the margin of the cell.

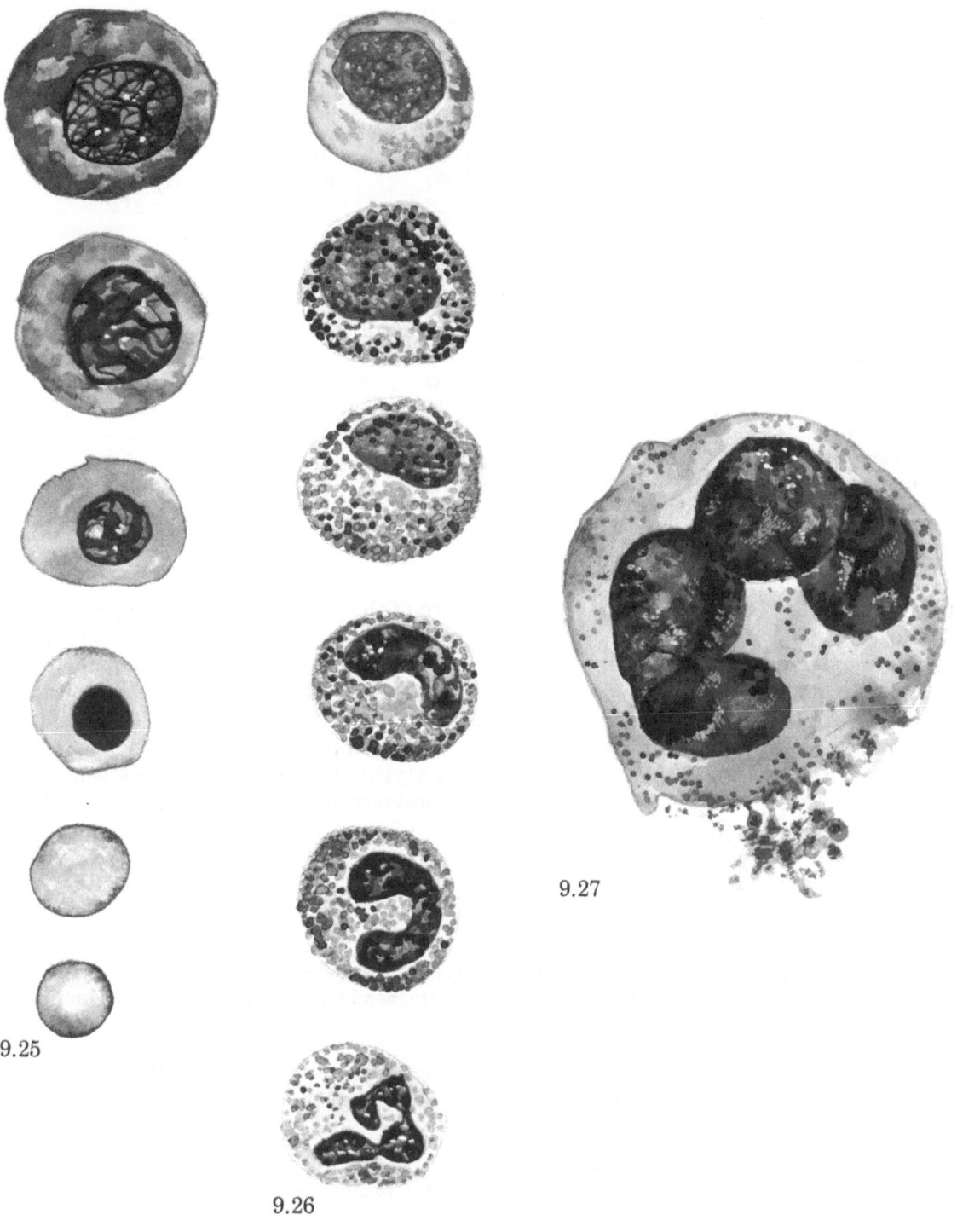

9.25

9.26

9.27

Table 9.1
Blood Counts in Various Conditions

	Normal Range	Chronic Lymphocytic Leukemia*	Acute Appendicitis*	Hypoplastic Anemia*
Leukocytes/mm³	5000–10,000	260,000	16,800	1200
Platelets/mm³	250,000–500,000	68,000	356,000	12,000
Hematocrit	30–56	28.6	47.0	21.2
Differential cell counts (no. of cells/100 leukocytes)				
Mature neutrophils	40–75	2	62	1
Band neutrophils	0	0	23	0
Metamyelocytes	0	0	1	0
Lymphocytes	20–45	97	12	93
Monocytes	2–10	1	2	1
Eosinophils	1–6	0	0	3
Basophils	0–2	0	0	2

* Data for these conditions courtesy of S. Goodnight

Disease

Blood and bone marrow are affected in many disease states. A few simple laboratory tests (see Table 9.1) are used very commonly, including in every hospital admission. This indicates their general usefulness in diagnosis and patient care.

Neoplasia may strike the hematopoietic system like other systems, and it may be of basic undifferentiated (stem) cells or of one or more of the differentiated cell types. Polycythemia rubra vera (primary excess of erythrocytes) is one example. Another is leukemia (literally, white blood; actually, a neoplasm of leukocytes), which may involve stem cells, monocytes, lymphocytes or granulocytes. Until a few years ago these conditions were always progressive, either slowly or quickly, and therefore eventually fatal. A primary reason for the difficulty in their control lies with the nature of the hematopoietic system. Mar-

Fig. 9.28. *Myeloid (granulocytic) leukemia,* section of bone marrow. Fat is being crowded out. Most of the cells are immature members of the myeloid series. Families are not apparent. ×175.

Fig. 9.29. *Myeloid (granulocytic) leukemia,* smear of blood. Most of the white cells are band polymorphonuclear leukocytes. Earlier stages (arrows) are also present. ×175.

Fig. 9.30. Section of *liver in myeloid (granulocytic) leukemia.* This disease originates in bone marrow and often affects all of the types of marrow cells to some degree. The liver is infiltrated with a collection of mature and immature cells of the granulocytic series (top). Two megakaryocytes are also visible, reflecting the multipotency of the stem cells. ×250. (Courtesy of K. Ireland.)

Fig. 9.31. *Carcinoma,* metastatic to bone marrow. The tumor cells are undifferentiated and not easily distinguished from marrow cells. There is no active bone marrow in the field. The undifferentiated tumor is quite cellular and it has caused the formation of new uncalcified (U) and heavily calcified (C) bone. This finding was an aid to understanding the patient's anemia. ×125.

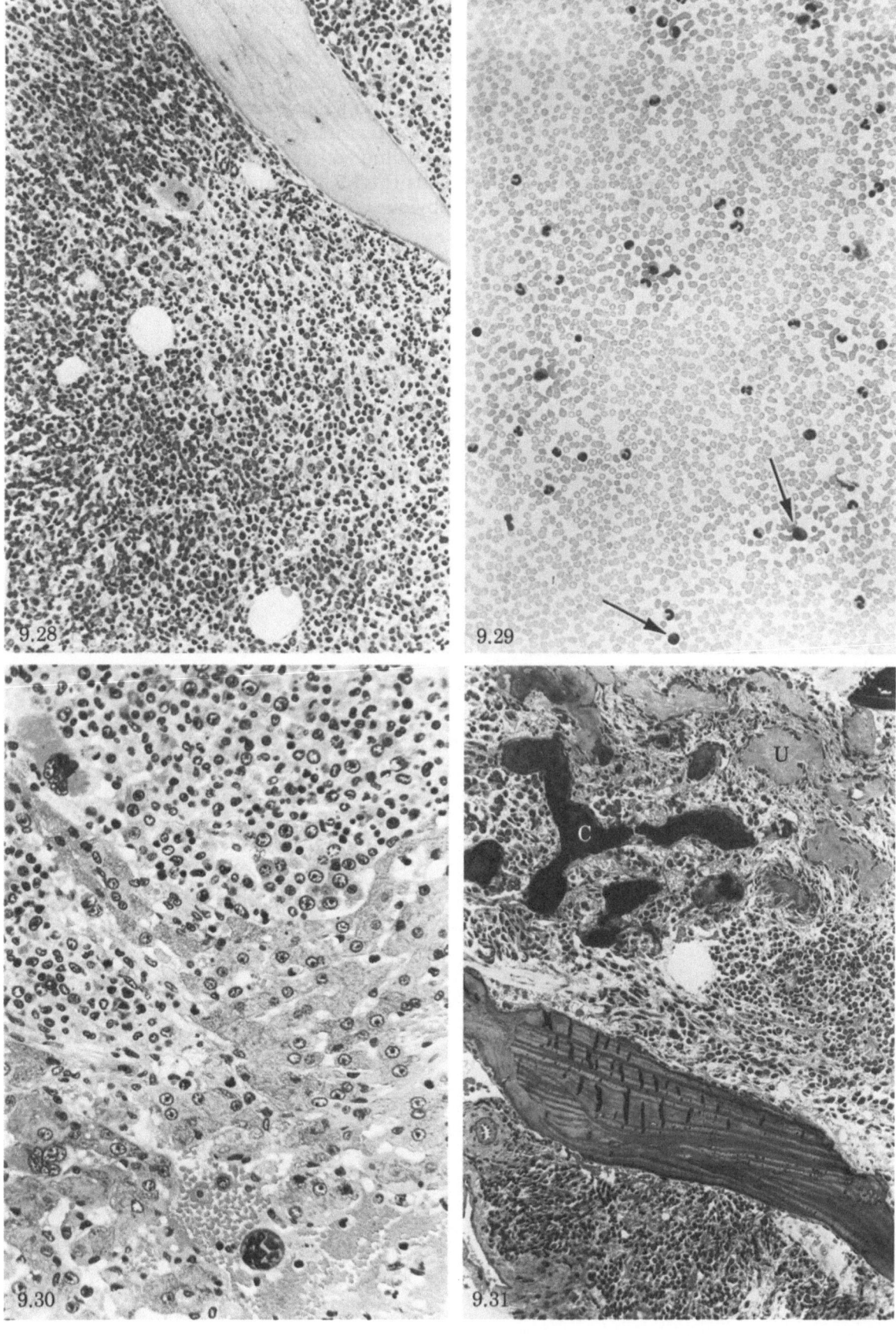

row is anatomically distributed rather generally in the axial skeleton—more like a tissue than an organ—and it feeds its products directly into the circulation. Therefore neoplasms of marrow (Fig. 9.28) are likely to be reflected in peripheral blood (Fig. 9.29), and to involve diffusely any or all tissues of the body (Fig. 9.30). As in other malignancies, the trouble they cause is by crowding out or overcoming some other cells. In leukemia erythrocytes and platelets tend to be affected. Anemia and thrombocytopenia are the results.

In other instances tumors originating in other organs may spread to the bone marrow and cause its malfunction, again because of crowding with metabolic inhibition of marrow cells (Fig. 9.31). Anemia is usually the most obvious consequence.

10 Lymphoid System

Introduction

The lymphoid system is an interrelated series of organs that protect the body from invasion by foreign substances. Its functions are integrated by humoral and cellular messages carried by blood and lymph. The structural complexity of the components of this system ranges from the relatively simple diffuse tissues in the lamina propria of the digestive tract to the complex parenchyma of the spleen. The common denominator is the lymphoid tissue, a morphologically homogenous but functionally heterogenous population of lymphocytes, associated with a delicate three-dimensional reticulum of cells or of cells and fibers (Fig. 10.1).

Lymphoid Tissue

The appropriateness of the location and structure of lymphoid tissue is understood when one is aware that it is specialized entirely for defense of the body against foreign bodies or substances. It is present: (1) as tonsils and diffuse lymphoid aggregates in mucous membranes of digestive and respiratory tracts, where materials from outside the body are processed and absorbed; (2) in lymph nodes, which by way of lymphatic vessels continuously sample and filter interstitial fluids from most tissues and organs; and (3) in large depots (spleen and thymus), which have special defense functions. Lymphocytes and macrophages respond to antigenic or other humoral signals from foreign materials, and have rapid access to nearly all tissues and organs via blood and lymphatic channels.

Strictly speaking, the cellular elements of the lymphoid system are lymphocytes, the plasma cells to which they give rise, and macrophages (Fig. 10.2). However, in carrying out the functions of this system, other cells are included, such as granulocytes and perhaps mast cells and others. This larger group of functionally related cells might more accurately be referred to as the immune system. Its functions are: (1) monitoring circulating body fluids; (2) recognition of abnormal cells such as cancer; and (3) identification of chemical messages coming from foreign invaders or damaged cells. The immune system then responds by producing an appropriate reaction involving: (1) antibody synthesis and secretion for systemic distribution; (2) assistance to other cells; and (3) the local release of agents to destroy invaders.

Structure of Lymphoid Tissue

Lymphoid tissue consists of a delicate stroma of reticular fibers and fixed cells, and a large population of more or less transient free cells.

The STROMA is a three-dimensional framework of reticular fibers supporting numerous *reticular cells*. The porosity of the stroma varies in different lymphoid organs and in different parts of the same organ depending on the relative density of the total cell population. The more dense this population the more open is the fiber framework.

The reticular cell population is a heterogeneous one. Presumably many of these cells are fibroblasts which form and maintain the reticular fibers. However, under certain conditions, some reticular cells are avidly phagocytic (fixed macrophages). Other reticular cells accumulate antigens that they process for reaction with antibodies. Those that accumulate antigens or carry out phagocytosis probably have an origin different from that of the fibroblasts. Like macrophages in other tissues, they are derived from monocytes of the blood and have originated in bone marrow.

FREE CELLS (Fig. 10.2). The population of free cells in lymphoid tissue consists of macrophages, lymphocytes, and plasma cells. One may also see other blood cells such as polymorphonuclear leukocytes of any type, but neutrophils are most common, followed by eosinophils. These appear readily in response to various stimuli.

Macrophages. Most of the macrophages are probably of bone marrow origin. These have been described in Chapter 4.

Lymphocytes are of two basic types established by colonization either from the thymus (T lymphocytes) or from bone marrow (B lymphocytes) (Fig. 10.3). The lymphocytes cannot easily be differentiated from each other on the basis of morphology. Some surface features visible by scanning electron microscopy differ. The principal distinguishing characteristics are immunologic.

Fig. 10.1. *Structure of lymphoid tissue.* This has reticulum in both the cords (C) and the sinuses (S). Reticulum stain. ×560.

Fig. 10.2. *Cells of lymphoid tissue* include lymphocytes (L), plasma cells (P), macrophages (M) and, in vessels, erythrocytes (E). ×560.

Fig. 10.3. *Origin and distribution of lymphocytes.* The yolk sac of the embryo is the origin of lymphocyte precursors which settle permanently in bone marrow and thymus. There are other fetal, mostly temporary, colonization sites. By the time the yolk sac is lost at birth the colonies are well established and serve as continuing sources of lymphocytes throughout life. Bone marrow continues to provide cells for gut (including tonsils), lymph nodes, spleen and thymus but also contributes B lymphocytes to the circulating blood. Thymus contributes T lymphocytes to gut, lymph nodes, spleen and circulating blood. Details of B and T cell distribution within the different lymphoid organs are described in the text.

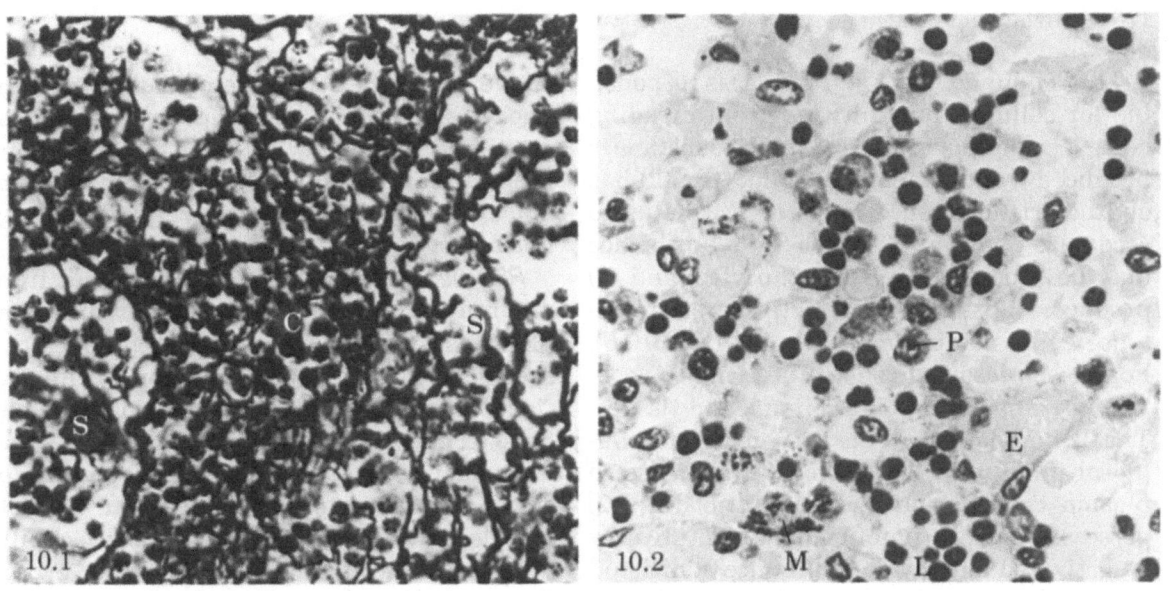

10.1

10.2

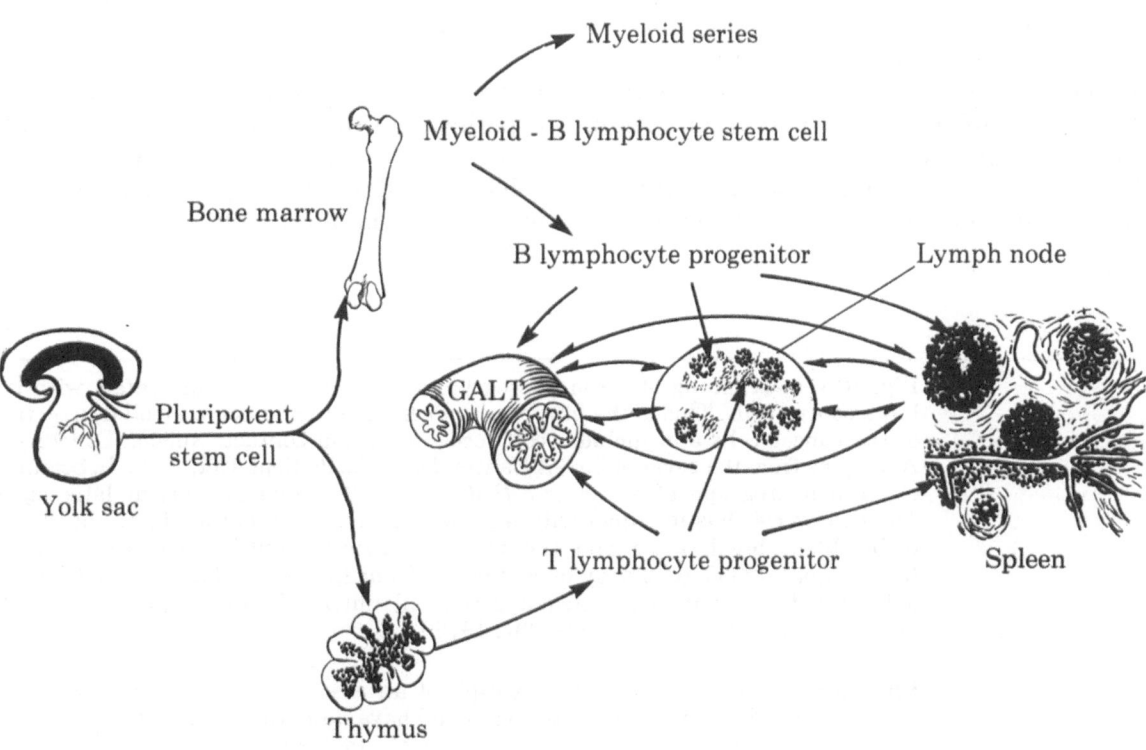

Myeloid series

Myeloid - B lymphocyte stem cell

Bone marrow

B lymphocyte progenitor

Lymph node

GALT

Pluripotent
stem cell

Yolk sac

T lymphocyte progenitor

Spleen

Thymus

10.3

The T lymphocyte (Fig. 10.4): (1) is responsible for cellular immunity, wherein invading cells are destroyed by cytotoxic substances produced by activated T lymphocytes; (2) has characteristic surface antigens; (3) helps to recognize some antigens so that antibodies may be produced by B lymphocytes; and (4) produces substances that activate other defense cells, notably macrophages (Fig. 10.5). For these reasons it constitutes a major problem in transplantation of organs and tissues. The B lymphocyte: (1) is responsible for humoral immunity. B lymphocytes give rise to plasma cells, which produce antibodies; (2) possesses surface immunoglobulins; (3) may be activated and divide to produce additional B lymphocytes and plasma cells (or their precursors, the plasmablasts).

Most of the lymphocytes usually found in blood and lymphoid tissue are small cells, 5–8 μm in diameter, with darkly staining, round or slightly indented nuclei. The cytoplasm is reduced to a thin basophilic rim. This is the form most commonly seen in blood. Larger lymphocytes may be found, particularly in lymphoid tissues and organs stimulated by the presence of foreign antigens. These larger cells represent stages in the production of immunologically and mitotically active cells. The structure of individual lymphocytes and their cellular derivatives is best examined in smears. In fixed tissue sections the nuclear chromatin pattern, cytoplasm, and cytoplasmic granules of lymphocytes may not be easily seen.

Plasma cells (plasmacytes) originate from differentiation of antigen-stimulated B lymphocytes and are specialized to produce the specific antibodies responsible for B cell function. They are variable in size and shape but have a characteristic overall appearance. The nucleus is eccentric, with large chunks of chromatin arranged in a clock-face or cartwheel pattern. The cytoplasm is basophilic (due to the large quantities of RER), except for a pale zone near one side of the nucleus occupied by the Golgi apparatus. Antibodies have been identified in the cisterns of the endoplasmic reticulum. Thus the plasma cell is a highly differentiated antibody-forming end cell and probably does not live longer than a few weeks.

Others. Lymphoid tissues, being exposed to a diversity of stimuli, and also serving as a pathway of movement of materials, naturally will contain a changing variety of other cells, particularly neutrophils, and, less often, eosinophils and mast cells.

Fig. 10.4. a: Scanning electron micrograph of a *T lymphocyte* in contact with two large cancer cells. This is the first phase of cell-mediated cytolysis (cell destruction) of the cancer cells and includes cell recognition and contact. ×6500. (Courtesy of A. Liepins from the cover of Ca—A Cancer J Clin. 30 (5) Sept–Oct, 1980.) **b:** Scanning electron micrograph of a *cancer cell* (C) and a *T lymphocyte* (T) at later stage. The cancer cell has few microvilli and has developed numerous large membrane blebs. Blebs break loose and the process continues until the cancer cell has fragmented. ×9300. (Courtesy of A. Liepins from Liepins A, Faanes RB, Choi YS, deHarven E. T-Lymphocyte mediated lysis of tumor cells in the presence of alloantiserum. Cell Immunol 36:331–334, 1978.)

Fig. 10.5. Scanning electron micrograph of an association of *lymphocytes and a macrophage.* The lymphocytes are round and have numerous microvilli. The macrophage is flat and spread out. It has large surface folds in some areas and is smooth in others. ×3900. (Courtesy of E. Unanue.)

Fig. 10.6. *Diffuse and nodular lymphoid tissue* in the wall of the intestine. Epithelium is at upper right. ×85.

Fig. 10.7. *Germinal center* (top) in a lymphoid nodule shows cellular enlargement, granular nuclei and nuclear fragmentation. These are indicators of cellular activity in response to infection. ×250.

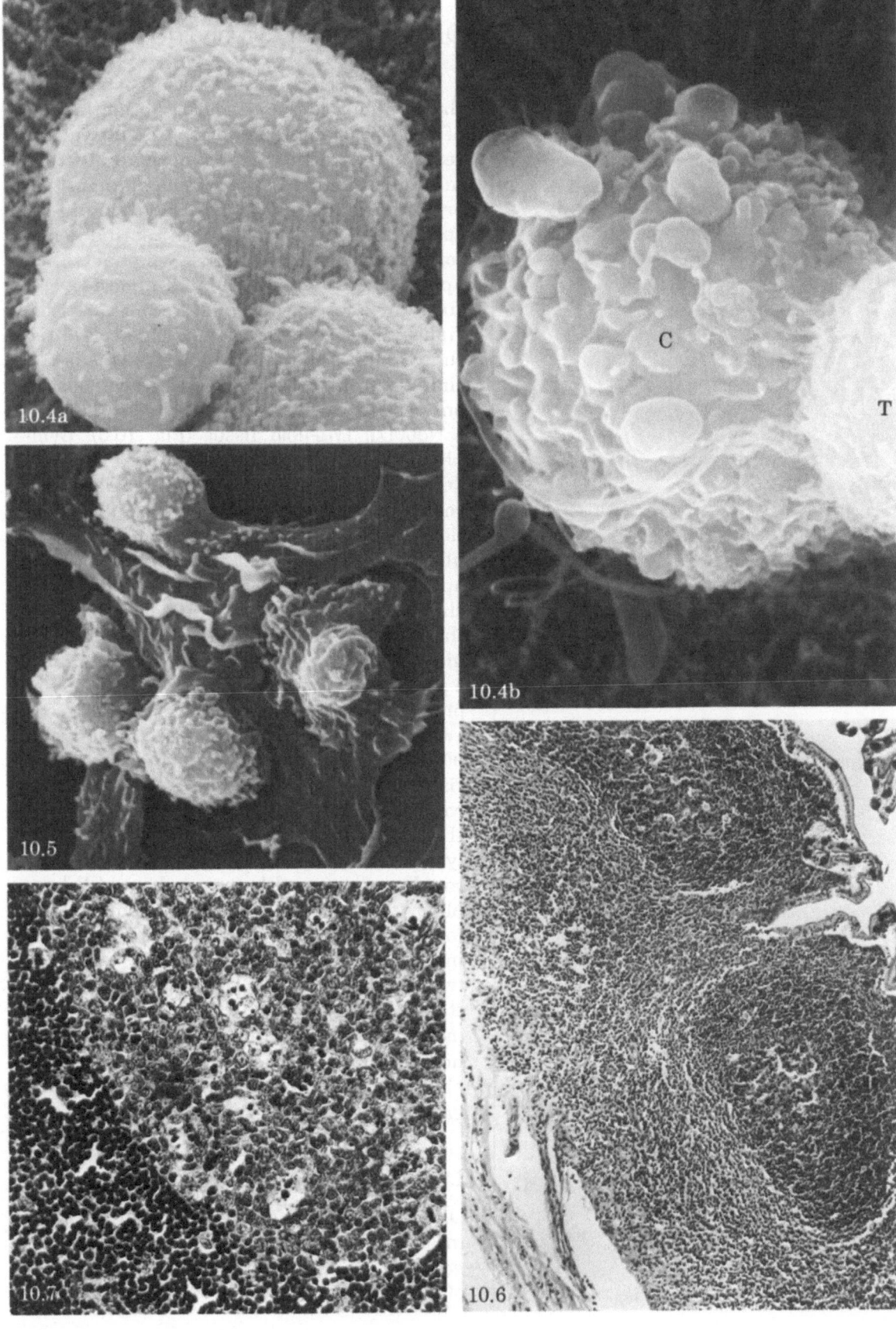

10.4a

10.4b

C

T

10.5

10.7

10.6

Organization of Lymphoid Tissue

DIFFUSE LYMPHOID TISSUE (Fig. 10.6) occurs in the lamina propria beneath the epithelium of mucous membranes of the digestive and respiratory tracts. It is also normally present in small amounts in the stroma of almost every organ and it may further develop in response to defense needs. With routine hematoxylin-eosin staining, diffuse lymphoid tissue appears as an area populated almost exclusively by lymphocytes, and grading at its periphery into the surrounding connective tissue without a discrete boundary. This is the simplest form of lymphoid tissue and consists only of lymphoid stroma and free cells.

NODULAR LYMPHOID TISSUE (Fig. 10.6). Lymphoid nodules are approximately spherical, dense aggregates of lymphocytes, usually surrounded by diffuse lymphoid tissue. The reticular stroma is very sparse in nodules. Nodules are not permanent structures; they may appear or disappear and undergo dramatic changes in response to immunologic needs of the organism. In histologic sections many nodules show a more lightly staining center with a peripheral ring of densely packed small lymphocytes. These lightly stained central areas are termed *germinal centers* (reaction centers) (Fig. 10.7). Germinal centers contain medium-sized and large lymphocytes, numerous macrophages, and occasional plasma cells, and show much mitotic activity. They develop in lymphoid nodules in response to a need for rapid production of large numbers of B lymphocytes. As such they are prominent in tonsils and in lymph nodes draining sites of infection. Germinal centers are areas of transformation of B lymphocytes to blast stages, which in turn divide and differentiate into antibody-producing cells. Thus lymphoid nodules are essentially aggregates of B lymphocytes; germinal centers are primarily aggregates of B lymphocyte precursors.

Lymphoid Organs

Organs of the lymphoid system are divided into two categories: (1) *primary lymphoid organs,* which are responsible for the initiation of differentiation of the T and B lymphocytes from lymphocytic precursors; and (2) *secondary lymphoid organs,* which are seeded with appropriate cell types from the primary lymphoid organs, and which continue to produce these cells. In fact, the secondary lymphoid organs are the principal source of continuing cell production and function in the adult.

Primary Lymphoid Organs

Primary lymphoid organs are characterized by a reticulum composed only of cells. There are no reticular fibers and the cells are of epithelial rather than mesenchymal origin. Apparently the differentiation of T and B lymphocytes is initiated by the action of these epithelial reticular cells. It is worth noting that these organs do *not* contain lymph nodules.

THE THYMUS (Figs. 10.8 through 10.11) is the primary or original source of T lymphocytes (the cells that provide for cellular immunity). If the fetal thymus is absent, T lymphocytes will not develop. The individual will not have *cellular immunity.* However, removal of the thymus from a newborn infant, as is sometimes desirable simply because it is in the way of thoracic surgical procedures (Fig. 10.8), usually carries no such risk, because the secondary lymphoid organs by this time have received their basic population of T lymphocytes. The secondary organs are then capable of producing T lymphocytes. However, the thymus (at least in laboratory animals) does produce a substance called thymosin, which has been shown to stimulate the differentiation of T lymphocytes.

Stroma. The thymus has a connective tissue capsule and incomplete partitions, the trabeculae (Fig. 10.9). Its bilateral origin is reflected in its right and left lobes, which are closely joined in the midline by connective tissue. Each lobe is partially subdivided into 15–20 lobules and these are further subdivided by finer trabeculae. Connective tissue elements are limited to the capsule and trabeculae; thus there are no reticular fibers within the structure as there are in other parenchymatous organs. The reticulum is composed entirely of *epithelial reticular cells* (Fig.

10.12) that have migrated here from the branchial pouches of the embryo.

PARENCHYMA. Sections of thymus show that each lobule has a darkly staining cortex of densely packed lymphocytes, and a more lightly stained medulla with fewer lymphocytes (Figs. 10.9 and 10.10).

Cortex. This zone, particularly in the newborn, carries a dense population of lymphocytes actively proliferating under the stimulation, not of antigens as in most lymphoid organs, but of the epithelial reticular cells. This active growth is necessary to provide the immense numbers of cells required to populate the other developing lymphoid organs with immunocompetent T cells. As yet unsatisfactorily explained is the very high frequency of cell death and phagocytosis in the cortex during the proliferation phase.

The principal blood supply to the thymic cortex is from arteries along the corticomedullary junction. Only capillaries extend from here into the cortex, and these do not permit passage through their walls of cells, antigens, or other macromolecules. Part of this *blood–thymus barrier* is probably provided by a pericapillary coat of epithelial reticular cells as well as by the structure of the capillary wall itself. These capillaries drain to postcapillary venules (Fig. 10.13) in the thymic medulla, where exchange of cells and macromolecules can occur. These vessels have an endothelium whose cells are more cuboidal than those of other normal blood vessels. Lymphocytes destined to leave the cortex by penetrating the lining of the postcapillary venule migrate to the medulla to do so.

Medulla. The lightly staining appearance of the medulla is due to the presence of fewer lymphocytes, with their densely staining nuclei and sparse cytoplasm, and of more reticular cells and macrophages with pale cytoplasm and euchromatic nuclei. Characteristic of the medulla are the scattered *thymic (Hassall's) corpuscles* (Fig. 10.12). Each corpuscle is a cluster of concentrically arranged, epithelial reticular cells bearing a striking resemblance to epithelial pearls characteristic of squamous (i.e., stratified squamous) carcinoma. The appearance of both the Hassall's corpuscles and the carcinoma probably repre-

180   Lymphoid System

sents the process of local differentiation of an epithelium deprived of a free surface.

INVOLUTION.   After establishment of populations of immunocompetent cells in other organs of the lymphoid system throughout the body, the thymus becomes insignificant immunologically except in emergencies when severe damage to other lymphoid organs requires their repopulation with T cells. Soon after birth the thymus begins to involute (Fig. 10.10). Apparently under the influence of adrenal and gonadal steroids the process continues and, over a course of several years, most of the organ is gradually replaced by fat (Fig. 10.11). For uncertain reasons involution is more rapid in many disease states. During the process of involution thymic corpuscles enlarge before eventually disappearing.

BURSA-EQUIVALENT.   In birds a cloacal mass of lymphoid tissue termed the bursa of Fabricius is the primary and original source of B lymphocytes. In mammals there is no single site of differentiation of B lymphocytes, and the B cells are said to originate from a "bursa equivalent." It may be that the induction of "B-ness" in mammals is initiated by prenatal association of B lymphocyte precursor cells with an epithelium at an unknown site. These new progenitor cells are then seeded elsewhere (for example, in bone marrow, gut, and lymph nodes), where their progeny in the adult continue to become B lymphocytes.

Fig. 10.8. *Normal thymus* (arrows) of a 7-month-old child. Heart (H), lungs (L). Figs. 10.9, 10.10, and 10.11 are all from normal thymus glands at the same magnification (×26) but at different ages.

Fig. 10.9. *Newborn.* Cortex (C), medulla (M).

Fig. 10.10. *Adolescent.* Thymic corpuscles are now prominent in the medulla. The cortex has atrophied somewhat.

Fig. 10.11. *Adult.* Only small amounts of lymphoid tissue with thymic corpuscles (arrow) remain.

Fig. 10.12. *Thymic corpuscles* and *epithelial reticular cells* (arrows). ×250.

Fig. 10.13. *Postcapillary venule* with large, rounded endothelial cells. Reticulum stain. ×560.

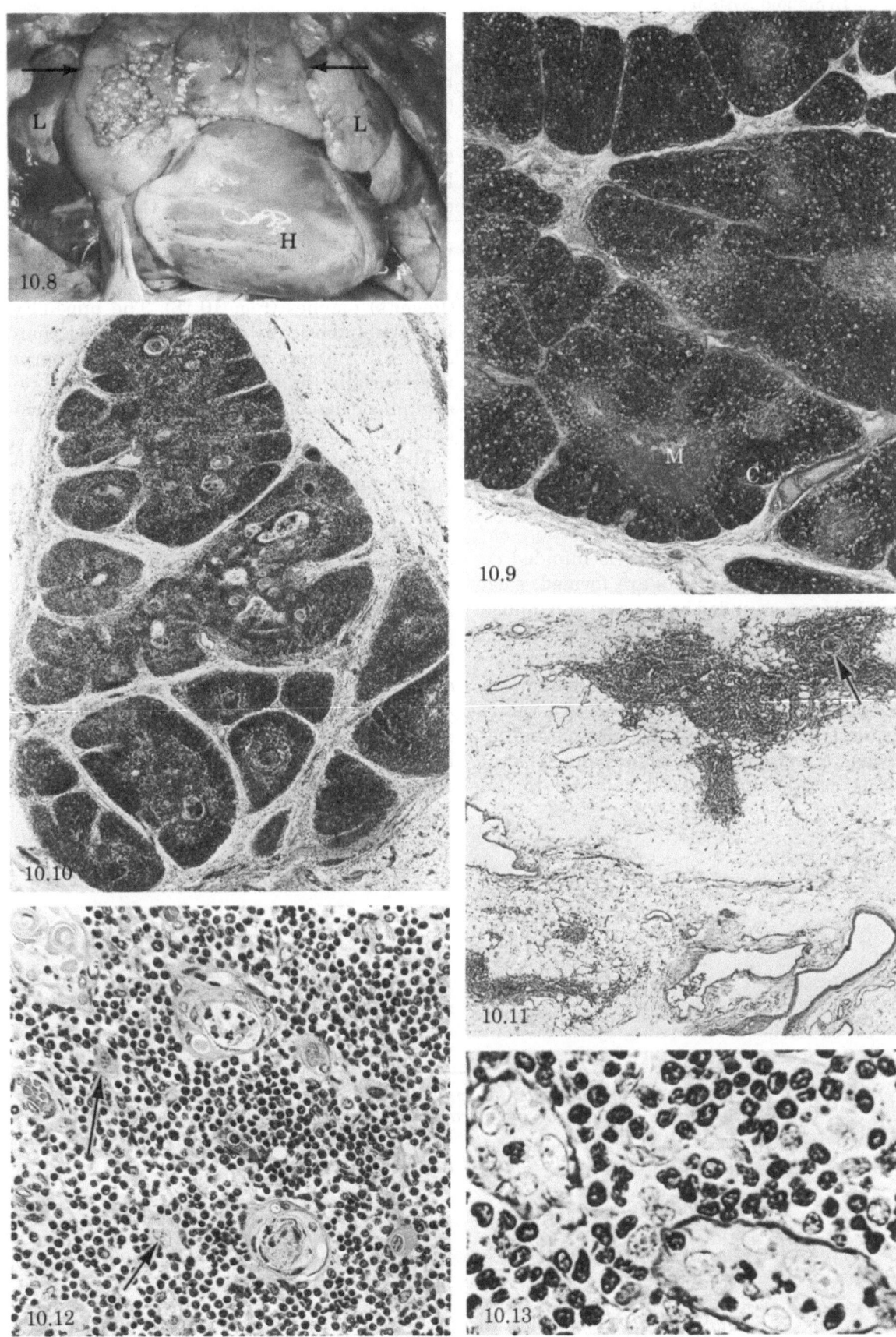

10.8

10.9

10.10

10.11

10.12

10.13

Secondary Lymphoid Organs

These include *tonsils* and other *gut-associated lymphoid tissues* (GALT), *lymph nodes,* and *spleen.* Although their development begins during fetal life, it is not completed until around the time of birth, when these organs are populated by mass immigration of lymphocytes. The B lymphocytes form the characteristic nodules and the T lymphocytes form parts of the uniform diffuse lymphoid tissue of these organs.

TONSILS AND GALT. Five tonsils (Figs. 10.14 through 10.16) are arranged so as to form a ring (Waldeyer's ring) around the origin of the pharynx from the oral and nasal cavities. There are paired palatine (Figs. 10.14 and 10.15) and lingual (Fig. 10.16) tonsils and a single median pharyngeal tonsil in the roof of the pharynx (called adenoids when enlarged). The tonsillar mucosa is infolded so that deep epithelial crypts are formed, each crypt being surrounded by nodules and diffuse lymphoid tissue in the lamina propria. The nodules commonly have large germinal centers. The parenchyma is supported by a mesh of reticular fibers. A thin connective tissue capsule is present with trabeculae extending between the crypts. Some glands and skeletal muscle commonly are seen external to the capsule in histologic sections. Lymphocytes may be seen within the tonsillar epithelium (Fig. 10.17). When tonsils are infected (Fig. 10.15), the inflammatory process often extensively erodes this epithelial layer, making it less recognizable, and increases the amount of lymphoid tissue, enlarging the tonsils.

Similar aggregates of diffuse and nodular lymphoid tissue also occur in the submucosa of the ileum. These are termed ileal lymphoid (Peyer's) patches (Fig. 10.18). The appendix is probably basically a lymphoid rather than a digestive organ. Here, the lamina propria is essentially replaced by lymphoid tissue resembling that of tonsils and ileal lymphoid patches.

The lamina propria of the entire digestive and respiratory tracts may be considered a portion of the lymphoid system. It contains large numbers of lymphocytes, frequently as nodules, all associated with a reticular stroma. This tissue together with tonsils, ileal lymphoid patches, and appendix is often referred to as the gut-associated lymphoid tissue (GALT). It has been suggested that all or part of the GALT may be the bursa equivalent of at least some mammals. However, this part of the lymphoid system develops only after birth. Its proliferation appears to be antigen-controlled, and it contains both T and B zones.

Fig. 10.14. *Normal child's faucial tonsil.* Stratified squamous epithelium covers the surface and lines crypts (arrows) that divide the lymphoid tissue. ×7.5.

Fig. 10.15. *Chronically inflamed faucial tonsil* with enlargement. ×7.7.

Fig. 10.16. *Lingual tonsil.* ×26.

Fig. 10.17. *A tonsillar crypt* shows distortion and loss of its epithelium in chronic tonsillitis. ×250.

Fig. 10.18. *Ileal lymphoid patch* (arrows) (low magnification of the same specimen as in Fig. 10.6). ×19.

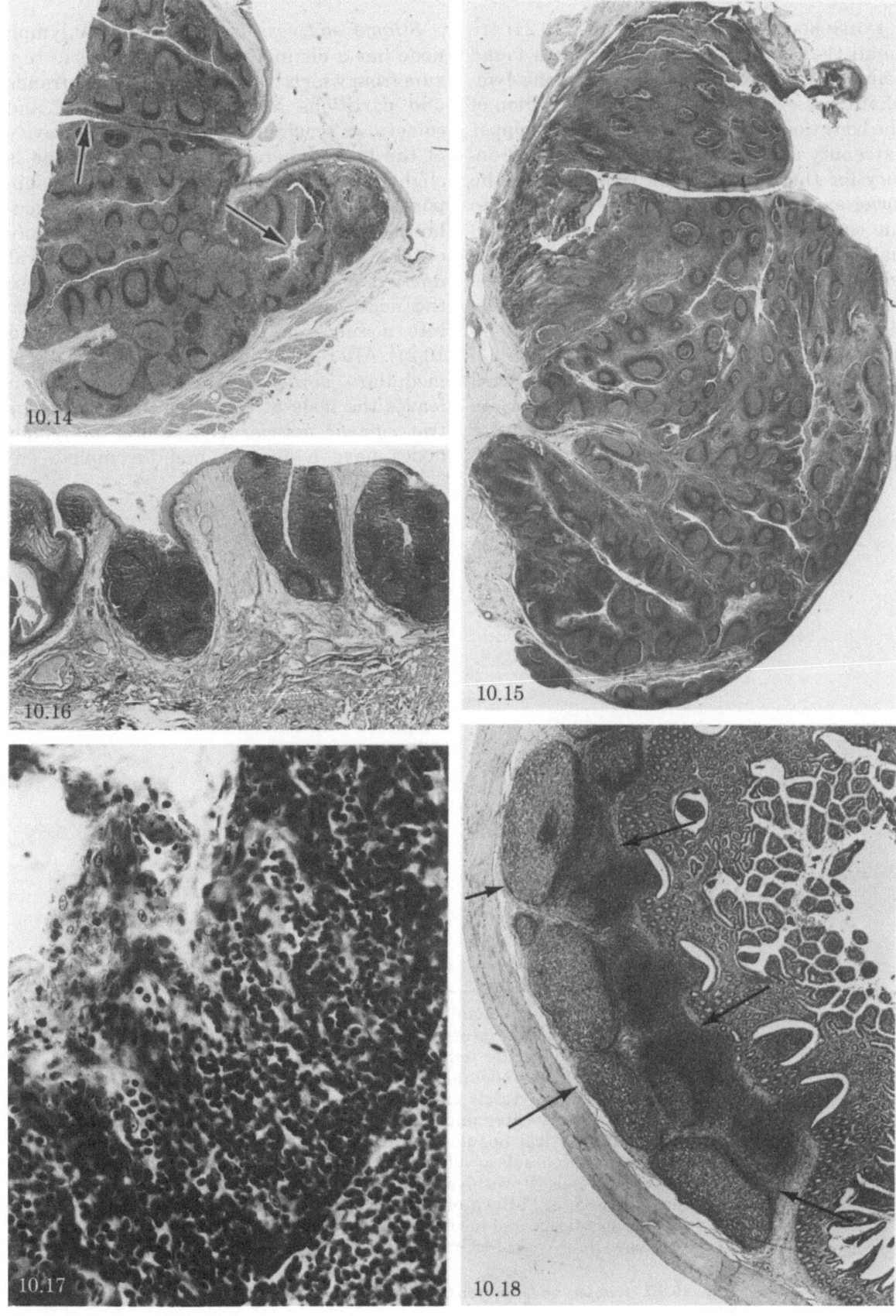

10.14

10.15

10.16

10.17

10.18

LYMPH NODES (Figs. 10.19 through 10.24) are small (1–25 mm), bean-shaped organs found commonly in groups at intervals along lymphatic vessels draining a particular region of the body (for example, the axilla for the upper extremity and breast, the root of the mesentery for the intestine, and the groin for the lower extremity). Lymph that is returning to the cardiovascular system from the interstitial space is filtered through lymph nodes, where its content of particulate and dissolved substance is monitored. Foreign or toxic materials are: (1) recognized and phagocytosed by macrophages; (2) destroyed by T cells; or (3) neutralized by antibodies that are produced by B cells and plasma cells. The appropriate immune response is triggered by the nature of the antigenic stimulation.

Stroma and vessels (Fig. 10.19). A lymph node has a distinctive connective tissue *capsule* from which *trabeculae* extend as strands and partitions into the node toward, and sometimes reaching, the *hilus* (the concavity of the bean) where the connective tissue is slightly thickened. The parenchyma is supported by a rich framework of delicate reticular fibers and reticular cells (*see above*). Many of these stromal cells are phagocytic. Several *afferent lymph vessels* bringing lymph into the node penetrate the capsule and empty into a *subcapsular sinus* (Figs. 10.19 and 10.21). After percolating through cortical and medullary *sinuses* (Fig. 10.22) the lymph leaves the node at the hilus through one or two *efferent vessels*. The sinuses of lymph nodes have a delicate and incomplete en-

Fig. 10.19. Drawing and photomicrograph in composite illustration of the structure of a *lymph node*. Each lettered segment illustrates a feature of lymph node architecture. **A:** The large *connective tissue assemblies*, i.e., capsule and trabeculae. **B:** The fine organization of the *reticulum*. Clear areas, without fibers, show the location of nodules. Lymphatic vessels enter at the periphery and leave at the hilus. **C:** *Blood supply*. Vessels enter and leave at the hilus. Capillaries make loops and nets around the cortical nodules and drain into medullary venous channels. **D:** *Photomicrograph*. Note subcapsular and medullary sinuses (arrows), cortical nodules (N), lymphatic vessels (V) with valves, diffuse lymphoid tissue of the thymus-dependent zone (T). ×35. **e:** Pattern of *lymphocyte distribution* showing nodule, diffuse cortical lymphoid tissue and medullary cords. (Based on Fig. 14.7 in Weiss L, Greep RO: Histology. New York, McGraw Hill, 1977.)

Fig. 10.20. *Lymph node in youth.* The section does not pass through the hilus. ×26.

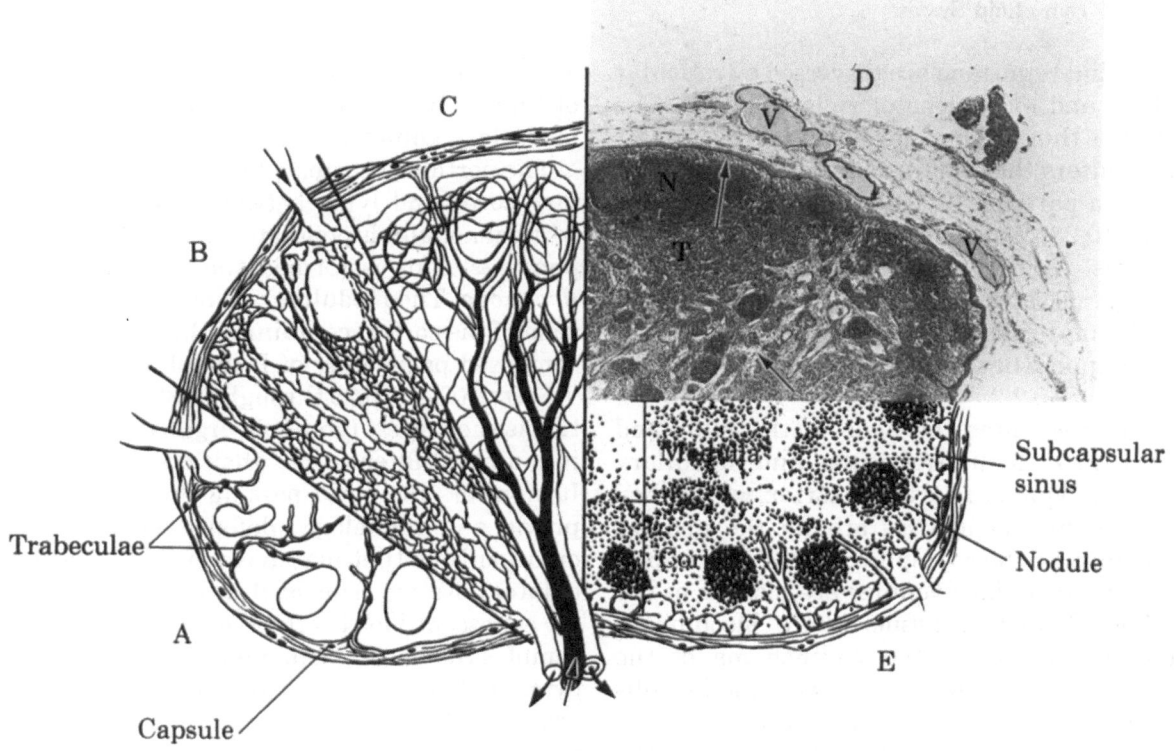

Trabeculae

Capsule

Subcapsular
sinus

Nodule

10.19

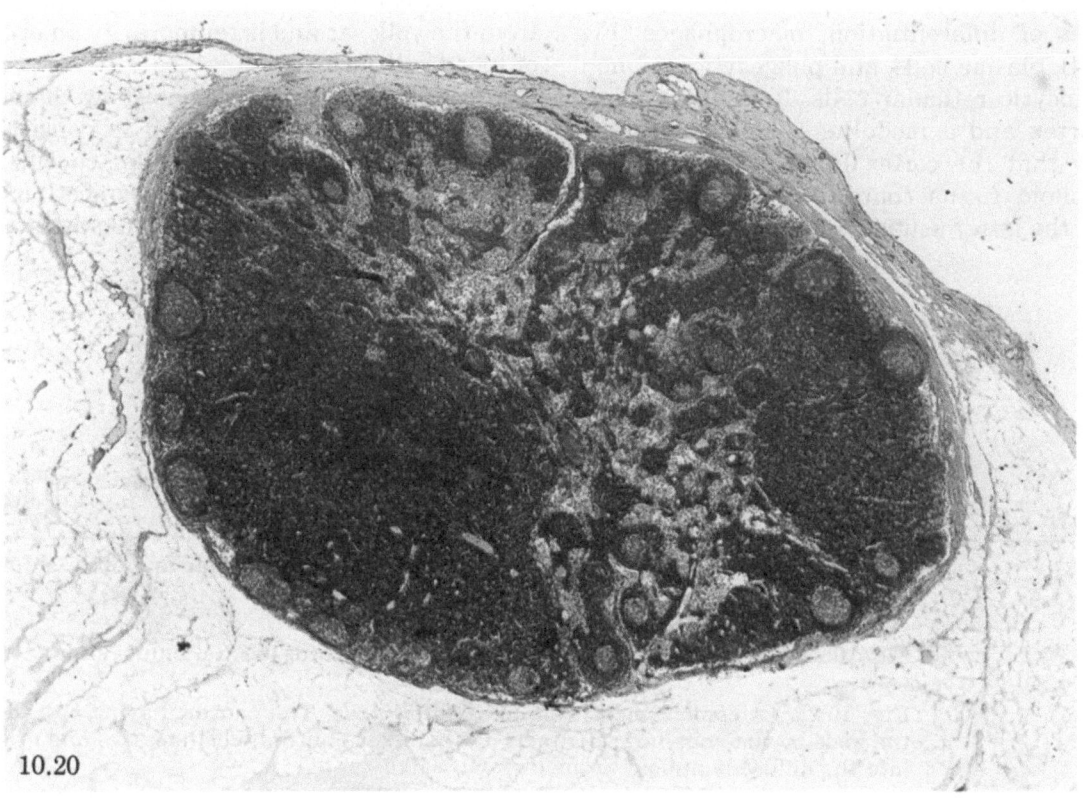

10.20

dothelial lining and are traversed by reticular fibers and extensions of reticular cells. The sinuses thus are not open channels but in fact true filters that capture large objects such as foreign particles (Fig. 10.24) and cancer cells (Fig. 10.23), which may be in passage in lymph vessels. An early indication of metastasis or spread of cancer is given by the presence of malignant cells in the lymph nodes draining the region where the primary cancer is growing (Fig. 10.23).

Arteries enter the node at the hilus and pass through the trabeculae and medullary cords of lymph tissue to the cortex, where they branch into capillaries around the nodules and in the diffuse lymphoid tissue. The important postcapillary venules are located in the diffuse lymphoid tissue where blood-borne lymphocytes enter the parenchyma of the node. As in the thymus, the endothelial cells of these vessels are cuboidal rather than simple squamous. Veins leave the node at the hilus.

Parenchyma. The lymphoid tissue of the node is a mixture of lymphocytes in various stages of differentiation, macrophages (Fig. 10.24), plasma cells, and phagocytic and non-phagocytic reticular cells. It is divided into a cortex and a medulla. Histologic sections show that the cortex has a layer of diffuse lymphoid tissue containing numerous nodules, the latter usually with germinal centers.

The medulla consists of strands and sheets of diffuse lymphoid tissue separated by the medullary sinuses.

The portion of cortex adjacent to the medullary cords and lying between them and the cortical nodules is populated mainly by T lymphocytes. This is termed the *thymus-dependent zone.* The medullary cords and the outer zone of the cortex, containing the nodules, are composed principally of B lymphocytes.

SPLEEN (Figs. 10.25 through 10.32). Although this is the largest lymphoid organ of the body, it is a blood filter rather than a lymph filter. It monitors the blood passing through it and provides immunologic defense against microorganisms that may have entered the circulatory system. This is also the "graveyard" for senescent blood cells (Fig. 10.31). It disassembles the hemoglobin molecules of erythrocytes and provides part of a mechanism for recycling the iron. Its elastic fibromuscular capsule permits considerable size change, but its function in humans as a regulator of blood volume is not as great as in other animals. In the fetus the spleen is seeded by stem cells from the yolk sac and is temporarily an organ of blood cell formation.

Stroma. Histologic sections show the capsule of the spleen (Fig. 10.25) to consist of dense connective tissue containing considerable numbers of elastic fibers and smooth muscle cells. It is of quite uniform thickness and

---

Fig. 10.21. *Reticulum stain* of a node demonstrates subcapsular and other sinuses (arrows). ×100.

Fig. 10.22. Higher magnification of *sinuses* (S) and cords (C). Reticulum stain. ×250.

Fig. 10.23. *Carcinoma metastatic to a lymph node.* The cancer, having spread to the node by the lymphatic channels (C), here has obliterated sinuses (S) and grows into the diffuse lymphoid tissue (arrow). ×100.

Fig. 10.24. *Anthracosis* (black pigment in a thoracic lymph node, see lower third of picture), a universal finding. Inspired carbon dust has been ingested by macrophages and transported by lymphatics to local nodes. ×85.

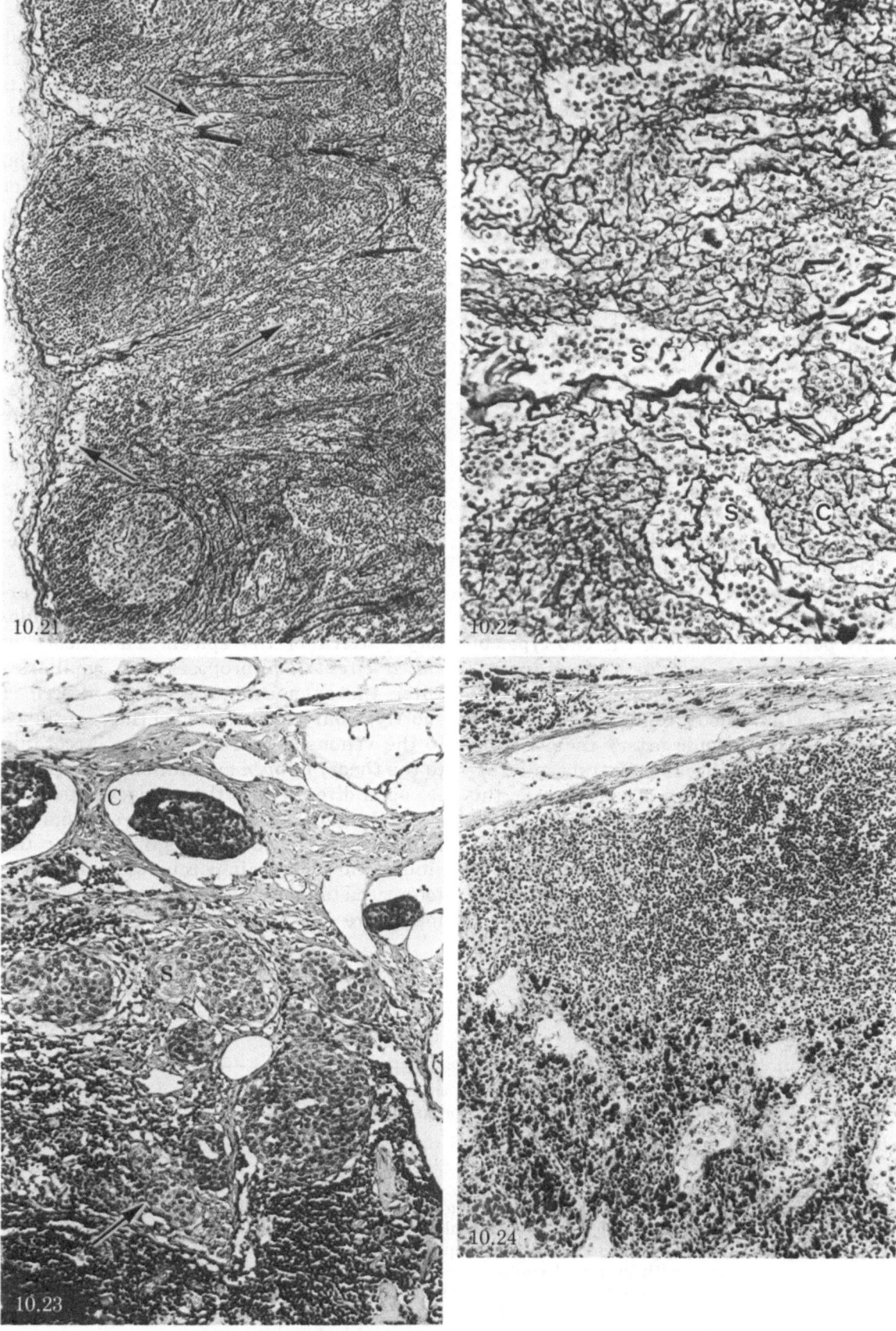

is covered on its surface by simple squamous epithelium (mesothelium). From the hilus trabeculae radiate toward the capsule to subdivide the organ partially. At the hilus arteries enter and veins and lymphatics leave. The lymphatic vessels are efferent only. They arise and run in the trabeculae; there are no lymphatic vessels in the parenchyma. Between and around the trabeculae there is an extensive spongework of reticular fibers supporting the parenchyma. The cellular components of the reticulum include a permanent resident population of phagocytic and nonphagocytic reticular cells.

Parenchyma and vessels (Figs. 10.26 through 10.30). To a greater extent than in most other organs, the blood vessels of the spleen are intimately related functionally to its parenchymal cells. Both structure and function of the organ are best understood in relation to the pattern of blood flow through it. These two components will therefore be described together.

The parenchyma of the spleen is a soft and mushy pulp. The names of the two types of *pulp, red,* and *white,* refer to the gross appearance and reflect the content of, respectively, red and white blood cells. The primary branches of the splenic artery radiate from the hilus in the trabeculae as trabecular arteries. Smaller branches of these enter the pulp as arterioles. Here they acquire a coat of lymphoid tissue (the periarteriolar lymphoid sheath, or PALS) (Figs. 10.26 and 10.27), composed largely of T lymphocytes. They are now termed *central arteries* or *white pulp arteries.* Lymphoid nodules, with and without germinal centers, and composed mainly of B lymphocytes, are scattered along the lymphoid sheath. The arteries pass tangential to these nodules or through their periphery. The term central artery refers to the position of the vessel relative to the lymphoid sheath, not the lymph nodule.

After branching several times, the central arteries lose their coating of lymphoid cells and divide into a tight cluster of branches, the so-called penicillar arteries, which are short and straight. They are very small and the endothelium has a thick basal lamina. Near the terminations of these vessels some of them have localized thick coats of macrophages. Here the basal lamina is thin and often incomplete or absent. This specialized region is termed the ellipsoid. Beyond the ellipsoid the vessels are capillaries or, sometimes, small arterioles.

There is some controversy about the arrangement from this point on in the circulatory pattern of the spleen. The theory of *closed circulation* proposes that capillaries enter the splenic sinuses, to be described shortly, from which the blood then continues to the venous side of the system. According to the theory of *open circulation* the capillaries open directly into the spongework of the red pulp and deposit blood there. From the red pulp the blood is thought to enter the sinuses through their porous walls and then to proceed to the veins. Possibly both arrangements are present.

Fig. 10.25. *Spleen.* Capsule (C), trabeculae (T), red pulp (R), and arteriole (arrow) with PALS, adjoining nodule and germinal center. ×36.

Fig. 10.26. *Red pulp,* arterioles and *PALS.* ×100.

Fig. 10.27. Diagram of the *circulation* and the principal *architectural features* of the *spleen.* Capsule (C), trabeculae (T), artery (A), vein (V). (1) trabecular artery; (2) artery leaves trabecula, acquires coat of lymphoid cells (PALS); (3) nodules, some with germinal centers, in PALS; (4) penicillar arteries; (5) arteriole opens into red pulp between sinuses, as in theory of open circulation; (6) arteriole opens into splenic sinus as in theory of closed circulation; (7) blood from sinus enters pulp vein; (8) blood from pulp veins enters trabecular vein.

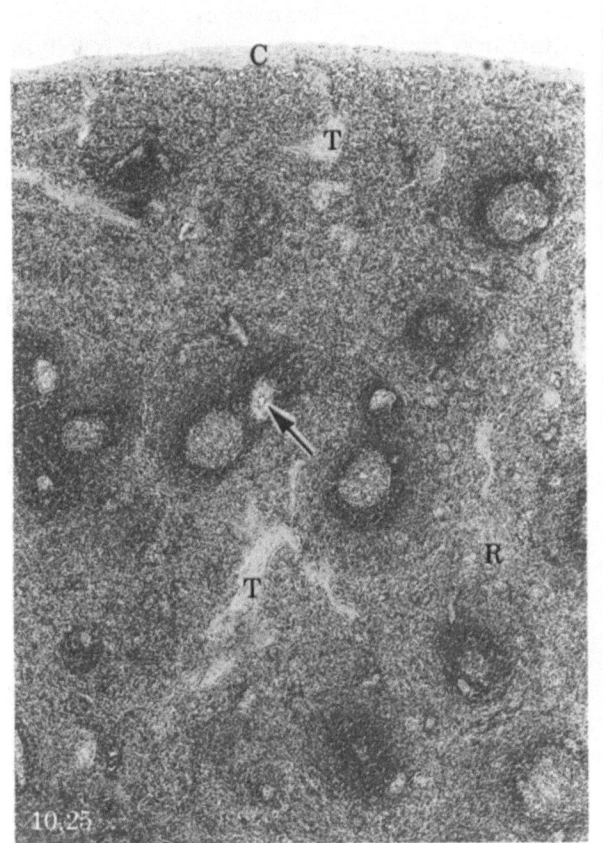

10.25

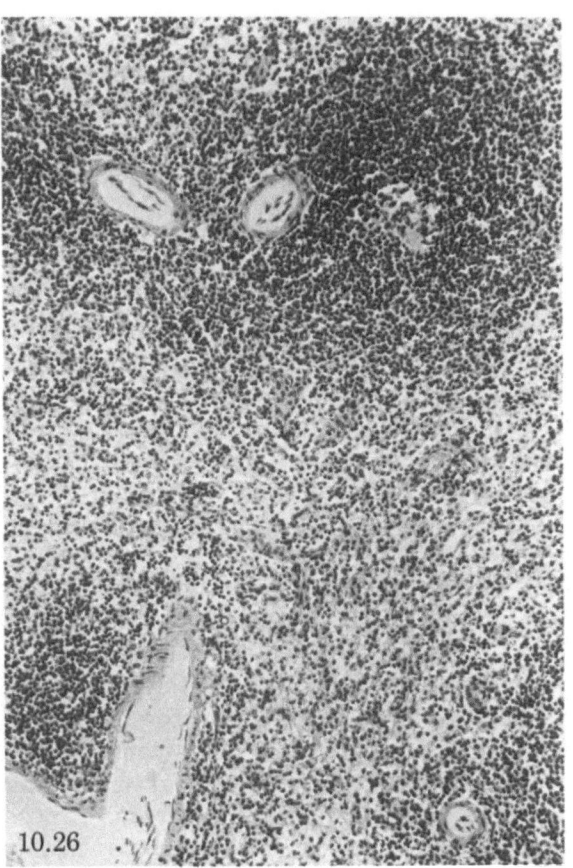

10.26

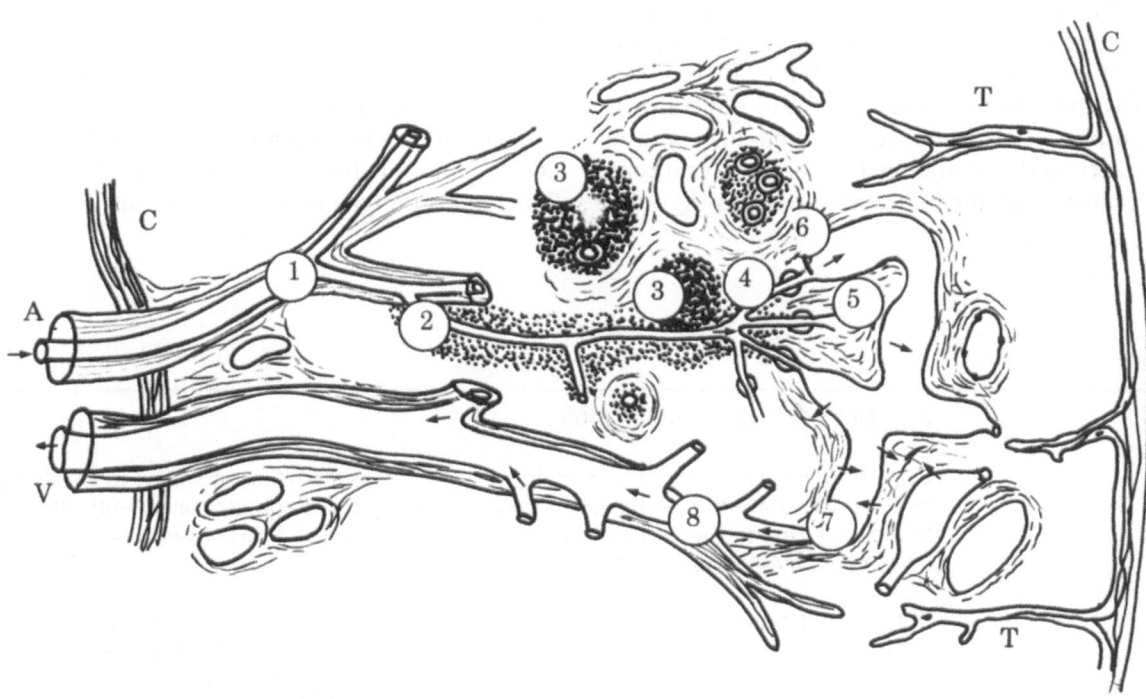

10.27

The *splenic sinuses* (Figs. 10.28 through 10.30) are irregular vascular channels in which the endothelium is in the form of long tapering cells arranged in the pattern of barrel staves with spaces between them On the outside of the sinuses are approximately circular "hoops" of reticular fibers. These hoops are interconnected by longitudinally placed reticular fibers. From the porous sinuses blood flows into the veins, which are without lymphoid sheaths and thus are surrounded directly by red pulp.

Pulp is a three-dimensional meshwork of reticular fibers and cellular stroma with red blood cells, lymphoid cells, and granulocytes. The pulp veins leave the red pulp and become trabecular veins, which are essentially channels in the trabecular connective tissue. They are without highly structured walls of their own. From here blood leaves the spleen in the splenic vein at the hilus. The areas of red pulp (Fig. 10.27) between the splenic sinuses are termed splenic cords (cords of Billroth). The term cord is somewhat misleading because, in a three-dimensional sense, these are actually sheets and masses of reticular stroma with the accompanying cell population. Only in a two-dimensional histologic section do some of them appear to be cords.

The *white pulp* consists of the periarterial lymphoid sheath and the scattered lymphoid nodules (Figs. 10.25 and 10.26). In the area of transition between white and red pulp the lymphocytes gradually become less numerous; thus the boundary between the two types of pulp is rather indistinct at high magnifica-tion. This area of transition is termed the marginal zone. This zone contains few lymphocytes, but many macrophages that are actively phagocytic (Fig. 10.31).

Enlargement of spleen, like that of lymph nodes, is detectable by physical examination, and connotes significant, potentially life-threatening, disease. While infectious illnesses are the most common causes of these enlargements, malignancies of the lymphoid system (lymphomas) and of circulating lymphocytes (lymphocytic leukemia) are also a major cause.

Neoplasms tend to recapitulate, but in a less than normally ordered manner, the form of the parent structure as they grow and increase its size. Malignant tumors of the lymphocyte lineage sometimes retain in a visibly striking way the distinction between diffuse and nodular structure (Fig. 10.32).

Functional considerations. Antigens brought to the spleen by the blood are trapped in the white pulp. They stimulate B lymphocytes in the nodules to proliferate and differentiate into antibody-producing plasma cells. The T lymphocytes in the periarterial sheaths proliferate in these areas and migrate to the red pulp to enter the sinuses and be carried away in the blood. Thus they become available for the needs of cell-mediated immune activities. Antigens that reach the nodules and the marginal zone appear to be bound in considerable quantities to reticular cells that have many unusually long and branched processes. These cells are termed dendritic cells. The macrophages of the spleen are particu-

Fig. 10.28. *Splenic sinuses.* ×400.

Fig. 10.29. Scanning electron micrograph of fractured surface of *spleen* of rat. Note *sinuses* with sieve-like walls and intervening red pulp of splenic cords. ×500. (Courtesy of T. Fujita in Fujita T, Tanaka K, Tokunaga J. SEM Atlas of Cells and Tissues. New York, Igaku-Shoin, 1981.)

Fig. 10.30. Scanning electron micrograph of a fractured surface of human *spleen.* Note sinuses (S) with elongated "barrel-stave" endothelial cells and intervening clefts, and so-called splenic cords (C) of red pulp between the sinuses. ×1000. (Courtesy of T. Fujita in Fujita T, Tanaka K, Tokunaga J. SEM Atlas of Cells and Tissues. New York, Igaku-Shoin, 1981.)

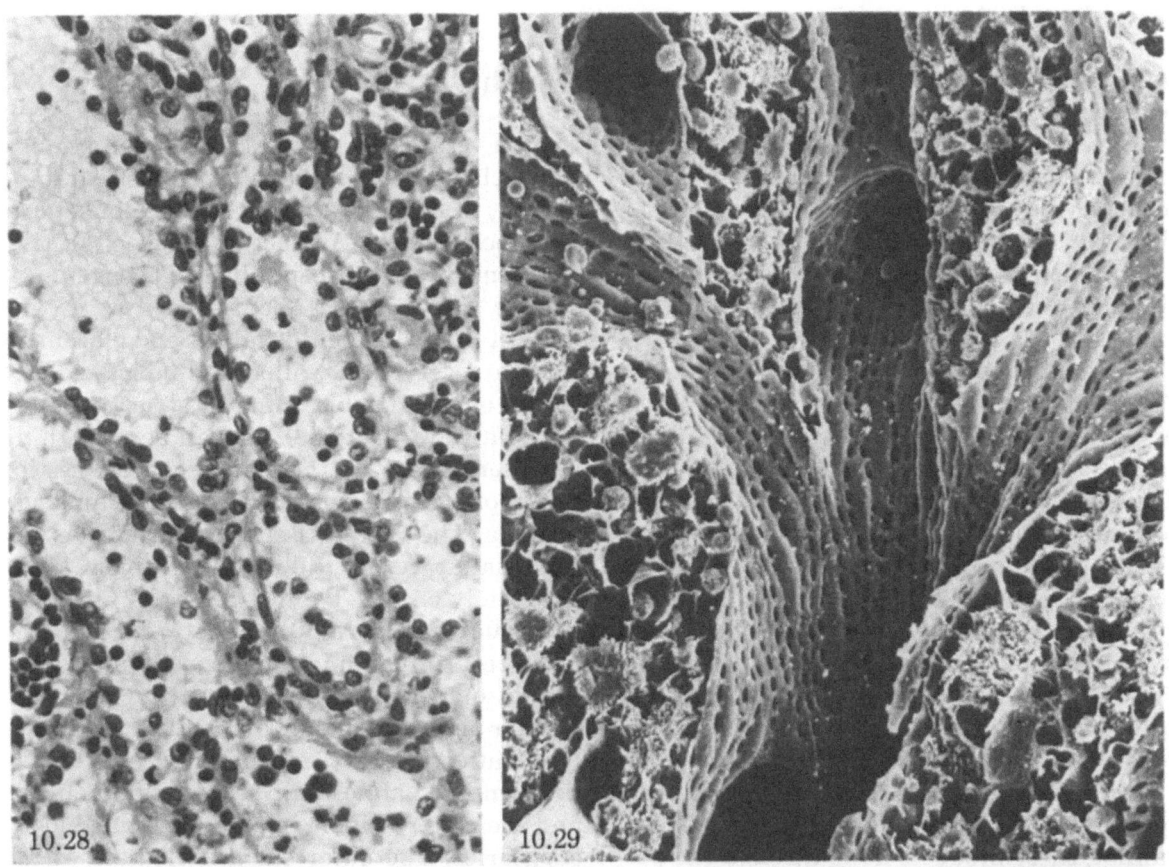

10.28

10.29

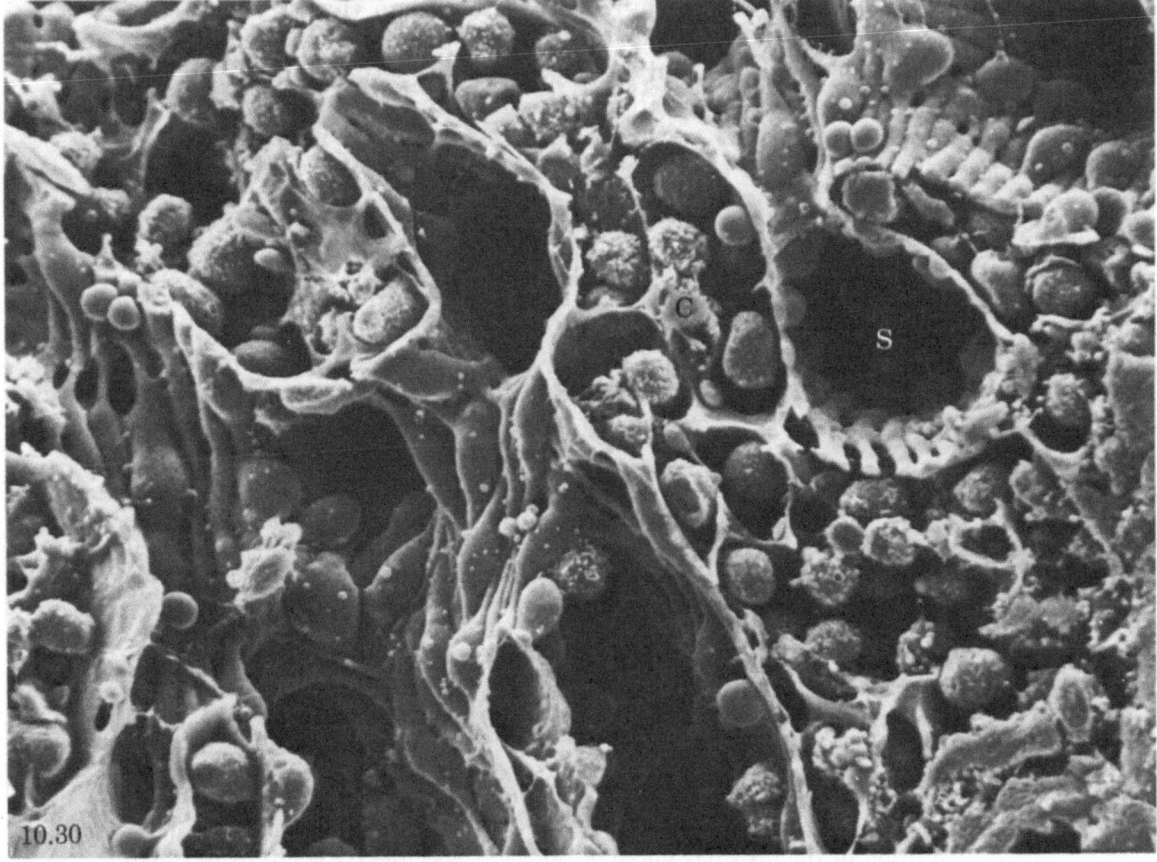

10.30

larly active in phagocytosing living foreign bodies such as viruses and bacteria. They also accumulate lipid droplets when there are unusually high levels of lipids circulating in the blood, as may be encountered in diabetes mellitus.

Lymphocytes coming from the blood into the spleen take up residence in the white pulp at least for a time.

An important function of the spleen already mentioned is the destruction of old erythrocytes (Fig. 10.31). These cells are more fragile and less flexible than the younger ones. Thus they are easily caught and broken down in the reticulum meshwork of the splenic cords. Cellular fragments are engulfed by phagocytosis and digested by the lysosome system of the macrophages. This is facilitated by the sluggish circulation in the cords. The digestive process lyses the hemoglobin and produces two important substances: (1) bilirubin, a hemoglobin derivative that does not contain iron; and (2) ferritin, which is an iron-protein compound. Blood from the spleen containing these products flows through the portal venous system to the liver where the bilirubin is further processed and excreted. The ferritin is not excreted but is passed on by the blood to the bone marrow where the iron is recycled in the production of new erythrocytes by this tissue.

The spleen is not necessary for life and its surgical removal, as for traumatic laceration, has only rather recently caused concern. Its various functions apparently can be taken over by other organs and tissues but not quite as well. The individual is more prone to infection.

Lymph Vessels

Lymph vessels (lymphatics) are endothelium-lined channels that begin as anastomosing nets or, in skin and gut mucosa, as blind ends. They occur in the connective tissue of all tissues and organs except: liver parenchyma, splenic parenchyma, bone marrow, CNS, coats of the eyeball, internal ear and placenta. They are very thin walled and delicate. The larger ones resemble veins in structure and have valves (Fig. 10.33), as well as very thin representations of the three characteristic layers of blood vessels, intima, media, and adventitia. They drain tissue fluid from the interstitial space. As they join and rejoin they ultimately become two main trunks, the thoracic duct and the right lymphatic duct. These ducts return lymph to the blood vascular system at or near the junctions of the internal jugular and subclavian veins. The smallest lymphatic vessels, the lymphatic capillaries, are composed almost entirely of endothelium and are more variable in diameter than blood capillaries. The outer surface of their walls are attached to the surrounding connective tissue by fine filaments that are perpendicular to the course of the capillary. These anchoring filaments apparently serve to keep the lumens of these somewhat flabby vessels open.

Circulation of Lymphocytes

Discussion of the circulation of lymphocytes requires a consideration of several matters already presented in this chapter. Some repetition may be helpful. Although the largest

Fig. 10.31. Three scanning electron micrographs of a *macrophage* enjoying an erythrocyte meal. About ×7600. (Courtesy of M. Bessis from Figs. XVI–5, 6, and 7 in Bessis M: Corpuscles—Atlas of Red Blood Cell Shapes. New York, Springer-Verlag, 1974.)

Fig. 10.32. *Malignant lymphoma* involving spleen. A: The tumor appears to involve only the white pulp. Nodules are irregular in outline and enlarged. ×23. B. From the area within the rectangle in A. Only immature cells are seen, but the nodule (at the bottom of the field) contains the least differentiated cells. There is one mitotic figure. ×560.

Fig. 10.33. *A lymphatic channel* with *valve*. This structure is visible in lower magnification in the previous photo of the same specimen, Fig. 10.19 E. ×100.

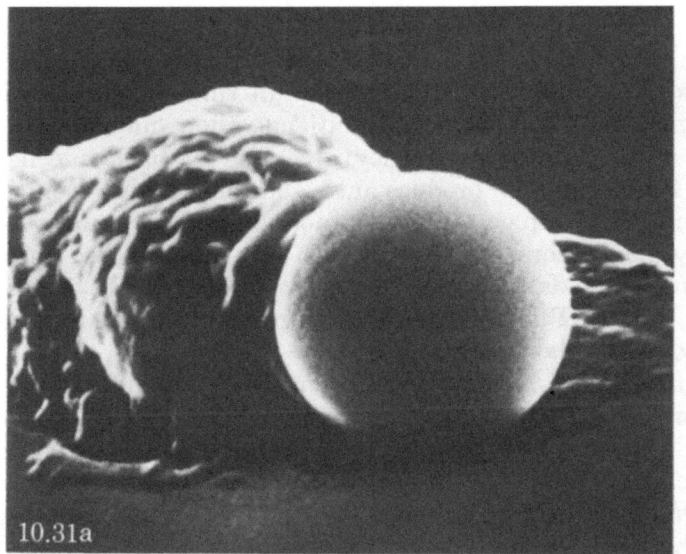

10.31a

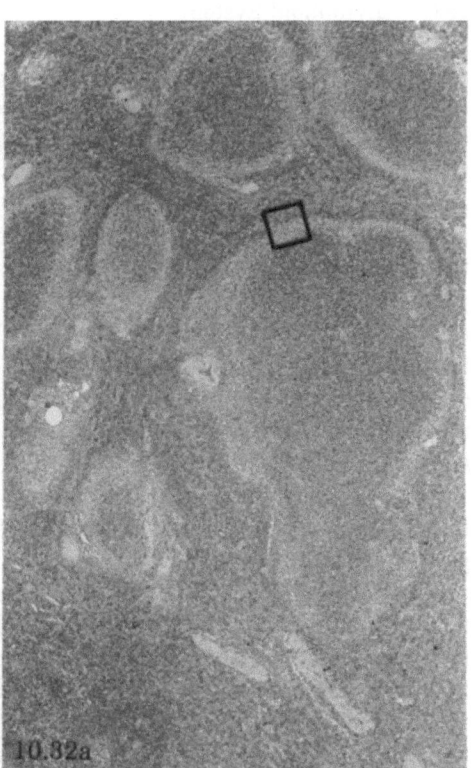

10.32a

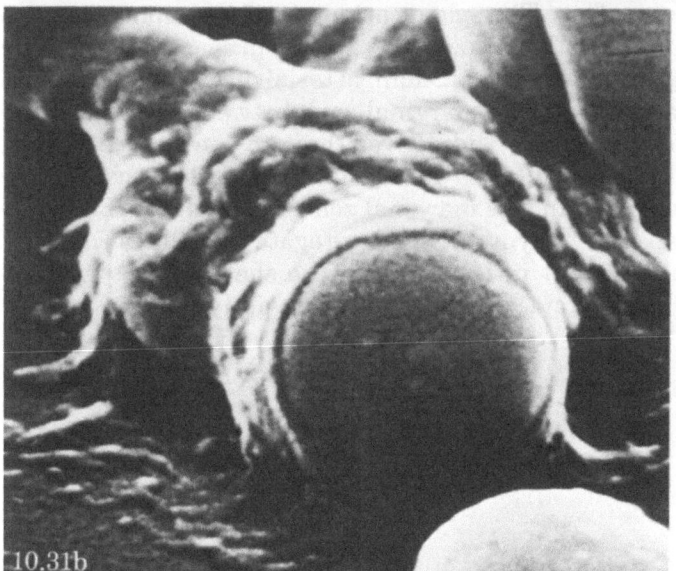

10.31b

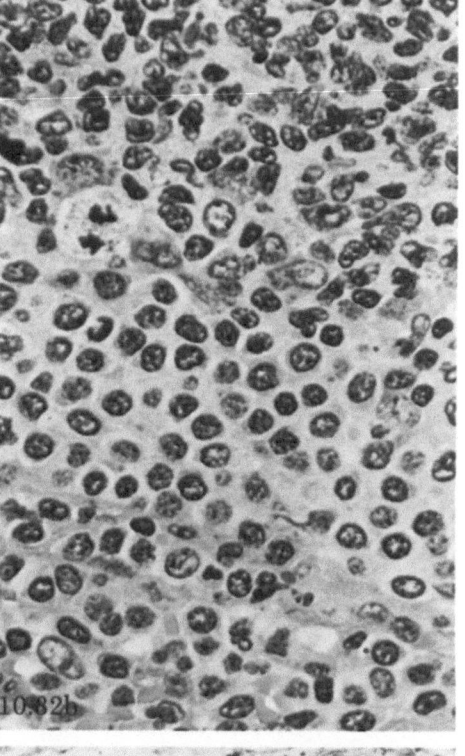

10.32b

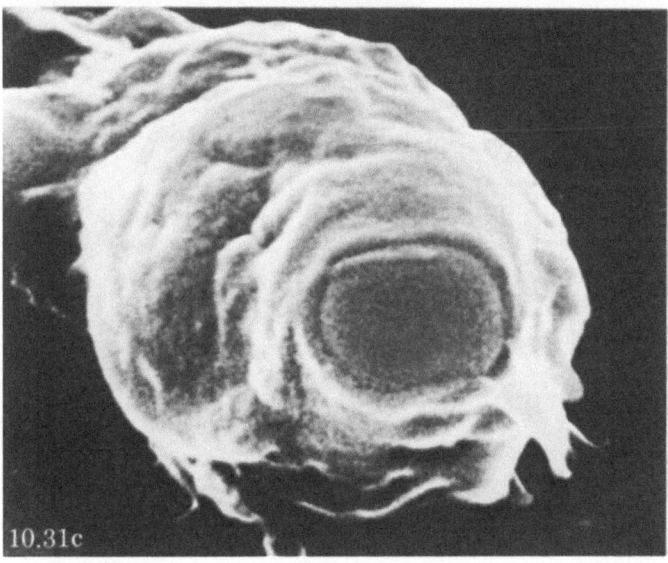

10.31c

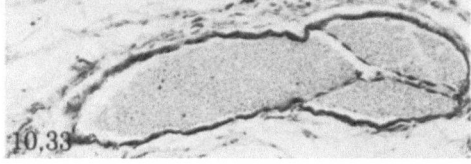

10.33

aggregations of lymphocytes are to be found in the above-described lymphoid tissues, these cells are always present to some degree in the connective tissue stroma of nearly all tissues and organs. A few lymphocytes, for example, occur at almost all levels of every portal tract in the liver. They are usually more plentiful in loose than in dense connective tissue. As we have seen in Chapter 9, small lymphocytes are a regular component of both circulating blood and bone marrow. This representation is quantitatively large when considered as a whole.

Small lymphocytes in the blood are carried to all tissues to destroy (usually) foreign antigens. Greater numbers are passed through the vessel walls and into the parenchyma of the lymphoid organs. They enter lymph nodes by two routes: (1) they may pass through the hilus via arteries to the capillaries. Many of them leave the blood stream by traversing the walls of the postcapillary venules of the diffuse (nonnodular) tissue of the deeper cortex; or (2) they may pass through the capsule via afferent lymphatics to the subcapsular sinus, and then to other sinuses, of the node.

B lymphocytes delivered to lymph nodes migrate to the nodules. In times of attack or stimulation by antigens their numbers increase and they give rise to plasma cells, which produce antibodies. If exposure to antigen continues, the nodules and germinal centers increase in size and number and they develop irregular and indistinct edges. Plasma cells become prominent in the medullary cords.

T lymphocytes remain in the diffuse lymphoid tissue, later gradually migrate into sinuses and eventually leave the node by efferent lymphatics. These channels flow into the major lymphatic ducts which empty into the large veins at the base of the neck.

The splenic artery carries lymphocytes into the spleen (the spleen has no afferent lymphatics). Small arterial branches terminate in the marginal zone between red and white pulp and deliver them to the tissues. T lymphocytes reside for varying lengths of time in this marginal zone and in the PALS, while B lymphocytes aggregate in nodules which lie at intervals along the sheath. Most lymphocytes leave the spleen via lymphatics.

11 Integument

Introduction

The integument (Fig. 11.1) consists of the skin and its associated appendages, the hair, nails, sweat glands, mammary glands, and sebaceous glands. The skin, the largest organ in the body, has an outer epithelial layer, the *epidermis,* adhering firmly to an underlying layer of dense, irregular connective tissue, the *dermis.* Beneath this is a soft flexible layer of fat and loose connective tissue, the hypodermis. The principal, and probably phylogenetically original, function of skin is to maintain a constant internal environment for the cells of the body, a culture medium, as it were, separated from the variable external environment. Loss or destruction of large areas of skin, as in burns, results in serious, often fatal fluid loss and changes in electrolyte balance and blood concentration. In addition, the uncovering of the underlying tissues exposes them to infections. Thus a major function of skin is protection from invaders as well as from gross physical insults. It also functions in excretion, temperature regulation, sensory reception, and photochemistry. It is flexible, elastic, self-sealing, and self-replacing. All of these properties are self-adjusting to environmental changes; instead of being worn away by friction, for example, skin thickens to form a callus.

The skin is an important source of diagnostic information for the physician. Its own myriad diseases are directly visible, and, in addition, subtle skin changes often reflect disease states in other systems of the body. Its texture, sensory innervation, and pheromone production play major roles in sexual activity. The pattern of epidermal ridges on plantar and palmar surfaces (dermatoglyphics) is unique to each individual and the basis for identification in criminology. Skin may be transplanted without rejection to burned or otherwise damaged areas of the same individual (autograft) and may be transplanted as a temporary emergency covering to burned areas in other individuals (allograft). It may also be transplanted between individuals of the same genetic constitution (isograft), such as highly inbred strains of laboratory animals or human identical twins.

Epidermis

Although there are differences in structural details in different regions of the body, the epidermis is always stratified squamous epithelium of the keratinized type. It is derived from the ectoderm of the embryo. Its layers will be described from deep to superficial to follow more clearly their structural and functional differentiation.

Layers of the Epidermis (Fig. 11.2)

The STRATUM BASALE (stratum germinativum, basal layer) (Fig. 11.2) is a layer of columnar or cuboidal cells, firmly anchored to the underlying connective tissue by hemidesmosomes. It is essentially composed of stem cells, which by their mitotic activity continually produce daughter cells to be pushed upward by their successors, become keratinized, and lost at the surface. The exfoliation of keratinized cells at the surface normally is precisely balanced by the mitotic activity of this deep layer.

STRATUM SPINOSUM (spinous layer) (Figs. 11.2 through 11.4) is a densely packed layer of many polygonal cells firmly joined by desmosomes. Some mitotic activity continues in this layer, particularly in its lower portions. The more superficial cells lose their ability to undergo mitosis as they begin to show signs of differentiation. They begin to synthesize pro-

teins, for the most part filbrillar in form. The numerous desmosomes and their associated tonofibrils give the cells a prickly or spinous appearance in the light microscope. The stratum basale and the stratum spinosum together constitute a layer referred to as the *stratum malpighii.*

THE STRATUM GRANULOSUM (granular layer) (Fig. 11.2) is the most superficial layer in which the cells contain nuclei. It is a thin stratum of one to several layers of cells containing noticeable granules. Some of these granules (keratohyalin) are not membrane-enclosed, and are thought to provide a matrix for the developing intracellular fibers of keratin. Others, enclosed by membranes, appear to undergo exocytosis and may provide an intercellular cementing substance or sealant for the more superficial layers of the epidermis.

THE STRATUM LUCIDUM (clear layer) (Fig. 11.2) is a narrow but sharply defined zone. Nuclei and other organelles have disappeared. Polymerized keratin nearly fills the cells and results in an apparent homogenous zone. The optical properties of the keratin and the changing cell membranes show no cell details at the light microscope level. This zone is often so narrow as to be indistinguishable.

STRATUM CORNEUM (keratinized or cornified layer) (Figs. 11.2 and 11.5). By the time the cells are pushed above the stratum lucidum, rapid polymerization of the keratin converts them to fibrous masses firmly bound to their neighbors. These are now dead cells with very few remnants of organelles even at the electron microscope level.

The process of exfoliation (Fig. 11.5) is inadequately understood. The relative thickness of the stratum corneum in different areas of the body may be a function of variation in the durability of the intercellular cementing substances. Generally, the shedding of the outer cornified cells is imperceptible, but occasionally large flakes of many cells are shed.

The epidermis, being in constant contact with the external environment, might be expected to show some characteristic reactions

Fig. 11.1. The basic *structure of the integument.*

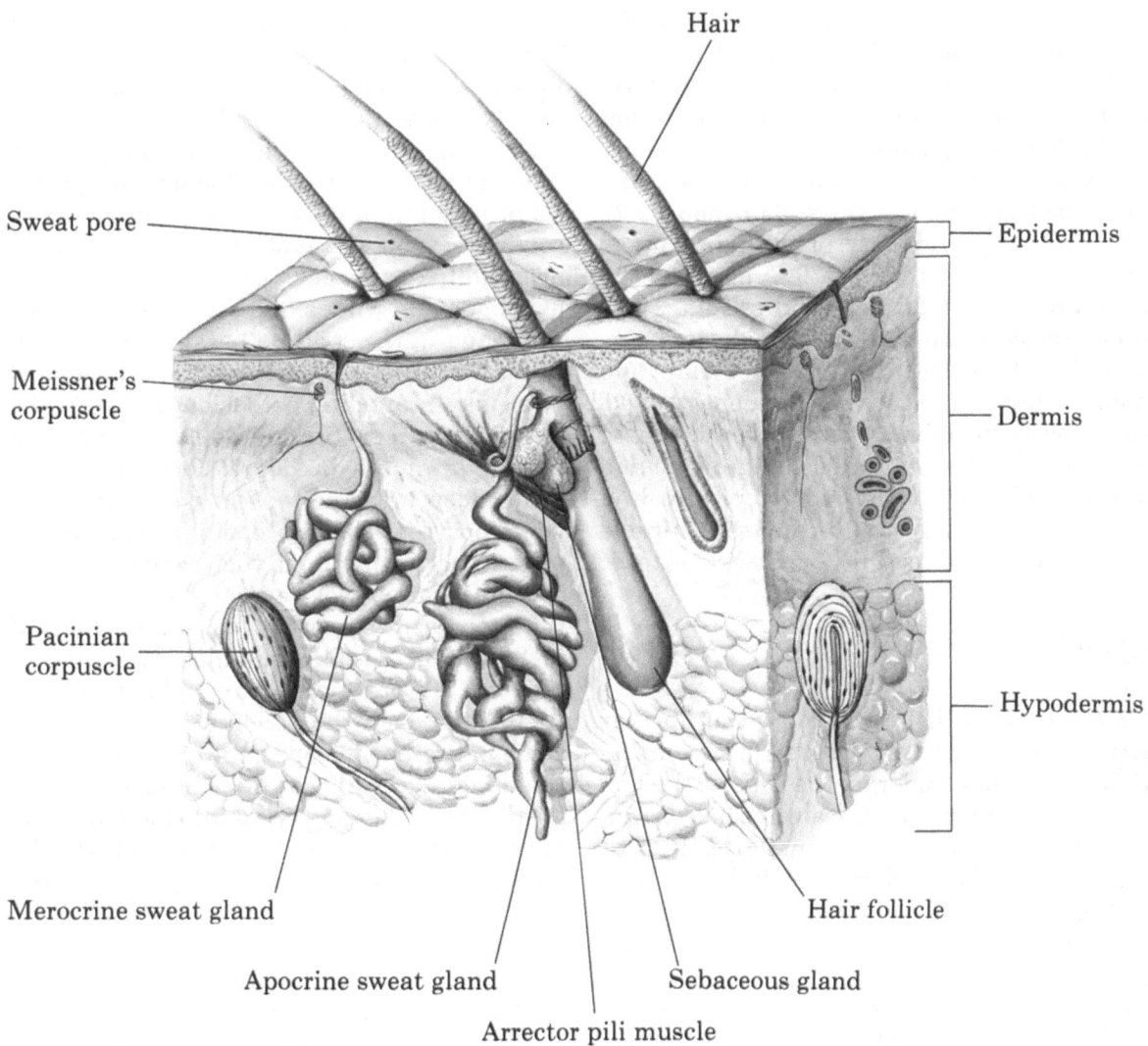

Hair

Sweat pore

Epidermis

Meissner's corpuscle

Dermis

Pacinian corpuscle

Hypodermis

Merocrine sweat gland

Hair follicle

Apocrine sweat gland

Sebaceous gland

Arrector pili muscle

11.1

in those individuals who have been exposed to a harsher surrounding milieu. This is in fact the case; the skin of the parts of the body that are more exposed to sun and wind (that is, the face, ears, and backs of the hands) are likely to develop in later life epidermal squamous cell carcinomas (Figs. 11.6 and 11.7). This is true particularly of the fair-skinned (perhaps because they are less protected by melanin), and of farmers and sailors. However, these tumors also, though less frequently, affect those with darker skin and many whose unusual environmental exposure has been limited to their youth. These malignancies are generally slow-growing and are preceded by both microscopically and grossly (that is, clinically) recognizable changes known as actinic, or solar, keratosis.

Other Cell Types

On the basis of their specific type of fibrillar protein and the complex process of keratinization which they undergo, the cells of the epidermis described thus far are termed *keratinocytes*. These, of course, constitute the vast majority of the epidermal cell population; however, scattered among these are at least three other cell types of significance. These probably arise elsewhere and secondarily take up residence in the epidermis.

MELANOCYTES (Figs. 11.8 and 11.9), as the name implies, are responsible for the synthesis of melanin, a dark brown pigment. They originate from the embryonic neural crest, eventually to appear in sections of adult skin as clear cells with small dark nuclei. They are found in the stratum basale and stratum spinosum. The cell body is somewhat rounded with long branching extensions between the neighboring keratinocytes. These cell processes terminate in depressions and sometimes deep invaginations in the wall of the keratinocytes. They do not have the desmosomes characteristic of their neighbors, but contain granules of several different forms that represent stages in the development of melanin. These cells accumulate tyrosine and convert it to 3,4-dihydroxy phenylalanine (DOPA) through the action of tyrosinase, an enzyme present in considerable quantities in this highly specialized cell. Through a series of steps DOPA is converted into melanin. The mature melanin granules are moved into the long cell processes and are injected by the

---

Fig. 11.2. *Layers of the epidermis:* stratum basale (A); stratum spinosum (B); stratum granulosum (C); stratum lucidum (D); stratum corneum (E). A coiled sweat duct passes through the epidermis. ×200. (Courtesy of W. Montagna and N. Roman.)

Fig. 11.3. *"Intercellular bridges"* (arrows) in the stratum spinosum. ×400.

Fig. 11.4. Cells of the *stratum spinosum* in an electron micrograph. Structures that appear in Fig. 11.3 to be intercellular bridges are seen here to be not bridges, but closely spaced intercellular junctions of the macula adherens type (long arrows). The intercellular spaces (short arrows) between the drawn out maculae accentuate the appearance of bridges. ×8500. (Courtesy of M. Webb.)

Fig. 11.5. Scanning electron micrograph of the *surface of the skin* of the anterior abdominal wall. Several creases may be seen crossing the field at various angles and numerous keratinized cells are partially loosened and in the process of being shed. ×150 (Courtesy of W. H. Fahrenbach.)

Fig. 11.6. Multiple *actinic keratoses and carcinomas*. The exposed skin is generally the most affected. (Courtesy of F. Storrs.)

Fig. 11.7. *Actinic keratosis.* Cellular changes in malignancy (nuclear variation, enlargement, and hyperchromatism) are apparent and the epidermis and dermis are distorted. However, interdigitations of the superficial dermis with epidermis are partially retained. ×65.

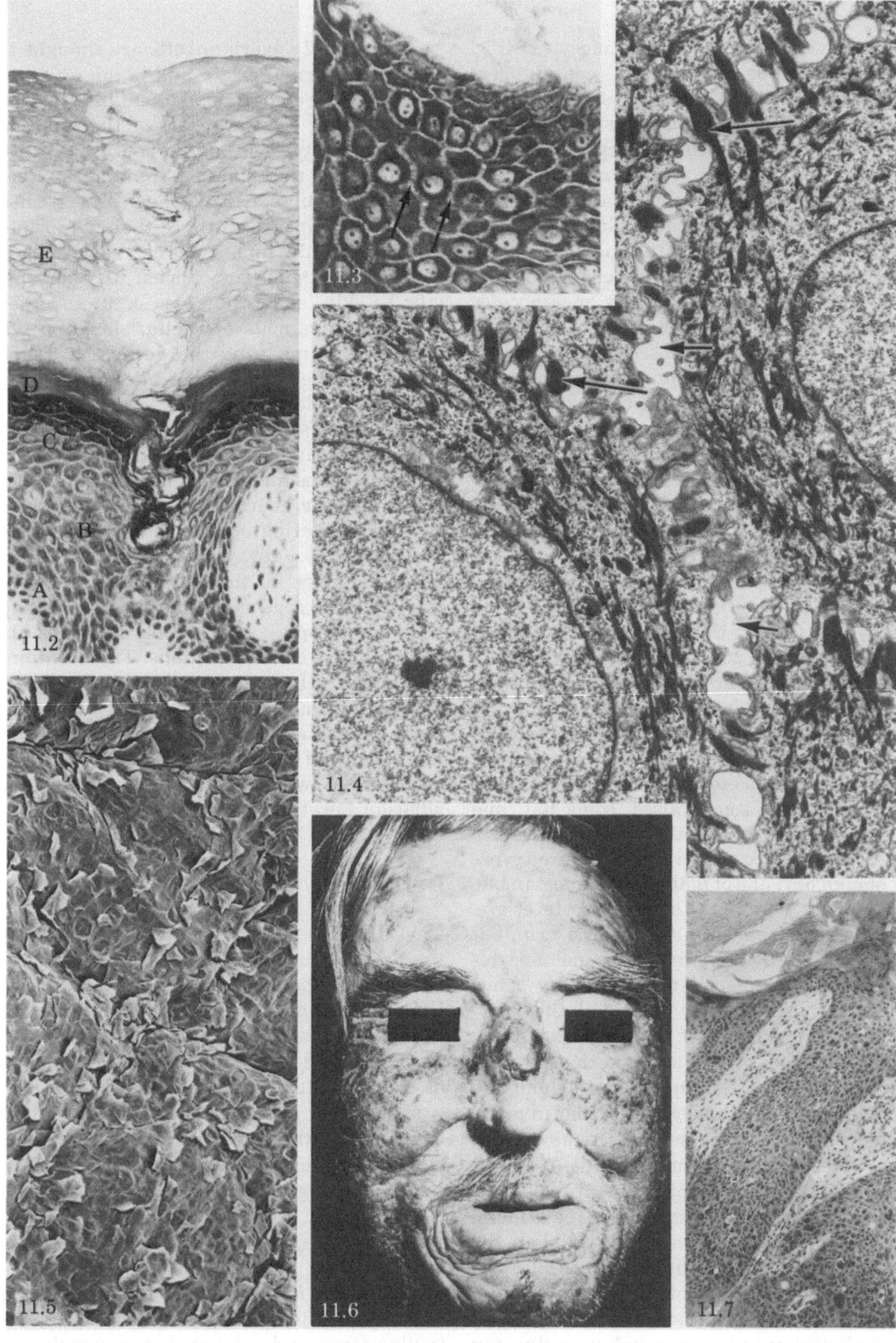

melanocytes into the keratinocytes (Fig. 11.10). Melanocytes actually contain less melanin than the keratinocytes (Fig. 11.11), which accumulate it avidly as soon as it is completely synthesized. The pigmentation of the skin is a reflection of the amount of melanin in the keratinocytes, the rate of melanin granule formation in the melanocytes, and the rate of turnover of the melanin in the keratinocytes. Although not easily seen in routine histologic preparations, melanocytes can be readily demonstrated by treating pieces of skin with DOPA (Fig. 11.8). Since only the melanocytes and not the keratinocytes have tyrosinase, these cells convert the DOPA to obvious deposits of the dark pigment. Tanning of the skin by sunlight involves an increase in the rate of melanin synthesis in the melanocytes, increase in rate of its transfer to keratinocytes, and darkening of melanin already present.

Melanocytes vary in number in different regions of the body and in different races. One study of skin from the thigh has shown numbers from about 1000 per mm² in whites, to about 1400 per mm² in blacks. They may be found in groups in the epidermis or in the underlying dermis as freckles or somewhat larger masses called *nevi* (singular, *nevus*). Every human has several, usually hundreds, of visible nevi, some raised, some flat, and some pigmented and others not (Figs. 11.12 and 11.13). There are several recognized types of benign nevi and of malignant tumors (melanomas; see Fig. 11.14) of melanocyte origin. These most commonly arise in the skin, but have arisen at other sites where melanocytes migrate. Pigment cell neoplasms are sometimes striking in their color, but they may also be unpigmented if melanogenesis is incomplete. Melanomas are notorious for becoming widely disseminated throughout the body. Reports of primary melanomas in many sites other than skin serve to remind us of the widespread distribution of neural crest cells with pigment-forming potential.

LANGERHANS CELLS are star-shaped cells found in the two deepest layers, especially in the stratum spinosum. Definite identification of the cells requires use of the electron microscope, with which characteristic small rod- or club-shaped membrane-bound granules can be observed. Langerhan cells are thought to be of mesodermal origin and to migrate into and out of the epidermis. Current information suggests that they are part of the immune system and function in the capture of antigens entering the epidermis from the environment. They subsequently transfer these antigens to lymph nodes, where the appropriate antibodies and lymphocytes can be developed to dispose of them. They appear to be not specific to skin, since they also occur in other stratified squamous epithelia, skin appendages, the thymus and the dermis. It seems likely that they will be shown to have important immunologic functions.

MERKEL CELLS are most numerous in the stratum basale and are scattered through the stratum spinosum. They probably arise from the embryonic neural crest and migrate into the differentiating epidermis of the embryo. They are almost always associated with naked nerve endings in the epithelium and are thought to be sensory in function. They have very few cytoplasmic filaments and thus appear as clear cells in sections. They contain, as seen with the electron microscope, numerous small membrane-bound granules, particularly along the surface in contact with the expansions of nerve endings. They possess desmosomes, which appear to attach them to adjacent keratinocytes.

Dermis

This is the sheet of connective tissue underlying and supporting the epidermis. It makes up most of the skin's thickness. Leather is the result of denaturation of dermis by the tanning process. It is quite variable in density, elasticity, and thickness in different regions of the body. It is subdivided into two parts, a superficial, *papillary* layer in immediate contact with the epidermis and a deeper, *reticular* layer of very dense, irregular connective tissue (Fig. 11.15).

The Papillary Layer

The *papillary layer* is usually somewhat loose and contains finer collagen fibers than the reticular layer and a much larger population of cells. It is termed papillary because of its finger-like extensions upward into the epidermis. From the papillary layer, small collagenous fibers extend upward and are cemented into the basal lamina of the epidermis. The papillary layer also contains numerous elastic fibers generally aligned parallel to the surface. The papillae are quite variable in structure; some are simple extensions of connective tissue only; some contain elaborate loops of capillaries (Fig. 11.16); and some, particularly in the digits, are ridge-like rather than finger-like. Nerve endings such as Meissner's corpuscles, end bulbs, and naked nerve endings are found in some of these papillae. Descriptions and functions of these structures are given in Chapter 7.

Reticular Layer

The *reticular layer* (Fig. 11.15) consists of dense, irregular connective tissue with more and larger fibers and fewer cells than the papillary layer. In general, these large bundles of connective tissue are parallel with the skin surface and are the basis for lines of tension in the skin known as Langer's lines. These are of some practical significance because they determine the amount of gaping of wounds and the stretching of scars. The process of healing is considerably assisted when surgical incisions are made parallel to these lines of tension rather than across them.

Throughout life, perhaps as part of the normal aging process, melanocytes normally and gradually migrate from the lower portions of the epidermis downward into the dermis. The dermis may also contain anastomosing bundles of smooth muscle cells (Fig. 11.17), particularly in its deeper portion. These may be found in the skin of the scrotum, perineum, penis, and areolae. Their contraction in response to thermal or sexual stimuli results in wrinkling and tightening of the skin in these areas. Other dermal smooth muscle associated with hairs will be described below.

Cells of the dermis and hypodermis include all of the usual varieties to be found in connective tissue generally. Commonly, additional local collections of cells occur, principally lymphocytes or neutrophils. When these aggregates are prominent enough to the trained eye they will be regarded as evidence of inflammation. Individual sensitivity to any of the innumerable substances with which skin may come into contact is extremely variable; the resulting inflammation, called contact dermatitis, may be severe.

Regional differences in skin appear to be controlled by the dermis. If dermis from the sole is grown in tissue culture with epidermis from a thin area such as the surface of the ear, this combination will result in the differentiation of epidermis characteristic of the sole. Similarly, sole epidermis cultured with ear dermis, results in the development of a thin epidermis with hair follicles characteristic of the ear.

Hypodermis (Figs. 11.15 and 11.18)

This also termed the tela subcutanea, is a layer of loose connective tissue which varies in thickness in different parts of the body and varies greatly in the amount of fat which it contains. Its connective tissue fibers are downward extensions of those in the dermis and their thickness and numbers determine the firmness with which skin is attached to deeper structures. Fat is usually abundantly present, occasionally to the extent that the layer may be termed a panniculus adiposus. In this layer also are located the lower ends of the larger sweat glands and of hair follicles. Many nerve endings occur here and this is a characteristic location for lamellated corpuscles (of Pacini) (Fig. 11.18).

Types of Skin

On the basis of difference in structure of the epidermis, there are two general categories of skin.

Thick Skin (Fig. 11.19)

This type is characteristic of palmar and plantar surfaces, in other words of friction surfaces. Here the epidermis may become 1 mm thick in the palms and 1½ mm on the soles.

Fig. 11.8. *DOPA reaction* showing *melanocytes* on the deep surface of the epidermis. The tissue has not been stained except with the pigment produced by the reaction. ×250. (Courtesy of W. Montagna and N. Roman.)

Fig. 11.9. *Melanocytes* (arrows) in the basal layers of the epidermis and the superficial dermis are visible because of their perinuclear clear zones. Melanin does not accumulate in melanocytes but is passed on to keratinocytes. ×400.

Fig. 11.10. *Melanocytes synthesizing melanin* granules for keratinocytes in the basal layer of the epidermis. The melanocyte accumulates tyrosine, synthesizes tyrosinase, and sequesters both compounds in melanosomes. Here tyrosine is converted to melanin. (After Fig. 19.5 in Junqueira L, Carneiro J, and Contopoulos A. Basic Histology. Los Altos, Lange Medical Publications, 1977.)

Fig. 11.11. *Pigment* in the basal layer of *keratinocytes* of dark skin. ×225.

Fig. 11.12. Three *pigmented nevi;* nipple of breast is at lower right. (Courtesy of F. Storrs.)

Fig. 11.13. *Nonpigmented intradermal nevus.* Clusters of small and regular melanocytes (nevus cells) are almost completely separate from the epidermis. ×110.

Fig. 11.14. *Melanoma.* The melanocytes are larger and less regular in grouping and individual appearance than in Fig. 11.13. Also some are in the epidermis. Pigment is present near the surface. ×110.

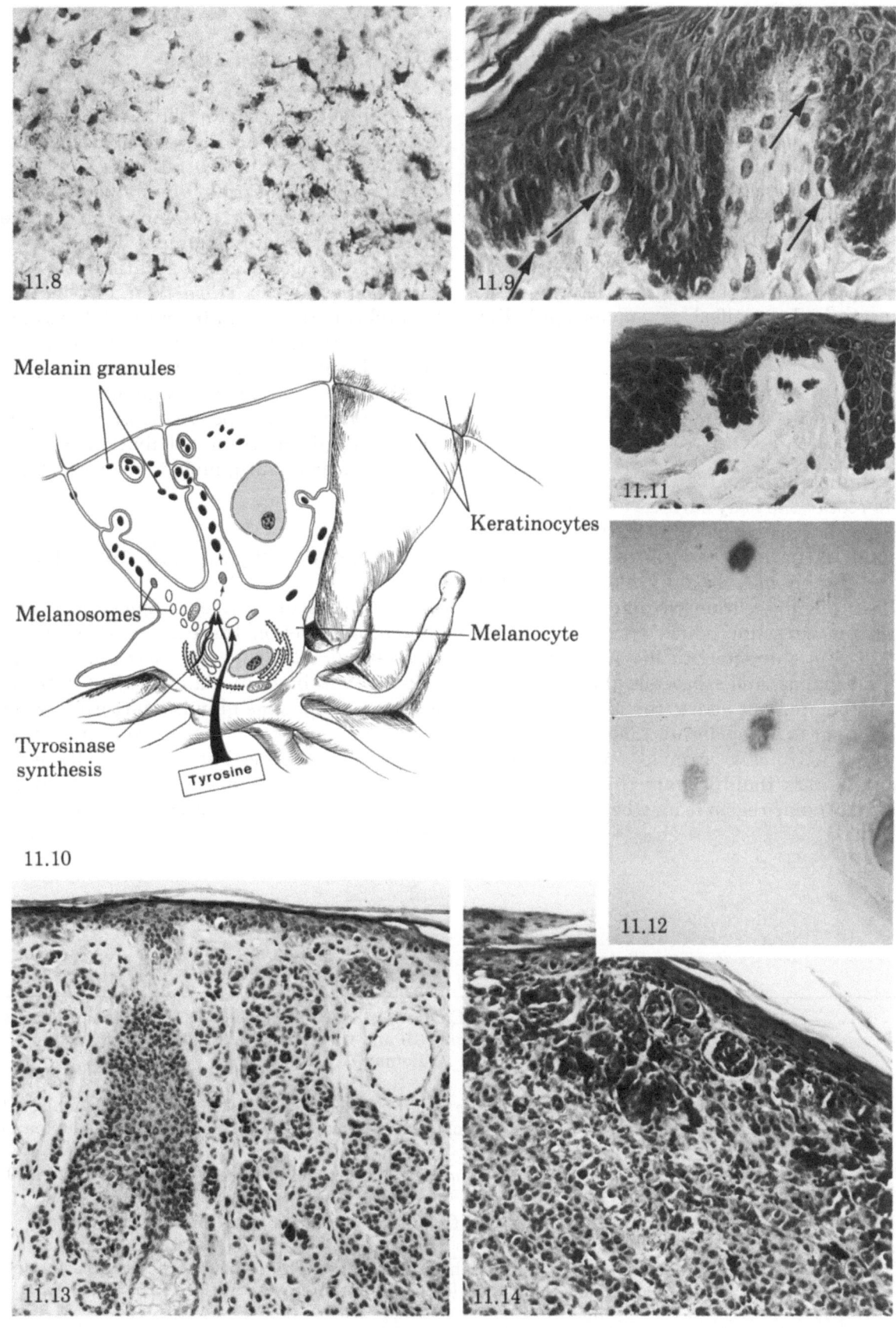

11.8

11.9

Melanin granules

Keratinocytes

Melanosomes

Melanocyte

Tyrosinase
synthesis

Tyrosine

11.10

11.11

11.12

11.13

11.14

Sweat glands are most numerous here (hence the sometimes liquid handshake and soggy socks). There are no hairs or sebaceous glands. Distinct patterns of grooves and ridges are visible on the surface and reflect the presence of underlying ridges of the dermis. The ducts of sweat glands open at the top of these epidermal ridges, and are seen in sections as spiral structures extending through the stratum corneum. All of the characteristic layers of keratinized stratified squamous epithelium are clearly seen in thick skin.

Thin skin

In thin skin (Fig. 11.20), which is found over the rest of the body surface, all of the epidermal strata are much thinner, the stratum lucidum is usually absent, and the stratum granulosum may be only one or two cells thick. The most dramatic difference is in the stratum corneum, which is here very thin. Thin skin characteristically possesses hairs, sweat glands, and sebaceous glands.

As pointed out above, the terms thick and thin refer to the epidermis. The dermis in thin skin is extremely variable; on the eyelid it may be less than 0.5 mm thick and in the interscapular region it may be 5 mm or more thick.

Cutaneous Appendages

The skin appendages (Fig. 11.21–11.34), or accessory skin structures, are all epidermal derivatives whose differentiation is probably stimulated and controlled by inductive properties of the dermis. In the embryo all of these structures originate as simple downgrowths of cords or ridges of basal keratinocytes into the dermis. At this stage their distribution is uniform. In the scalp most will become hairs and some, sweat glands; on the palms all will become sweat glands; elsewhere, most will become sweat glands, some hairs. Differential growth of the body surface will result in loss of uniformity in distribution since no new hairs or sweat glands are formed later on.

Sweat glands (Figs. 11.21 and 11.22)

On the basis of histologic appearance and method of secretion, there are two basic types of sweat glands. They are *merocrine* (traditionally but inappropriately called eccrine) glands and *apocrine* glands. Merocrine sweat glands are present on the entire body surface except for very special areas such as the margin of the lip, the ear drum, and some portions of the genitalia. The merocrine type plays an important role in thermoregulation by provid-

Fig. 11.15. *Layers of the skin.* Epidermis (A), papillary dermis (B), reticular dermis (C), hypodermis (D). Sweat glands (S) and their ducts (arrows) are indicated. ×27. (Courtesy of W. Montagna and N. Roman.)

Fig. 11.16. Blood vessels of the papillary dermis are shown in a section subjected to the alkaline phosphatase reaction. ×60. (Courtesy of W. Montagna and N. Roman.)

Fig. 11.17. Bundles of *smooth muscle* fibers (arrows) in skin of the scrotum. ×100.

Fig. 11.18. *Pacinian corpuscle* (P) and *sweat glands* (S) in the hypodermis. ×35.

Fig. 11.19. *Thick skin* from the heel. The heavy cornified layer (bracket) is perforated by sweat ducts and retains surface ridges. Contrast with Fig. 11.20. ×34.

Fig. 11.20. *Thin skin.* The terms thick and thin refer to the epidermis, mainly the cornified layer (bracket). ×35.

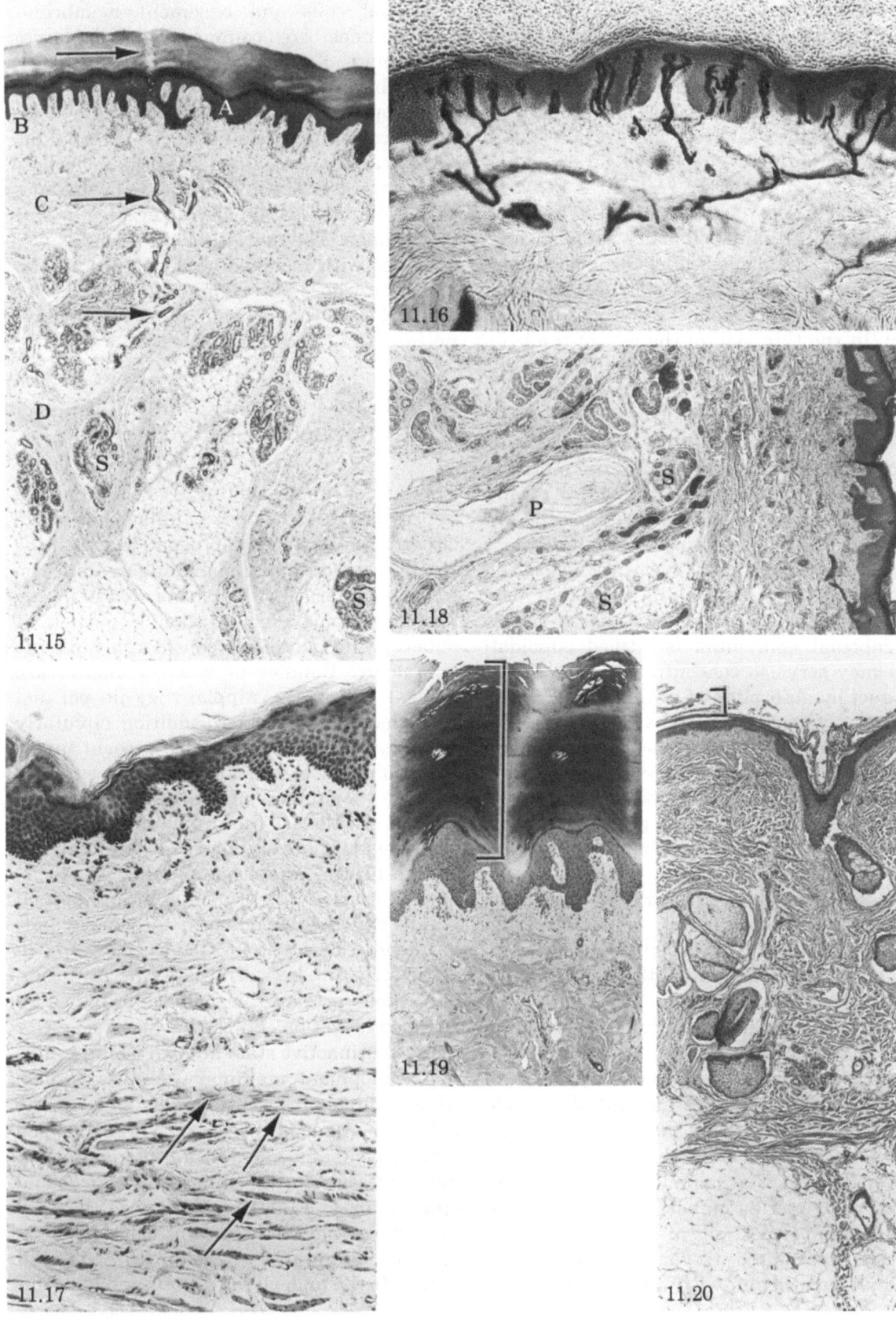

ing a moist film for evaporative cooling. They are particularly responsive to nervous stress. The thermoregulatory and stress responses differ in the pattern with which they are turned on. In stress, palms and soles commonly start to sweat first, whereas in response to heat, sweating begins on the forehead and gradually spreads to the rest of the body.

MEROCRINE SWEAT GLANDS (Fig. 11.21) are the simple, coiled tubular glands with long, relatively straight ducts, which are most commonly seen in sections of skin. As has been pointed out, they are most numerous in thick skin. In the thin skin of the rest of the body they average over 200 per cm². This is a far greater density than other animals possess. The coiled secreting portion of the gland may be located at different levels in different portions of the body, varying from the more superficial portion of the dermis down to and into the hypodermis. The secretory cells are of two types, one secreting a watery product containing various substances in solution, the other producing a mucoid glycoprotein. The sweat gland duct is composed of two layers of cuboidal epithelium (stratified cuboidal) and may serve to concentrate the secretory product by absorption of water. These glands have a noticeable basement membrane. Between the epithelium and the basement membrane are located myoid or myoepithelial cells that have been assumed to function in expressing secretion from the glands; however, it has also been proposed that they are passively supportive structures. They do appear to possess some ultrastructural features characteristic of smooth muscle cells. Merocrine glands open directly on the surface of the skin. They are functioning at birth and are innervated by cholinergic nerves.

APOCRINE SWEAT GLANDS (Fig. 11.22) are large sweat glands located in the areolae of the breasts, in the axillae, the labia majora, and the anal region. These are also initially simple coiled tubular glands but they have very large and closely packed coils which develop diverticula. The ducts are similar in structure to those of merocrine glands, but usually open into the upper portions of hair follicles. The glands are composed of simple cuboidal or columnar epithelium with well-developed myo-

epithelial cells and basement membrane. The lumens are commonly much larger than those of the merocrine glands. These glands begin to function only at puberty. They are supplied by adrenergic nerves.

The ceruminous glands of the external auditory canal are modified sweat glands whose secretions are mixed with those of sebaceous glands to produce the characteristic ear wax or cerumen. The margin of the eyelid is also provided with modified sweat glands (glands of Moll), whose secretions are swept across the surface of the cornea in blinking and have an important protective function.

Breast and Mammary Gland (Figs. 11.23 through 11.26)

The skin of the nipple (Fig. 11.25) and areola is provided with dermal papillae that reach closer to the surface than usual, thus making capillaries more superficial and providing the rose color characteristic of this area in immature individuals. Pigmentation begins here at puberty and increases considerably during pregnancy. Bundles of smooth muscle are present within the nipple; they lie parallel to the lactiferous ducts. In addition, circularly arranged muscle bundles are present under the epidermis of the nipple and around its base. These bundles provide the mechanism for the erection of the nipple during sexual excitement. There are many sebaceous glands on the nipple. The circular area, or *areola*, at the base of the nipple contains special glands which are modified mammary glands or modified sweat glands. They are intermediate in structure between these two categories, and their presence is indicated by small rounded elevations on the surface.

In their inactive state and particularly during development, mammary glands are somewhat similar to sweat glands. Indeed, the mammary gland is a series of 15 to 25 modified sweat glands imbedded in fat and dense connective tissue. In the embryo the ectodermal epithelium, in a line on each side of the body extending from the axilla to the groin, thickens considerably and develops the potential to invade the underlying dermis and hypodermis and become glandular. In the human, at one pair of points along these lines, such an ingrowth occurs as a group of cell cords. Each cord constitutes the precursor of an eventually large, compound tubular gland in which the hollowed out cord becomes the duct, the deeper ends of which eventually develop into secretory alveoli. The connective tissue of the dermis and hypodermis keeps pace with the growing duct rudiments to form the stroma of the completed gland. The stroma occurs as dense partitions and strands of connective tissue which separate the original lobes from each other and further subdivide each lobe into many lobules. While the *inter*lobular connective tissue is of the dense irregular variety with scattered masses of fat cells, the *intra*lobular connective tissue is of a delicate loose type with numerous cells (Fig. 11.23).

At birth, both sexes have distinct mammary glands with alveoli and occasionally some temporary secretion because of the maternal hormones to which they are exposed during intrauterine life. In males development ceases when rudimentary ducts have formed; in females development continues. Because of the complexity of endocrine control of breast function related to reproduction, only the basic histologic structure of the mammary gland will be described here.

Most of the enlargement of a mammary gland in females at puberty is accounted for by increase in the amount of fat in the stroma. Some is provided by growth of the lactiferous ducts and the development of small, tubular alveolar rudiments within the lobules. In the mammary gland of a sexually mature, nonpregnant woman the epithelial glandular components are widely scattered lobular clusters of ducts with occasional indications of rudimentary alveoli. In the usual histologic section these may be so widely scattered as to be easily overlooked. Most of the section appears to be composed of dense, irregular connective tissue and fat. The gland at this stage is referred to as an *inactive* or *resting mammary gland* (Fig. 11.23). After the reproductive period (after the menopause) the breast undergoes some atrophy of epithelium, a slight increase in connective tissue and some reduction of fat.

Sebaceous Glands

These are simple or branched alveolar glands of varying size and complexity (Fig. 11.27). They are classified as holocrine because their secretion is made up of remnants of dead cells. Each alveolus is an oval sac with a short duct lined by stratified squamous epithelium which opens into the neck of the hair follicle in most instances, but which may open directly onto the surface of the skin. The alveoli are completely filled with the distended cells derived from the differentiation and death of cells proliferated in their walls. Peripherally the cells are small and more or less cuboid with occasional mitoses. As they are pushed toward the interior of the alveolus they become progressively larger as a result of accumulation of a complex mixture of triglycerides, free fatty acids, and cholesterol. The nuclei of these cells become pyknotic, shriveled, and small. The secretion of these glands is called *sebum*. Its accumulation renders the skin and hair greasy and soft, and prevents drying. It seems likely that sebaceous glands also produce pheromones, which may be involved in chemical communication between individuals. The more pleasant odor of human skin after washing away the accumulated products of bacterial degradation of skin detritus is apparently provided by sebum.

Hair

Hairs (Figs. 11.28 and 11.29) are elongated columns of fused cornified or keratinized cells of the epidermis. Each hair projects from its own tubular invagination of the epidermis into the dermis. At its deep extremity this tubular sheath expands into a bulb which is deeply indented at its bottom by a dermal papilla of well vascularized connective tissue (Fig. 11.29). The epidermal cells over this dermal papilla proliferate, become fused together and pushed upwards as a cylinder through the tube provided by the root sheaths. Cells produced by the stratum basale over the very apex of the papilla are carried up in the center of the hair as its medulla. These cells eventually shrivel and separate and the intercellular

Fig. 11.21. *Merocrine sweat glands* (G) and *ducts* (D). Myoepithelial cells (arrows) form the outer layer of the gland wall. ×250. (Courtesy of R. Sauter.)

Fig. 11.22. *Apocrine sweat glands.* ×250. (Courtesy of W. Montagna and N. Roman.)

Fig. 11.23. *Breast.* The lobular collections of small ducts are invested with delicate connective tissue. ×36.

Fig. 11.24. Diagram of the structure of the *breast.*

Fig. 11.25. *Nipple* with ducts (arrows). ×5.5.

Fig. 11.26. *Mammary dysplasia* with a variety of different changes, including many cysts. This is a common cause of lumps in the breast.

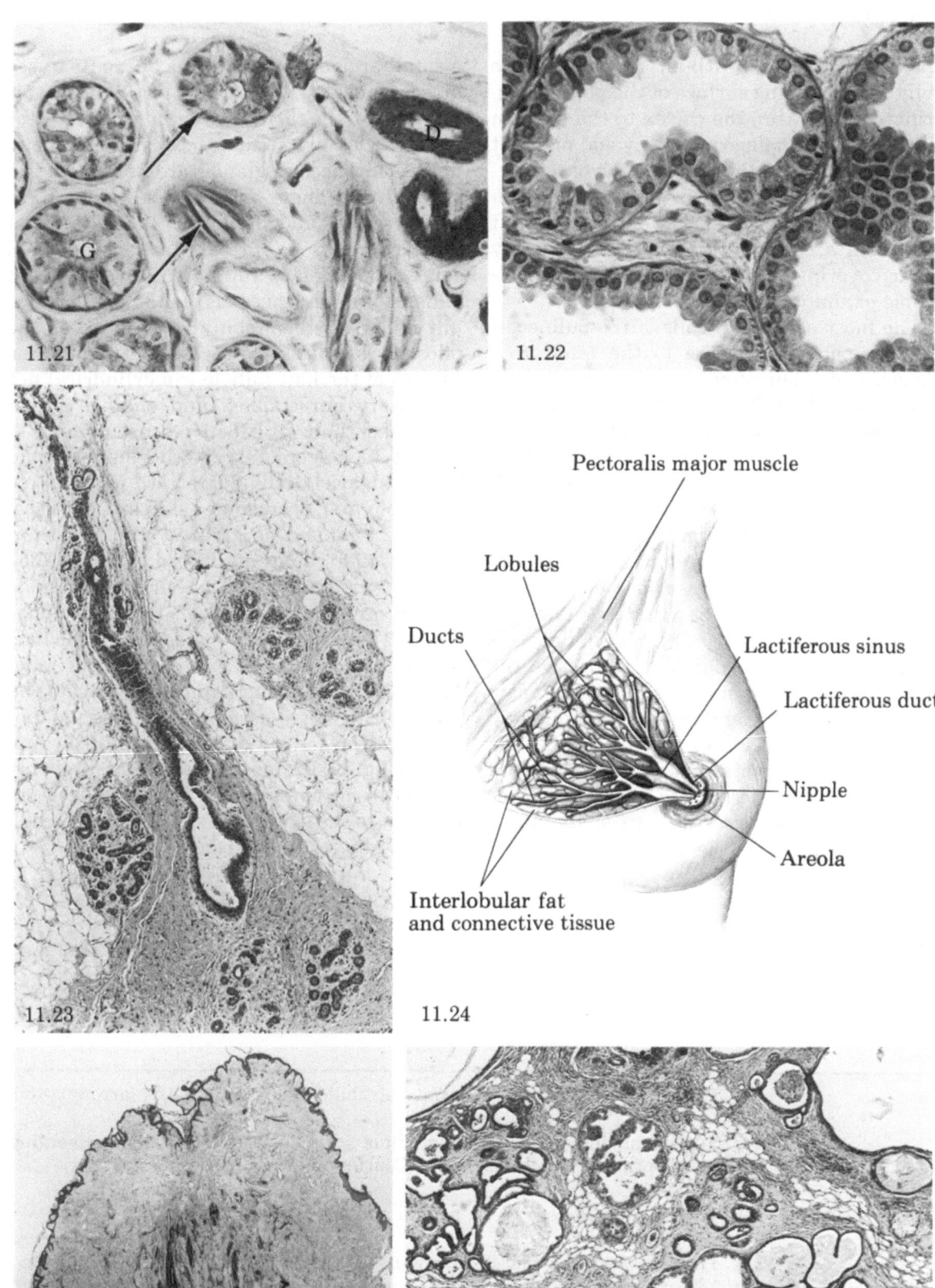

11.21

11.22

11.23

11.24

Pectoralis major muscle

Lobules

Ducts

Lactiferous sinus

Lactiferous duct

Nipple

Areola

Interlobular fat
and connective tissue

11.25

11.26

spaces become filled with air. Stratum basale cells on the sloping surface of the papilla contribute, as keratin, the cortex to the hair. In this area also, melanocytes may add pigment to provide color to the hair. On the outer surface of the hair cortex the flattened keratinized cells are elongated parallel to the shaft and form a cuticle. This provides the scaly outer covering which can be seen on microscopic examination of a whole hair.

The most peripheral cells of the bulb coating the papilla give rise to the inner root sheath which surrounds the deeper portions of the hair shaft. The sheath is a temporary structure whose cells disintegrate and separate from the hair cuticle so that the hair lies free in the upper portions of the follicle unattached to the sheaths around it. The wall of the follicle itself, the long tubular invagination of the epidermis, is continuous with the malpighian layer of the surface epithelium. There is a distinct basement membrane around the follicle between its epithelial components and the surrounding connective tissue. Attached to one side of this dense connective tissue sheath and extending obliquely upwards to the papillary layer of the dermis are bundles of smooth muscle. These are the *arrector pili* muscles (Fig. 11.30) whose contraction tends to raise the hair shaft into a vertical position and at the same time pull

a small area of the epidermis above its upper attachment down to form a pit. We call this dimpling of the surface goose bumps. Arrector pili muscles are innervated by sympathetic nerves. Sebaceous glands are commonly located in the angle between the hair follicle and arrector pili muscles, so that their contraction tends to press these glands and squeeze out their secretion. This arrangement of hair follicles, sebaceous glands and arrector pili muscles is commonly referred to as the pilosebaceous unit. Closely applied to the outer surface of the hair follicle is a cylindrical net of sensory nerve fibers and endings which make each hair an effective sense organ.

Most teen-agers respect the disease acne (acne vulgaris). Individuals with more active sebaceous glands and oilier skin are more susceptible to this. The greatest risk is during puberty and young adulthood. The familiar raised, red, lumpy and sometimes pustular lesions occur mostly on the face and upper trunk. They begin with a plugging of the hair follicle by lipid-impregnated keratin (Fig. 11.31). Bacterial infection may aggravate the process, causing hyperemia, swelling and tenderness. The follicle may rupture or be ruptured (Fig. 11.32); most ruptures are probably caused by attempts to force the obstructing plug out to the skin surface. A larger, parafollicular, abscess may ensue.

Fig. 11.27. *Sebaceous glands* (S) about hair follicles and *hair shafts* (arrows). ×85.

Fig. 11.28. Scanning electron micrograph of *scalp*. Two hairs are shown emerging from neighboring hair follicles. ×200. (Courtesy of W. H. Fahrenbach.)

Fig. 11.29. *Hair follicle* (F) with papilla and hair shafts. ×55.

Fig. 11.30. *Arrector pili* muscle (arrows). ×35.

Fig. 11.31. *Acne vulgaris,* inflammation of the pilosebaceous apparatus. ×36. (Courtesy of S. Kessler.)

Fig. 11.32. *Acne* with parafollicular *abscess* due to rupture of the follicle wall. Moral: Don't squeeze your zits. ×80. (Courtesy of S. Kessler.)

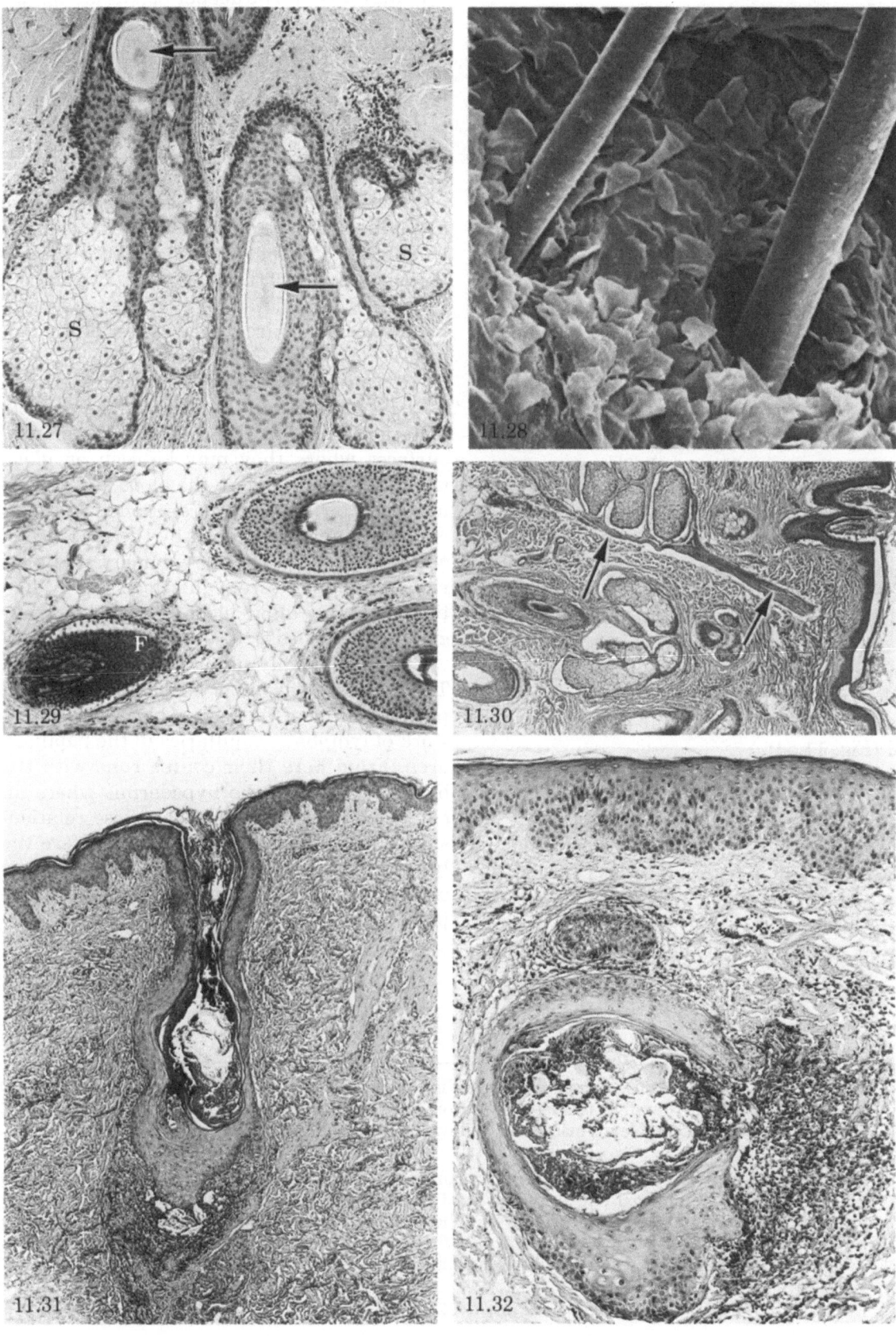

Nails

Nails (Figs. 11.33 and 11.34) are cornified, hard scales derived from the skin over the distal phalanges. The body of the nail is the attached, laterally curved, uncovered part of the structure which on each side bends down into the lateral nail groove. The free edge is unattached and extends distally over the tucked in stratum corneum of the fingertip. Much of this accumulated stratum corneum (hyponychium) is scraped away in the process of cleaning the nails. The nail root is the buried proximal portion. The fold of skin which buries the root is the proximal nail fold. Epithelial growth and differentiation produce a thickened nail matrix under the root. The proliferation of this matrix and its keratinization result in growth of the nail. The process produces quantities of a substance termed hard keratin, which is high in sulfur content and firmly polymerized to prevent desquamation. The nail grows in a distal direction, sliding over the malpighian layer of the nail bed. The nail bed itself is not involved in the process of nail formation; this process is limited to the nail matrix. Longitudinal dermal ridges rather than papillae are present and extend from the root to the distal end of the nail bed (Fig. 11.34).

Blood Vessels and Lymphatics

Arterial supply to the skin (Fig. 11.35) is distributed through two plexuses, one at the plane between hypodermis and dermis, and one at the plane between the papillary and reticular layers. The deeper plexus is supplied from major vessels in the hypodermis. Blood from the deep plexus flows downward through capillaries into the hypodermis. Branches from the deep plexus also course through the reticular layer of the dermis to the more superficial plexus. From the superficial plexus vessels ascend into the connective tissue papillae. Each papilla has one arterial vessel ascending into it and one venous channel leaving it. Venous drainage of the skin is through a series of three plexuses, two of them intimately associated with the two arterial plexuses and a third in the center of the dermis.

Arteriovenous anastomoses (Figs. 8.39 and 8.40) are frequent in the skin and are particularly noticeable in thick skin of the plantar surfaces where they may be seen as *glomi* (singular-glomus). Here the blood vessels connecting arteries and veins are coiled and their walls are much thickened by the presence of epithelioid cells. They are important in peripheral temperature regulation since by dilation they may allow blood to bypass superficial capillary beds.

The skin is richly supplied with lymphatics. They originate as blind vessels in the dermal papillae which drain into a horizontal meshwork of lymphatic capillaries in the papillary area. From here their course runs with the blood vessels into the hypodermis where an extensive plexus is present in close relationship to the plexus of blood vessels. Here the lymphatic vessels have valves and follow the characteristic regional pathways to the appropriate aggregate of lymph nodes.

Fig. 11.33. Distal segment of a digit to show the structure of a *nail* in relation to its surrounding tissues. (Based on Fig. 11.51 in Elias H., Pauly J. and Burns E. Histology. New York, John Wiley and Sons, 1978.)

Fig. 11.34. *Nail* shown in a scanning electron micrograph. All soft tissues have been removed and only the hard keratin nail plate is shown. The nail has been cut transversely and viewed obliquely to show the cut edge and the grooves on the lower surface which, in life, fitted into the longitudinal ridges of the nail bed. ×150. (Courtesy of W. H. Fahrenbach.)

Fig. 11.35. *Blood vessels of the skin.*

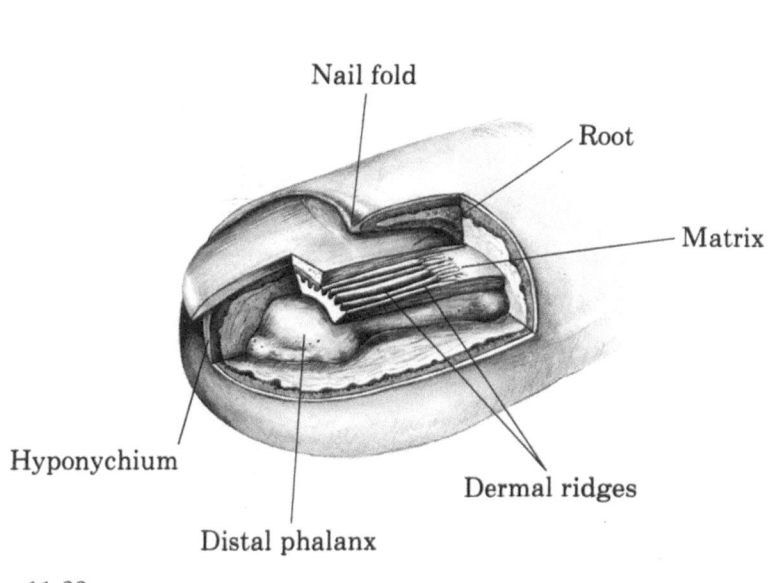

Nail fold

Root

Matrix

Hyponychium

Dermal ridges

Distal phalanx

11.33

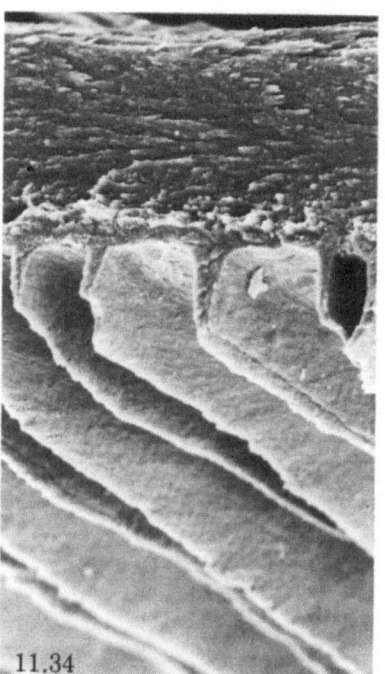

11.34

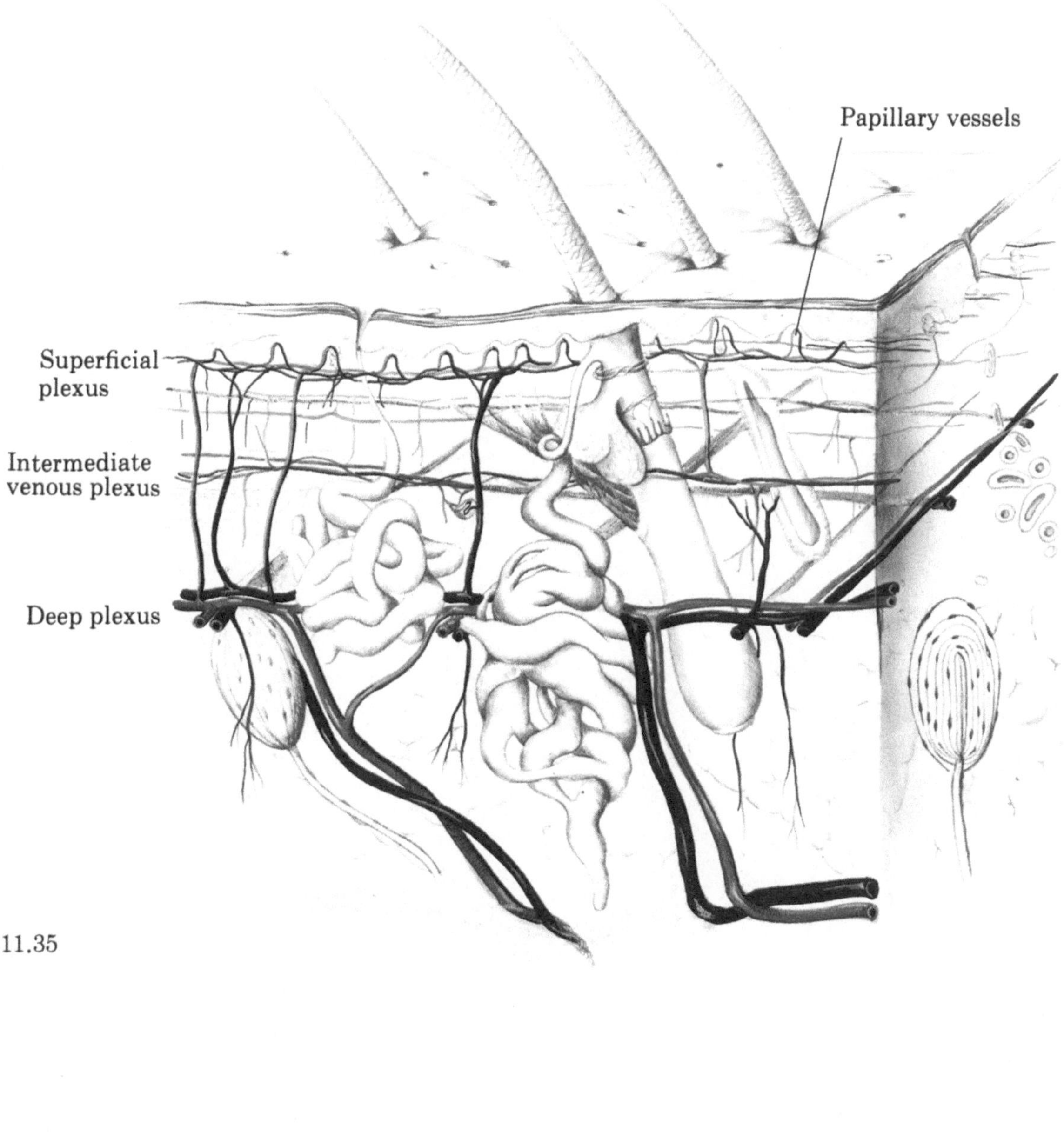

Papillary vessels

Superficial plexus

Intermediate venous plexus

Deep plexus

11.35

12 Digestive System, Tubular Portion

General Features of Structure and Function

The digestive system consists of (1) a convoluted 26-foot epithelium-lined tube (Fig. 12.1), and (2) a number of associated glands derived by evagination and extended growth of the epithelium into or through the other layers of the tube. This chapter deals with the first of these two major subdivisions.

Functional Organization

The digestive system is essentially an automated food processor that obtains substances required for growth and energy from ingested food. It contains arrangements for mechanical and chemical modification of its contents. Food placed in the *oral cavity* is quickly assessed by complex physical and chemical sensory processes for acceptability, requirements for mastication, amount of salivary dilution of salts, acids, and other items needed and amount of moistening required for dry materials. The appropriate program for mastication time, salivary mixing, bolus formation, and swallowing is then set in motion. After these first steps are taken, the bolus is passed on to the *pharynx*, the last point at which voluntary rejection can occur. As might be expected, this chamber contains striated (voluntary) muscle in its walls. From here food passes to the *esophagus*, which, by the action of both striated (voluntary) and smooth (involuntary) muscle in its walls, conducts it without modification through the chest into the abdomen, where most of the digestive organs are located. The esophagus passes food into the *stomach*, where it accumulates in the upper end in a more or less solid mass. The stomach mixes the food with enzymes and, after liquefying and hydrolyzing it at a pH of approximately 2, passes it on, a small amount at a time, to the *small intestine*. Here, appropriate enzymes are added to the gut contents from liver, pancreas, and mucosal glands (in amounts determined by advance information through endocrine and nervous mechanisms). Digestion is continued and most of the absorption of the products of digestion also occurs in the small intestine. From here, indigestible material is passed into the *colon*, where it is formed into fecal masses by dehydration. The addition of a lubricating mucous coating facilitates passage and eventual discharge through the *anus*.

Basic Structural Plan

It is apparent from the preceding brief functional summary that different levels of this tube have different purposes. As might be expected, they also have differences in structure, but a pattern persists throughout (Fig. 12.2). This fundamental pattern, except in the oral cavity, consists of four concentric layers. From the innermost to the outermost these are: *mucosa, submucosa, muscularis,* and *serosa* or *adventitia.*

THE MUCOSA (mucous membrane) consists of three concentric sublayers. The innermost is an *epithelium* that faces the lumen. In the digestive system this is normally either non-keratinized stratified squamous or simple columnar. It is a moist, flexible sheet of cells through which precursors of all the materials to be used in body functions must pass. Its delicacy makes the mucous membrane particularly vulnerable to damage and invasion. It is in direct contact with ingested materials, from which it must selectively absorb appropriate components.

Beneath the epithelium, and extending into any folds or projections a given region may possess, is the *lamina propria,* a supporting layer of loose connective tissue. This contains a large variety of cells, many of which are concerned with immunologic and other protective functions. Appropriately for these functions it often has localized accumulations of diffuse and/or nodular lymphoid tissue. Except in the mouth and pharynx, the deepest

Fig. 12.1. General anatomic organization of the *digestive tube;* digestive glands have been omitted. Most of the tube is compactly arranged in the abdominal cavity. The esophagus, without digestive function, simply conducts food through the thorax, which is occupied by components of other systems.

Fig. 12.2. Tissue architecture of the *digestive tube.* The various configurations of the mucosa and the three different locations of glands which exist in different organs of the tube are assembled in this diagram. In the background the tube is shown entering the abdominal cavity and being suspended from the abdominal wall by a double layer of the peritoneum, the mesentery. The layer of peritoneum covering the surface of the tube is the serosa. If the gut is directly applied to some other organ or to the wall of the abdomen, as shown in the foreground, the serosa is absent and the external coat is the adventitia.

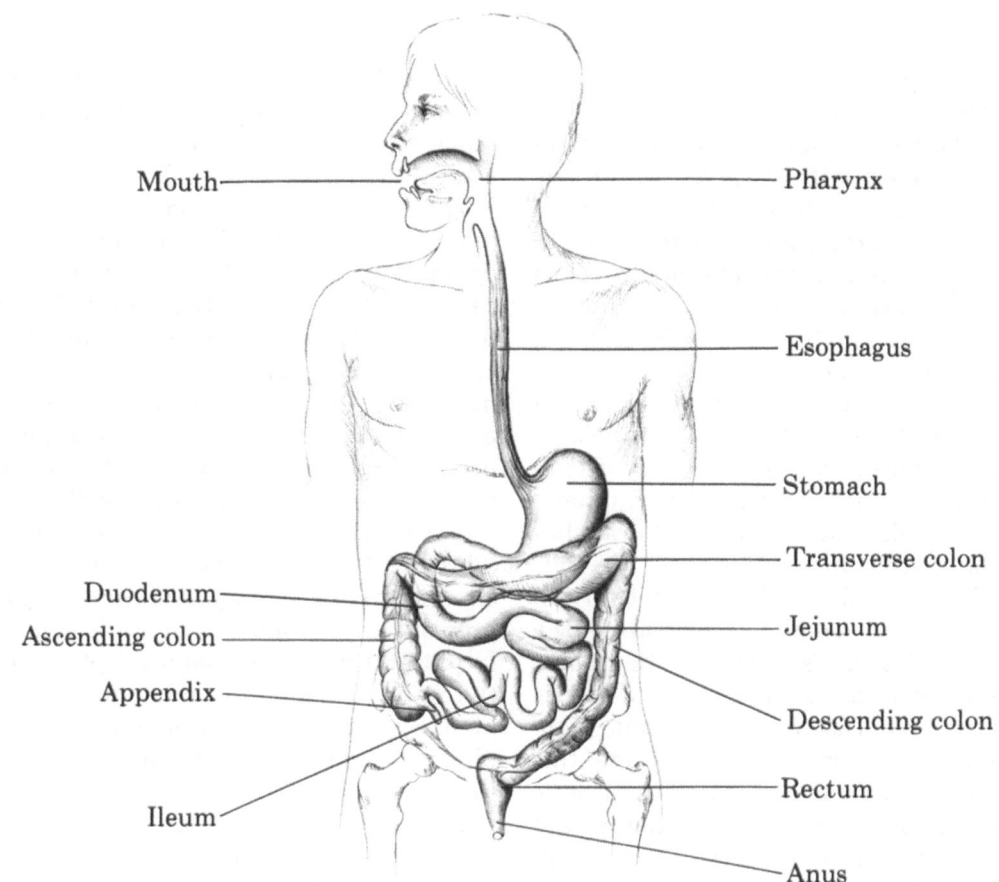

Mouth

Pharynx

Esophagus

Stomach

Transverse colon

Duodenum

Jejunum

Ascending colon

Appendix

Descending colon

Ileum

Rectum

Anus

12.1

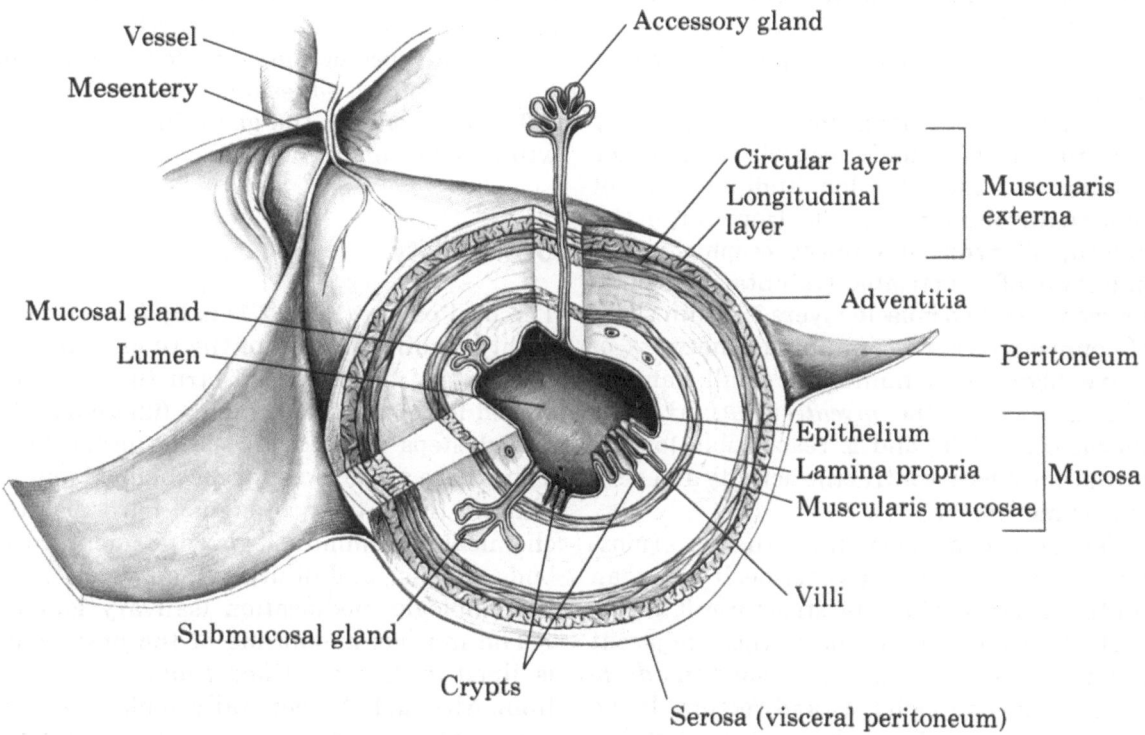

Vessel

Mesentery

Accessory gland

Circular layer
Longitudinal layer

Muscularis externa

Adventitia

Mucosal gland

Lumen

Peritoneum

Epithelium
Lamina propria
Muscularis mucosae

Mucosa

Submucosal gland

Villi

Crypts

Serosa (visceral peritoneum)

12.2

mucosal layer is a thin layer of smooth muscle, the *muscularis mucosae*.

The mucosa is the most variable layer of the digestive tract with respect to its histologic organization. It shows at each level of the system an arrangement appropriate to the function of that particular organ. Thus the principal diagnostic features distinguishing, for example, small intestine from colon, are to be found in the mucosa.

THE SUBMUCOSA, the next most peripheral layer, is one of distensible loose connective tissue. It contains a variable amount of lymphoid tissue and rich networks of lymphatic and blood vessels from which small branches supply the mucous membrane.

The submucosa also includes a network of nerves and small ganglia, constituting the *submucous* (Meissner's) *plexus,* the motor components of which control the muscularis mucosae and, at least to some extent, glandular secretion. Nerve fibers entering this plexus are preganglionic parasympathetic and postganglionic sympathetic fibers (see Chapter 7). These constitute the extrinsic innervation of the gut. The plexus itself, made up of neurons and connecting strands of nerve fibers, contributes to the intrinsic innervation of the tube. The other portion of this intrinsic innervation is the myenteric plexus (of Auerbach) (*see below*).

THE MUSCULARIS EXTERNA (often called simply the muscularis) usually consists of an inner circular and an outer longitudinal layer of smooth (involuntary) muscle. However, in the mouth, pharynx, and upper esophagus the muscle is of the striated (voluntary) variety. Between the two muscle layers is a thin sheet of connective tissue containing a network of nerve fibers with numerous small ganglia. This constitutes the *myenteric* (Auerbach's) *plexus* (Fig. 12.3), and is responsible for the initiation of local contractile activity and peristaltic movement.

THE SEROSA OR ADVENTITIA, the outermost layer, is of loose connective tissue. If the organ is attached to neighboring structures it blends with the connective tissue of these adjacent organs, and the layer is then termed an *adventitia,* as in the esophagus and rectum. If the tube is not bound to other organs, but lies in the abdominal cavity, attached by a mesentery to the body wall (Fig. 12.2), the connective tissue is covered by a layer of simple squamous epithelium and the layer is termed a *serosa* (Fig. 12.4).

The serosa, being smooth and lubricated, allows easy movement of the different organs against each other. This advantage, however, can be lost permanently as a result of an inflammatory process, as in peritonitis (Fig. 12.5), if this inflammation is followed by its natural sequel, fibrous adhesions between organs (Fig. 12.6). Abdominal surgery, with the necessary handling and retraction of tissues, may cause enough irritation of this delicate surface to cause the production of fibrous scar (fibrosis). Sometimes there may result only one or two fine stringy adhesions, or just one area of the peritoneal cavity may be involved. In patients who have had multiple operations the entire peritoneal cavity may be obliterated. Some of the fundamentals of this complex process of repair of injury are discussed in Chapter 20.

This fibrous obliteration of the peritoneal space is not necessarily a cause of any trouble at all but, on the other hand, it may threaten life. A single fibrous band may sharply kink the bowel and result in a point of obstruction as the band contracts with scarring. In some cases acute obstruction may occur years after formation of the adhesion.

The segments of the gastrointestinal tract will now be considered individually.

Oral Cavity

The oral cavity (Fig. 12.1) is by far the most highly modified region of the tubular part of the system, since special structures are required for each of its complex functions. The initial steps in food processing occur here. Thus there are devices for mechanical manipulation (lips, teeth, tongue, hard palate), chemical and immunologic assessment (taste buds, tonsils), and dilutional, enzymatic, and immunologic modification (salivary glands).

The mucous membrane of the oral cavity is lined with a stratified squamous epithelium. Although it is generally nonkeratinized, it may possess some degree of keratinization in those areas that are most often irritated or abraded. The submucosa is not sharply demarcated from the mucosa and may be absent in such areas as the hard palate and upper surface of the tongue. These later structures, along with the teeth, constitute the shearing and crushing surfaces of the food mill. In the hard palate the lamina propria blends with the periosteum; in the tongue it penetrates between the bundles of muscle.

The submucosa contains numerous clusters of mucous, serous or mixed (mucoserous) glands that constitute the minor salivary glands. Indeed, these are so numerous that it is difficult to prepare a section of oral mucosa that does not contain some of them. An important function of these and the major glands is the continuous moistening of the mucous membrane (for further details of the major glands see Chapter 13).

Lips

The lips (Fig. 12.7) are histologically a zone of transition from keratinized (epidermal) to nonkeratinized (mucosal) stratified squamous epithelium. The red margin is the zone where the keratin becomes less dense than on the skin. It is also more hydrated (therefore more transparent), and the connective tissue papillae become taller and carry capillary loops closer to the surface than in the skin. These three features explain the redness of the unpainted lip. Cancer of the lip is illustrated in Fig. 12.8.

Teeth

Teeth (Fig. 12.7) are rooted in the maxillary and mandibular bones. The deciduous, or baby, teeth and the permanent teeth are histologically similar. A tooth is basically a hollow column of hard *dentin*, 80% of which consists, as in bone, of calcium in the form of crystals of hydroxyapatite. The central cavity is termed the *pulp chamber* and has an opening, the *apical foramen,* at its deeper end. Blood vessels and nerves enter this foramen and pass through a narrow *root canal* into the connective tissue of the pulp chamber. A layer of cells termed *odontoblasts* coats the inner surface of the dentin and lies between

it and the pulp. Their function is to form and maintain dentin. The dentin contains countless long, narrow *dentinal tubules* radiating from the pulp chamber; each contains a cytoplasmic extension of an odontoblast, the *odontoblast process* (Fig. 12.9).

The *crown* projects into the oral cavity through the oral mucosa (in this area termed the *gingiva* or gum). *Enamel* coats the crown and is by far the hardest substance in the body. During development of the tooth it is secreted by ectodermal epithelial cells called *ameloblasts* in the form of tightly packed, long, thin prisms that become heavily calcified (enamel is 99% inorganic). Since the ameloblasts do not persist after a tooth is completed (contrary to the dentin-forming odontoblasts), enamel cannot be replaced if damaged by decay (caries) or trauma.

The *root* is set in an *alveolus* (socket) in the bone of the jaw. Roots are coated with bone-like substance called *cementum.* Bundles of collagen, with one end embedded in the cementum and the other in the periosteum of the alveolus, hold the tooth firmly in place and probably absorb some of the shock of the great pressures produced by the biting and chewing process. Collectively these anchoring bundles constitute the *periodontal ligament* (Fig. 12.10).

An almost universal problem is the disease periodontitis (Fig. 12.11), which is associated with inadequate oral hygiene. The resulting destruction of periodontal ligament causes loss of teeth and the infection may become life-threatening.

The cementum that coats the roots is similar in structure and composition to bone. Its thin areas near the crown are acellular, but toward the apex it becomes thicker and the *cementoblasts* that form it become entrapped in lacunae as *cementocytes* in much the same way that osteoblasts become osteocytes.

The Tongue

THE TONGUE (Fig. 12.12) is an organ for tasting and manipulating food as well as for speaking. It therefore has chemical sensors (*taste buds*), striated muscle, and mucosal projections (*papillae*).

Fig. 12.3. The *myenteric plexus,* a system of nerves (N) and ganglion cells (G) between layers of muscularis. ×250.

Fig. 12.4. The *serosa,* including mesothelium (arrow) and connective tissue (C), overlying *muscularis* (M). ×100.

Fig. 12.5. *Acute peritonitis.* All layers are infiltrated with neutrophils. The loose connective tissue (C) of the serosa is swollen by edema. Features of a vein (V) are partially obliterated by the inflammatory process. M, Muscularis. This occurred in a case of appendicitis. ×100.

Fig. 12.6. *Fibrous peritoneal adhesions,* binding the loops of bowel together in a single mass (arrows). This is a late complication of peritonitis. In addition to causing episodes of acute intestinal obstruction, which may constitute acute emergencies, such adhesions may make surgery difficult.

Fig. 12.7. *Lip, gum, and tooth* in a section through the lower jaw.

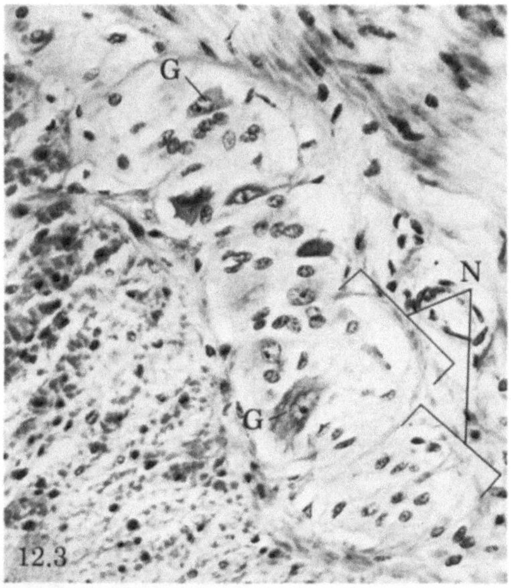

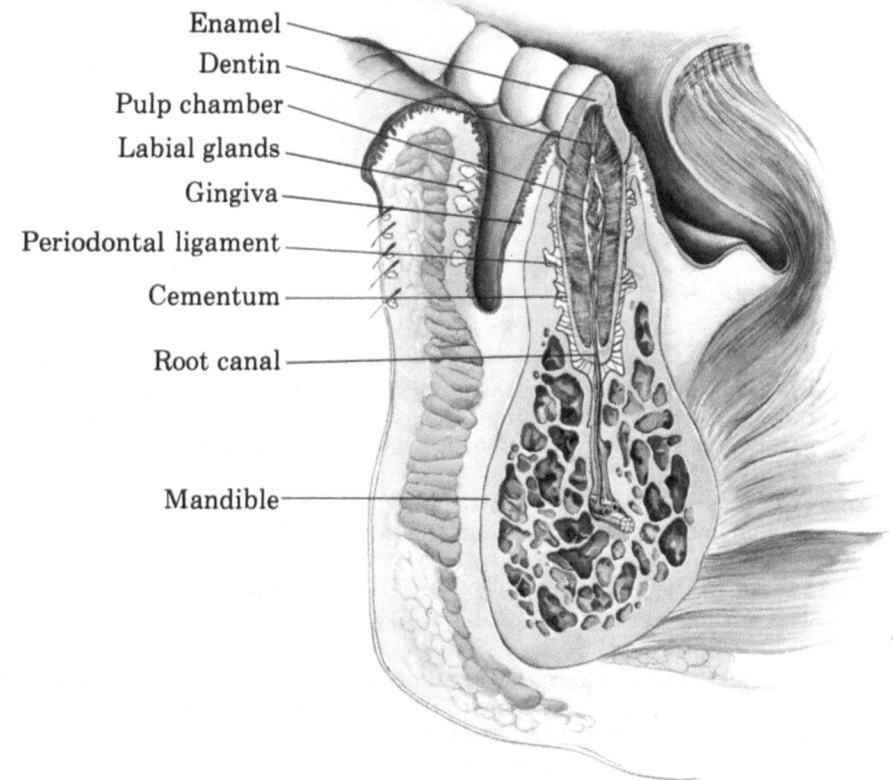

G
N
G
12.3

C
M
12.4

C
V
M
12.5

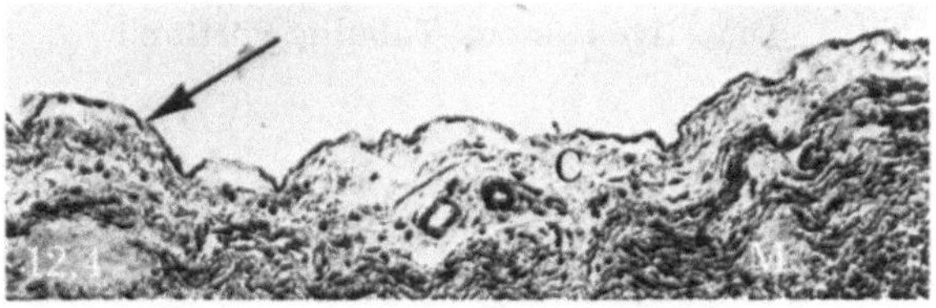

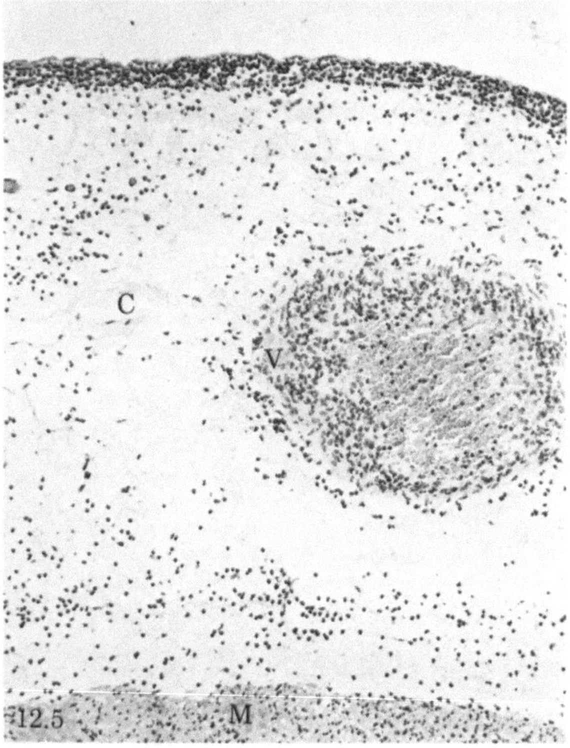

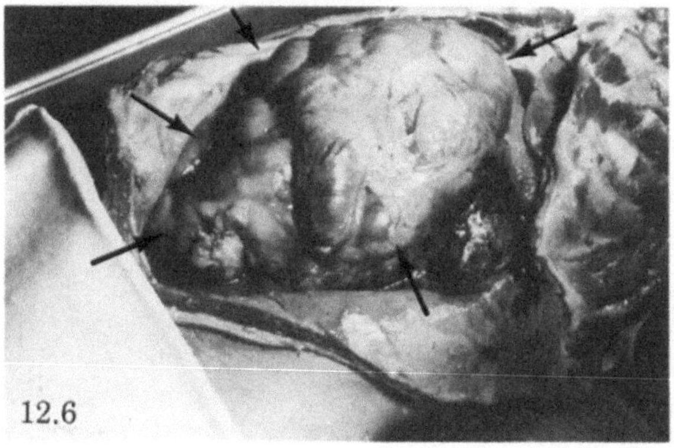

12.6

Enamel
Dentin
Pulp chamber
Labial glands
Gingiva
Periodontal ligament
Cementum
Root canal
Mandible
12.7

Fig. 12.8. *Epidermoid carcinoma of lip.* The tumor appears to have originated at the top of the lower lip (top). It has obliterated the mucosal epithelium on this surface. The limit of the tumor is easily identified (arrows). ×5.5.

Fig. 12.9. *Odontoblast processes* (arrow), extending from odontoblasts (0) in the pulp chamber, into the dentinal tubules (D). ×400.

Fig. 12.10. *Periodontal ligament* (arrows) fixes the tooth (T) to the bone (B) in the wall of the socket. ×85. (Courtesy of M. Bartley.)

Fig. 12.11. *Periodontitis,* the result of inadequate oral hygiene. Debris (De) accumulates next to the tooth (T) beneath the surface of the gingiva (G) calcifies and becomes adherent to the cementum. Epithelium (long arrow), accompanied by inflammatory cells (short arrows), migrates down from the surface, gradually destroying the periodontal ligament and loosening the tooth. ×25. (Courtesy of M. Bartley.)

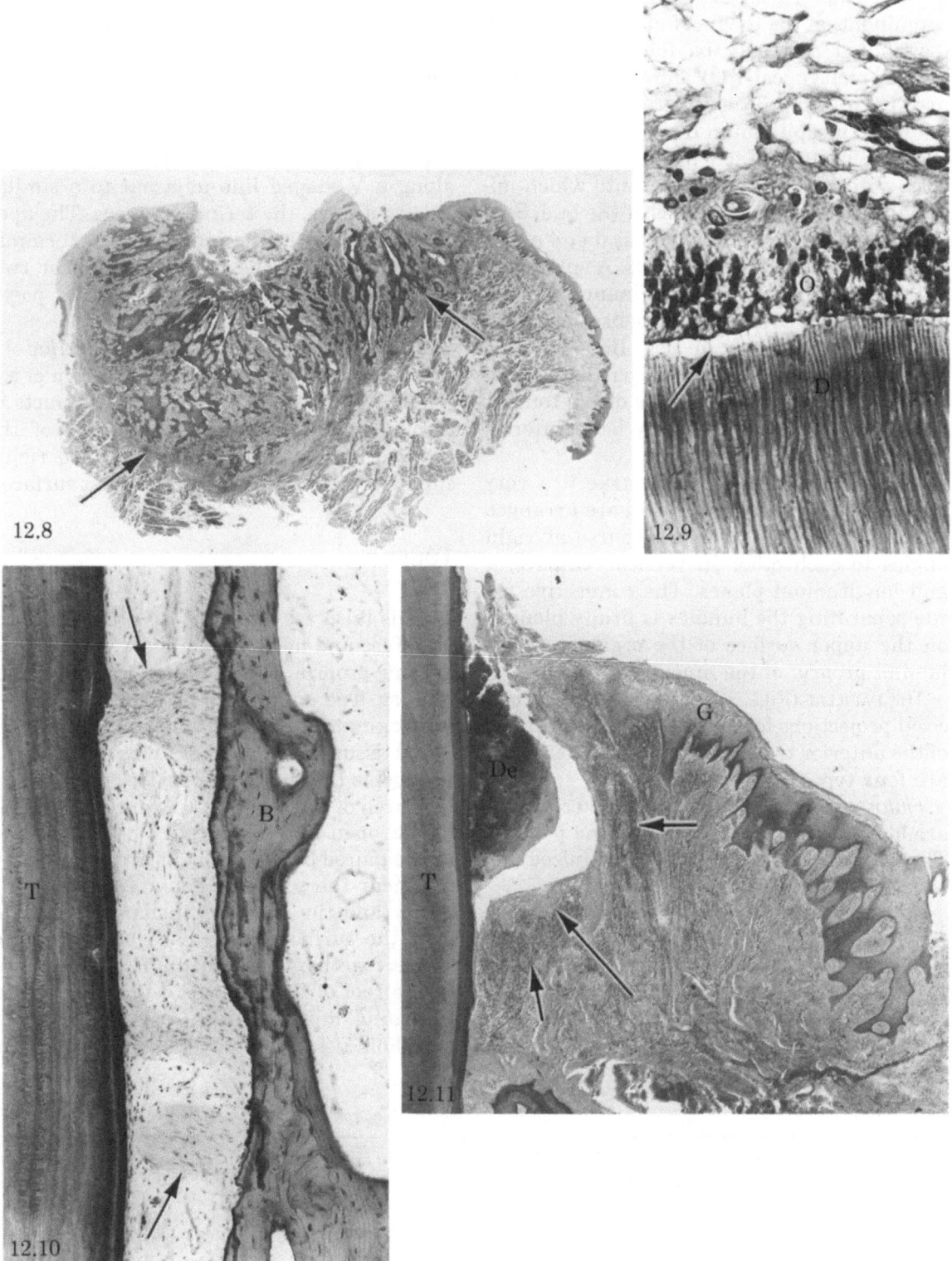

TASTE BUDS (Figs. 12.13 and 12.15) are most prominent on the tongue, but are also widely distributed and may be found in the soft palate, pharyngeal wall and epiglottis. They are barrel-shaped structures that extend through the epithelium from basal lamina to the free surface. Each has an opening, the *taste pore*, at the free surface into which microvilli project from the cells of the bud. Sensory nerve endings enter the basal end of the bud and ramify around its cells. A single bud is thought to respond predominantly to only one of the four primary taste sensations, that is, sweet, salty, bitter, or acid. Buds for each of these four have their own particular pattern of location on the surface of the tongue. A map of these locations may be of interest to wine-tasters.

THE MUSCLES of the tongue make it a very mobile organ, since their fibers are arranged in numerous bundles which course at right angles to each other in vertical, transverse and longitudinal planes. The connective tissue separating the bundles is firmly blended on the upper surface of the organ with the lamina propria of the mucosa.

THE PAPILLAE (Figs. 12.12 and 12.14) are mucosal projections located on the upper surface of the anterior two-thirds of the tongue. There are four types:

Filiform papillae are the most numerous and are long (about 2 mm), tapering, and pointed. Their epithelium is partially keratinized and therefore whitish in color.

Fungiform papillae are, as the name implies, mushroom-shaped. Their epithelium is non-keratinized and they therefore appear as small red spots. Some are provided with taste buds.

Vallate papillae (Fig. 12.15) are broad and circular in surface view, do not project above the surface, and are bounded by a deep moat and a circular ridge (vallum). In the walls of the moat are numerous taste buds. The fluid in the moat is provided by serous glands through ducts opening into its bottom. There are about a dozen vallate papillae arranged along a V-shaped line adjacent to a similar shaped groove, the terminal sulcus. The apex in this V is directed posteriorly. The terminal sulcus separates the papillate anterior two-thirds of the tongue from the tonsillar posterior one third.

Numerous *foliate* (leaf-like) *papillae* lie along each side of the posterior portion of the tongue. They overlap like shingles. Ducts of serous glands open in the bottoms of the grooves between them and they are richly supplied with taste buds on their flat surfaces.

TONSILS

Tonsils (also see Chapter 10) are aggregates of diffuse and nodular lymphoid tissue in the lamina propria of the oral and pharyngeal mucosa. The epithelium covering each tonsil is invaginated deeply into the underlying lymphoid tissue in the form of numerous branching crypts that increase considerably the surface area of the organ. A few ducts of mucous glands open into the crypts.

The paired *palatine* tonsils are placed laterally near the posterior boundary of the oral cavity and the *lingual* tonsils are scattered over the surface of the back of the tongue. These, together with a median tonsillar group in the roof of the pharynx and numerous intervening minor masses, provide a ring of lymphoid tissue (Waldeyer's ring) around the

Fig. 12.12. *Posterior surface of tongue and epiglottis.* Note vallate (V) and fungiform (arrows) papillae.

Fig. 12.13. *Taste buds* (arrows) cut in various planes. ×100.

Fig. 12.14. Tongue with three major varieties of *papillae,* vallate (V), fungiform (Fu), filiform (Fi).

Fig. 12.15. *Vallate papilla (V).* Serous glands (S) secrete into the trench, presumably affecting the function of the taste buds. ×38.

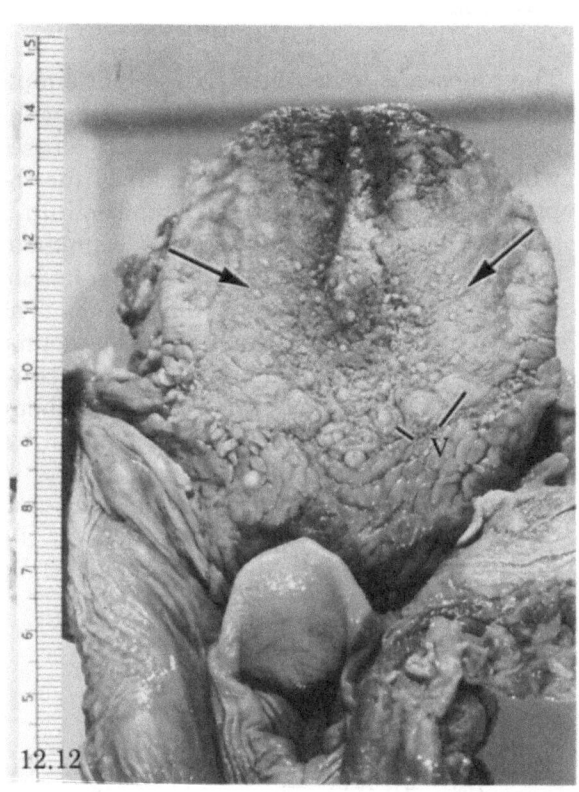

12.12

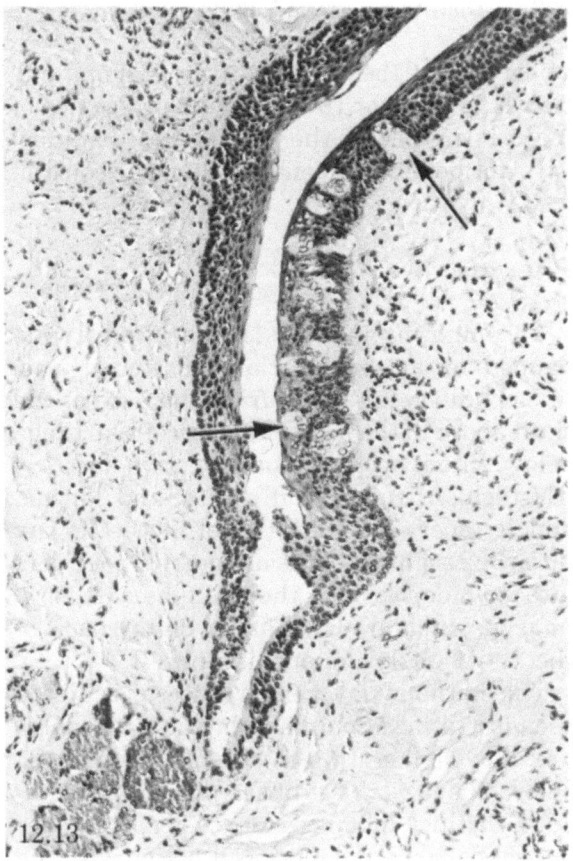

12.13

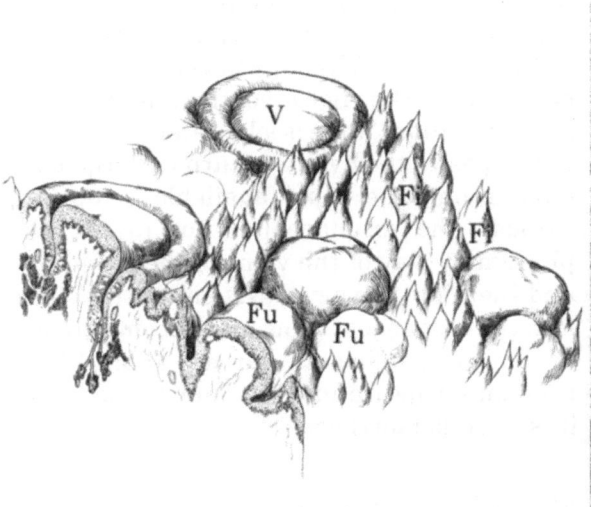

12.14

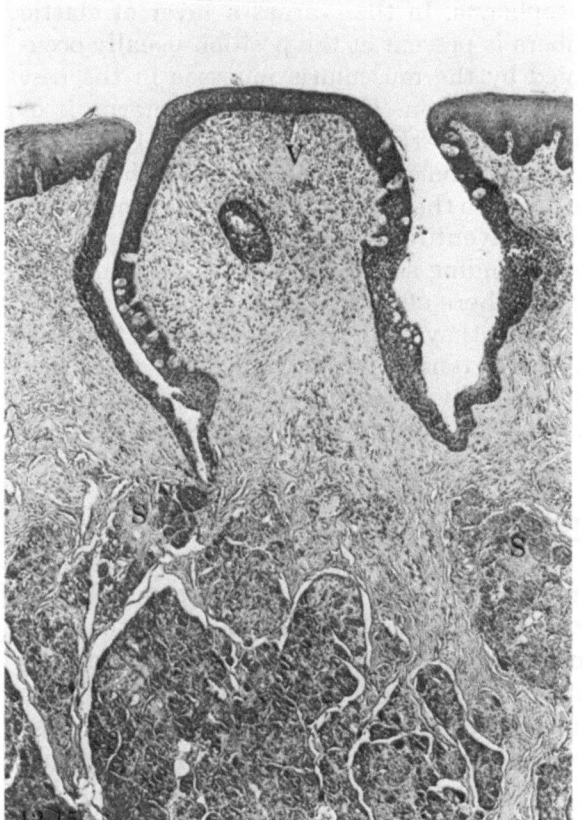

12.15

upper end of the digestive tract. Their function is to monitor the antigenic properties of materials entering the tube and to manufacture antibodies for their immunologic control.

Pharynx

The pharynx (Fig. 12.1) is a laterally expanded or anteroposteriorly flattened, saclike chamber extending from the base of the skull above to the level of the cricoid cartilage below. Into it opens the nasal cavity, auditory (Eustachian) tubes, oral cavity, and larynx, and it tapers below the level of the larynx into the esophagus. It is divided without definite boundaries into the nasopharynx, oropharynx, and laryngopharynx on the basis of the major chambers opening into it.

The epithelial layer of its mucosa is ciliated pseudostratified columnar in the nasaopharynx and nonkeratinized stratified squamous below this level. Most of the pharynx is without a distinct submucosa, except in its upper lateral portions and near its junction with the esophagus. In these areas a layer of elastic fibers is present at the position usually occupied by the muscularis mucosae in the rest of this system. The muscularis externa is of irregularly arranged bundles of skeletal muscle, the pharyngeal constrictors. These continue into the upper portion of the esophagus. The adventitia which binds the pharynx to surrounding structures is fibrous and strong and is here often termed a fibrosa.

Since they lie in the nasopharynx, the *pharyngeal* tonsils (termed adenoids when enlarged) have their crypts lined with pseudostratified ciliated columnar epithelium.

Esophagus

Beginning at the upper end of the esophagus the basic pattern of the digestive tube becomes more apparent (Fig. 12.16a) and remains so throughout the rest of the system. Here the muscularis mucosae appears first in the position of the elastic layer of the pharynx and the muscularis externa gradually becomes clearly organized into inner circular and outer longitudinal layers.

Mucosa

The mucosa is folded into six to eight simple longitudinal folds that extend throughout the length of the esophagus. These are erased when the circular muscle is relaxed for the passage of a bolus of food. The epithelium is generally nonkeratinized stratified squamous (Fig. 12.17). The lamina propria often has areas of diffuse lymphocytic infiltration. The muscularis mucosae is thickest in the esophagus (Fig. 12.16b) and may sometimes show inner circular and outer longitudinal fibers. At the upper end of the tube there are a few mucosal mucous glands similar to those in the pharynx. At its lower end, there are mucosal mucous glands similar to those in the cardiac portion of the stomach; hence the name *cardiac glands*.

Submucosa

Occasional mucous glands are present in this layer (Fig. 12.16b). They are usually fairly regularly spaced throughout the length of the tube, but are extremely variable in size and number among individuals. Their ducts, as seen in sections, are often widely dilated along part of their course, appearing to be cystic. In the submucosa also are located the larger blood vessels, lymphatics, and the submucous (Meissner's) plexus of nerves.

In cases of advanced cirrhosis of the liver, the flow of portal venous blood through this organ from the digestive tract may be obstructed. Blood then seeks alternate routes and bypasses the liver to return to the general circulation. One route available is upward through the esophageal hiatus in the diaphragm by way of the veins of the esophagus and then into the caval system. In this situation the esophageal veins may become greatly distended (esophageal varices) (Fig. 12.18); they may rupture into the lumen and result in severe hemorrhage.

Muscularis Externa

In the upper quarter or fifth of the organ this layer (Figs. 12.16a and 12.18) contains skeletal muscle representing a downward extension of the pharyngeal constrictors. This gradually becomes replaced by smooth muscle arranged in the usual pattern of inner circular and outer longitudinal layers. At the lower end of the esophagus the smooth muscle constitutes a physiologic sphincter that normally prevents regurgitation of stomach contents. There is hardly any histologic difference from that of the other smooth muscle of the gut, but here the muscle generally remains contracted except when food is passing downward.

Adventitia and Serosa

A loose connective tissue layer (adventitia) binds the organ to neighboring structures such as the aorta and the trachea. Below the level of the diaphragm, as the esophagus approaches its termination at the stomach, it is coated with peritoneal epithelium; thus here it is a serosa.

Stomach

The stomach is in general a gourd-shaped sac (Figs. 12.1 and 12.19), but demonstrates a wide range of form depending on its physiologic state. The esophagus empties into the right side of the expanded upper portion; the junctional zone between these two organs is termed the *cardia*. That portion of the sac above and to the left of the esophageal orifice is the *fundus*. The main portion of the stomach, the *body*, tapers to the *pylorus*, which is the narrow part of the gourd. The duodenum continues from the pylorus.

With respect to food manipulation, the organ behaves as if divided into upper and lower halves. The upper half is principally a food reservoir where semisolid material is held as it is received from the esophagus. Enzymes and hydrochloric acid are added and churning movements mix the contents. In the low pH provided, acid hydrolysis occurs and the digestion process continues. About a liter of gastric fluid is added after a meal's accumulation and the lower half of the stomach then contains a fluid suspension and solution of en-

zymes and partially digested food. This *chyme* is passed to the duodenum, a small quantity at a time, by peristalsis of the lower half of the stomach. Muscular activity throughout the stomach is so coordinated that volume changes during filling or emptying take place with little if any change in internal gastric pressure. As emptying progresses, muscle continues to contract and the mucosa throughout the organ is buckled into six to eight longitudinal folds termed *rugae*.

Mucosa

In addition to the rugae which have cores of submucosa, the general mucosal surface of the stomach is uniformly "quilted" with small, rounded domes of mucosa termed *gastric areas* (Fig. 12.20). Each of these is a few millimeters wide and separated from its neighbors by shallow trenches. At the microscopic level the mucosal surface is everywhere provided with invaginations to its surface epithelium, termed *gastric pits* or *foveolae* (Figs. 12.21 and 12.25). These number about 20,000/cm². Several glands open into the bottom of each pit.

A simple columnar epithelium lines the surface of the stomach and its pits. This is made up of *mucous surface cells* (Figs. 12.21 and 12.25). These differ from the goblet cells to be seen at lower levels of the system, both in their form and in the chemical makeup of the mucus precursors they contain. In this type of cell mucus does not appear to accumulate in the form of a single large droplet, but is continuously secreted onto the free surface, where it forms a protective barrier against the strong acid of the stomach contents. In the deeper portions of the gastric pits the cells are smaller, appear to be less highly differentiated and contain smaller amounts of mucus precursors. Autoradiographic studies indicate that the cells of the epithelial lining have a very high turnover rate and are replaced approximately every 3–5 days. The cells at the bottoms of the pits divide, migrate toward the surface, differentiate as they move and replace the cells lost into the lumen. The same zone of undifferentiated cells also provides replacements for cells dying or otherwise lost

Fig. 12.16. *Esophagus.* **a:** Mucosa (M), submucosa (S), muscularis externa (Me), and adventitia (Ad). ×24. **b:** Higher magnification of **a.** Note epithelium (E), lamina propria (L), muscularis mucosae (Mm), submucosa (S), submucosal gland (G), and duct (D). ×100.

Fig. 12.17. Scanning electron micrograph of *esophageal mucosal surface* showing desquamating surface cells. Because the epithelium is not keratinized nuclei are visible (arrows). ×200. (Courtesy of M. Webb.)

Fig. 12.18. *Varices of the esophagus.* Submucosal and other veins (V), seen here filled with blood, have enlarged and multiplied because of an obstruction to the normal flow of venous blood from the gut to the liver. ×17.

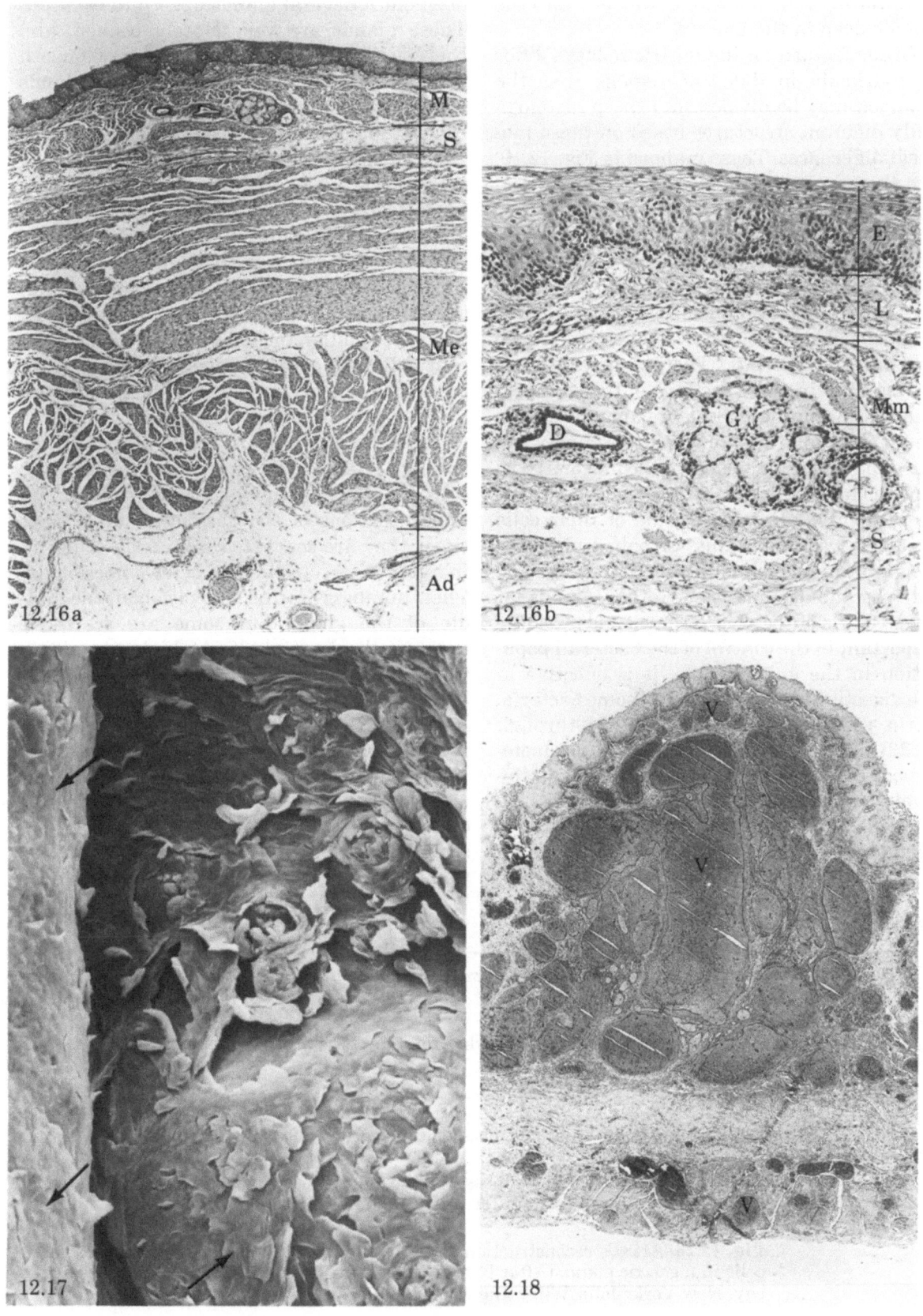

12.16a

12.16b

12.17

12.18

deeper in the glands. In this instance the differentiating cells migrate downward into the glands deep in the mucosa.

Other features of the gastric mucosa differ so markedly in different regions that the stomach may be divided into three histologically different structures based on these mucosal differences. These mapped in Fig. 12.19, are the (a) *cardia*, (b) *fundus and body*, and (c) *pylorus*.

CARDIA. In this area the mucosa is the thinnest to be found in the stomach. The gastric pits are short, widely spaced, and therefore fewer in number. Simple or branched tubular glands, coiled at their lower ends, open into the bases of the pits. The glands are more sparse than in other sections of the stomach, and there is a relatively large amount of connective tissue in the lamina propria between the glands. The glands are of the mucous type, but also have occasional enteroendocrine cells (*see below*), and at least some of their cells produce lysozyme. This carbohydrate-splitting enzyme, which is also secreted by some salivary glands and some other glands at lower levels of the digestive tract, is probably important in the control of the bacterial population in the gut contents. It is effective in the digestion of the cell walls of some bacteria.

THE FUNDUS AND BODY (Figs. 12.21 through 12.23) are anatomically two regions, but histologically one. Here the gastric pits are relatively shallow, constituting from one-fifth to one-fourth of the thickness of the mucosa. The remainder of the layer of mucosa is filled with long, relatively straight, closely packed, parallel *gastric glands* that often branch at their deep ends. Several glands open into each pit. These glands are very closely packed, and there is little lamina propria. Slips of smooth muscle extend upward between the glands from the muscularis mucosae. Gastric glands contain four types of cells: *mucous neck cells, parietal cells, chief cells*, and *enteroendocrine cells*.

Most of the mucous neck cells (Fig. 12.22) are located in the narrow necks of the gastric glands near their junction with the gastric pits, but they are also present in smaller numbers throughout the upper third of the glands. They are smaller and darker than surface mucous cells and contain apical secretory granules with mucus precursors different from those of other mucous cells.

Parietal cells (oxyntic cells) (Figs. 12.21 through 12.23) are large, strongly eosinophilic cells, and are particularly numerous in the upper portions of the gastric glands. Sometimes they are separated from each other by individual, or clusters of a few, neck cells. Their numbers drop off sharply about the middle of the gland, but some are scattered through the lower half. At high magnifications of the light microscope they have a "fried egg" appearance, with the yolk represented by the nucleus and the white by the cytoplasm. They often appear to be squeezed to the periphery of the gland by neighboring mucous or chief cells, hence the adjective parietal. With the electron microscope they are seen to have an extensive, complex invagination of apical cytoplasm lined with numerous

Fig. 12.19. *Geography of the stomach.* The height and width of the folds vary with the degree of distention.

Fig. 12.20. *Gastric mucosa* showing raised gastric areas (A) varying in length, but each is about 0.5 mm in width.

Fig. 12.21. *Mucosa of the gastric corpus* showing the characteristic mixture of cell types. Note pits (Pi) and mucous, parietal (arrow) and chief (C) cells. ×85.

Fig. 12.22. *Glands* of the mucosa of the *corpus* with parietal (P), chief (C) and mucous (M) cells. Jones stain for reticulum and mucus. ×400.

Fig. 12.23. Artist's reconstruction of a *parietal cell.* Inset shows chief and parietal cells in a gastric gland. (After Fig. 12.36 in Elias H., Pauly J.E., Burns E.R. Histology. New York; John Wiley and Sons, 1978.)

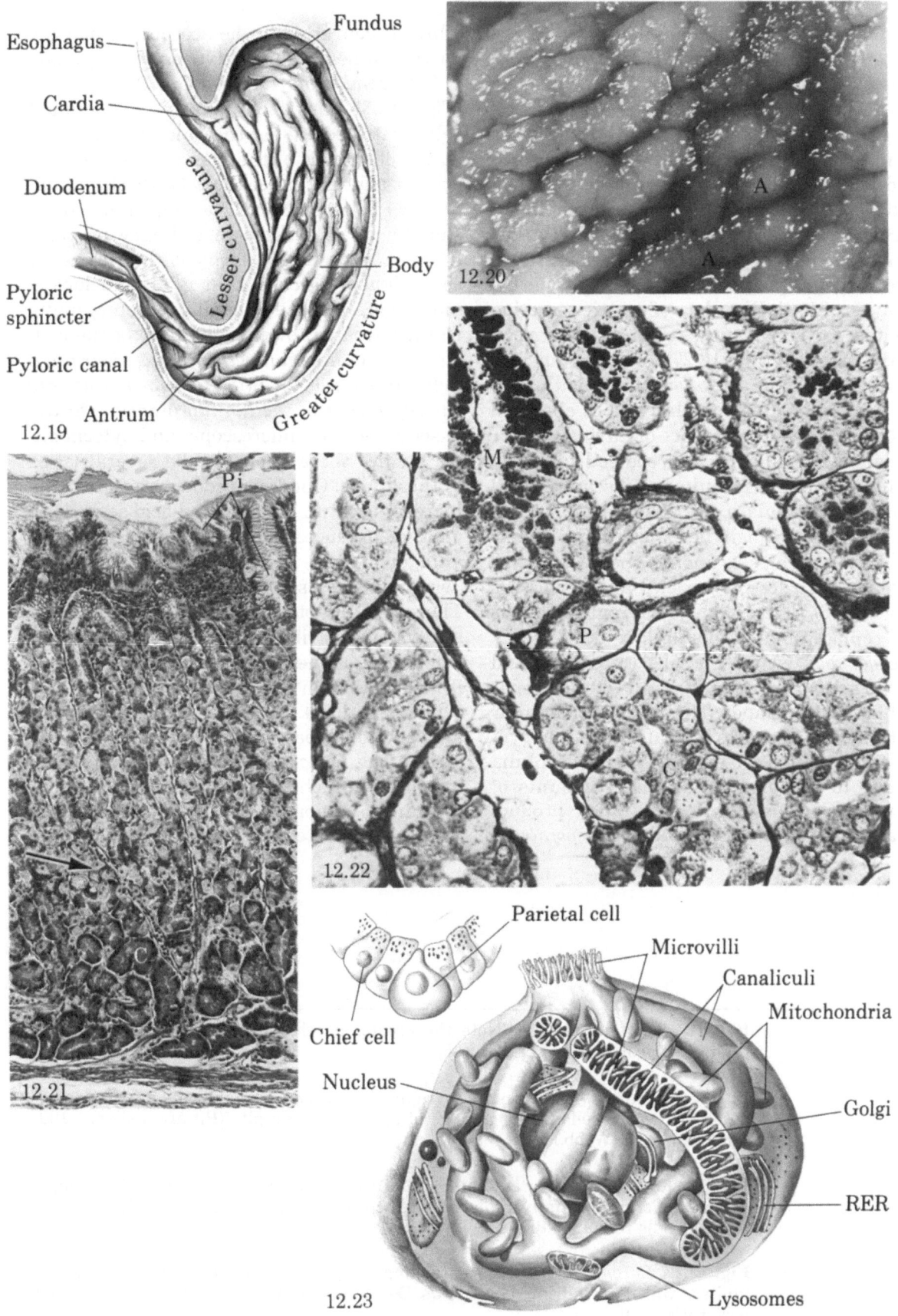

Esophagus

Fundus

Cardia

Duodenum

Lesser curvature

Pyloric
sphincter

Pyloric canal

Antrum

Body

Greater curvature

12.19

12.20

A

A

M

P

C

Pi

C

12.21

12.22

Parietal cell

Microvilli

Canaliculi

Mitochondria

Chief cell

Nucleus

Golgi

RER

Lysosomes

12.23

microvilli. This invagination is termed the *secretory canaliculus* (Fig. 12.23). The cytoplasm contains numerous large mitochondria, indicating that their metabolic activities require considerably more energy than those of most cells. Parietal cells produce 0.16 *M* hydrochloric acid and a glycoprotein called *intrinsic factor*. The acid is responsible for the low pH of gastric juice (0.9 to 2.0) that converts inactive proteolytic enzymes to active forms and provides the medium for acid hydrolysis of food. Disorders of gastric secretion related to acidity may result in ulceration of the stomach (Fig. 12.27) or duodenum.

Intrinsic factor (*see above*) binds with vitamin B_{12} to make a complex that is absorbed in the ileum. In the absence of intrinsic factor the vitamin cannot be absorbed and a B_{12} deficiency occurs. This results in a disease termed pernicious anemia, a disorder of red blood cell maturation. As might be expected, the gastric mucosa in pernicious anemia shows extensive atrophy with loss of parietal and chief cells (Fig. 12.26). These highly differentiated cells are replaced by mucous neck cells.

Chief cells (zymogenic cells) (Figs. 12.21 and 12.22) are the predominant cells of the deeper half of gastric glands. They are low columnar in form, with features typical of cells that synthesize proteins for export. Their basophilia is due to the presence of large amounts of rough endoplasmic reticulum. Their product is an inactive enzyme precursor, *pepsinogen,* which is converted in the acid medium of the gastric lumen to an active protease *pepsin.*

Enteroendocrine (argentaffin, APUD) *cells* (Figs. 12.37 and 12.38) appear as individual cells scattered among the chief cells near or at the deep ends of the glands. They require special staining procedures (with chromium or silver salts) for identification, but can occasionally be recognized in ordinary preparations because their polarity is the reverse of the neighboring cells; that is, the nucleus is more apical and the Golgi and secretory material are located towards the base of the cell. *As they are endocrine cells, most of their products are passed not into the lumen, but into the capillaries of the lamina propria.* On the basis of electron microscopic and cytochemical studies there appear to be several types of these cells. One type produces gastrin (this increases gastric motility and acid secretion); another produces enteroglucagon (an insulin antagonist) and another produces serotonin (which induces smooth muscle contraction). There may be others. Enteroendocrine cells are widely distributed throughout the stomach and intestines and additionally discussed in the section on small intestine.

IN THE PYLORUS (Fig. 12.24) the gastric pits are very deep, reaching halfway from the surface to the muscularis mucosae. The glands are short, branched, tubular, and mucous and contain occasional enteroendocrine cells. They also secrete lysozyme.

Fig. 12.24. *Pyloric mucosa.* Note the greater depths of the gastric pits (Pi) here than in the corpus (Fig. 12.21). ×85.

Fig. 12.25. Scanning electron micrograph of *gastric mucosa* showing a surface composed of mucous cells (M). Openings of several gastric pits (Pi) are visible. ×190. (Courtesy of M. Webb.)

Fig. 12.26. *Chronic gastritis* (section from the corpus of the stomach). The glands are atrophic and partially replaced with chronic inflammatory cells. No chief or parietal cells remain. ×85.

Fig. 12.27. *Chronic gastric ulcer* extending completely through the muscularis, the limits of which are indicated by arrows. Dense connective tissue (scar) has prevented perforation. ×6.

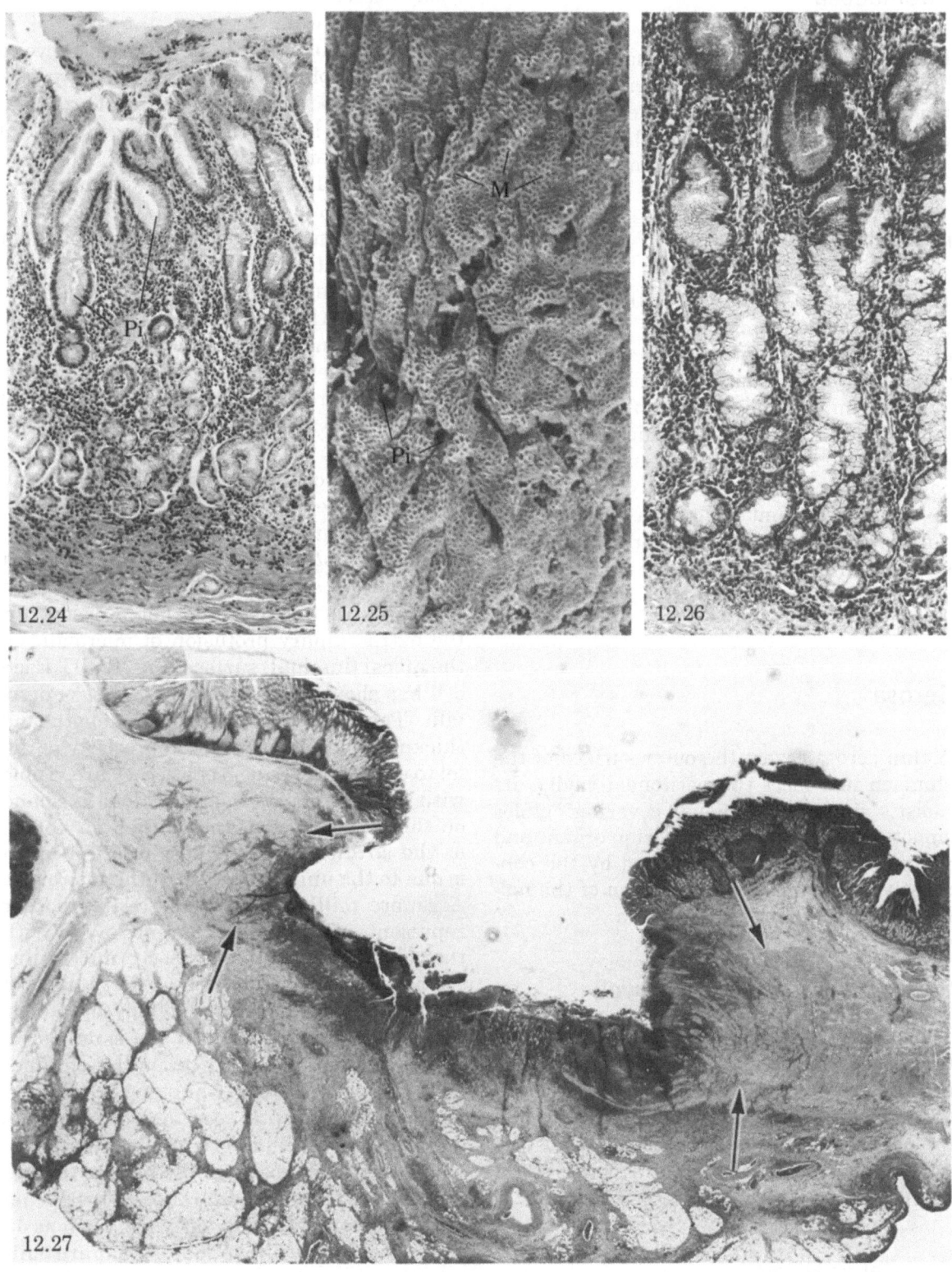

12.24

12.25

12.26

12.27

Submucosa

In this layer are located the usual larger blood and lymph vessels and a sparse submucous nerve plexus. The submucosa contains more numerous mast cells and lymphoid cells than it does at other levels of the gut.

Muscularis Externa

This has three, rather than the usual two, layers of smooth muscle, and their bundles are less highly organized. The outer layer is generally longitudinal, the middle circular, and the inner oblique. The middle circular is the most regular and is thickened at the pylorus to form the pyloric sphincter. This sphincter normally assures the delivery of the appropriate amount of stomach content to the duodenum. The small diameter of the lumen at this point makes the pylorus a site where slight distortion in the lumen may cause obstruction.

Serosa

A thin serosa covers the outer surface of the stomach and faces the peritoneal cavity. Its moist, simple squamous covering glides smoothly over that of neighboring organs and permits the movement required by the constantly changing size and position of the hollow parts of the digestive system.

Small Intestine (Small Bowel)

This portion of the digestive tube, about 6 meters in length, begins at the pylorus and ends at the ileocecal junction (Fig. 12.1). Its digestive and absorptive functions are integrated by neural and hormonal controls, most of which originate within the digestive system itself.

General Features

Although the small intestine is subdivided into three regions or divisions (duodenum, jejunum, and ileum) the basic tubular plan already described (Fig. 12.2) is apparent in any section of its wall.

THE STRUCTURE OF THE MUCOSA, just beyond the pyloric sphincter, changes abruptly; this is the pyloroduodenal junction. Three features appear here: *villi, intestinal crypts* (of Lieberkuhn) and *plicae circulares*.

Villi (Figs. 12.28 through 12.33) are small (0.5–1.5 mm) mucosal projections into the intestinal lumen. They are present throughout the small intestine. They vary from leaf-shaped in the upper portion (duodenum) to finger-like in the lower portion (ileum). In histologic sections they are diagnostic of small intestine. They increase the absorptive surface area approximately six times that which would be provided by a similar tube without them.

The simple columnar epithelium of the villi contains three types of cells: *absorptive* cells, *goblet* cells, and *enteroendocrine* cells.

The *absorptive* cells are by far the most numerous. They are of typical columnar form and not structurally remarkable except for the extraordinary profusion of microvilli on the apical (luminal) surface (Fig. 12.31). Each cell has about three thousand of these microvilli. They are very uniform in length and thickness, closely packed and precisely parallel to each other. In aggregate they are visible with the light microscope in sections as a band on the free surface of the epithelium known as the *striated border,* whose uniform width is due to the uniform length of the microvilli. A square millimeter of this striated border represents about 200 million microvilli. With the electron microscope each microvillus seems to be covered with a fuzzy coat of branching, tree- or shrub-like, glycoproteins. Although most digestion in the small intestine is carried out in its lumen by enzymes from the pancreas (see Chapter 13), this surface coat apparently contains components which serve as binding sites for substances which are to be absorbed directly or further broken down before absorption. This breakdown is accomplished by enzymes (such as disaccharidases and dipeptidases) that are built into the plasmalemma of the microvilli.

There is a group of diseases characterized by the single term *malabsorption.* In some cases genetic defects are responsible. Damage to microvilli and abnormalities of their enzymes are possibly involved. The intestinal mucosa may undergo marked distortion (Fig. 12.34), which is sometimes reversible.

Mechanisms of cellular intake include *diffusion* down the gradient from lumen to blood and *active transport* (including *pinocytosis*) across the cell membranes. Throughout most of the life span, this latter process takes in well-digested food products. However, in the infant, where passive immunity is to be developed by the pinocytotic intake of maternal milk-borne antibodies, undigested proteins may be absorbed. Thus an infant may produce antibodies to some dietary proteins absorbed in this manner and subsequently be allergic to them.

Free fatty acids and monoglycerides resulting from the digestion of triglycerides by pancreatic lipase are emulsified by bile in the intestinal lumen and absorbed as micelles into the cytoplasm of the columnar cells. In the SER they are reassembled into triglycerides. The Golgi apparatus then builds these into complex glycolipoproteins and packages them as membrane bound droplets (*chylomicrons*). The droplets pass first by exocytosis into the space between the epithelial cells, then basally through the basement membrane into the lamina propria where they enter the central lymphatic channel (*lacteal*) of the villus.

As described in Chapter 3, *goblet cells* (Figs. 12.35 and 12.36) are unicellular, mucus-secreting glands. Here in the intestine they are scattered among the absorptive cells. Relatively sparse in the duodenum, they gradually become more abundant in the ileum. To reiterate further, the cup-shaped apical region of a mature goblet cell is packed with droplets of mucigen. The nucleus is crowded toward the base of the cell and is often flattened. The close packing of the droplets and their thin membranes produce an appearance in the light microscope of one large drop occupying the upper portion of the cell. The product, *mucin,* a concentrated protein-polysaccharide complex, is hydrated when secreted to form *mucus.* This viscous lubricant protects the lining of the gut from its destructive contents. The protein component of mucigen is synthesized in the RER. The formation of polysaccharides, their linking to protein and their sulfation apparently occur in the Golgi apparatus. Release of the mucus is by exocyto-

sis of fused droplets. This is apparently a continuous process throughout the 2–4-day lifespan of the cell.

Enteroendocrine cells (argentaffin cells, APUD cells) (Figs. 12.37 and 12.38), appropriately to their internal secretory function, rest on the basement membrane and taper toward the lumen, which they may or may not reach. Their products are released from the deep surface into the lamina propria and its vessels. These hormones are distributed throughout the body, but only certain tissues respond.

In the duodenum several types of enteroendocrine cells are present. One produces *secretin,* which acts on the pancreatic ducts to control the pH and ionic makeup of the pancreatic secretion. This allows neutralization of acid materials coming from the stomach. It also permits the appropriate digestive enzymes to be activated and alkaline hydrolysis to occur. Another cell type produces a gastric inhibitory polypeptide. Others produce *cholecystokinin* (pancreozymin) in response to the entrance of stomach contents from the pylorus. This substance stimulates contraction of the gall bladder and release of enzymes from the pancreatic secretory cells. Still others, not limited to the duodenum, produce *somatostatin* (see Chapter 16) and probably other substances not yet identified. As in the stomach, a glucagon-like compound (see Chapter 16) is secreted here.

The lamina propria forms a core for each villus (Figs. 12.32 and 12.33). It has large numbers of lymphocytes, plasma cells, eosinophils, and macrophages, all residing in a meshwork of reticular and small collagenous fibers. Local aggregations of diffuse lymphoid tissue may be seen. Each villus contains, in addition to a network of capillaries, a central lymphatic channel termed a *lacteal,* into which absorbed fats are passed. This begins blindly near the tip of the villus and drains into the larger vessels of the submucosa. Parallel to the lacteal are strands of smooth muscle which contract the villus several times per minute, acting as a pump to force absorbed materials from the lacteal into the larger channels. These muscle strands are extensions from the muscularis mucosae.

Intestinal crypts (of Lieberkuhn) (Fig. 12.32) are simple, straight, tubular, glandular invaginations of the mucosa. Their mouths lie at

Fig. 12.28. *Small intestine* showing plicae (P), their fuzzy coating of villi, and circular (large arrow) and longitudinal (small arrow) layers of the muscularis. ×7. (Courtesy of P. Stenzel.)

Fig. 12.29. Scanning electron micrograph of inner surface of *small intestine.* ×100. (Courtesy of M. Webb.)

Fig. 12.30. Longitudinal section of *small intestine* with plicae (P), villi (V), submucosa (S), and circular (large arrow) and longitudinal (small arrow) layers of muscularis externa. ×8.

Fig. 12.31. Electron micrograph of *intestinal epithelium.* Note microvilli (arrow), lamina propria (Lp), and endothelium (E). ×2500. (Courtesy of R. S. Connell.)

Fig. 12.32. *Small intestine* with three basic features: villi (V); crypts (C); and goblet cells (arrows). ×100.

Fig. 12.33. Cross-section of a *villus* showing striated border (arrow), lacteal (La) and vein (Ve). ×400.

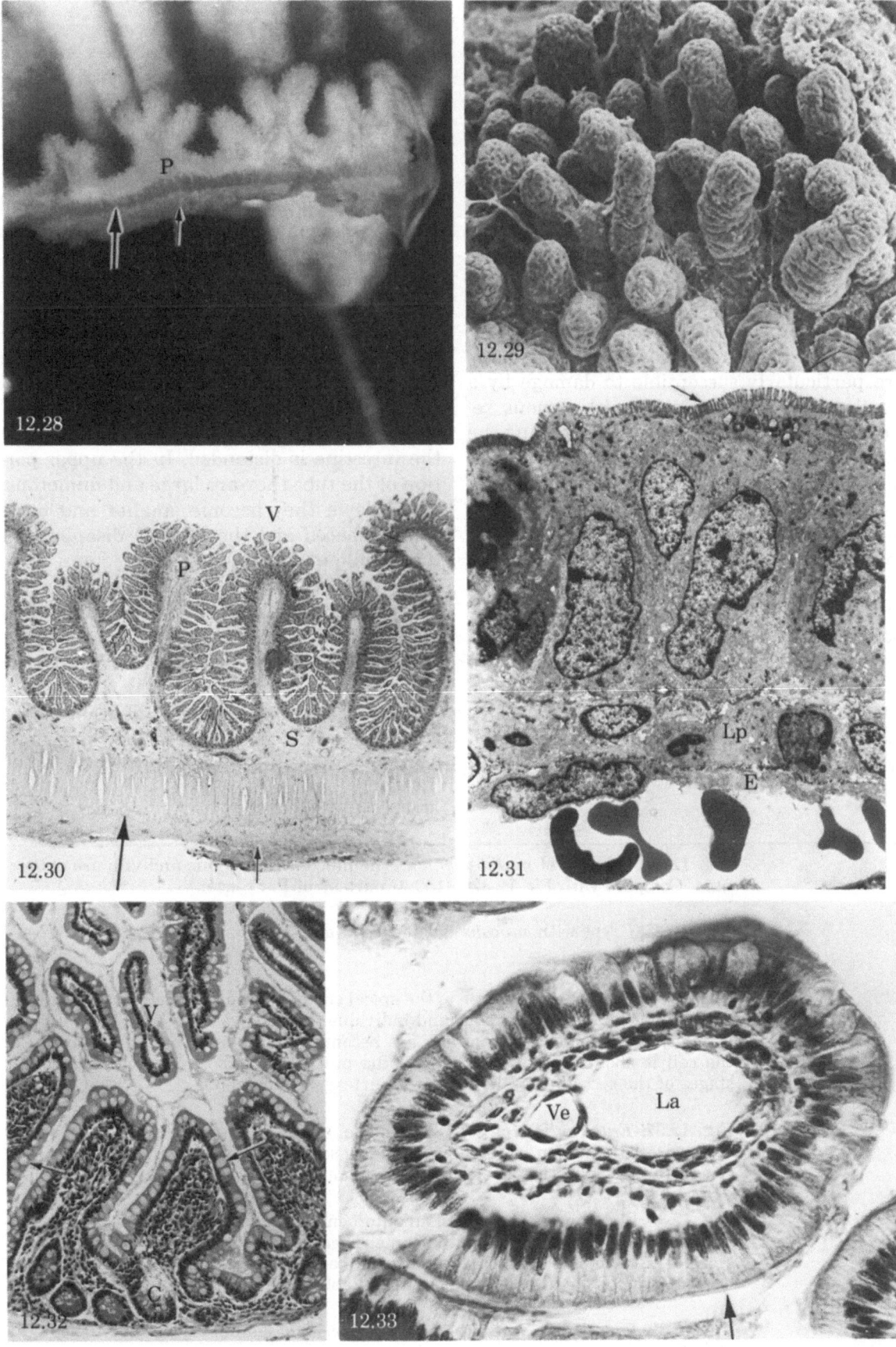

12.28

12.29

12.30

12.31

12.32

12.33

the bases of the villi and they extend nearly to the muscularis mucosae. Their lining epithelium is similar to that of the surface epithelium of the villi except that two additional cell types are present in the bottom of the crypts. Of primary importance are the *undifferentiated cells* which divide to produce replacements for epithelial cells shed from the villi. The differentiating cells resulting from this mitotic activity migrate upward; they are shed near the tip of the villus about five days after the mitosis which produced them. Since these stem cells are actively dividing, they are particularly susceptible to damage by a number of noxious agents, with serious results. The devastating impact of shedding the intestinal epithelium without replacing it may well be imagined. Major symptoms of radiation sickness and some of the side effects of cancer chemotherapy are due to damage to dividing cells in the intestinal crypts.

The Paneth cells (Fig. 12.39), found in groups in the deepest portions of the intestinal crypts, contain numerous, usually large, secretory granules which stain intensely with eosin. Although they are rather striking cells, very little is known about their function. They have a higher than usual content of zinc, and lysozyme has been detected in their granules.

They are probably involved in the control of the bacterial population of the digestive tract, but this is not known with certainty. They have a lifespan of about 30 days, much longer than that of other cells of the mucosal epithelium.

Plicae circulares (Figs. 12.28, 12.30, and 12.40) are transverse, crescent-shaped folds of mucosa projecting up to 1 cm into the lumen of the small intestine. Each extends part way around the intestine and its ends overlap with those of its neighbors. Some may completely encircle the lumen in a spiral fashion. The center support of each fold is a ridge of submucosa. These are permanent, surface-increasing structures that do not flatten when the intestine is distended. In the upper portion of the tube they are large and numerous; lower down they become smaller and more widely spaced and they finally disappear in the middle or lower ileum.

The lamina propria of the small intestine occupies the space between the epithelium and muscularis mucosae, wrapping the intestinal crypts and extending as cores into the villi.

The muscularis mucosae, as at other levels, is the deepest layer of mucosa and marks its boundary with the submucosa.

Fig. 12.34. Changes of *malabsorption*. The mucosa is atrophic and villi are obliterated. Compare with Fig 12.32. ×150. (Courtesy of P. Stenzel.)

Fig. 12.35. Crypt with *mucous* (goblet) *cells* and *lamina propria*. ×320. (Courtesy of R. Sauter.)

Fig. 12.36. Electron micrograph of the apical end of a mature *goblet cell* of intestinal epithelium. The membranes around individual mucous vesicles have broken down in many places and their contents are becoming confluent. The apical surface of the cell is about to open and release the mucus. Neighboring cells are in other stages of the secretory cycle. ×4250. (Courtesy of M. Webb.)

Fig. 12.37. *Enteroendocrine cells.* The nuclei (large arrows) are on the side of the cell nearest the lumen of the gland and the secretory granules (small arrows) are closest to the connective tissue. Toluidine blue stain. ×520. (Courtesy of B. Naylor.)

Fig. 12.38. Electron micrograph of an enteroendocrine cell from an intestinal crypt. Below and to the left, toward the lumen, are nuclei of two epithelial cells. The secretory granules of the enteroendocrine cell are located between nucleus and basal lamina (B). ×7400. (Courtesy of M. Webb.)

Fig. 12.39. *Paneth cells* with granules in the bases of jejunal crypts. ×400. (Courtesy of R. Sauter.)

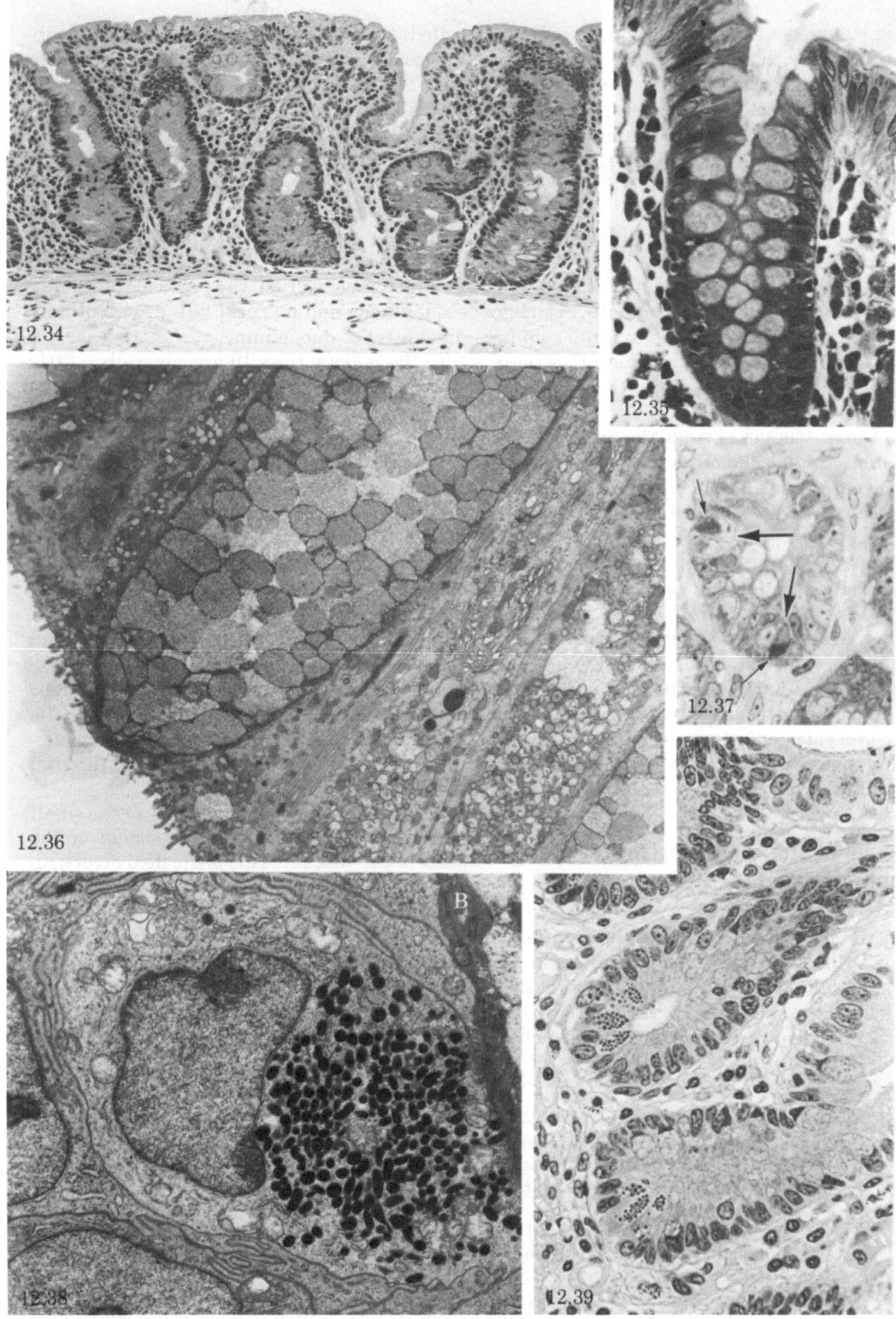

12.34

12.35

12.36

12.37

12.38

12.39

THE SUBMUCOSA is a layer of connective tissue containing a rich plexus of blood vessels that have penetrated through the muscularis externa and that send branches through the muscularis mucosae into the lamina propria. The submucous plexus of nerves is also located here. The larger lymphatic vessels in this zone form meshes around lymph nodules and through the diffuse lymphoid tissue. They anastomose profusely and the larger ones accompany the blood vessels out of the system. They then enter regional lymphatic drainage patterns. In the upper duodenum the submucosa contains mucous glands that are strictly limited to that level. They will be discussed below.

In the MUSCULARIS EXTERNA the basic pattern of inner circular and outer longitudinal muscle layers obtains. The connective tissue sheet between them is occupied by the myenteric plexus.

SEROSA. The outer surface of the muscle is coated with a layer of loose connective tissue which is covered in turn by a layer of simple squamous epithelium (mesothelium) facing the fluid of the peritoneal cavity. The serosa is continuous with the mesentery along the line of its attachment to the gut wall. The mesentery, being in turn attached to the posterior abdominal wall, provides access for vessels and nerves.

Special Features of the Three Levels of Small Intestine

In the DUODENUM (Fig. 12.40) as mentioned above, villi of the upper small intestine are flat, broad, long, numerous and closely packed. In the submucosa of the upper portion of the duodenum are groups of branched, coiled, tubular, mucous glands, the only submucosal glands below the level of the esophagus. They open into the bases of the crypts. These are the *duodenal glands* (of Brunner) (Fig. 12.40). They produce a neutral or alkaline secretion that is mixed with the strongly acid stomach contents. This serves to protect the duodenal mucosa and to promote digestion by pancreatic enzymes which have a higher pH optimum than do gastric enzymes. In a histologic section, the presence of submucosal glands and mucosal villi are absolutely diagnostic of duodenum.

In the JEJUNUM the villi are generally a little shorter and less closely packed. There are no specific diagnostic features for this level of the small intestine.

In the ILEUM the villi are still shorter, finger-shaped and even more widely spaced. In the lamina propria along the antimesenteric side of the ileum are 20–30 large, elongated *lymphoid patches* (of Peyer) (Fig. 12.41). Each is composed of two or three dozen lymphoid nodules embedded in diffuse lymphoid tissue. A patch may be 1 or 2 cm in width and several centimeters in length. Their presence in a section is diagnostic of ileum, but not all sections of ileum will happen to include them. The ileum empties into the left side of the cecum, the dilated beginning of the colon, through the ileocecal valve.

A frequent congenital anomaly of the small bowel is the persistence of a portion of the stalk of the yolk sac. This is the ileal diverticulum (of Meckel) (Fig. 12.42). It is located on the antimesenteric border of the ileum, a couple of feet above the ileocecal valve. The sac may have in its wall mucosa typical of the body of the stomach, with parietal and chief cells (Fig. 12.42b), and these may secrete enough acid into the gut to cause ulceration

---

Fig. 12.40. *Duodenum.* **a:** Note villi (V), muscularis mucosae (arrow), submucosal (Brunner's) glands (G), and muscularis externa (Me). ×19. **b:** Mucosal and submucosal glands and muscularis mucosae (Mm). ×85.

Fig. 12.41. *Ileal lymphoid* (Peyer's) *patch,* a collection of nodular and diffuse lymphoid tissue in the lamina propria and submucosa. ×19.

Fig. 12.42. *Meckel's diverticulum* of the ileum, with gastric mucosa and branching structures, some of which may be villi. **a:** ×2.5. **b:** ×85. (Courtesy of P. Stenzel.)

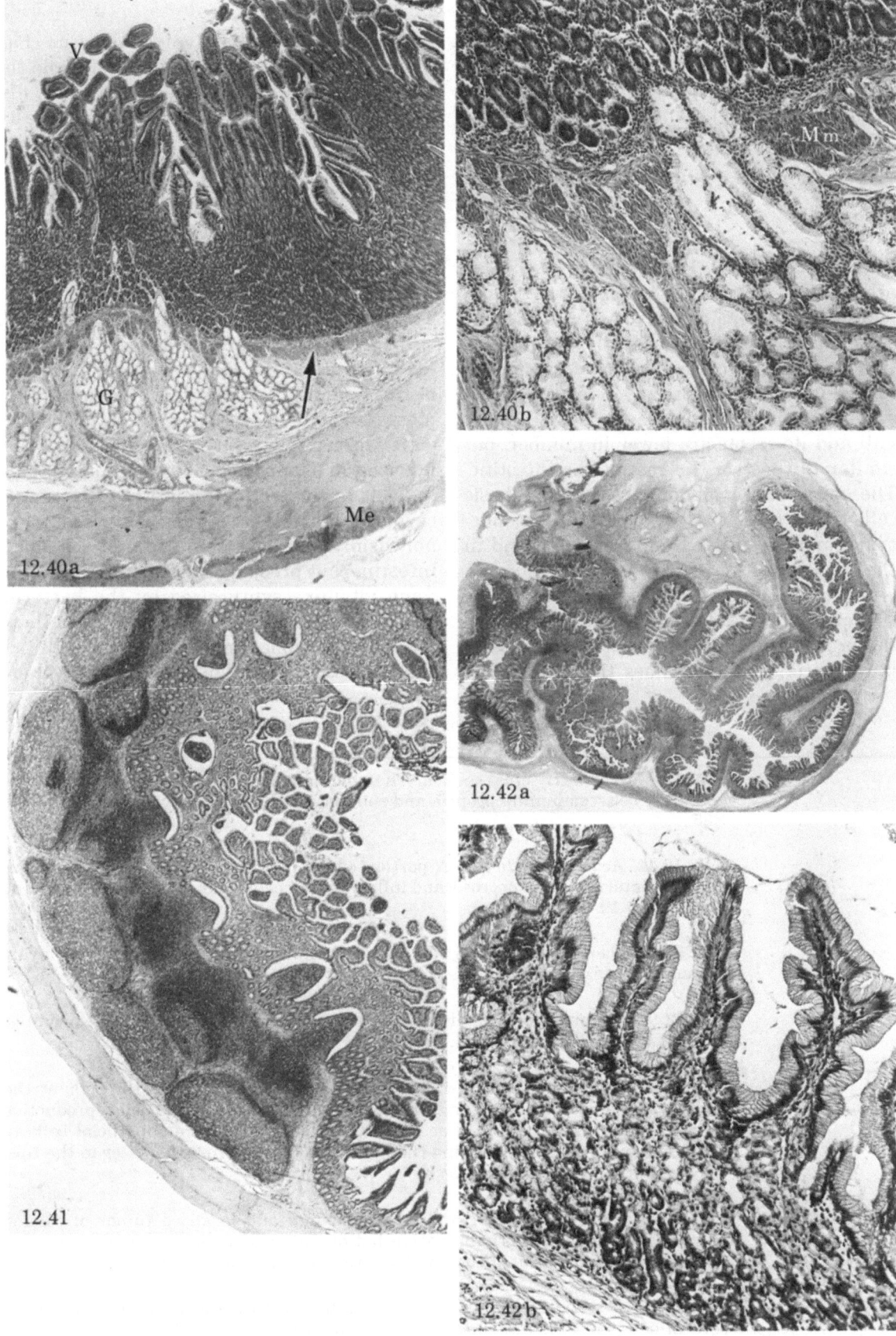

12.40a

12.40b

12.41

12.42a

12.42b

and clinically severe hemorrhage. In some cases exocrine pancreatic tissue may be found in the wall of the diverticulum. Embryologic explanation for these surprising combinations is lacking.

Appendix

The appendix (Figs. 12.1, 12.43, and 12.44) is a blind evagination of the cecum. Although nonfunctional as a digestive organ it has the same basic, four-layered, histologic organization as the rest of the digestive tract. The lumen is small and usually irregular in its cross-sectional outline. The mucosa has no villi and its crypts are fewer in number, but similar to those of the rest of the intestine. The epithelium includes the same five basic cell types (absorptive, goblet, enteroendocrine, undifferentiated and Paneth) found in the small intestine. The muscularis mucosae is thin, incomplete and difficult to visualize. The characteristic feature of the appendix is the prominent infiltration of the entire lamina propria, and sometimes the submucosa, by diffuse and nodular lymphoid tissue (Fig. 12.43). However, in later life, as lymphoid tissue generally loses prominence, this may disappear. The organ might be termed an intestinal tonsil and probably should be considered a lymphoid organ. Its immunologic functions are not currently understood (see Chapter 10).

Large Intestine (Colon, Large Bowel)

The large intestine (Figs. 12.1, and 12.45 through 12.49) prepares undigested materials for elimination. It does this by dehydration of the luminal contents into lubricated fecal masses. The dehydration is accomplished by water absorption through the mucosa, and the lubrication by mucus from the numerous goblet cells in the epithelium of the surface and crypts (Fig. 12.46). The absorptive cells are not visibly different from those of the small intestine, but probably absorb only water and some vitamins synthesized by the bacteria. No enzyme-producing cells appear, and there are only occasional enteroendocrine cells. No Paneth cells are present but, of course, there

---

Fig. 12.43. *Appendix,* cross-section. The abundant lymphoid tissue obliterates the boundary between lamina propria and submucosa. Some submucosal fat is present. ×35.

Fig. 12.44. *Acute appendicitis.* A portion of the mucosa is visible (top) but this is abruptly interrupted by necrosis and inflammatory cells (leukocytes), which pervade all layers. ×19.

Fig. 12.45. *Colon.* There are no villi and epithelium is mucus-secreting. Two layers of muscularis externa are present in this section. ×17.

Fig. 12.46. Scanning electron micrograph of inner *surface of colon* showing openings of crypts. ×100. (Courtesy of M. Webb.)

Fig. 12.47. *Radioautograph* of rat *colonic mucosa.* In this photo the cells at the bases of the glands, having taken up radioactive thymidine, reflect their reproductive rate. Samples taken a short time later would show the more superficial cells to contain these granules, indicating the migration of cells from the bases to the tips. ×560. (Courtesy of T. Richards.)

Fig. 12.48. *Adenomatous polyp.* This is a benign and localized tumor of colonic mucosa. Being benign, it is not invasive, but remains superficial and tends to develop a stalk because of repeated tugging by peristaltic movement. ×7.5.

Fig. 12.49. *Diverticulosis.* The mucosa has herniated through the muscularis at several points but remains intact. There is no perforation. ×2.7.

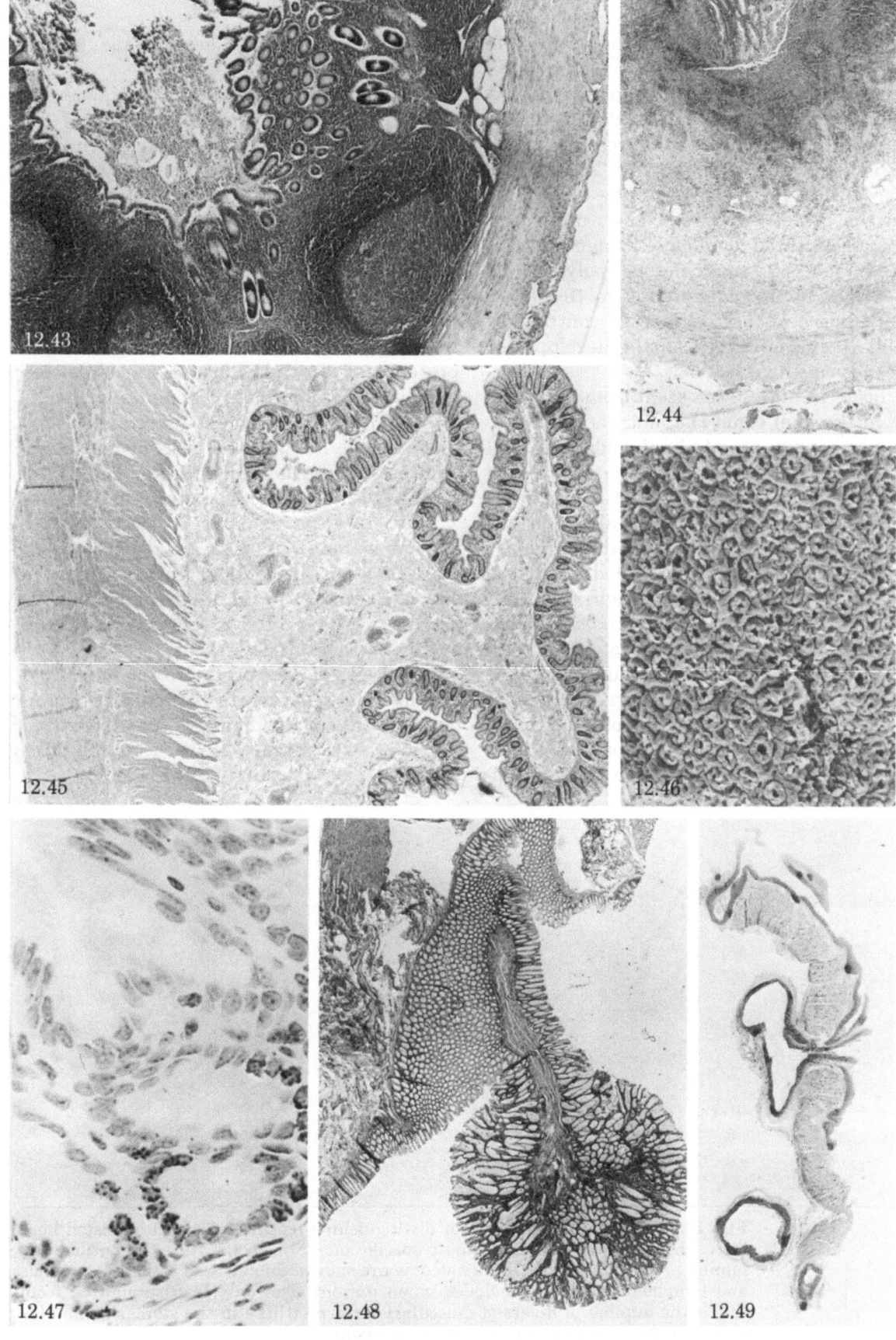

12.43

12.44

12.45

12.46

12.47

12.48

12.49

are undifferentiated cells in the bottoms of the crypts. These are the source of replacement for the entire epithelium (Fig. 12.47).

There are no villi in the colon; in histologic sections the mucosa somewhat resembles that of small intestine with the villi "shaved off" (Fig. 12.45). However, the crypts are deeper and the goblet cells much more numerous.

Small localized nodules of benign but neoplastic mucosa, adenomatous polyps (Fig. 12.48), are a frequent finding in the colon. There has been a good deal of controversy about their significance in the development of cancer of the colon.

Plicae circulares are absent from the colon, but in the anal canal the mucosa has five to ten permanent, longitudinal folds, the anal columns (of Morgagni). The lower end of each of these folds is connected to its two neighbors by semilunar folds, the anal valves. At the level of these valves the epithelium changes from simple columnar to stratified squamous. In the anal canal the lamina propria contains a rich plexus of veins. This plexus has a dual drainage: (1) into the portal system through the inferior mesenteric vein and; (2) into the caval system through the internal pudendal and internal iliac veins. Thus obstruction of either of these routes may overload the plexus and, as in the esophagus, cause the develop-

ment of varicosities, here termed hemorrhoids.

The lamina propria of the colon generally contains numerous lymphoid cells and frequent lymph nodules which may extend into the submucosa.

The muscularis externa is unique in that the outer longitudinal muscle is not usually a continuous sheet, but tends to be gathered into three longitudinal bands, the taenia coli. In the anal region the circular layer is much thickened to serve as the internal sphincter.

Another common finding in the colon is the presence of multiple herniations of mucosa and submucosa through the muscularis (Fig. 12.49). These are known as diverticula. They may become inflamed—a risk for any blind-ended structure, including the appendix. Peritonitis, with or without rupture, may result.

The serosa, particularly in the transverse colon, has frequent, small, stalked projections (appendices epiploicae) which vary greatly in size and number in different individuals. In aggregate they probably represent a fat (reserve energy) storage system.

It is easy to forget or ignore the individual features that allow one to distinguish the various segments of the digestive tube from each other. The key features, fewer than might be expected, are summarized in Fig. 12.50.

Fig. 12.50. *Overview* of the *gut* for distinguishing features. The details listed here for each portion are only the most specific ones. In each figure the epithelium, lamina propria, and muscularis mucosae are shown. Submucosal structures (glands and lymphoid tissue) are included when present. The only feature omitted from this is the number of layers of muscularis externa (three in the stomach, one plus an incomplete one in the colon, otherwise two).

A. Esophagus

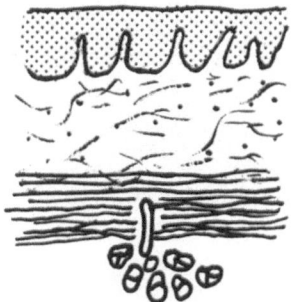

Stratified squamous
epithelium

Few submucosal glands

Prominent muscularis
mucosae

B. Gastric corpus

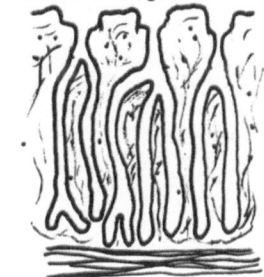

Pits

Mucosal serous glands
with mixture of cell types
(not shown here)

C. Pylorus

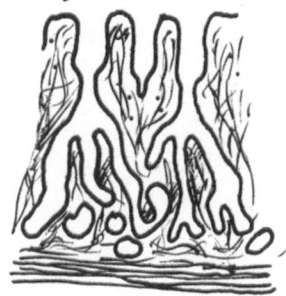

Deeper pits

Mucosal mucous glands

D. Duodenum

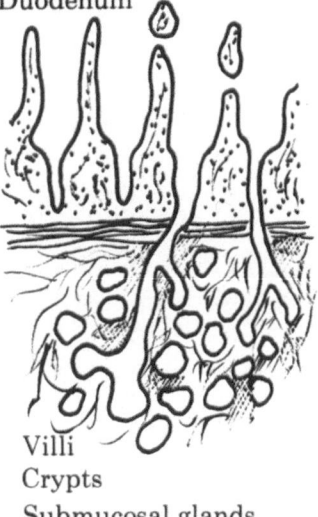

Villi
Crypts
Submucosal glands

E. Jejunum

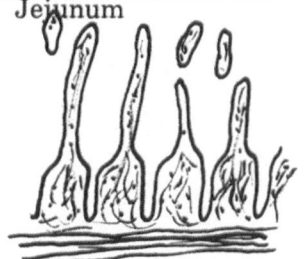

Villi
Crypts

F. Ileum

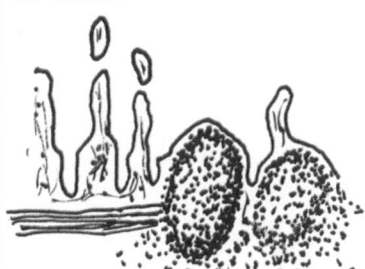

Villi
Crypts
Lymphoid patches

G. Appendix

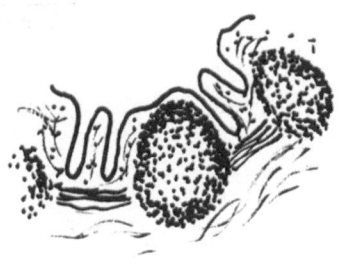

Few crypts

Much lymphoid tissue

H. Colon

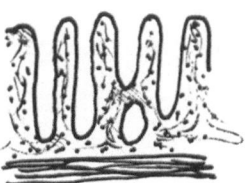

Crypts

Many goblet cells

12.50

13 Digestive System: Glandular Portion

Introduction

The numerous, small, *intrinsic glands* of the digestive system located in the mucosa or submucosa of the gastrointestinal tube (e.g., the minor salivary glands, gastric glands, duodenal submucosal glands, etc.) have been described in the previous chapter. An additional series of glands, too large to be accommodated within the wall of the tract, develop by evagination of the mucosal epithelium entirely through the wall into adjacent tissues such as the facial connective tissue and the mesenteries of the duodenum. In each instance the original outgrowth remains as the major duct and the much-branched ends develop into large masses of secretory acini or, in the liver, cords and sheets of glandular tissue. These, the *extrinsic glands*, are the major salivary glands, pancreas, and liver.

Salivary Glands

There are three pairs of major salivary glands: parotid, submandibular, and sublingual (Fig. 13.1). They produce their secretions in response to the presence or anticipation of food, in contrast with the widely distributed minor salivary glands. The latter secrete nearly continuously, although the amount of their secretion may vary in time.

General features

ORGANIZATION.   All of the major salivary glands are compound acinar or tubuloacinar (see Chapter 3). They consist of several lobes separated by thin connective tissue sheets (Fig. 13.2). Extensions of this connective tissue in the form of septa penetrating each lobe subdivide it into numerous lobules, and further extensions from the septa surround each acinus and duct with a delicate connective tissue investment. The density of the connective tissue capsule enclosing the entire gland differs somewhat among the three.

SECRETION.   There are two types of secretory cells, serous and mucous (Fig. 13.3). The cytoplasm of mucous cells show a characteristic foamy appearance and the nucleus is flattened and basally located. The serous cells contain secretory granules and produce a solution of salts, enzymes, and other proteins. Saliva is the viscid fluid made up of this solution, mixed with mucus and containing desquamated epithelial cells and lymphocytes. About 1.4 liters are produced each day, 25% of which is from the parotid glands, 70% from the submandibular glands, and 5% from the sublingual glands. Movement of this secretion into the duct system is assisted by the contraction of myoepithelial (basket) cells whose numerous processes surround each acinus like the fingers of a hand grasping a baseball. This secretory activity is principally controlled by sympathetic and parasympathetic innervation. Nerve endings penetrate the basal lamina of the acini and terminate among the epithelial cells. The secreted solution is modified by the ion pumps in the epithelium of the ducts and emptied into the oral cavity, where it is mixed with food. In addition to its wetting and softening action, saliva begins the hydrolysis of carbohydrates by the action of salivary amylase.

DUCTS

Structure.   The salivary gland ducts are generally classified on the basis of location and structure. It may be useful to review the section on glands in Chapter 3 at this point.

The *intralobular ducts* are located within the substance of each lobule and surrounded by secretory tubules and acini (Figs. 13.2, 13.5 through 13.8). These differ in structure along their course and, as seen in sections, are of two varieties. Beginning at the acinus or the mucous secretory tubule is the *intercalated duct,* composed of simple squamous or low cuboidal epithelium without granules or other special features. The next segment, considerably larger, is the *striated duct* (Figs. 13.4 and 13.6B), so called because of the noticeable striations in the basal portion of the cells of its simple columnar epithelium. Striations indicate basal membrane infolding and alignment of mitochondria along these folds. The nucleus is displaced apically and tends to be central or higher in position.

The *interlobular ducts* (Figs. 13.5 through 13.7) lie in the septa between adjacent lobules and are formed by junction of intralobular ducts. They have a tall columnar epithelial lining and are clearly differentiated from intralobular ducts only by their investment of connective tissue. Lobar ducts are formed by junction of several interlobular ducts and

---

Fig. 13.1. The three *major salivary glands*. Note that the sublingual gland is in reality an association of several small glands, each with its own short duct.

Fig. 13.2. *Salivary gland* lobules with interlobular (large arrow) and intralobular (small arrow) ducts. ×24.

Fig. 13.3. *Mucous* (M) and *serous* (S) *cells* in a salivary gland. ×400.

Fig. 13.4. Cellular *organization of salivary glands*. Serous and mucous acini may occur separately, or mucous tubules may be capped by serous crescents (demilunes). In the ducts the epithelium changes from the thin squamous type of the intercalated ducts to tall columnar with basal striations in the striated ducts, to ordinary columnar and, finally, at or near the exit, to nonkeratinized stratified squamous.

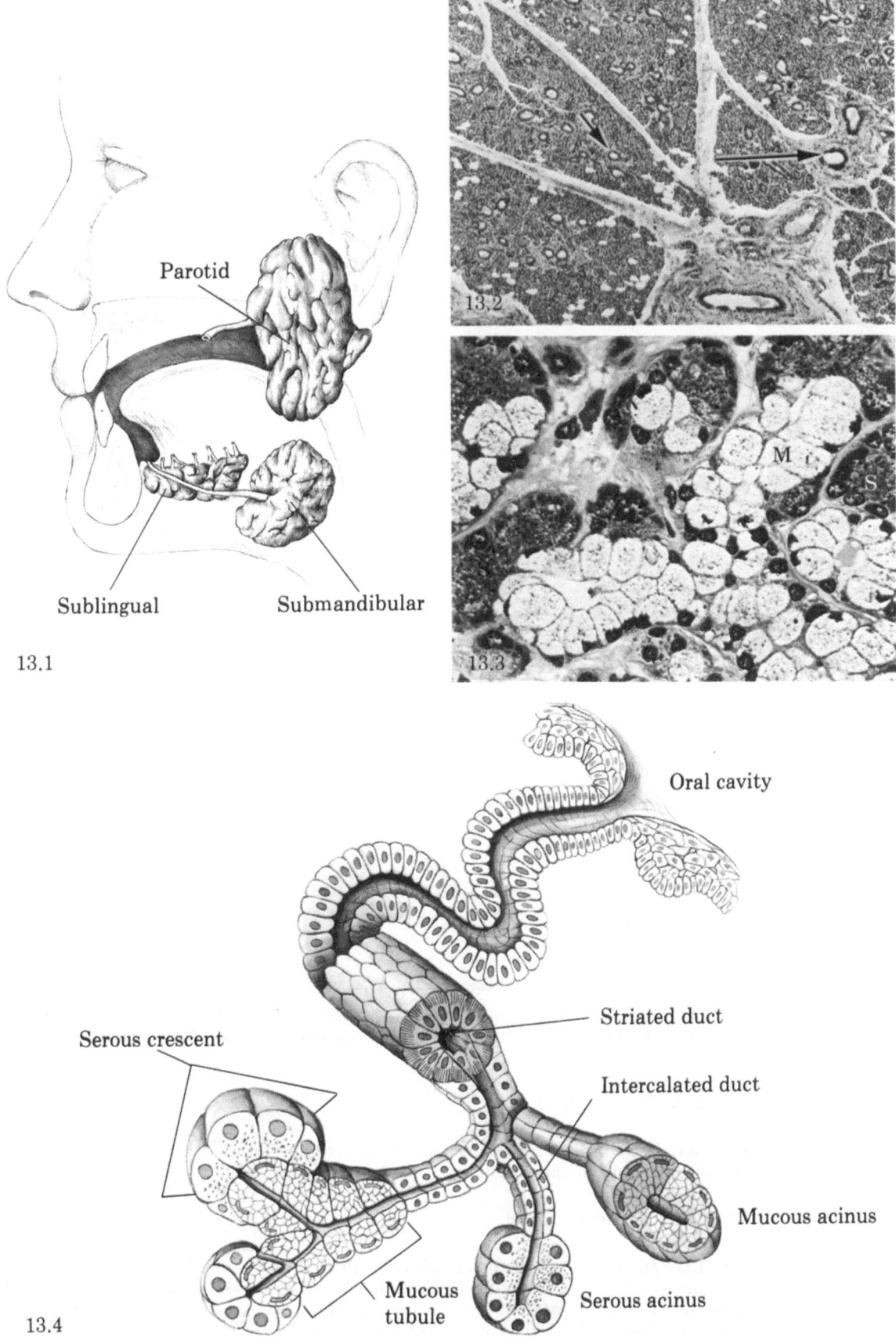

Parotid

Sublingual

Submandibular

13.1

13.2

13.3

M

S

Oral cavity

Striated duct

Intercalated duct

Mucous acinus

Serous crescent

Mucous tubule

Serous acinus

13.4

Figs. 13.5 through 13.7 show the salivary glands at low magnification (×24) on the left (**A**) and high magnification (×130) on the right (**B**). See text for specific features.

Fig. 13.5. *Parotid* gland.

Fig. 13.6. *Submandibular* gland. Cytoplasmic granules in the serous cells are emphasized by the basic fuchsin stain.

Fig. 13.7. *Sublingual* gland.

Fig. 13.8. *Mumps.* **a:** All of the glands are enlarged due to the inflammation which has spread into the loose connective tissue of the sides of the lower face and upper neck. **b:** Arrows indicate exudate in duct. Much of the architecture of the parotid gland is obliterated. ×250. (Courtesy of J. Kussy and the Department of Pathology, St Gabriel's Hospital, Little Falls, Minn.)

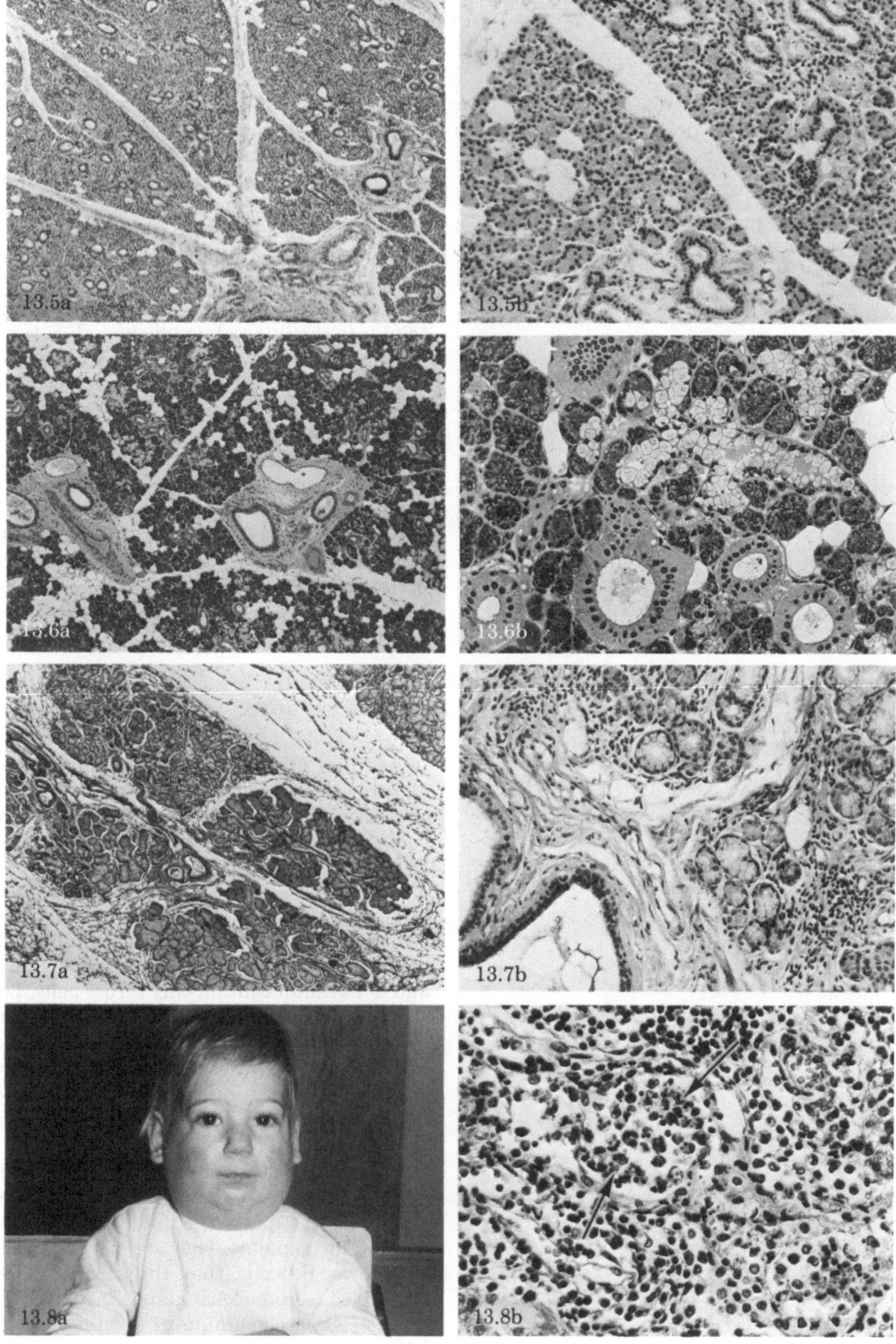

there is a gradual transition of the epithelium from simple columnar to stratified cuboidal or stratified columnar. In the main duct, the final outflow channel, the epithelium is stratified or pseudostratified columnar and eventually changes to stratified squamous just before its termination in the oral cavity.

Function. In addition to their obvious function of conducting, the ducts in the salivary glands also control electrolyte levels in the fluid they are carrying. As it is passed from acini into the intercalated ducts, saliva is apparently isosmotic with blood. The cells of striated ducts (Fig. 13.4), resemble cells of the renal tubule, and seem to have some functional similarities as well. Here sodium is actively reabsorbed and potassium excreted. Thus, by the time the saliva reaches the interlobular and larger ducts, it is hypotonic. In these activities striated duct cells respond to two hormones, aldosterone and antidiuretic hormone (ADH), which have important effects on kidney tubular function as well (see Chapter 15).

Special Features

In addition to the common denominators of all three glands, each has its own special characteristics that relate to functional differences and provide diagnostic features in histologic sections.

THE PAROTID GLANDS (Figs. 13.1 and 13.5), the largest of the salivary glands, are flattened pads of tissue located under the skin in front of each ear. They are compound acinar glands and in the adult contain only serous cells. The serous cells secrete a starch-hydrolyzing enzyme called salivary amylase (ptyalin). Histologic sections show: (1) a parenchyma of one cell type; (2) numerous intralobular ducts; (3) numerous scattered individual, or small clusters of, fat cells; and (4) a thin capsule.

THE SUBMANDIBULAR GLANDS (Figs. 13.1 and 13.6) are paired, compound tubuloacinar glands located under the middle third of the body of the mandible. They are more compact, with fewer fat cells, than the parotids. They are mixed (seromucous) glands in which the serous cells predominate in a ratio of about 16 to 1. Most of the mucous cells are in the tubular portions of the secretory units (Fig. 13.3). The serous cells form acini or occasionally cap the ends of mucous tubules as serous demilunes (of Gianuzzi). These cells have rounded nuclei and basophilic granular cytoplasm as a result of the presence of abundant rough endoplasmic reticulum (RER) and zymogen granules. Serous cells of demilunes are reported to contain lysozyme. The other serous cells produce moderate amounts of amylase. The glands contain about the same proportion of striated ducts as do the parotids. The ducts (Wharton's) open beneath the tongue near the frenulum. There is a delicate capsule.

THE SUBLINGUAL GLANDS (Figs. 13.1 and 13.7) are compound tubuloacinar glands lying in symmetrical positions beneath the tongue. There are usually at least twice as many mucous as serous cells. Most of the latter are arranged in demilunes capping the long, tortuous, branched mucous tubules. There are fewer intralobular ducts, perhaps half the number found in the other two glands. Very few of them are striated, and intercalated ducts are rare or absent. There are several interlobular ducts, all of which finally open into the mouth near the opening of the submandibular duct. The lobes and lobules are more widely spaced, with considerable connective tissue in the septa, but there is no discrete capsule.

Pathology

The salivary glands, like all organs and tissues, are subject to a broad range of diseases. One of the more familiar is mumps, an acute viral inflammatory condition (Fig. 13.8).

Pancreas

This large and important gland lies behind the stomach and is fused transversely to the posterior abdominal wall. It is an association of two distinctly different glands, one exocrine and one endocrine (Figs. 13.11 and 13.14). Each of these has separate and practically independent functions, although they are closely related anatomically. This arrange-

ment will be contrasted with that of the liver (*see later*), which is also both exocrine and endocrine.

Development

The pancreas develops from the fusion of two rudiments that arise separately as dorsal and ventral epithelial outgrowths from the gut at the level of the future duodenum (Fig. 13.9A). Each retains a lumen connecting with the gut. Rotation and differential growth of the gut tube bring the two rudiments together (Fig. 13.9B). The dorsal rudiment becomes the body and the tail of the pancreas; the ventral rudiment becomes the head. The duct of the ventral rudiment taps that of the dorsal and provides the principal, and often the only, duct of the definitive pancreas. The duct of the dorsal rudiment may persist as an accessory duct (Fig. 13.9C).

Occasionally the ventral rudiment, instead of growing to the right and dorsally, may spread around both sides of the gut to fuse with the dorsal rudiment. This produces a ring-shaped pancreas entirely surrounding and constricting the duodenum, a serious congenital malformation called annular pancreas (Fig. 13.10).

Histologic Organization

The *exocrine pancreas* (Figs. 13.12 and 13.13) is a serous gland that produces enzymes for digestion of food within the intestine. The *endocrine. pancreas* consists of a group of cell clusters scattered through the substance of the exocrine pancreas (Figs. 13.11 and 13.14).

THE EXOCRINE PANCREAS is a compound acinar gland arranged in numerous lobules and lobes along a large main duct.

The stroma of the pancreas is made up of loose connective tissue that extends into the parenchyma from an indistinct and tenuous capsule. The septa are often incomplete and the lobules are thus frequently only partially separated. Groups of lobules are gathered into indistinct lobes by broader sheets of connective tissue. Blood vessels, nerves, and lymphatics lie in the interlobular connective tissue and send branches into the lobules parallel to the duct system.

Parenchyma. The secretory units of the pancreas are acini (Figs. 13.12 through 13.14) made up of columnar serous cells that are usually compressed toward one end into a pyramidal form. There are no basket cells. They show all of the features of cells manufacturing proteins for export. When seen with the light microscope, each cell shows an apical portion occupied by large numbers of zymogen granules, and a basal portion containing the nucleus and strongly basophilic cytoplasm. Often this basal region appears striated because of the parallel alignment of the RER and large numbers of mitochondria. The intense basophilia is a reflection of large amounts of RER. This is perhaps the heaviest concentration of RNA in any human cell, indicating an extraordinary rate of protein-synthesizing activity.

The secretion of the acinar cells is an alkaline solution of proenzymes and enzymes. The former are trypsinogen and chymotrypsino- gen, both precursors of protein endopepti- dases. The latter are ribonuclease, deoxyribo- nuclease, carboxypeptidase, amylase, and lipase. Control of enzyme concentration and of pH of the acinar cell secretion lies in the innervation and in hormones brought to the gland in its blood supply. Autonomic nerve fibers end around and within the epithelium of the acini.

Hormonal control resides in the products of two types of enteroendocrine cells (see Chapter 12) in the duodenal epithelium. One of these types produces *secretin* in response to a fall in the pH of duodenal contents. This fall is brought about by the presence of stomach contents or of bile acids in the duodenum. Secretin is carried to the pancreas in blood and stimulates the secretion of bicarbonate by the cells of intercalated ducts. A more dilute enzyme solution results.

The second hormone, *cholecystokinin*, also blood-borne, stimulates the release of secretory granules from the exocrine pancreas and thus increases the concentration of enzymes in pancreatic secretion.

Fig. 13.9. *Development of the pancreas* in ventral view (above) and cross-section (below). **A:** Dorsal and ventral rudiments with directions of migration indicated. **B:** Duodenum has shifted to the right and rotated clockwise. The right side of the duodenum also grows considerably more than the left, a process that serves to enlarge the cross-sectional area and at the same time to bring the ducts of the two rudiments relatively closer to each other. The ventral pancreas actually shifts about 270° from its original position. **C:** There is further differentiation and the ducts are rearranged.

Fig. 13.10. *Annular pancreas.* A ring of pancreatic tissue surrounds the duodenum. This restricts the size of duodenal lumen and may cause its obstruction, requiring surgery in the newborn. ×3.3. (Courtesy of S. Marshall.)

Fig. 13.11. *Exocrine* and *endocrine (arrows)* pancreas. ×24.

Fig. 13.12. Pancreatic acinus with *centroacinar* cells (arrows). ×560.

Fig. 13.13. Diagram to explain the appearance of *centroacinar cells* in a section. The section cut in plane a-a would suggest that the acinus contains cells in its lumen. The lumen, if it is to be seen at all, is of course that of the intercalated duct, not of the acinus. A section cut at b-b would show no duct cells and would conform to the usual concept of acinus.

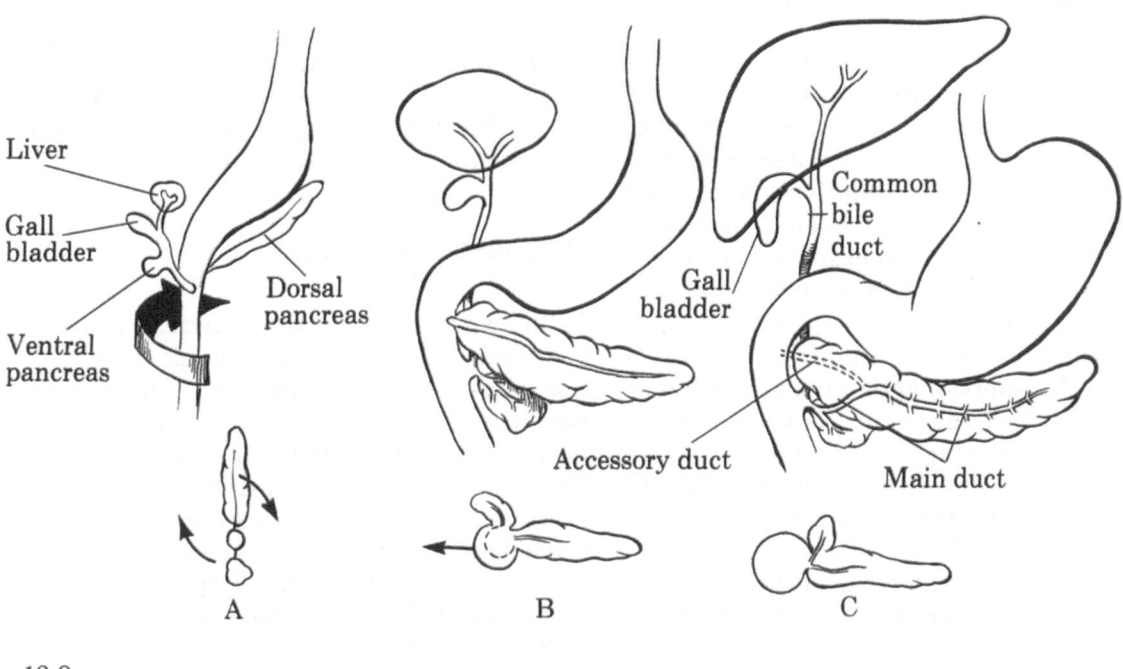

Liver

Gall
bladder

Ventral
pancreas

Dorsal
pancreas

Common
bile
duct

Gall
bladder

Accessory duct

Main duct

A

B

C

13.9

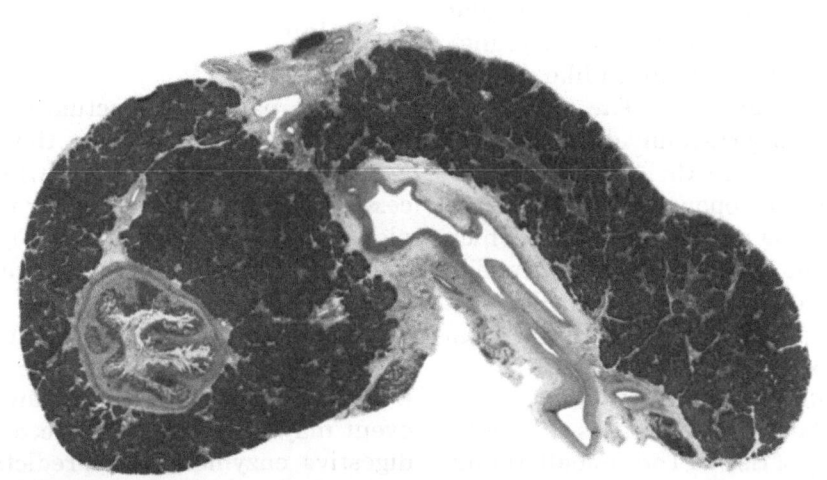

13.10

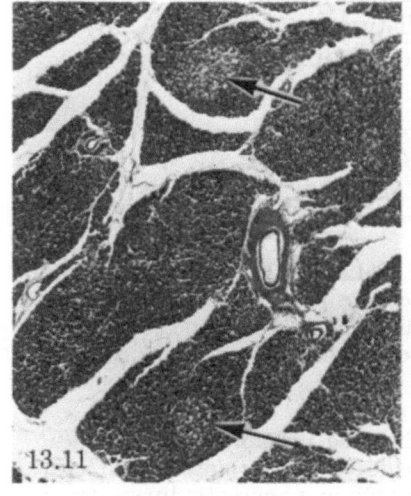

13.11

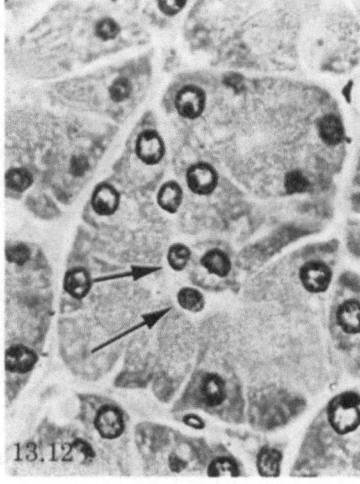

13.12

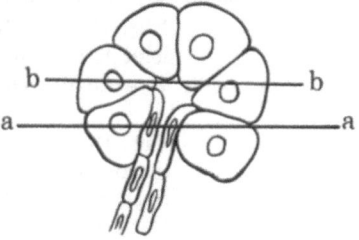

13.13

b

b

a

a

The duct pattern in the pancreas is quite different from that of the salivary glands. Striated ducts are absent and the only intralobular ducts are of the intercalated type (Fig. 13.14), lined by clear, relatively unstained, squamous or low cuboidal, epithelial cells. These ducts are long and branched. At its origin, an intercalated duct is tucked into the acinus, partially lining its lumen. Thus, in examining histologic sections, an observer may get the impression that the acinar lumen contains one or more cells if the section is cut at such an angle that it does not happen to show the continuity of these cells with the duct. These are termed *centroacinar cells* (Figs. 13.12 and 13.13).

The largest intercalated ducts leave the lobules and enter interlobular septa where the epithelium becomes columnar (but not striated). Occasional goblet cells and enteroendocrine cells are present. The interlobular ducts drain into the main duct (of Wirsung), around which they are arranged like needles on a twig of a spruce tree. The main duct and the larger interlobular ducts contain small mucous glands in their connective tissue. The main duct opens on the duodenal papilla through the ampulla of Vater, which it shares with the common bile duct. In addition to the main duct, there commonly is an accessory duct (of Santorini), that has a separate opening into the duodenum.

The ENDOCRINE PANCREAS is composed of a population of about 1 million islets of Langerhans totaling 1 g of tissue. These small, round, richly vascularized clumps of cells are unevenly scattered throughout the substance of the exocrine pancreas (Fig. 13.14). They are more numerous in the body and tail of the gland than in its head. They produce hormones involved in complex metabolic control systems to be considered in Chapter 16.

Diagnostic Features

In histologic sections the pancreas is easily confused with the parotid gland, since both are lobulated, compound acinar glands with one type of secretory cell. The features diagnostic of pancreas are: (1) absence of striated ducts, (2) presence of centroacinar cells, (3) presence of islets of Langerhans, (4) strong basal basophilia and coarse apical granules in the secretory cells, and (5) (particularly in young individuals) relative absence of fat cells.

Pathology

Since the pancreas is actually two separate organs it is not surprising that certain diseases affect one organ only, while some processes might damage both. For instance, simple atrophy of either portion (Fig. 13.15) may occur. The reasons for this specificity are seldom clear.

Another process that illustrates one of the particular functions of the pancreas results from its focal destruction. In pancreatitis, this event may release into the local area all the digestive enzymes, with predictable results. A histologic characteristic of this is fat necrosis, which is distinctive microscopically as well as grossly (Fig. 13.16).

Fig. 13.14. Schematic drawing of the *structure of the pancreas*. At the right an islet is shown with cells removed from its upper portion to demonstrate its rich vascularity. One acinus, with its intercalated duct, has been hemisected.

Fig. 13.15. *Atrophy* of exocrine pancreas. Atrophy makes the islets of Langerhans (arrows) stand out practically unsupported by exocrine pancreas. The latter has been reduced to a small fraction of its original bulk and largely replaced by fat. Patients usually do not have symptoms relative to this atrophy, perhaps because the process is gradual and they adjust to it. ×80.

Fig. 13.16. *Pancreatitis.* The tissue is partially digested by pancreatic enzymes. Necrosis of fat (bottom) is grossly opaque and white due to the formation of sodium stearate from the cleavage of triglycerides, presumably by pancreatic lipase, from necrotic cells. ×85. (Courtesy of K. Schmidt.)

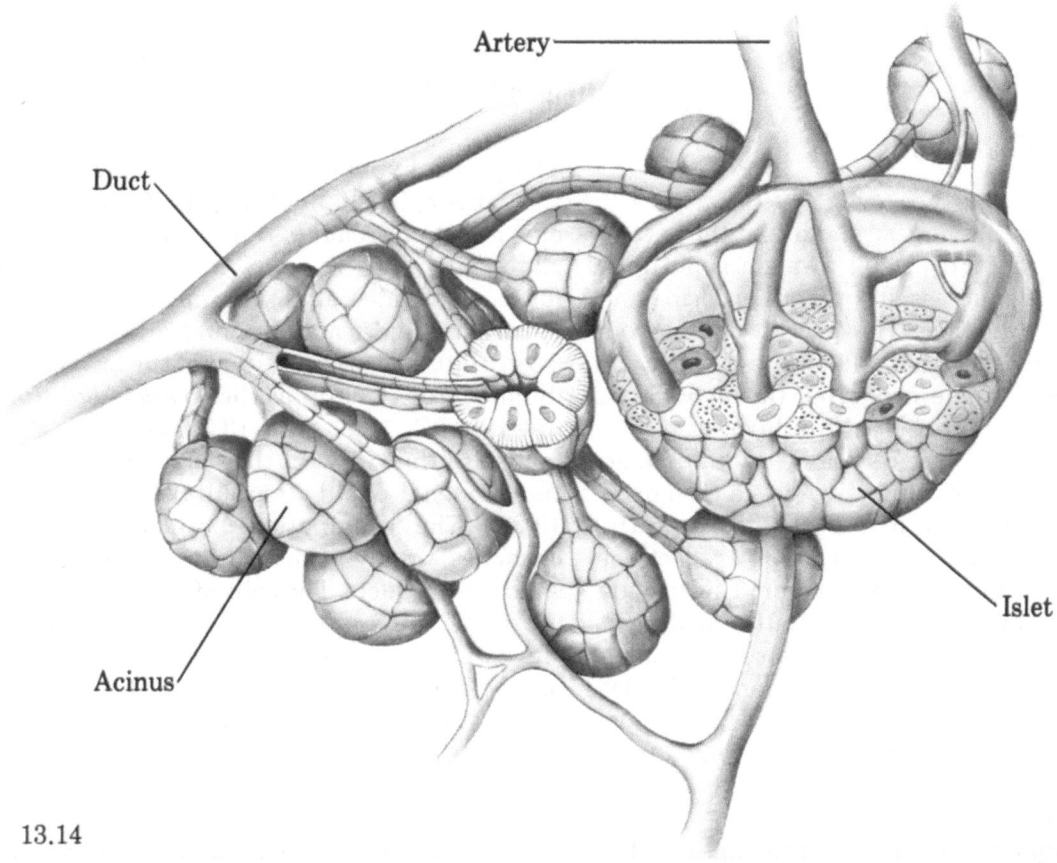

13.14

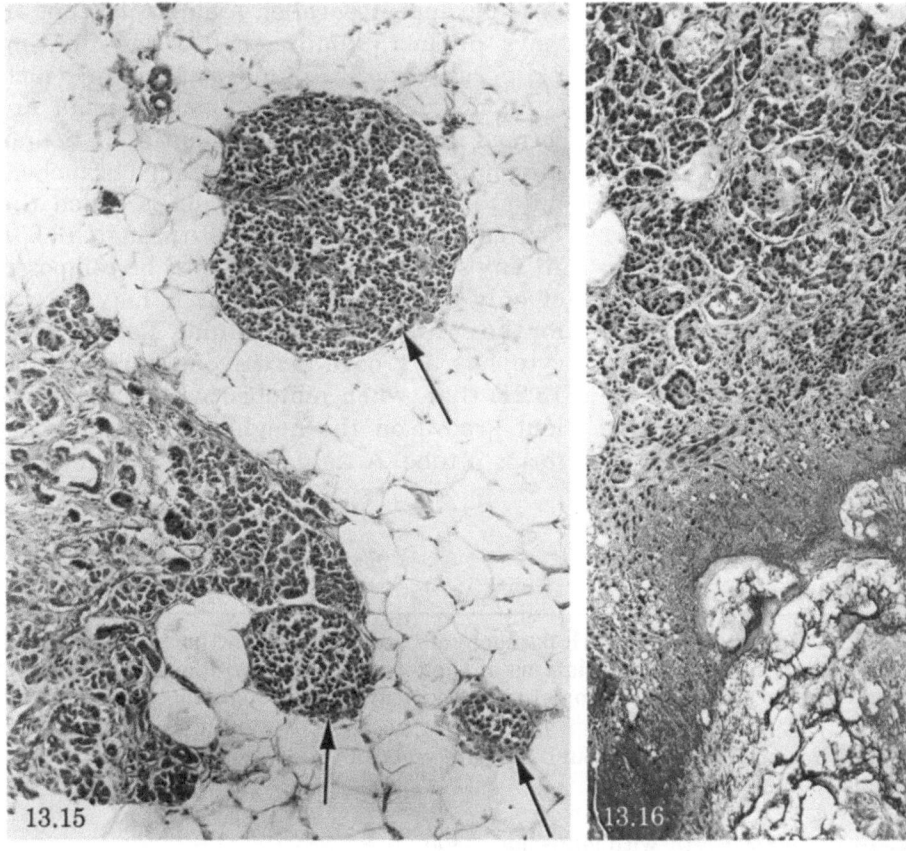

13.15

13.16

Liver

General Features

The liver is the largest gland and the second largest organ in the body; it weighs about 1500 g. Like the pancreas, it has both exocrine and endocrine functions. However, it differs from the pancreas in that all of these functions reside in a single cell type, the *hepatocyte*. The liver is covered by a thin layer of peritoneum similar to the serosa of the intestines, that is, a layer of connective tissue with overlying mesothelium. It is suspended from the diaphragm and abdominal wall by reflections of this covering peritoneal layer. The capsule extends into the gland, partially dividing it into four lobes. The liver secretes bile through a system of ducts into the duodenum. It also secretes a number of products into the blood. Most of the liver's blood supply comes from the gastrointestinal tube via the portal vein (Fig. 13.17).

In keeping with its exocrine nature, the liver has a hilus (the porta) through which its main ducts pass, along with its afferent blood vessels (portal vein and hepatic artery). From the porta the connective tissue of the capsule ramifies through the liver as strands containing the branches of portal vein, hepatic artery, bile duct, lymphatic vessels, and nerves. This much-branched strand of connective tissue with its contents is termed the *portal tract* (Fig. 13.18). A common, though less appropriate, name, since there are obviously more than three structures present, is *portal triad*. The efferent veins (Fig. 13.19) leave the liver via a different part of the organ and empty into the inferior vena cava.

Development and Structure of the Liver and Bile Ducts

The parenchyma of the liver is derived from the same epithelial outgrowth of the embryonic gut that produces the ventral pancreatic rudiment (Fig. 13.9A). As the outgrowth forms, it divides almost immediately into a pancreatic bud (caudally) and a hepatic bud (rostrally). The original stem of the branching (biliary) tree remains as the *common bile duct* (Figs. 13.9C, 13.17, and 13.32) (*see later*) attached to the gut with the pancreatic duct at the duodenal papilla (ampulla of Vater) (Fig. 13.33). The evagination branches and rebranches many times into smaller and smaller bile ducts. The cells of the last tubular branches differentiate into anastomosing sheets, called *laminae;* laminae are composed of single layers of secretory cells, the *hepatocytes*. The finest twigs of the biliary system (Fig. 13.20) run in the laminae between hepatocytes. The laminae are irregular, anastomosing, overlapping, and perforated. The perforations are called lacunae. Sometimes the laminae appear parallel. A single, but not always distinct, lamina, called the limiting plate, is wrapped around each portal tract.

As noted above, glandular elements are formed in which the equivalent of an acinar lumen is an intralaminar, much-branched, minute channel. This channel is called the *bile canaliculus* (Figs. 13.20 through 13.23). At any single level its wall may be composed of only two hepatocytes but it may extend for the entire length of a lamina. Each hepatocyte has a groove across one surface (Fig. 13.21) that, when matched with the equivalent groove on the neighboring hepatocyte, forms a tube. A tight junction (zonula occlu-

---

Fig. 13.17. Drawing of liver with parenchyma removed to show portal and hepatic venous trees and (inset) the relations of their terminal twigs. Blood from the gut enters the liver through the portal vein and leaves it through the hepatic veins.

Fig. 13.18. A cross-section through a *portal tract* of the liver. Bile duct (B), artery (A), and vein (V). ×400.

Fig. 13.19. *Central vein* with sinusoids. ×400.

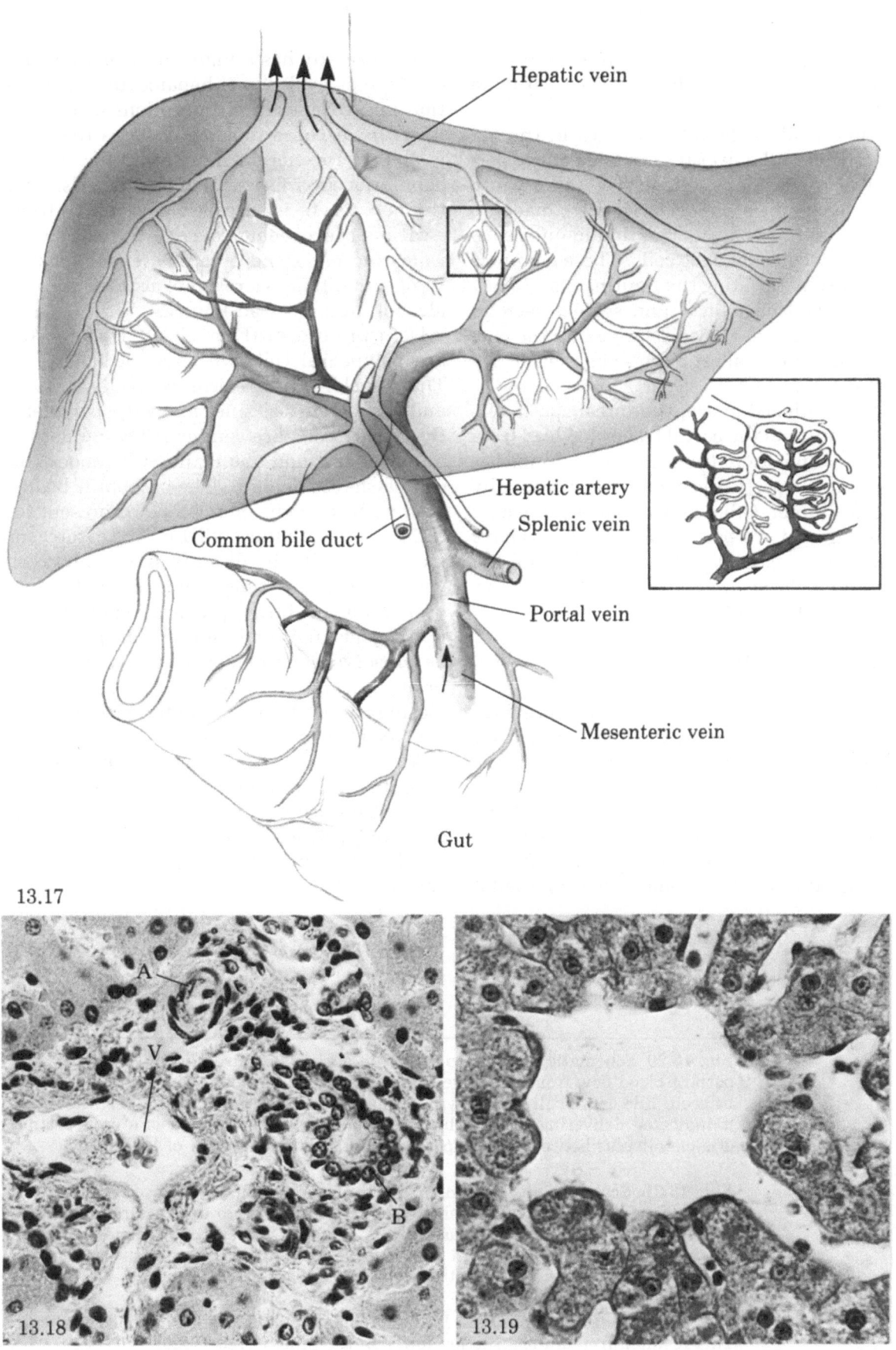

Hepatic vein

Hepatic artery

Splenic vein

Common bile duct

Portal vein

Mesenteric vein

Gut

13.17

13.18

13.19

dens) (Fig. 13.23) along each side of the grooves seals the two halves of each tubule together.

Almost all of the bile passages in the parenchyma of the liver (i.e., outside of the portal tracts) are bile canaliculi. They empty into minute channels (canals of Hering), made up of a mixture of hepatocytes and undifferentiated, low cuboidal duct cells. These channels are short, perforating the limiting plate. They are small, thin-walled, and seldom seen in routine sections. They discharge into the cholangioles, the smallest biliary channels in the portal tracts.

As mentioned above, the intrahepatic bile ducts course in the portal tracts and lead from the cholangioles to the right and left hepatic ducts at the porta. In so doing they gradually become larger. Often more than one bile duct will be found in a portal tract. The ducts have a simple cuboidal or columnar epithelial lining and a fibrous wall with rare smooth muscle fibers (Fig. 13.18).

The Hepatocyte

As one might have surmised from previous sections of this chapter, the hepatocyte is an unusual and special cell. For one thing it is probably the most versatile cell in the body, having several important, indeed vital, functions. This might seem to indicate that it is highly differentiated. However, in addition, the hepatocyte, like some other epithelial cells, normally has a high turnover rate; one easily finds evidence of hepatocyte degeneration and regeneration in sections of normal liver. In response to some diseases the liver is able to regenerate most of its hepatocyte population in a few weeks. Not surprisingly, the hepatocyte is susceptible to injury from a variety of exogenous causes (e.g., toxic chemicals) and endogenous causes (e.g., hypoxia). Its degeneration as a result of acute or chronic alcohol intake is well known.

LIGHT MICROSCOPY (Figs. 13.19). Hepatocytes are polyhedral cells with rounded margins. Their nuclei are spherical, centrally located, and variable in size since many are polyploid. Binucleate cells are common. The numerous mitochondria and abundant SER render the cytoplasm eosinophilic. The basophilic bodies seen with the light microscope respresent localized accumulations of RER. The cytoplasm may, especially in disease, have empty or vacuolated areas where lipid droplets have been dissolved during preparation of the section. Lipids and other stored substances can be preserved and demonstrated with appropriate special techniques. Glycogen, for example, may be easily demonstrated with the periodic acid-Schiff (PAS) stain.

At least one surface of every hepatocyte is in contact with a sinusoid. At least one surface shares a bile canaliculus with a neighbor; and, commonly, at least one is closely applied to another neighbor without special surface features.

Fig. 13.20. Schematic drawing to illustrate portions of three *hepatic laminae.* The path of blood flow from portal vein through two sinusoids to the central vein can be seen. Bile canaliculi are shown. A small terminal branch of the hepatic artery is indicated delivering arterial blood to a sinusoid. Below, left, is a cross-section of a canaliculus between two hepatocytes. (Based on the work of H. Elias.)

Fig. 13.21. Scanning electron micrograph of the fractured surface of a piece of *liver.* The fracture cleaved parenchymal cells (P) so as to open a branching bile canaliculus (BC) and three sinusoids (S). ×2500. (Courtesy of A. Jones in Jones AL, Schmucker DL: Progress in Hepatology—Current concepts of liver structure as related to liver function. Gastroenterology 73:833–851, 1977.)

Fig. 13.22. *Obstructive jaundice.* Plugs of inspissated bile fill and distend canaliculi. This resulted from an obstruction lower in the biliary tree. ×520.

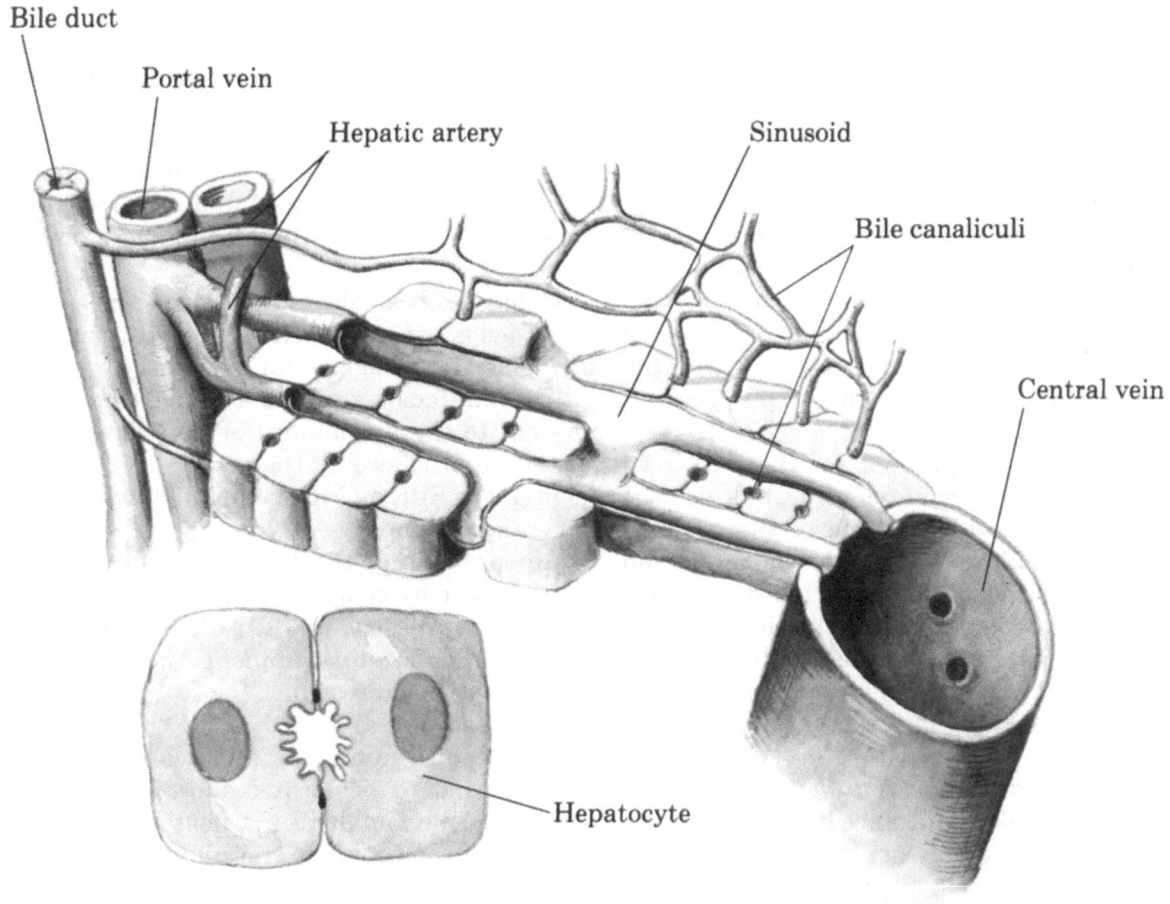

Bile duct

Portal vein

Hepatic artery

Sinusoid

Bile canaliculi

Central vein

Hepatocyte

13.20

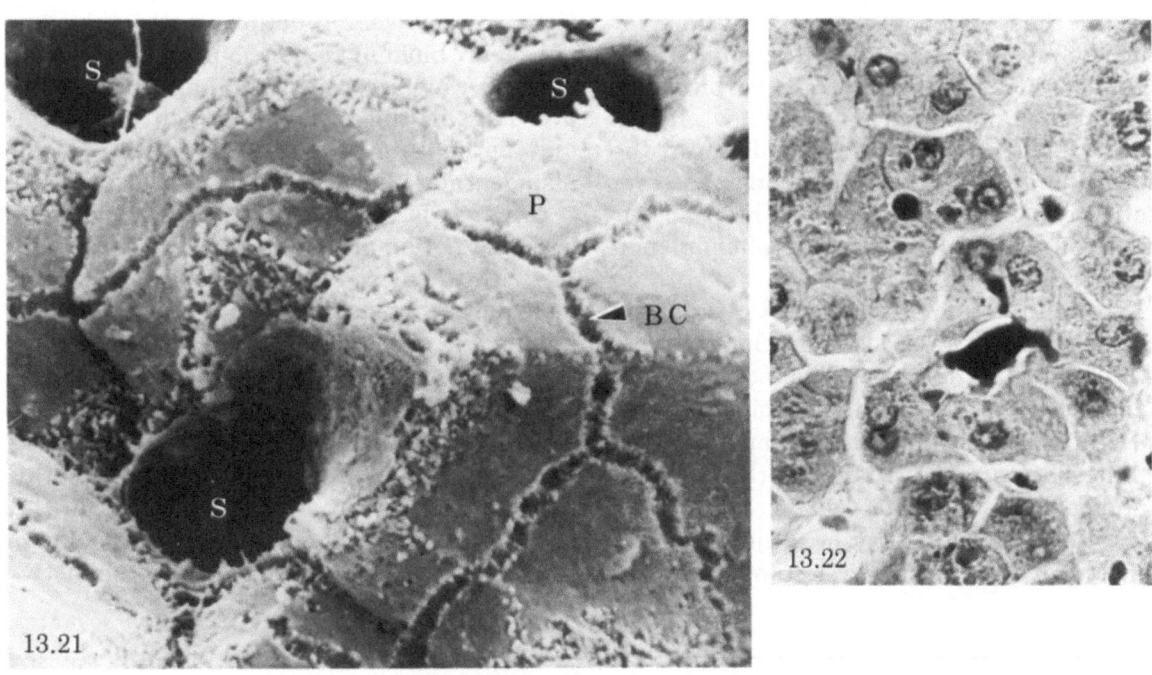

S

S

P

BC

S

13.21

13.22

ELECTRON MICROSCOPY (Fig. 13.23). Electron micrographs of hepatocytes show more of the usual organelles and inclusions than most other cells possess. We will discuss here only those involved in liver-specific functions.

Mitochondria number a thousand or more per cell, largely because of the amount of energy required for membrane transport and for the elaborate organic chemistry involved in the synthesis and degradation of the numerous substances that these cells process.

Rough endoplasmic reticulum (RER) synthesizes not only proteins for the cell's own structural and enzymatic needs, but also the albumin of the blood, some of the proteins involved in blood-clotting mechanisms, and most of the globulins of the blood. Proteins for export are completed in the Golgi but not stored as secretory granules or droplets. Instead they are directly, and more or less continuously, secreted into the blood (endocrine secretion).

Smooth endoplasmic reticulum (SER) of the hepatocyte is of significance in an astonishing variety of liver functions. The amount of SER varies greatly and changes rapidly in response to materials in the blood. SER contains enzymes responsible for oxidation, hydroxylation, or methylation of various compounds and/or their conjugation with sulfate or glucuronide. For example, by the conjugating action of glucuronyl transferase, barbiturates and antihistamines are inactivated. In response to the presence of these drugs in the blood, the amount of SER may increase dramatically. Such an increase is the basis for increased drug tolerance. This phenomenon is clinically useful.

Let us digress for a moment to exemplify this last point. Jaundice is caused by an excess of bilirubin in the blood. This compound is a product of degraded hemoglobin and it is normally processed by the liver and excreted in bile. The administration of barbiturates to jaundiced patients induces an increase in SER and thus in the quantity of conjugating enzymes, and the rate of excretion of the biliru-bin is increased with resulting reduction of the jaundice.

SER is also responsible for the polymerization of glucose to glycogen, and for its storage. Glycogen is depolymerized and released into the circulation when the blood glucose level falls.

Cholesterol is also synthesized and free fatty acids are esterified to triglycerides for cytoplasmic storage as fat droplets.

The bile acids secreted through the duct system to the duodenum for digestive functions are produced by the synthesis of cholic acid in the SER and its conjugation with taurine and glycine.

Lipoproteins of the blood are synthesized in the liver by cooperative function of RER (protein synthesis) and SER (lipid synthesis). The Golgi apparatus completes the assembly and secretion processes.

Golgi saccules arranged in the characteristic stacks are numerous and scattered, but groups tend to be located most frequently near the bile canaliculi or near the nuclei. In view of the constant and high level of the secretory activities of hepatocytes, these are of considerable importance to liver function.

Lysosomes and peroxisomes are numerous, and generally seem to have a peripheral location. Their specific functions in the liver are not clear, but under hormonal and other influences they apparently manage autophagic processes in the turnover of cell organelles and perhaps in hepatocyte turnover. They also degrade phagocytosed material.

Glycogen is, of course, a storage form of glucose and not an organelle. However, it is visible with the electron microscope as electron-dense granules usually occurring in clusters among the cisterns of SER. The glycogen in the liver constitutes an important pool for deposit or withdrawal of glucose to maintain a constant level of blood sugar. This is a critically important function since glucose is the principal energy-producing compound in the body. The amount of glycogen in the pool varies with nutritional condition, physical activity, and time of day.

Fig. 13.23. Electron micrograph of a portion of four *hepatocytes* surrounding a canaliculus (C). Glycogen (G), lysosome (L), Golgi (Go), RER (R), mitochondrion (M). ×14,600. (Courtesy of R. Brooks.)

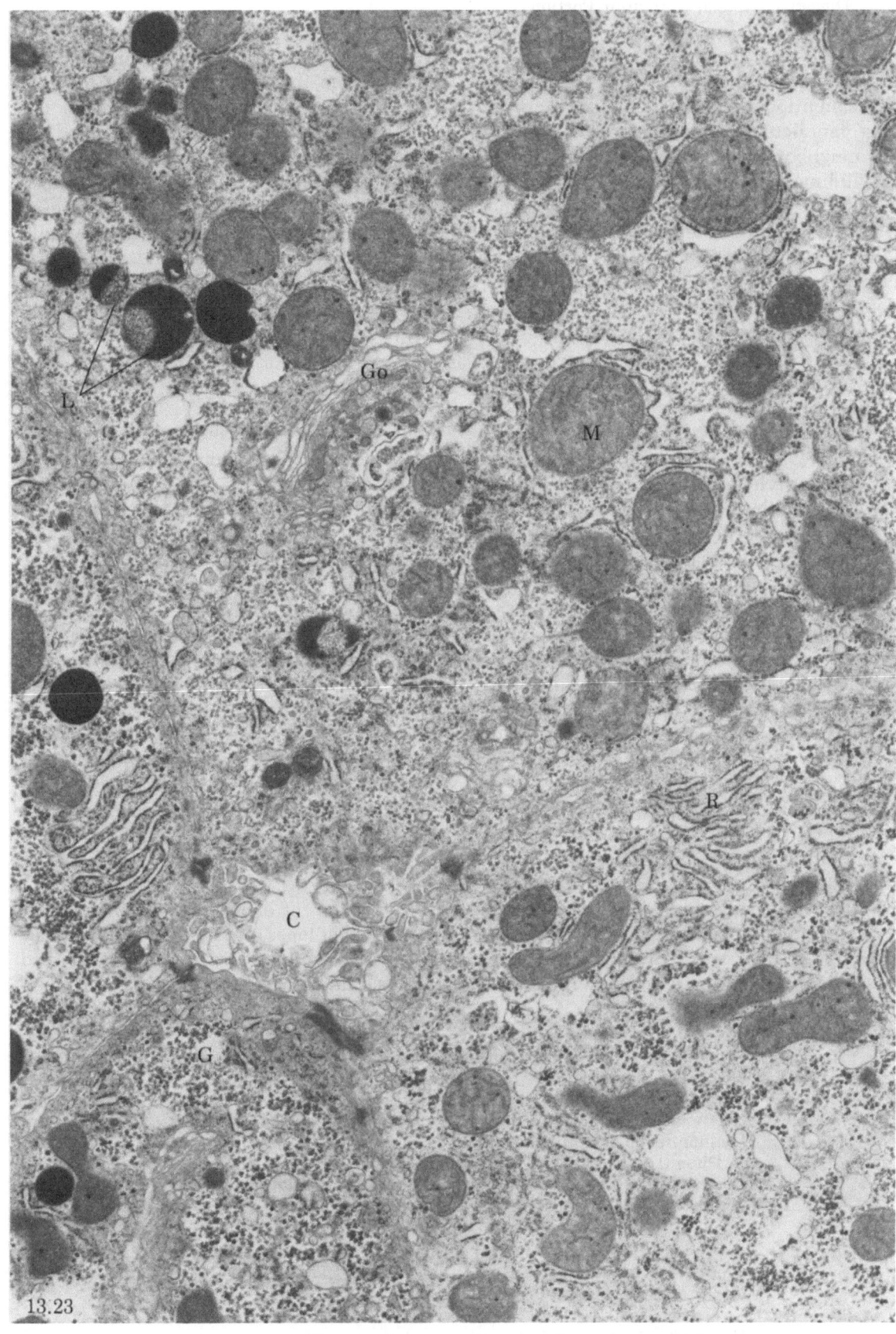

13.23

The features of the plasmalemma of the hepatocyte vary on the different surfaces of the cell. As mentioned above, the surface carrying a bile canaliculus is closely applied to that of its neighboring hepatocyte and has a strip of occluding junction along each side of the canaliculus. There are also scattered desmosomes and gap junctions. The bile canaliculus itself has a few short microvilli. The cell surface facing the sinusoidal endothelium is provided with numerous microvilli of irregular height and thickness. A glycocalyx is present.

Sinusoids

The liver requires a rich capillary network (Figs. 13.19, 13.24, and 13.28) to sustain its functions, especially the endocrine ones. This network, and the blood within it, surround and bathe each of the hepatic laminae. These capillaries are called sinusoids because they are variable in diameter and are lined by a discontinuous endothelium that has large fenestrations without diaphragms. The basal lamina is incomplete and often missing over large areas. Only the cells of blood are held back; the plasma flows readily through the wall and into the *perisinusoidal space* (of Disse). The perisinusoidal space is occupied by microvilli of the hepatocytes and by scattered fine reticular fibers (Fig. 13.24).

In addition to the flat endothelial cells, large, stellate *hepatic macrophages* (Kupffer cells) (Figs. 13.24 and 13.25) are present in the walls of the sinusoids. These are not flattened and thus they often extend into the lumen. Their processes also extend into the perisinusoidal space. They are not different from the macrophages seen in other organs and tissues of the immune system. They avidly phagocytose particulates brought from the gut as well as senescent and disintegrated red blood cells. From the latter they break hemoglobin into iron and bilirubin. The iron is stored as hemosiderin (Fig. 13.25) to be used again in erythrocyte formation, and the bilirubin is passed via the perisinusoidal space to hepatocytes. In response to unknown signals, the size of the macrophage population varies with the need for its services.

Liver Function, Lobules, and Disease

The liver's many endocrine functions will now be considered. These include the processing of practically all of the foods absorbed from the gut (blood from which drains only to the liver), the storage of glycogen, the detoxification of various undesirable materials, and the production of many vital components of blood and certain factors important to other body parts. It is no wonder that the liver is the largest gland in the body, especially when the amounts of these materials are considered.

To accomplish all of its tasks the liver needs: the system of excretory bile ducts, canals, and canaliculi mentioned above; a rich sinusoidal network allowing close association between blood and hepatocytes, like other endocrine glands; and a system that permits the continuing regeneration and replacement of dying hepatocytes.

As is typical of exocrine glands, the liver is composed of lobes and lobules. But the liver lobules are confluent with each other and their boundaries are arbitrary if not imagi-

Fig. 13.24. Scanning electron micrograph of *liver*. A hepatic lamina (P) has been cleaved to expose half of a canaliculus (BC). The sinusoids (S) are connected through an opening (lacuna) in the lamina. The upper sinusoid contains two leukocytes (L). A large Kupffer cell (K) extends from one sinusoid to the other through the lacuna. ×3300. Arrows indicate fenestrations connecting the sinusoid with the space of Disse (D). (Courtesy of P. Williams and A. Jones in Jones AL, Schmucker DL, Renston RH, Murakami T: The architecture of bile secretion—A morphological perspective of physiology. Dig Dis Sci 25:609–629, 1980.)

Fig. 13.25. *Kupffer cells* (arrows). The section has been stained for iron. It is from a patient with excessive destruction of erythrocytes (hemolytic anemia). Iron is also present in many of the hepatocytes. ×400.

Fig. 13.26. A *classic lobule* with portal tracts. ×90.

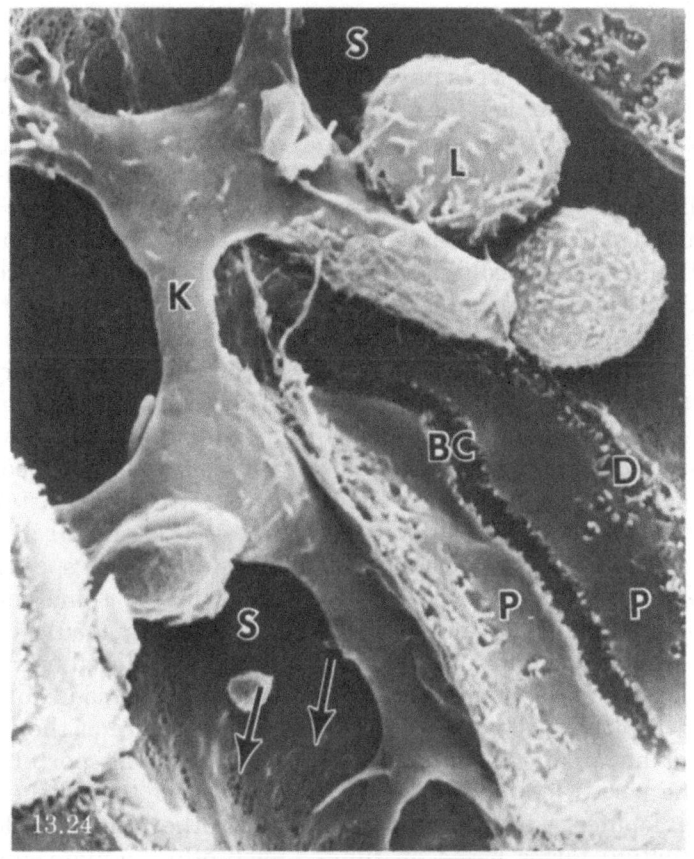

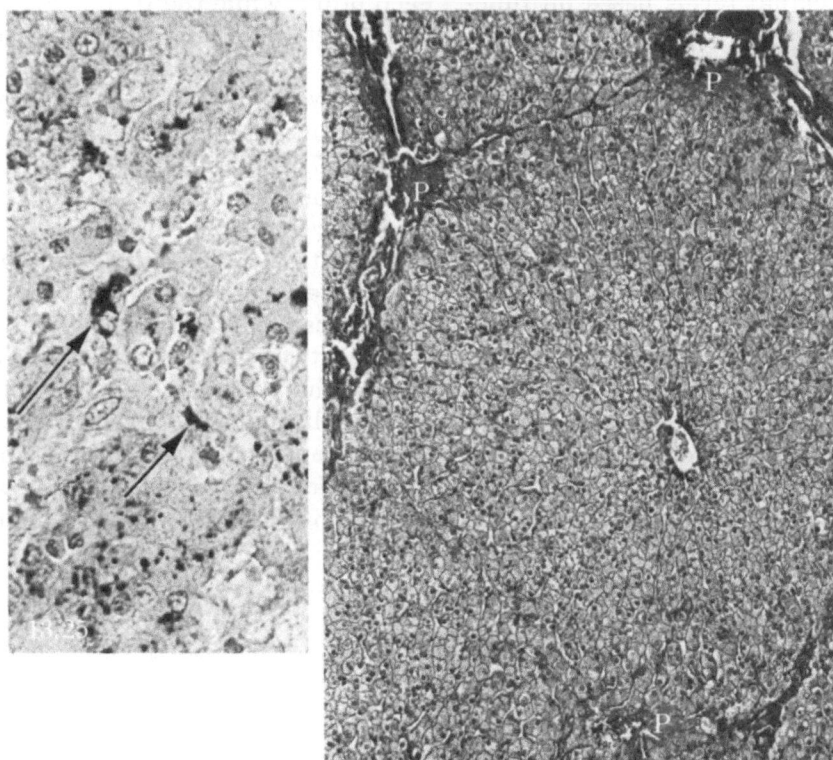

nary. There is controversy as to what a liver lobule really is, but two basic types have been described. The classic lobule (Figs. 13.26, 13.27) is a mass of liver tissue about 3 mm in diameter; it has a central vein (Fig. 13.19) around which laminae of hepatocytes appear to be radially arranged. The central vein collects the blood that has been perfused through the sinusoids; from central veins blood flows into progressively merging and larger channels to enter the inferior vena cava near the heart. The classic lobule has three to six portal tracts (Fig. 13.18) set about its periphery; these feed blood into the sinusoids. So blood flows from the periphery to the center of the classic lobule, and bile flows in the opposite direction, into the bile ducts of the portal tracts (Fig. 13.20).

The portal lobule (Figs. 13.26 and 13.27) is a unit (if only in concept) of a size similar to that of the classic lobule, but its center is the portal tract; the draining veins (which we and many others have called "central") are peripheral in the portal lobule. We want to stress that liver lobules, whether classic or portal, are conceptual terms based on function. Liver lobules do not have anatomic boundaries. Both blood and bile are able to find alternate routes via adjoining lobules when an intralobular obstruction occurs.

A hepatic lamina is usually wrapped around each portal tract. This lamina is called the limiting plate. Canals of Hering pass through it.

Specimens of liver, by both gross and histologic examination, often show two different appearances to the parenchyma in the same case and at the same time. This contrast is present quite evenly throughout the organ and it has a striking pattern. The contrast may result from any of several functional or pathologic states. The congestion of the liver associated with chronic heart failure has become well known as "nutmeg liver" (it hap-

pens to look like the cut surface of a whole nutmeg). The two contrasting zones are the pericentral one (surrounding the central vein), in which the parenchymal cells are dead or dying, and the periportal one, where the cells are healthier (Fig. 13.28a). The pericentral cells, being further from the source of supply of blood with its oxygen and other nutrients, are the first to suffer (Fig. 13.28b). The extent of the zone of degeneration varies according to the severity of its cause.

Not surprisingly, patterns similar to nutmeg liver may be produced by injecting a liver with two different-colored materials separately through portal and hepatic venous routes (Fig. 13.29). If one looks critically at either diseased specimens or injected ones, one will see some round areas conceivably representing lobule centers, but also many similarly colored ones that are serpentine or branching. This is due to the branching treelike structure of the two vascular systems of the liver, the portal and the central (Fig. 13.17). The tops of the two trees point toward each other, and are closely intertwined with each other, while the trunks extend in opposite directions. Using this model one can understand why the shape of the lobule, seen in just two dimensions in histologic sections, varies considerably.

About 70% of the blood delivered to a lobule comes from the portal vein, which is carrying blood received from the capillary network of the intestinal mucosa. The remainder of the blood in a lobule comes from the hepatic artery. Thus blood leaving the liver has passed through two capillary beds: that of the gastrointestinal mucosa and that of the liver. Hence, all material absorbed from the intestine (except lipids, which are transported by lymphatics to the caval system) traverses the liver before passing into the general circulation.

Fig. 13.27. Schematic reconstruction of one complete *classic hepatic lobule* and a portion of another. Five portal tracts and two central veins are shown. (Based on the work of H. Elias.)

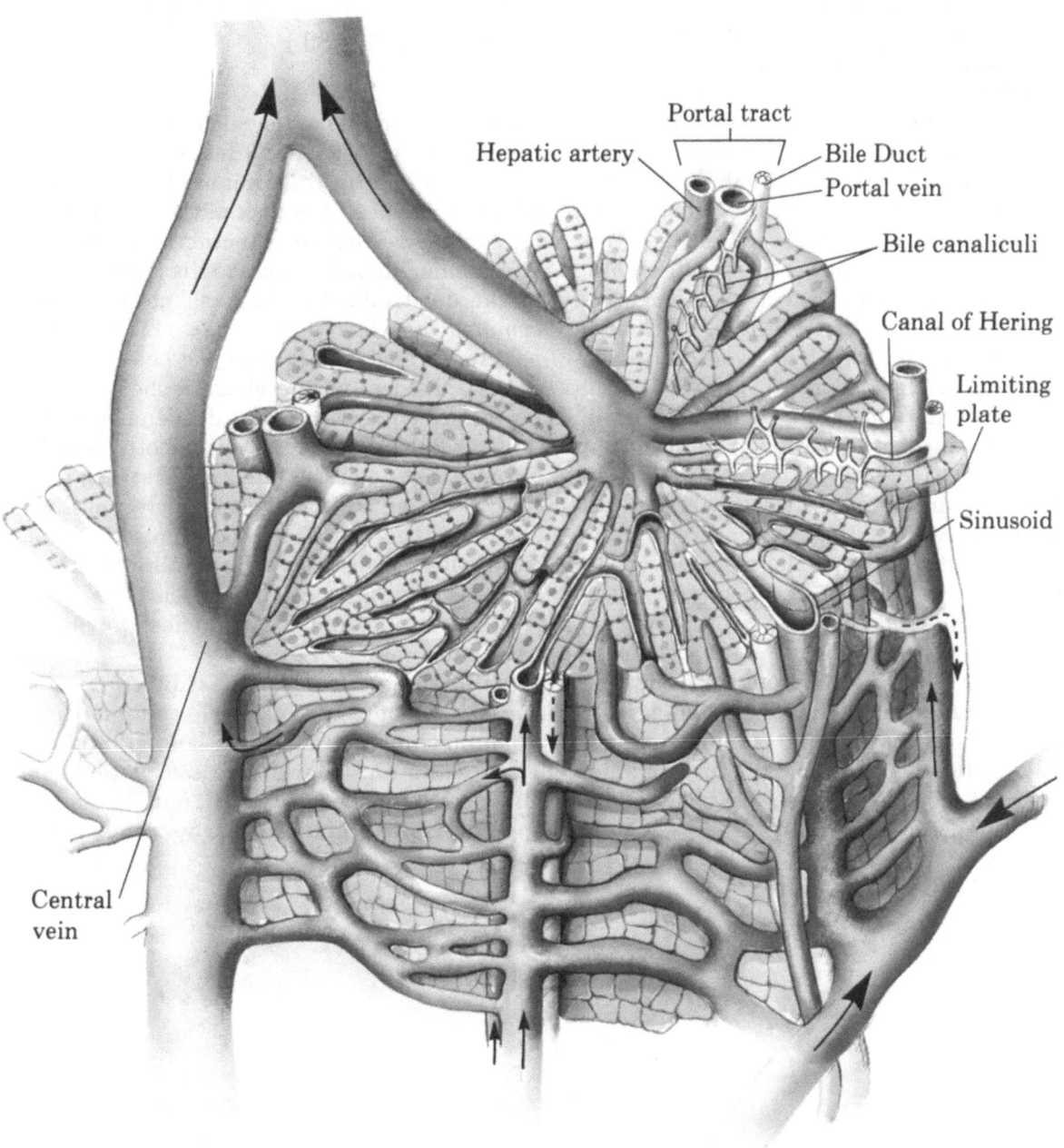

Portal tract

Hepatic artery

Bile Duct

Portal vein

Bile canaliculi

Canal of Hering

Limiting plate

Sinusoid

Central vein

13.27

Cirrhosis is a common liver disease that has several different causes, of which alcohol abuse is the most common and best known. To discuss the pathogenesis of this complex condition would be inappropriate here, but it is easy to point out the importance of the disrupted lobular architecture that characterizes this ailment. Basically the problem is a repetitive series of attacks on hepatocytes, their supporting framework and intervening sinusoids and canaliculi, with a progressive, disorderly regeneration of these. The lobule (either classic or portal) is eventually completely rearranged (Fig. 13.30). This occurs throughout the entire organ. Blood, instead of percolating slowly through sinusoids in close association with its target, the hepatocytes, is shunted more directly from portal to emissary vessels. Hepatocytes are supplied only indirectly and in some cases not at all. Canaliculi are also obstructed. In view of the numerous functions of the liver previously mentioned it is not difficult to see that many abnormalities can result from this condition. Jaundice (due to obstruction of bile canaliculi), increased susceptibility to infection, and tendency for easy bleeding and bruising (due to lack of clotting factors), are some of the more common ones.

Extrahepatic Biliary System (Figs. 13.9, 13.17, and 13.31)

DUCTS. Two main stems leave the porta of the liver as the right and left hepatic ducts. These join to form the common hepatic duct, which is joined by the duct of the gallbladder (*cystic duct*). From the junction of the cystic and common hepatic ducts to the termination in the duodenum the duct is known as the *common bile duct* (Fig. 13.32). This and the pancreatic duct usually join just before entering the duodenum and share a short, intramural segment within the duodenal papilla (Fig. 13.33). A sphincter of smooth muscle around the end of the bile duct is strong and controls its emptying. This sphincter (of Boyden), together with the smooth muscle of the papilla itself, constitutes the papillary sphincter (of Oddi). The papillary muscle is not particularly strong, and does not effectively hold back pancreatic secretion.

All of these ducts are lined by a mucous membrane composed of simple columnar epithelium supported by a thin lamina propria. There is no muscularis mucosae. A tenuous and inconstant sheet of smooth muscle is present that is not organized into discrete layers.

Fig. 13.28. "*Nutmeg liver*." The portions of parenchyma that surround the portal tracts (portal zones) and those about the central veins (central zones) are sharply contrasted because of the necrosis of the cells in the central zones. This was due to heart failure. **a:** ×35. **b:** Area within rectangle in **a.** Central vein (above) and portal tract (below). ×150.

Fig. 13.29. Simultaneous injection of light and dark colored substances into the *portal and central veins* produces a pattern similar to that of nutmeg liver. This is due to the interdigitation of the tops of the two trees shown in Fig. 13.17. ×35.

Fig. 13.30. *Fatty cirrhosis* in alcoholism. The normal lobular pattern has been entirely replaced. Portal tracts have extended around nodules. Blood is shunted away from parenchymal cells, which show marked accumulation of fat. ×85.

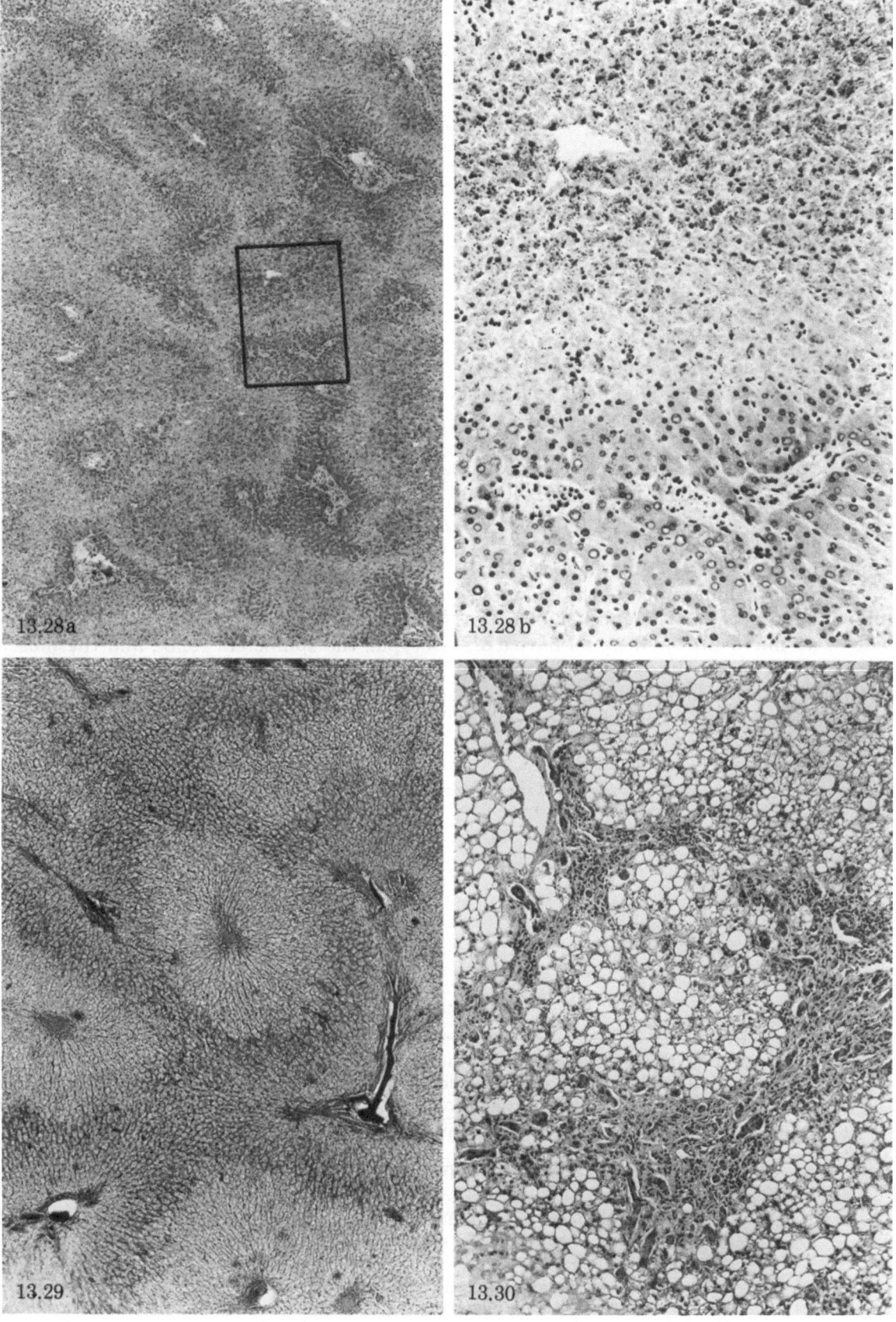

13.28a

13.28 b

13.29

13.30

The wall contains a moderate number of mucous glands. This muscularis becomes thicker at the lower end of the common bile duct and its lowermost part becomes the biliary sphincter.

THE GALLBLADDER is an elongated, tapering sac, about 10 cm in length and suspended from the posterior surface of the liver (Figs. 13.17 and 13.31). It is bound to the liver by an adventitia and covered on its free, unattached surface by a serosa. Its function is to store and concentrate bile secreted by the liver. It releases bile in response to neurologic and humoral stimuli. It consists of a body, a neck, and a cystic duct. The neck and cystic duct are twisted and kinked in such a way that the mucosa forms a spiral valve (of Heister). The muscularis is commonly thicker here than in the gallbladder itself, and mucous glands are present.

The mucosa (Fig. 13.34) is composed of branching and anastomosing folds of simple columnar epithelium supported by a loose cellular lamina propria. The epithelium is provided with microvilli, but does not have a distinct striated border. In sections, the pockets found under these folds often give the false impression of glands. Sometimes these spaces enlarge and, particularly in older individuals, extend deeply into the lamina propria and even through the muscularis. They do not occur in gallbladders of very young persons, and, although of common occurrence, may represent a pathologic change.

The epithelium is important in the concentration of bile. Its cells are joined by tight (occluding) junctions. Sodium is actively pumped from the cells into the intercellular space deep to the tight junctions. This establishes an osmotic gradient that pulls water from the lumen of the gallbladder into the space and from there into the connective tissue and blood vessels of the lamina propria.

There is no muscularis mucosae and thus no true submucosa.

Muscularis externa. Normally the muscle layer of the gallbladder is a thin but distinct, irregularly organized layer of overlapping sheets of smooth muscle. The fibers are generally oriented in a spiral, oblique pattern.

When dietary fats enter the duodenum, cholecystokinin is released from the intestinal crypts, the sphincters relax, and the muscle of the gallbladder contracts. These actions propel bile to the duodenum, where it emulsifies fats.

Fig. 13.31. X-ray of the extrahepatic *biliary system* demonstrated by injection of contrast agent into it. Gallbladder (G), cystic duct with spiral valve (Cy), common duct (C), intraduodenal portion (I) of common duct, duodenum (D). (Courtesy of the Department of Diagnostic Radiology, Oregon Health Sciences University.)

Fig. 13.32. *Common bile duct* from a child. ×90.

Fig. 13.33. *Duodenal papilla.* The termination of the common duct is narrow and surrounded by smooth muscle (arrow). ×5.5.

Fig. 13.34. *Gallbladder.* There is no muscularis mucosae and therefore no division of the connective tissue underlying the epithelium into lamina propria and submucosa. Junction of connective tissue and muscle is indicated by arrows. ×90.

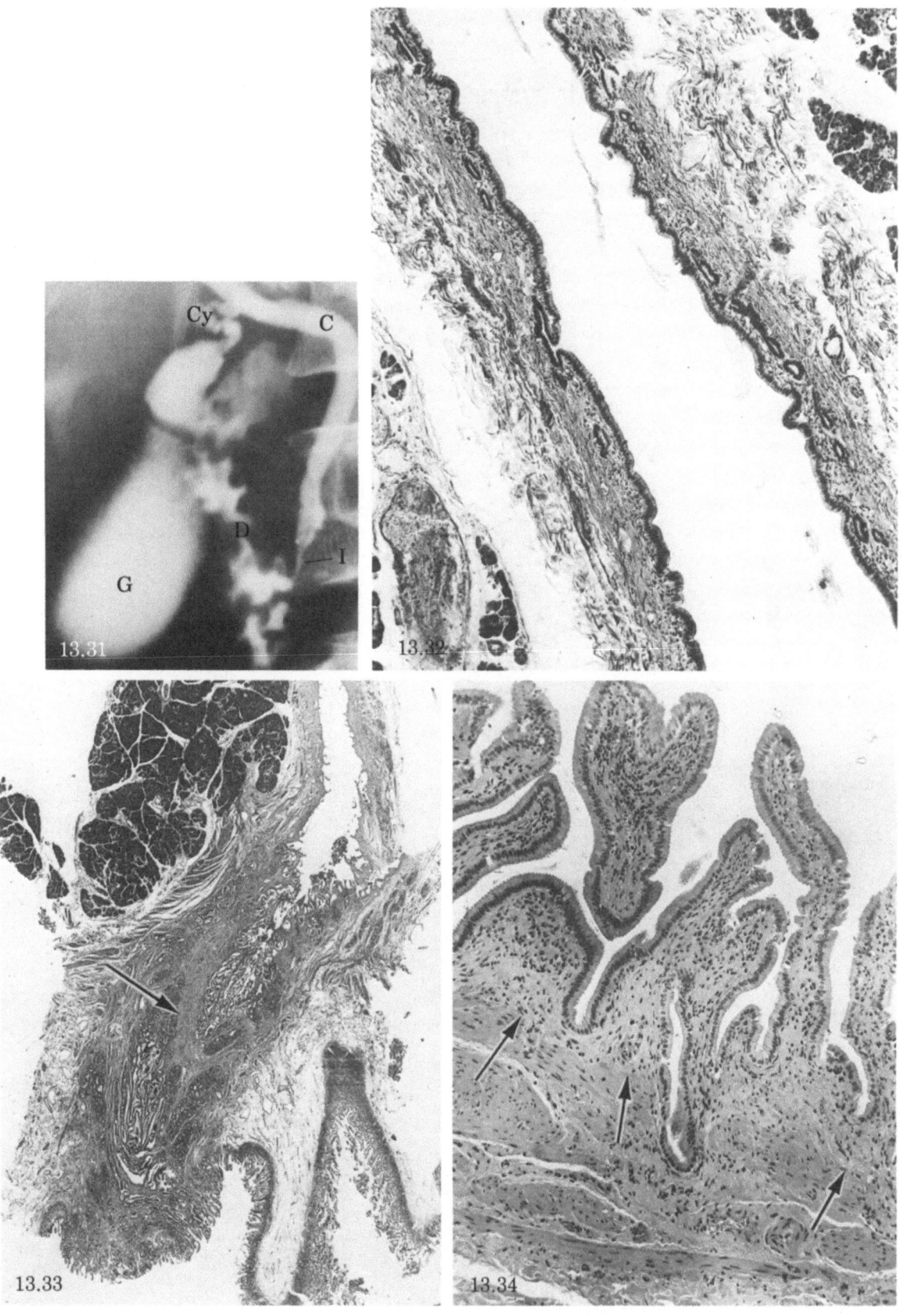

14 Respiratory system

Introduction

The main function of the respiratory system is to supply oxygen to the blood and eliminate carbon dioxide. The system (Fig. 14.1) must admit a maximal amount of air through a narrow inlet and a minimal volume of passageways. It must also distribute this air to the largest possible surface for gas exchange with blood. To do this the system has two functionally different parts, a *conducting portion* and a *respiratory portion*. The conducting portion includes nasal cavities with their associated olfactory mucosa (Fig. 14.2), paranasal sinuses, pharynx, larynx, trachea, bronchi, and bronchioles. It conducts air to the respiratory portion. The respiratory portion is composed of respiratory bronchioles, alveolar ducts, alveolar sacs, and some 300 million alveoli. Here gases are exchanged between air and blood. Table 14.1 lists some measurements of these components.

In addition to guiding air in and out of the lungs, the conducting portion provides mechanisms for removing particulate debris and adjusting the temperature and humidity of the inspired air. The respiratory part of the system contains an average of 70–80 m² of extremely thin, delicate membrane that separates the inspired air from the blood and allows the exchange of adequate volumes of oxygen and carbon dioxide. The necessary presence of a moving column of air has made possible the coincidental evolution of a structure that may be biologically unnecessary but is very useful, the larynx. (Figs. 14.3 and 14.4).

Anatomic features of the two portions of the system clearly differ, and diseases affecting them cause different physiologic abnormalities. For example, partial obstruction of

Table 14.1

	Larynx and Trachea	Bronchi	Bronchioles	Respiratory Bronchioles	Alveolar Ducts and Alveoli
Length, mm	220	130	5	4	3
Cross-sectional area at a single level, cm²	2	14	79	281	700,000
Volume, ml	80	71	43	865	3,000
Number of successive branchings in a single path (see text)	0	14	3	3	6
Number of structures at:					
most proximal level	1	2	1,000	121,000	832,000
most distal level		609	46,000	514,000	299,000,000

Data are from Thurlbeck WL, Wang NS: The structure of the lungs. In Middicombe JD (ed): Review of Science, Physiology Series One, Vol. 2, Respiratory Physiology. Baltimore, University Park Press, 1974.)

the smaller distal airways seriously affects many patients by limiting the passage of gases in and out. Conversely, thickening of the respiratory membrane, when sufficiently extensive, cripples others by limiting the exchange of gases. Clinical recognition of these conditions often demands specific tests for impairment of the conducting or respiratory functions.

Prevention of disability depends on the integrity of most, if not all, of the component layers of the airways. Loss of smooth muscle in a bronchial wall results in dilation (bronchiectasis) and consequent complications. Replacement of the normal bronchial mucosa with stratified squamous epithelium, as is commonly found in cigarette smokers, impedes the upward transport of mucus and for-

eign particles by cilia (mucociliary escalator) to the larynx. These substances are trapped and therefore accumulate in the lung. Other diseases affect the respiratory membrane by thickening it (as in interstitial fibrosis), by destroying it (as in emphysema), or by filling up the air spaces (as in bacterial pneumonia).

Conducting Portion

Nasal Cavities, Paranasal Sinuses, and Pharynx

The nasal cavities are a more or less symmetrical pair separated by a bony septum. The vestibule is the anterior portion of each

Fig. 14.1. *Orienting diagram.* The airways in the area labeled respiratory tissue are shown enlarged. The pleural cavities are collapsed spaces between the lung and the rib cage and other contiguous structures. They entirely surround each lung except at its hilum.

Fig. 14.2. *Olfactory epithelium.* The differentiating features are: the several layers of nuclei; a broad clear zone representing the apical portions of the columnar cells; and the ducts of the numerous mucosal (Bowman's) glands. ×320. (Courtesy of R. Quinton-Cox.)

Fig. 14.3. *Frontal section of lateral wall of larynx.* **A:** True vocal fold (cord). **B:** False vocal fold (cord). **C:** Vocal ligament. **D:** Ventricle. **E:** Vocalis muscle. **F:** Thyroid cartilage. ×12.

Fig. 14.4. *Anterior view of larynx.* The right half of the drawing is of a frontal section.

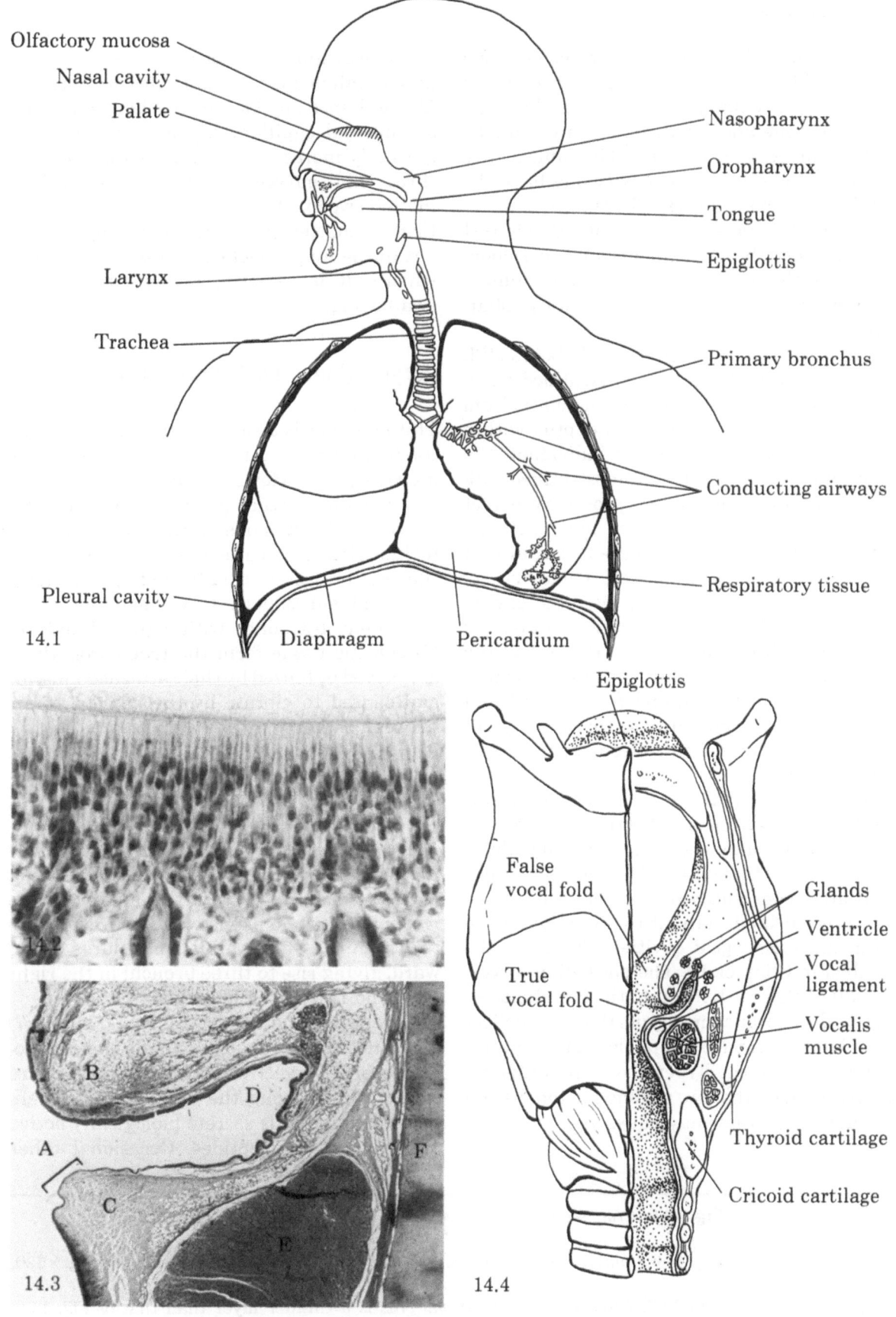

Olfactory mucosa
Nasal cavity
Palate
Larynx
Trachea
Pleural cavity
Diaphragm
Pericardium

Nasopharynx
Oropharynx
Tongue
Epiglottis
Primary bronchus
Conducting airways
Respiratory tissue

14.1

14.2

14.3

A   B   C   D   E   F

Epiglottis

False
vocal fold

True
vocal fold

Glands
Ventricle
Vocal
ligament
Vocalis
muscle

Thyroid cartilage

Cricoid cartilage

14.4

cavity; it lies within the skin-covered nose and has flexible walls. The remaining portions of the nasal cavities are surrounded by rigid walls of bone and cartilage and are lined by a thin mucous membrane. The sinuses are simply extensions of the cavity and have the same component layers. There is no submucosa; the lamina propria and its glands rest directly on the periosteum and perichondrium in the nose and sinuses and on muscle and other supporting structures in the pharynx.

Near the nostril each vestibule bears stiff, coarse hairs and keratinized stratified squamous epithelium. Further in, the epithelium is nonkeratinized. At various depths within the nasal cavities of different individuals the epithelium changes to pseudostratified ciliated columnar with mucus-producing goblet cells. Basal (reserve) cells do not reach the surface. This epithelium characterizes almost all of the conducting portion. Olfactory epithelium (Fig. 14.2), high in the nasal cavity, is relatively thick and cellular and it appears more specialized than that in the rest of the respiratory system. Numerous serous and mucous glands in the lamina propria assist in maintaining the humidity so that drying will not damage the delicate deeper portions of the system.

The portion of the nasal cavity posterior to the nasal septum is called the nasopharynx (Fig. 14.1); it contains several mucosal nodules of lymphoid tissue called adenoids. Larger and more constant lymphoid masses, tonsils, are present bilaterally at the junction of the oral and pharyngeal cavities. These are described in Chapter 10. The epithelium covering all of these extends into the lymphoid tissue as deep, branching crypts that may collect cellular debris. Such lymphoid accumulations are the site of the hyperplasia and other reactive changes that are common in tonsils and adenoids and that may cause their enlargement.

The warming of inspired air and the trapping of inhaled foreign particles are considerably enhanced by two means. One is the rich submucosal capillary plexuses; the other is a greatly increased surface area provided by three thin, curved turbinate bones. Ciliary motion sweeps the mucus and entrapped particulate matter, which is potentially dangerous to the lungs, backward into the pharynx, whence it is removed by expectoration or swallowing.

Larynx (Figs. 14.3 and 14.4)

This chamber is also lined almost entirely by conducting epithelium. Its wall contains some mucous glands. However, the true vocal cords and sometimes other portions have a mantle of stratified squamous epithelium. The walls include striated muscle and the laryngeal cartilages; the latter usually undergo calcification and subsequent bony metaplasia (replacement by bone) with aging. Bands of fibroelastic tissue form the true cords; these are moved or tensed by their attached muscles and caused to vibrate by the passage of air between them.

Trachea (Fig. 14.5) and Bronchi (Figs. 14.8 through 14.10)

The trachea is a thin-walled tube extending from the base of the larynx to a point where it divides into two primary bronchi. These enter the lungs at the hilus, and course downward, giving rise to three bronchi in the right lung and two in the left lung.

Conducting epithelium (Figs. 14.6 and 14.7) also lines these conduits. Small enteroendocrine (APUD) cells with clear cytoplasm are interspersed among the basal cells. The enteroendocrine cells secrete biologically active amines and polypeptides. Occasional other

Fig. 14.5. *Cross-section of trachea.* The posterior wall is at the bottom.

Fig. 14.6. *Conducting epithelium,* its basement membrane and lamina propria. ×520.

Fig. 14.7. *Bronchiolar epithelium.* This is a thinner layer than that of Fig. 14.6. **A:** Ciliated cells. **B:** Nonciliated cells. **C:** Basal cells. ×8000. (Courtesy of M. Webb.)

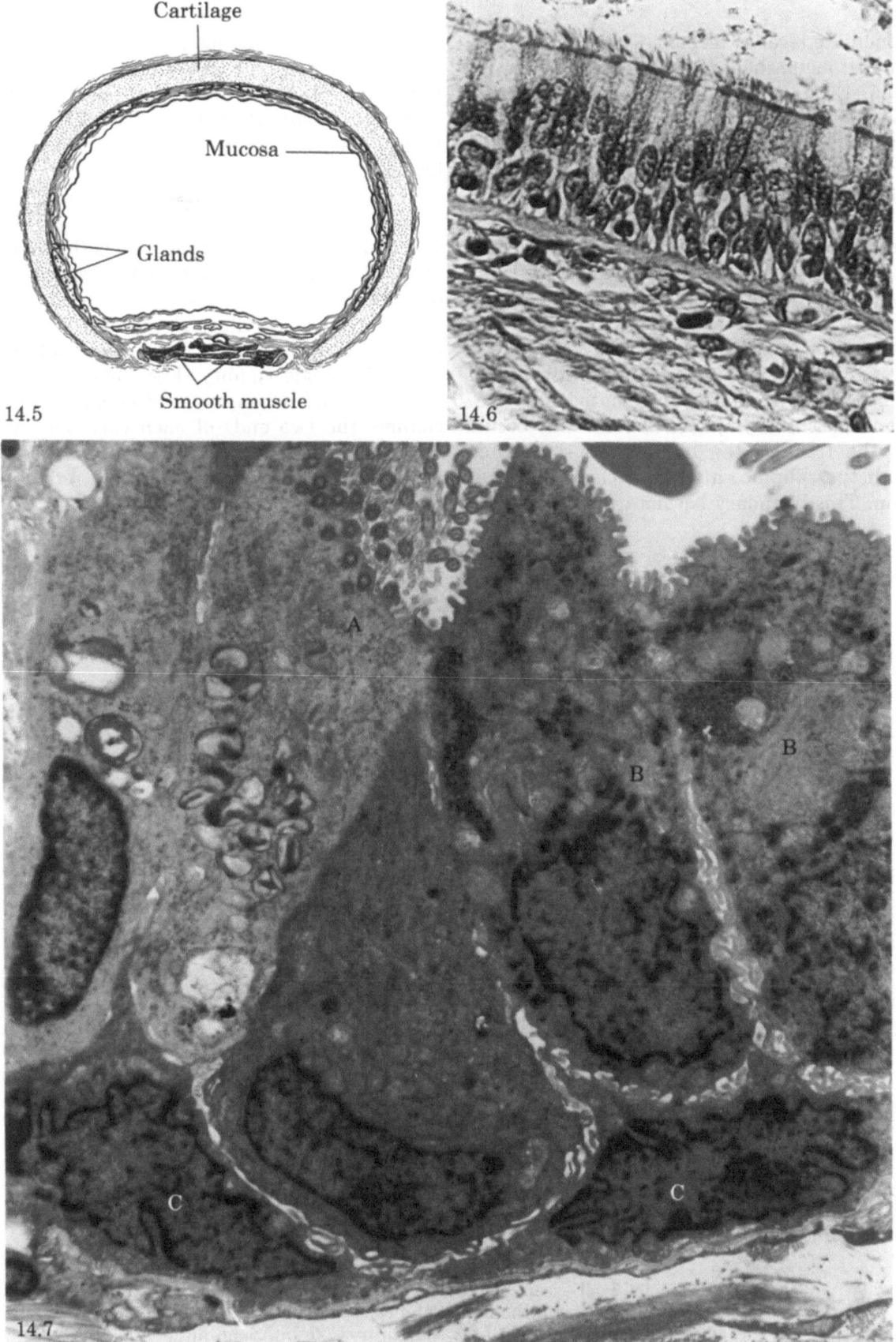

Cartilage

Mucosa

Glands

Smooth muscle

14.5

14.6

14.7

A

B

B

C

C

nonciliated cells, termed Clara cells, have small tongue-shaped projections into the lumen. Electron microscopy may be required for the identification of both of these cell types. The functions of both are unclear. The normal basement membrane is thicker than that underlying other epithelia (Fig. 14.6).

The lamina propria is a loose vascular connective tissue, which is infiltrated with a variety of cell types. It is similar to the same layer in the gut. The cells include lymphocytes, plasma cells, and macrophages. All these cells have important protective functions as the first line of defense against air-borne pathogens. They are diffusely distributed, but occasional discrete lymphoid nodules may occur. In the trachea, the lamina propria blends with the submucosa without clear demarcation. This boundary becomes more apparent

in the bronchi, being marked by a well-developed muscularis mucosae. This is in the form of bands of smooth muscle that run in inner and outer layers (Fig. 14.8). They are most highly developed in medium-sized and small bronchi.

The submucosa, external to the muscle, is a loose connective tissue containing small vessels and mucous and serous glands (Fig. 14.8 and 14.9). The glands also contain enteroendocrine cells.

The C-shaped cartilage rings of the trachea and the less regular cartilage plates of the bronchi provide rigidity (Figs. 14.8 through 14.10). In the trachea, bands of smooth muscle connect the two ends of each cartilage. All of these structures except the mucosa are invested with a rich network of fine reticular and elastic fibers.

Fig. 14.8. *Bronchial wall.* **A:** Smooth muscle. **B:** Mixed (mucoserous) gland. **C:** Cartilage. ×100.

Fig. 14.9. *Cross-section of a bronchus from a case of fatal asthma.* **A:** Hypertrophy of outer circular layer of smooth muscle. **B:** Hypertrophy of inner longitudinal bands of smooth muscle; this has caused folding of the mucosa. **C:** Some of the copious viscid mucus. The mucus secretion and muscular contraction are intermittent or spasmodic. It should therefore be clear why this is a reversible bronchial condition. Administration of appropriate drugs helps to relax the muscle, liquefy the mucus, and relieve the obstruction. ×11. (Courtesy of W. G. Brady.)

Fig. 14.10. *Adenocarcinoma* arising in a bronchus. **a:** The tumor replaces most of the bronchial wall except the cartilage plates. Obstruction of the bronchus results from both narrowing of the lumen and replacement of the normal epithelial lining. The rectangle indicates the area seen in **b.** ×7.5. **b:** Adenocarcinoma (upper right) contrasted with normal glands (lower left). ×100.

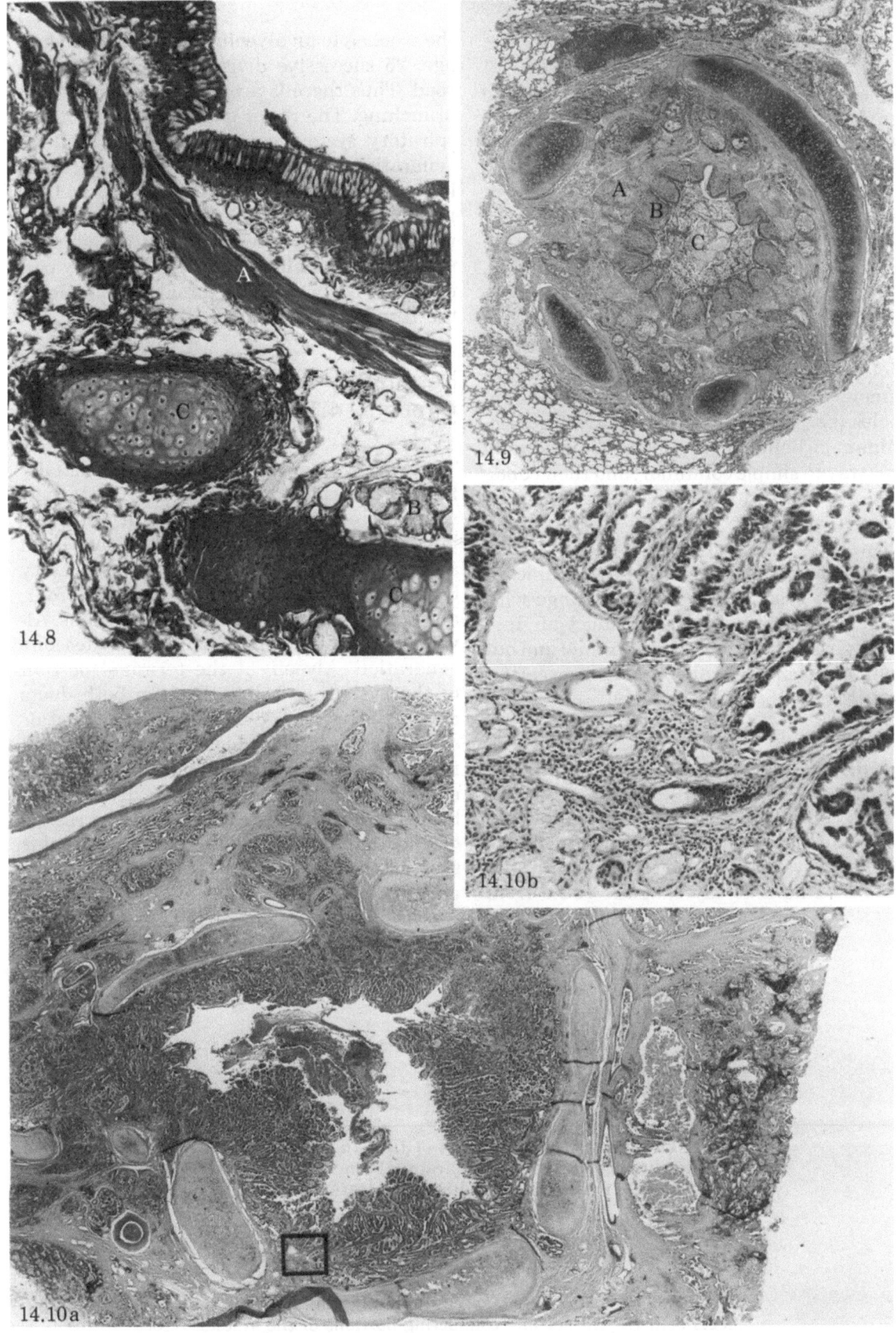

14.8

14.9

14.10b

14.10a

Bronchioles (Fig. 14.11)

Bronchi divide into smaller bronchi that lead into bronchioles. Each bronchiole branches into five to seven terminal bronchioles. These are the last airways completely lined with conducting epithelium (Figs. 14.6 and 14.7). They lead into respiratory bronchioles (*see below*). All the airways gradually and smoothly taper as they branch, like a tree, in a fashion similar to that of arteries and nerves throughout the body. The absence of cartilage distinguishes bronchioles from bronchi. Bronchioles are normally not more than 1 mm in diameter. In progression down the bronchioles (i.e., distally), the pseudostratified columnar epithelium with goblet cells gradually gives way to simple columnar, and then cuboidal, epithelium without goblet cells; cilia and submucosal glands are also present proximally and gradually disappear distally. None of this epithelium permits any significant transfer of gases across it for exchange with blood. It lines airways that conduct air into the respiratory epithelium (*see below*) and out again. It is therefore called *conducting epithelium* (Figs. 14.6, 14.7 and 14.19).

Respiratory Portion

There is an average of 25 or 26 generations of dichotomous and trichotomous branchings of the airways down to the terminal unit, the alveolus. This is to say that the route from the trachea to an alveolus passes, on the average, 25 successive divisions, or forks in the road. Thus there is a phenomenal amount of branching. The respiratory portion of the respiratory system contains 25–40% of these generations. The distance between branchings becomes shorter distally so that the lung parenchyma in histologic section appears more like a fine lacework than a system of tubes. The first airway of the respiratory portion (i.e., beyond the terminal bronchiole) is the respiratory bronchiole (Fig. 14.11).

Respiratory Bronchioles (Figs. 14.11 through 14.13, 14.20)

These are so named because they are partially lined by respiratory epithelium and their walls are interrupted by the openings of alveolar ducts and individual alveoli. There is an average of three generations of respiratory bronchioles. Alveolar ducts, next in order, also have an average of three generations. Alveolar sacs follow and usually have just one generation. Alveoli, at the terminal portion of the system bud directly from both ducts and sacs; there are 8–10 of these per duct or sac. Smooth muscle, which becomes more and more sparse distally, is found in alveolar ducts at the orifices of the sacs or alveoli that branch from them. Except for the presence of smooth muscle, alveolar ducts and alveolar sacs are much the same (Figs. 14.14, 14.15, and 14.20).

Fig. 14.11. *The respiratory portion of the lung.* **A:** Terminal bronchiole (the end of the conducting portion). **B:** Respiratory bronchioles. **C:** Alveolar duct. **D:** Alveolar sac. **E:** Alveoli. **F:** Pleura. **G:** Pulmonary arteries. ×40.

Fig. 14.12. *Atelectasis* (collapse of lung). The air spaces are reduced in size and nonfunctional. ×100.

Fig. 14.13. *Pneumonia.* Air spaces contain cellular inflammatory exudate. This affects both respiratory and conducting portions of the system. ×100.

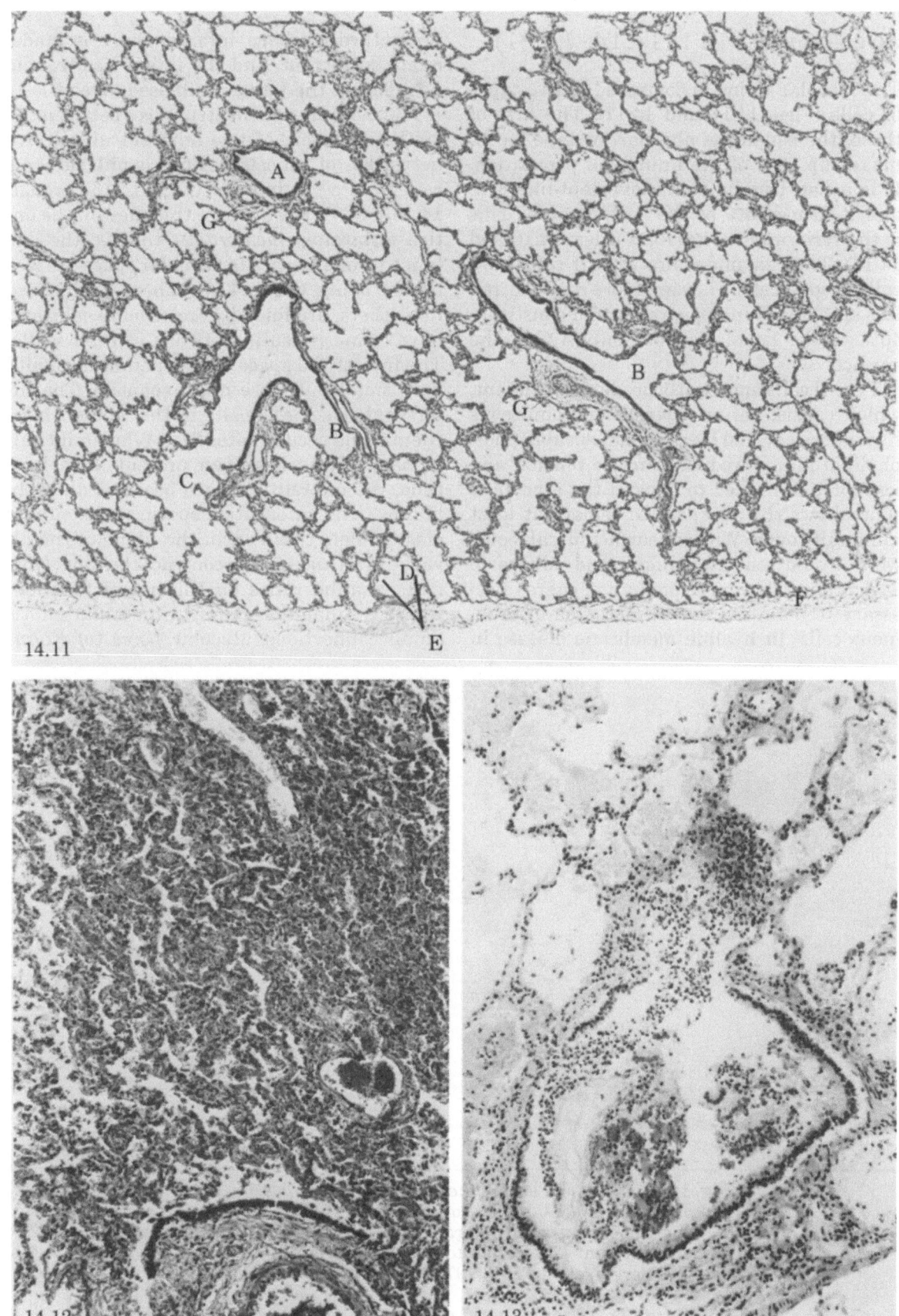

14.11

14.12

14.13

Alveoli (Figs. 14.11, 14.14, 14.21)

The alveolar lining is composed of two types of cells (Figs. 14.14 and 14.17). The first of these, the squamous alveolar, or type I cell, makes up 60% of the lining cell population. It is a flat, usually thin, pavement-like cell, and it forms 96% of the surface area. This is the *respiratory epithelium* (Figs. 14.16 and 14.17). The remainder are type II cells, also called septal cells. They are more rounded and less specialized in appearance and constitute 40% of the population but only 4% of the surface.

Type II cells apparently produce surfactant, which consists of an aqueous proteinaceous hypophase covered by a monomolecular phospholipid film. It reduces surface tension and less force is needed to expand the alveoli; it thus allows the air space to remain at least minimally open. Without surfactant, alveolar walls would tend to collapse and adhere to each other to lower the amount of energy necessary to maintain the surface area of squamous cells. In hyaline membrane disease in premature newborn infants, there is inadequate surfactant, and the infant has trouble in inflating the totally collapsed alveoli.

The most prominent structures between the epithelial layers of two adjacent alveoli are networks of anastomosing capillaries arranged in a single layer (Figs. 14.16 through 14.18, 14.23). The average thickness of the entire *respiratory membrane*—that is, the distance from air space to vascular space—is less than 0.5 μm (Fig. 14.17). These capillaries, like others, are lined by endothelial cells and have a fine reticulin network in their walls. The interstitial space about them is normally very small but loose and expansile. The intersital space is the site in the lobule where edema fluid accumulates first. When mild pulmonary edema has been present for a long time, the interstitial space becomes diffusely fibrous. The interstitial space also contains elastic fibers that run in the plane of the alveolar wall and tend to contract the lung. Normal exhaling relies on this recoil function, whereas inhalation requires muscular effort. Small connections, alveolar *pores (of Kohn)*

Fig. 14.14. *Functional unit of the lung.* Diagram indicating the cellular components. **A:** Conducting epithelium. **B:** Smooth muscle. **C:** Capillary. **D:** Type II pneumocyte. **E:** Type I pneumocyte. **F:** Interalveolar pore. **G:** Macrophages. (Based on Fig 21–36 by S. Sorokin: The Respiratory System. Weiss L and Greep R: Histology, 4th ed. New York, McGraw-Hill, 1977.)

Fig. 14.15. *Alveolar duct and alveoli.* ×49.

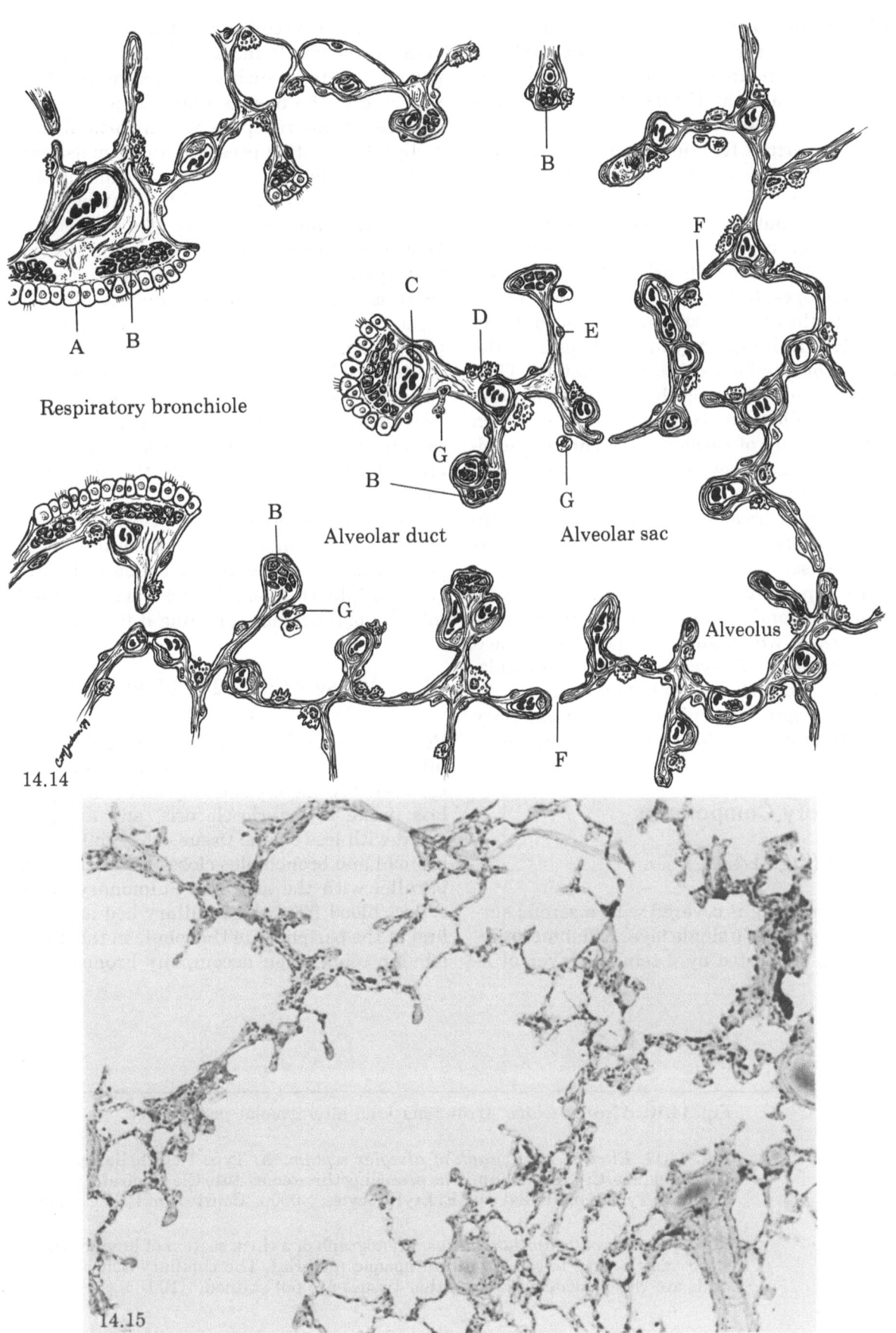

Respiratory bronchiole

Alveolar duct

Alveolar sac

Alveolus

14.14

14.15

(Figs. 14.14, 14.16, and 14.21), exist between alveoli. They serve as an alternate pathway around obstructions in small airways and thereby reduce the threat of either overdistention or collapse.

An important functional component of the lung is the alveolar macrophage (Figs. 14.14 and 14.23). A few of them may be found in any section but they are present in large numbers under certain circumstances (such as bronchitis). These cells originate, as do other macrophages, from the bone marrow and migrate to the alveolar spaces from blood. From the alveolar lumen they normally pass up the airway on the "mucociliary escalator." They often contain visible carbon or dust particles and are called dust cells, which are common in the sputum of patients with chronic respiratory disease. They also travel in lymphatics and settle in hilar lymph nodes. Collections of them may occur either interstitially or intraalveolarly, and more of them appear as needs arise.

We repeat for emphasis: the two exceptional anatomic features of the respiratory membrane, which allow it to exchange such large volumes of oxygen and carbon dioxide, are its huge surface area (70 m² in the adult) of both respiratory epithelium and capillary endothelium, and the thinness of the membrane.

Accessory Components

Pleura (Fig. 14.11)

The entire lung is covered with a serous surface composed of a single layer of flat mesothelial cells supported by a tenuous layer of fibrous and elastic connective tissue. This is the visceral pleura. It faces a similar layer, the parietal pleura, which is applied to the chest wall and to the mediastinum. Together they enclose the pleural space, which normally has a slightly negative pressure and a moist surface, but almost no fluid. Thus, normally this is only a potential space like that between the bladder and the casing of a basketball. However, various fluids or air may collect in this space under certain circumstances. If there is a large collection it may totally collapse the lung (atelectasis). In other cases the pleural space and the mesothelium may be obliterated by fine or heavy fibrous adhesions. These are scar tissue and they result from previously active disease, such as bacterial pneumonia or tuberculosis, which has travelled the short distance from the air spaces to the pleura.

The visceral pleural membranes separate the lobes of the lung except at the hilus. There is also a layer of loose connective tissue underlying the pleura. From this layer septa extend into the parenchyma, dividing it into lobules.

Blood Vessels (Figs. 14.11 and 14.27)

Pulmonary blood vessels enter and exit at the hilus. The arteries are similar to other arteries, but are more delicately structured, are less prone to arteriosclerosis, and are provided with less elastic tissue. They follow the bronchi and bronchioles closely, branching in parallel with the airways. Pulmonary veins collect blood from the capillary bed and run first at the periphery of the lobule in the interlobular septa, then accompany bronchi and

Fig. 14.16. *Alveolar walls.* Arrows mark an interalveolar pore. ×400.

Fig. 14.17. *Electron micrograph of alveolar septum.* **A:** Type I epithelial cells. **B:** Basal laminae. **C:** Endothelium. The preceding three constitute the respiratory membrane. **D:** Type II epithelial cell. **E:** Erythrocytes. ×6000. (Courtesy of R. S. Connell.)

Fig. 14.18. *Alveolar capillary plexus.* Photograph of a thick section of lung in which blood vessels were injected with an opaque material. The capillary-rich alveolar walls are clearly demonstrated. Other tissues are not stained. ×100.

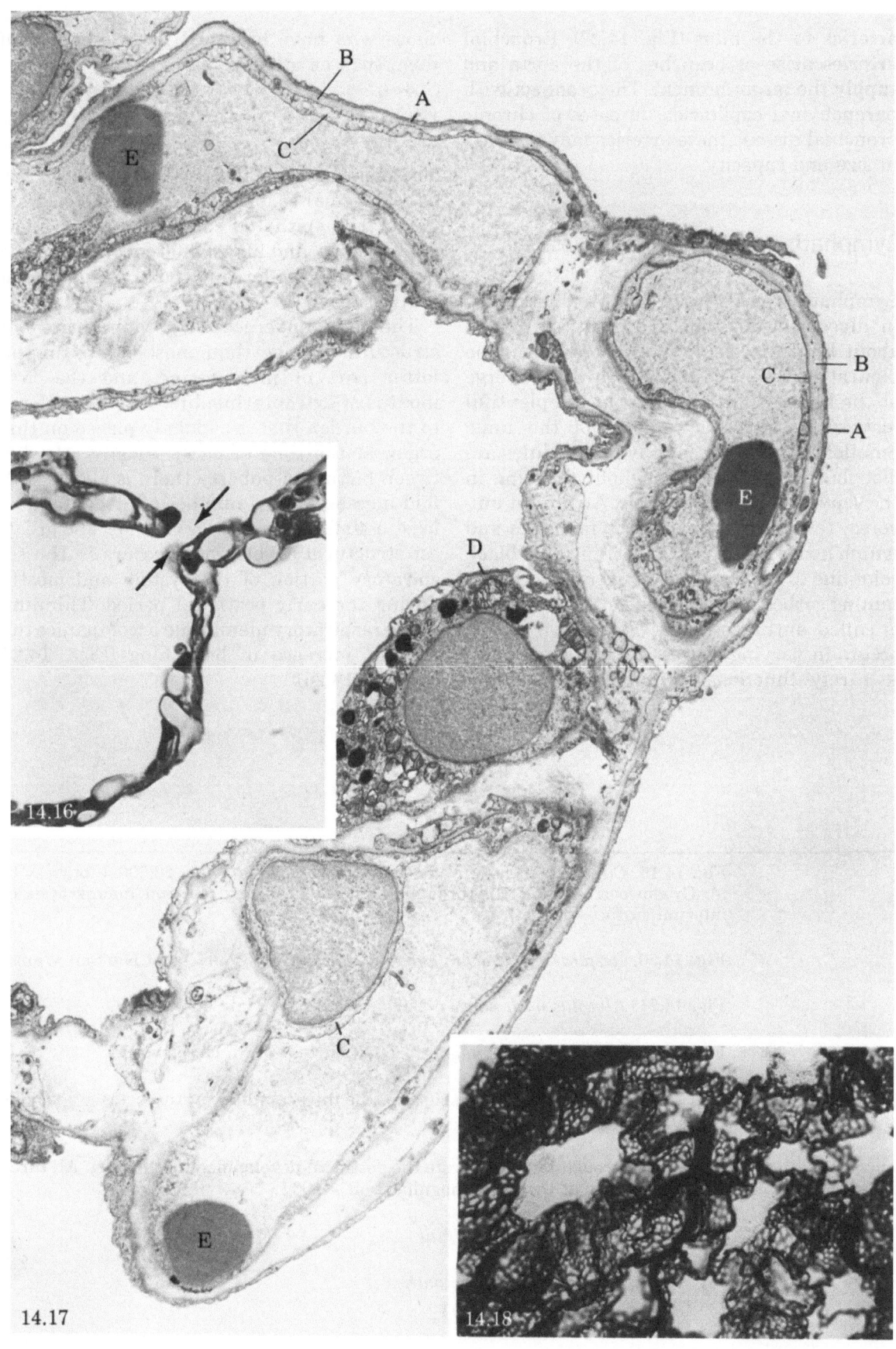

14.16

14.17

14.18

arteries to the hilus (Fig. 14.27). Bronchial arteries arise as branches of the aorta and supply the larger bronchi. They connect with parenchymal capillaries. In cases of chronic bronchial disease these arteries may increase in size and capacity.

Lymphatics and Lymphoid Tissue

Lymphatic vessels have not been identified in alveolar walls, but are plentiful in and about bronchial walls and just beneath the pleural surface. These channels all converge at the hilus. Hilar lymph nodes are plentiful just within and just outside of the lung. Smaller lymph nodes and lymph nodules are distributed liberally throughout the lung in the septa and bronchial walls. An almost universal feature of pulmonary lymphatics and lymph nodes is the grossly striking blue-black color due to the presence of macrophages containing carbon and other dusts. The condition is called anthracosis (see Fig. 10.24) and it occurs in varying degrees or depths of color. It rarely functionally impairs any except those who have breathed large amounts of dust, such as miners.

Development

The nasal cavities and paranasal sinuses are of ectodermal origin, arising from the stomadeum. The epithelial components of the larynx, trachea, and lungs differentiate from the outgrowth of the foregut and are endodermal derivatives.

The lung undergoes a greater degree of structural change than most organs in the latter part of intrauterine, and the first months of extrauterine, life. This fact relates to the burden that is suddenly placed on this organ at the time of birth. At any rate, between birth and puberty there is about a 10-fold increase in the number of alveoli and at least a 40-fold increase in volume. The greatest structural development occurs in the respiratory portion of the system and mostly during the early postnatal period. Thinning of the respiratory membrane accompanies the marked increase in branching (Figs. 14.24 through 14.26).

Fig. 14.19. *Ciliated and nonciliated bronchial epithelial cells.* ×2600. (Courtesy of M. Greenwood.) Figs. 14.19 through 14.23 are scanning electron micrographs of internal surfaces of the lung.

Fig. 14.20. *Respiratory bronchiole and alveoli.* ×220. (Courtesy of Nai-San Wang.)

Fig. 14.21. *Alveolus with pores.* ×2200. (Courtesy of Nai-San Wang.)

Fig. 14.22. *Alveolar macrophage.* ×8350. (Courtesy of M. Greenwood.)

Fig. 14.23. *Alveolar wall.* The shapes of the intracapillary erythrocytes are visible. ×7100. (Courtesy of M. Greenwood.)

Figs. 14.24 through 14.26 illustrate the postnatal development of the lung. All three photographs are at the same magnification, ×100.

Fig. 14.24. *Lung of newborn infant.*

Fig. 14.25. *Lung of child of 7 months.*

Fig. 14.26. *Lung of adult.*

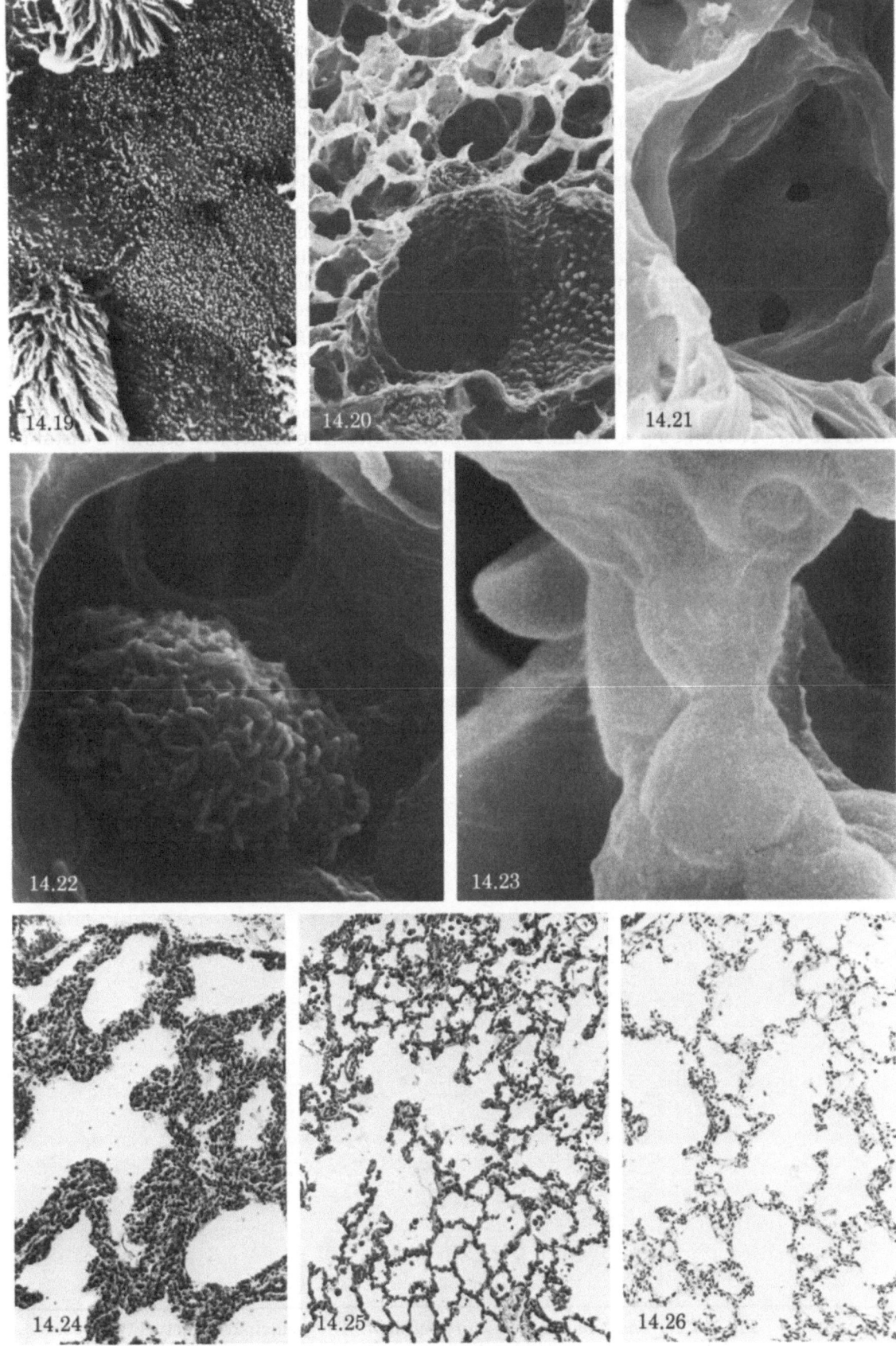

Organization of Structural Units in the Lung

Each lung has one mainstem bronchus, one main pulmonary artery, and two main pulmonary veins. Each of the two or three lobes has a single branch or tributary of each of these and contains from two to five nearly constant bronchopulmonary segments. The positions of the bronchopulmonary segments are important to pulmonary surgeons and bronchoscopists, but not to others.

Labeling of specific smaller lung units is meaningless until one reaches the level of the *lobule,* which averages slightly more than 1 cm in diameter. There being a minimum of wasted space in the system, lobules are fitted compactly and assume various shapes, but are for the most part pyramidal. Lobules are ordinarily not easily identified in the lung but under certain conditions their outlines, the interlobular septa, may be accentuated and make them visible. Fluid migrates from the alveolar walls to these septa in cases of incipient pulmonary edema. Chest X-ray may reveal septa thus thickened, an early sign of heart failure. The lobular bronchiole and vessels enter and leave at the apex of the pyramid. This bronchiole is, on the average, of the fourteenth generation of branching. The lobule is about 75% enclosed by fibrous tissue septa.

The lobule contains three to five terminal bronchioles. The structural elements distal to the terminal bronchiole constitute the functional (i.e., respiratory) part of the lung.

Fig. 14.27. *The bronchopulmonary segment.* The principal structural components from tertiary bronchus to alveoli. The area in the circle has been enlarged. Lymphatics and nerves are omitted.

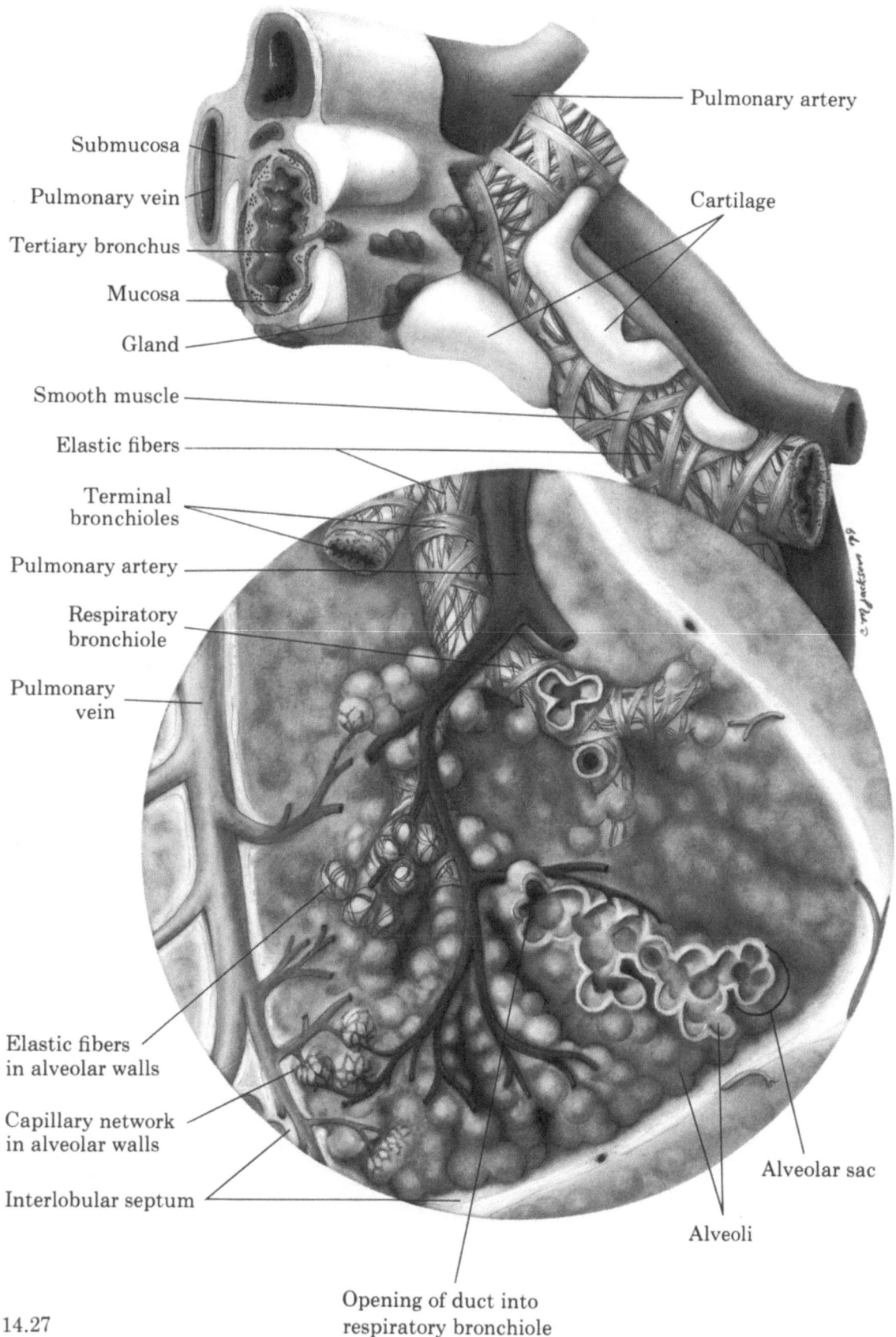

Pulmonary artery

Submucosa

Pulmonary vein

Tertiary bronchus

Mucosa

Gland

Smooth muscle

Elastic fibers

Terminal
bronchioles

Pulmonary artery

Respiratory
bronchiole

Pulmonary
vein

Cartilage

Elastic fibers
in alveolar walls

Capillary network
in alveolar walls

Interlobular septum

Alveolar sac

Alveoli

Opening of duct into
respiratory bronchiole

14.27

15 Urinary System

Introduction

The urinary system consists of four organs that function cooperatively in the removal of wastes from the blood and in their elimination from the body (Fig. 15.1). These four organs and their respective functions are: (1) *kidneys:* complex filtration and ion-exchange systems to remove wastes, metabolites, excess water and electrolytes from the blood, producing urine; (2) *ureters:* ducts to carry this fluid to temporary storage in the bladder; (3) *bladder:* a distensible, muscular storage tank with a neurally controlled emptying mechanism; (4) *urethra:* a duct for the delivery of urine to the exterior. In the male, urethral functions are shared with the reproductive system.

Kidneys

General Features

Each of the paired kidneys is a complex, encapsulated, tubular gland consisting of about 1 million tubular *nephrons* and their associated collecting tubules (Fig. 15.3b). The nephron (*see later*) is a long convoluted tube, the proximal, blind end of which is invaginated by a tuft of capillaries, to form a *renal corpuscle.* As blood circulates through the capillaries, plasma is filtered through their walls into the tubule. During its course down the tubule this filtrate is modified by the selective removal and addition of ions and water. This process serves to maintain the appropriate volume, electrolyte balance, and pH of body fluids. Electrolytes and water needed by the body are reabsorbed, and the excess, along with metabolic wastes, continues through the collecting ducts. This modified filtrate finally passes into the ureter as urine, a complex aqueous salt solution of metabolic wastes.

The fetal kidney is distinctly divided into about a dozen lobes by inward extensions of its capsule. Reduction of the internal connective tissue and fusion of the lobes during development obscures this embryonic lobation so that the adult organ usually has a smooth outer surface and the lobar structure is apparent only when the kidney is opened. Examination of the cut surface of a frontal section of a whole kidney (Fig. 15.2) shows a thick C-shaped band of parenchyma enclosing a space, the *renal sinus,* which opens at the *hilus.* Into this sinus is fitted the branched, funnel-shaped upper end of the ureter, which is here termed the *renal pelvis.* The sinus is also the passageway for the major renal vessels.

The parenchyma is divided into distinct cortex and medulla (Fig. 15.3). The cortex forms the outer layer, lying under the connective tissue capsule and, as the *renal columns* (of Bertin), extends into the medulla, dividing it into about a dozen *medullary pyramids.* The base of each pyramid abuts on the cortex and streaks of medullary tissue may be seen extending from the base of a pyramid outwards into the cortex. These extensions are the *medullary rays.* The rounded apex of each pyramid projects, as a *papilla,* a short distance into one of the eight or so subdivisions of the renal pelvis termed *minor calyces.* Each minor calyx is fitted over a papilla like a small funnel. Although it is not apparent in most sections, a single papilla in actuality represents fusion of the apices of two or three neighboring pyramids. The surface of each papilla is perforated by one or two dozen pores. Each pore is the opening of a major collecting duct (of Bellini). Through these ducts urine from the tubules of the parenchyma passes into a minor calyx, then into one of two or three major calyces and finally into the ureter. The ureter conducts the urine to the bladder for temporary storage.

Fig. 15.1. Basic anatomy of the *urinary system.*

Fig. 15.2. Cut surface of a *kidney.* Pyramid (P), cortex (C), renal column (R), pelvis (Pe), papilla (Pa).

Fig. 15.3. a: Large microsection of a *kidney* with multiple abscesses (arrows) in acute pyelonephritis. These are areas of destruction of the tissue by bacteria; they involve both cortex and medulla. A calyx is marked (Ca). **b:** A segment of the same section with a nephron and its collecting tubule marked. Since it is impossible to follow the entire course of a nephron in a single section this is an idealized depiction.

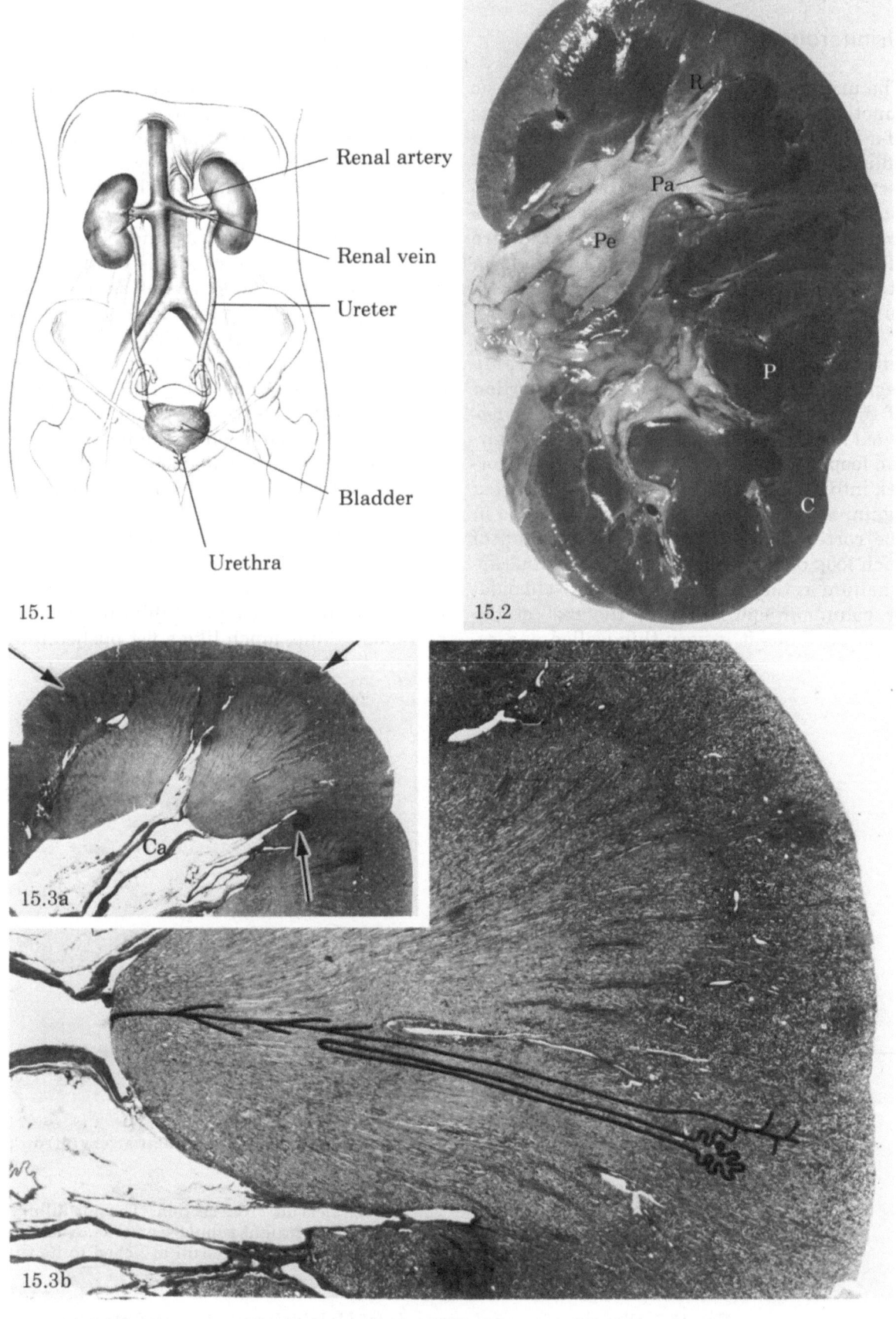

Renal artery

Renal vein

Ureter

Bladder

Urethra

15.1

15.2

15.3a

Ca

15.3b

Uriniferous Tubule

The uriniferous tubule (Fig. 15.4) is the basic functional unit of the kidney. Each consists of a nephron, which produces the filtrate and adjusts its chemical components, and a collecting tubule, which concentrates this solution by removal of water. These components have different embryonic origins, and failure of their primordia to differentiate or to form structures that make proper connection, results in serious or fatal congenital defects.

The invaginated upper end of the nephron with its tuft of blood vessels is the *renal (Malpighian) corpuscle*. The long tubular portion of the nephron consists of a *proximal convoluted tubule* located in the cortex; a long hairpin loop (*Henle's loop*) extending from the cortex into the medulla and back into the cortex again; and a *distal convoluted tubule* also in the cortex near the corpuscle. A portion of each loop of Henle is formed of squamous epithelium rather than of the usual cuboidal or columnar epithelium of the rest of the nephron. Thus it is very thin-walled and re-

ferred to as the *thin segment*. The distal convoluted tubule is continuous with a *collecting tubule*. Each collecting tubule is shared by several nephrons that join it much as the limbs of a fir tree join the trunk. The main stem of each collecting tubule system extends into the medulla, together with neighboring tubules and limbs of Henle's loop, eventually to open at the papilla into a minor calyx. Each medullary ray of the cortex is composed of several collecting tubules as well as ascending and descending limbs of Henle's loops. A medullary ray together with surrounding nephrons that are connected to its tubules constitutes a *renal lobule* (Figs. 15.5 and 15.6).

THE NEPHRON. The structure and basic functions of each subdivision of the nephron will be described in the sequence in which the filtrate is formed and passed through the tubular system.

The renal corpuscle (Fig. 15.7) has both vascular and epithelial components.

The *vascular component* is a tuft of capillary loops invaginating and dilating the end of a long tubule, much like a fist pushed into

---

Fig. 15.4. A typical *uriniferous tubule* with its nephron and collecting tubule. The arterial blood supply to the glomerulus is also shown.

Fig. 15.5. A segment of cortex with three *medullary rays*. Interlobular artery (arrow); lobule (bracket). ×34.

Fig. 15.6. Several *renal lobules* (dashed circles) in cross-section. The medullary rays are columns of collecting tubules and some straight tubule segments. A lobule is composed of a medullary ray and the surrounding glomeruli attached to its tubules. ×35.

Fig. 15.7. Diagram of a *renal corpuscle* (of Malpighi) and associated structures.

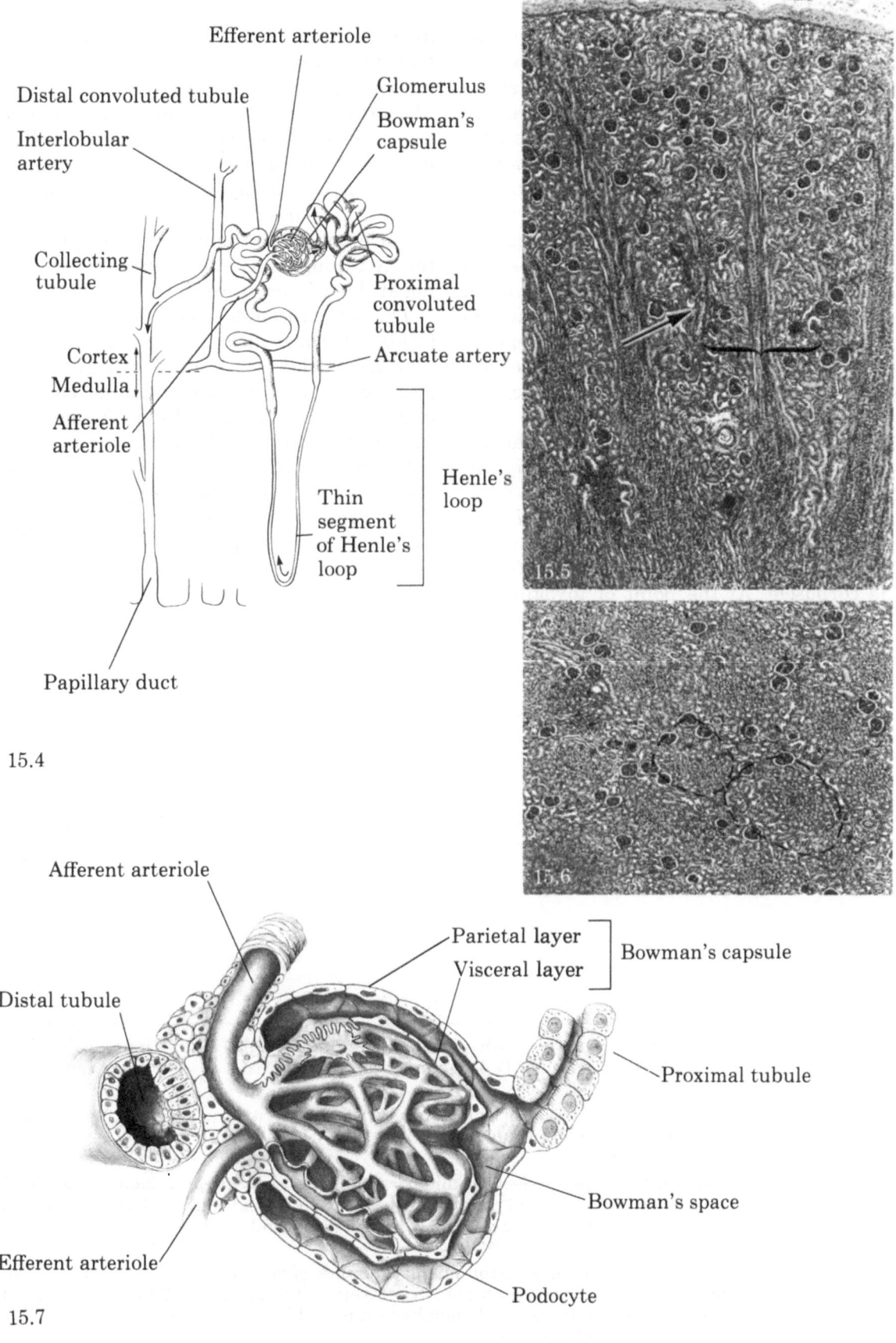

Efferent arteriole

Distal convoluted tubule

Interlobular artery

Glomerulus

Bowman's capsule

Collecting tubule

Proximal convoluted tubule

Cortex

Medulla

Arcuate artery

Afferent arteriole

Henle's loop

Thin segment of Henle's loop

Papillary duct

15.4

15.5

15.6

Afferent arteriole

Parietal layer

Visceral layer

Bowman's capsule

Distal tubule

Proximal tubule

Bowman's space

Efferent arteriole

Podocyte

15.7

the blind end of a long narrow balloon. The tuft of vessels receives blood from a single *afferent arteriole* and is drained by a single *efferent arteriole*. These two vessels are in close contact with each other and this area where they enter the corpuscle is termed its *vascular pole* (Figs. 15.8 and 15.9). Each of the individual capillary loops, which arise by branching of the afferent arteriole, carries with it, in the process of invagination, a portion of the thin squamous epithelial wall of the nephron. Thus the vascular endothelium is in close contact with the tubular epithelium, as if the fingers of the fist described above had become separated so that each finger is covered by a membrane.

The *epithelial component* of the renal corpuscle, collectively called *Bowman's capsule,* consists of two facing layers of simple squamous epithelium. The outer or *parietal layer* is continuous with the epithelium of the proximal tubule at the *urinary pole* (Fig. 15.8) of the corpuscle. At the point of invagination by the blood vessels, the parietal layer is folded back over the vascular tuft as a *visceral layer* of epithelium usually referred to as the *glomerular epithelium.* The cluster of capillary tufts and its visceral covering epithelium is termed the *glomerulus.* Between the visceral and parietal layers of Bowman's capsule is the *capsular* or *urinary space.* This space is continuous with the lumen of the proximal tubule through a narrow funnel-shaped opening at the urinary pole (Figs. 15.10 and 15.11).

The filter through which fluid from blood passes into the urinary space from the glomerular capillaries is composed of three layers (Fig. 15.12): vascular endothelium, basal lamina, and visceral epithelium. The endothelium of the capillary loops is very thin and is fenestrated. Its pores are more numerous than in capillaries of other organs, and pore diaphragms are generally absent. This layer effectively holds back blood cells and platelets but allows free access of plasma to the basal lamina.

Fig. 15.8. *Glomerulus* with vascular pole (upper right) and urinary pole (lower left). ×300. (Courtesy of D. Houghton.)

Fig. 15.9. *Vascular pole* of a glomerulus with afferent arteriole (arrow), juxtaglomerular apparatus and macula densa (M). ×300.

Fig. 15.10. Scanning electron micrograph of the *visceral epithelium* of Bowman's capsule. Foot processes of podocytes are shown on the external surface of a glomerular capillary. ×6000. (Courtesy of W. H. Fahrenbach.)

Fig. 15.11. Scanning electron micrograph of a *glomerular capillary* that has been broken open and viewed on end. The layers of the filter and Bowman's space (B) can be seen. The fenestrated endothelium is visible lining the vessel. ×9000. (Courtesy of W. H. Fahrenbach.)

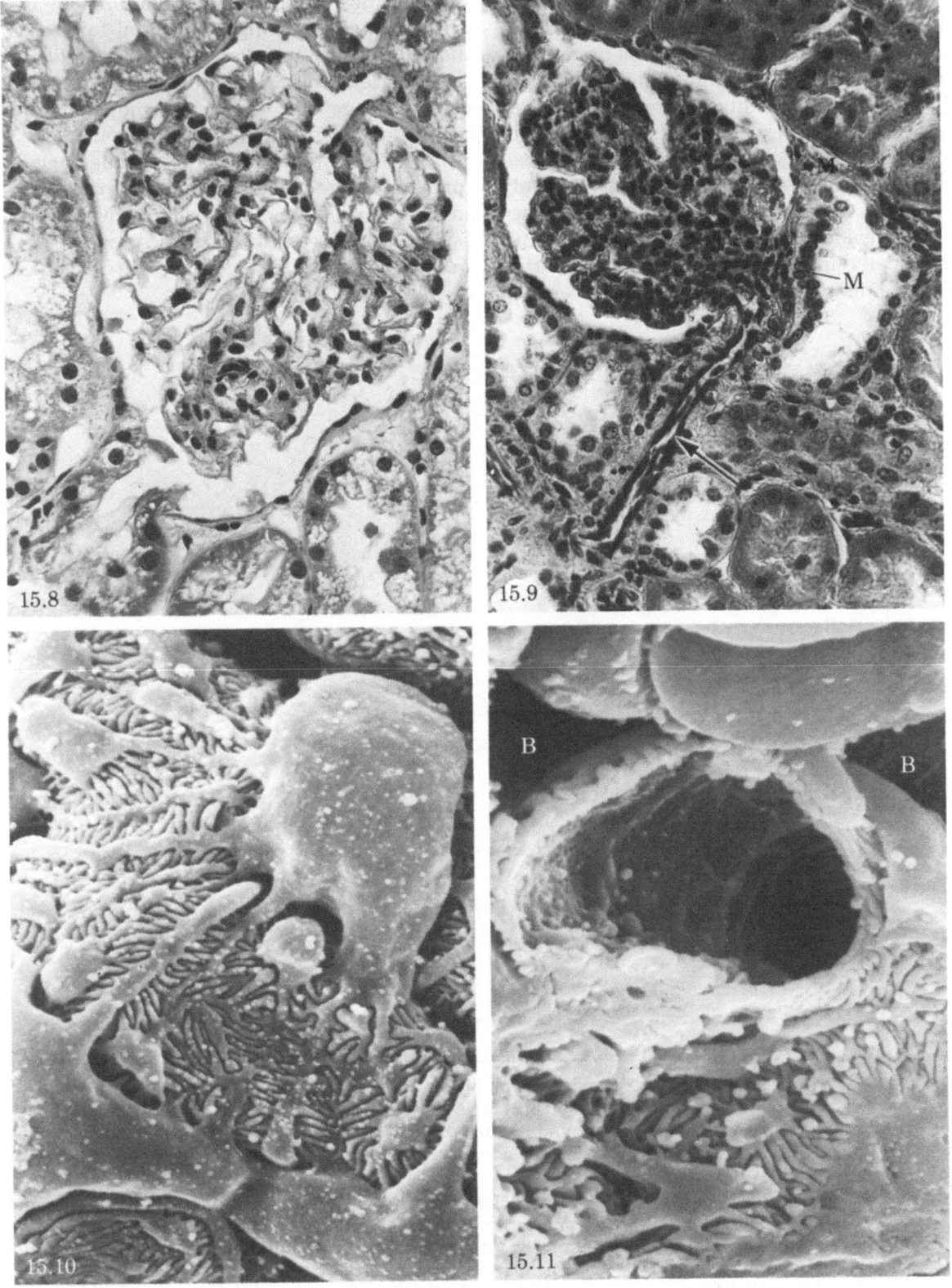

15.8

15.9

15.10

15.11

The middle layer of the filter is an unusually thick basal lamina (Fig. 15.12). This layer theoretically represents the fused basal laminae of the epithelium and endothelium. Although it is not visibly different from other such laminae, it is apparently biochemically complex. With the electron microscope, each surface of the basal lamina appears relatively less dense than the middle layer, and there is some evidence that these two surfaces are chemically different. In some diseases pathologic changes may occur in only one layer (Fig. 15.13). Since both the endothelium and epithelium have openings, the basal lamina is the only continuous component of the filtration barrier. This portion of the barrier prevents passage of most plasma components of molecular weight greater than about 68,000 daltons. Thus the filtrate (provisional urine) contains solutes of lesser molecular weight, such as glucose and electrolytes. Molecular weight, osmotic and hydrostatic pressures, as well as electrostatic pore charge, are involved in the filtration process.

Fig. 15.12. Electron micrograph of a section of a glomerulus to show the structure of the *filter* through which plasma is passed from capillary lumens (L) into Bowman's space (B). Fenestrated endothelium, basal lamina (arrows) and podocyte foot processes are seen. ×12,750. (Courtesy of M. Webb.)

Fig. 15.13. *Membranous glomerulonephritis.* **a:** An electron micrograph of a section of the glomerular filter. The basal lamina (arrows) is thickened by dense masses of deposit on its epithelial side (on the right in the photo). The sharply and regularly interrupted layer corresponds to what is seen in **b.** This has acquired the term picket-fence. Labels as in Fig. 15.12. ×14,600. (Courtesy of R. Brooks and D. Houghton.) **b:** *Picket-fence change* (arrow) in the same specimen as in **a.** ×300. (Courtesy of D. Houghton.) **c:** *Immunofluorescence* photograph showing the heavy granular deposits outlining the glomerular capillaries. ×450. (Courtesy of D. Houghton.)

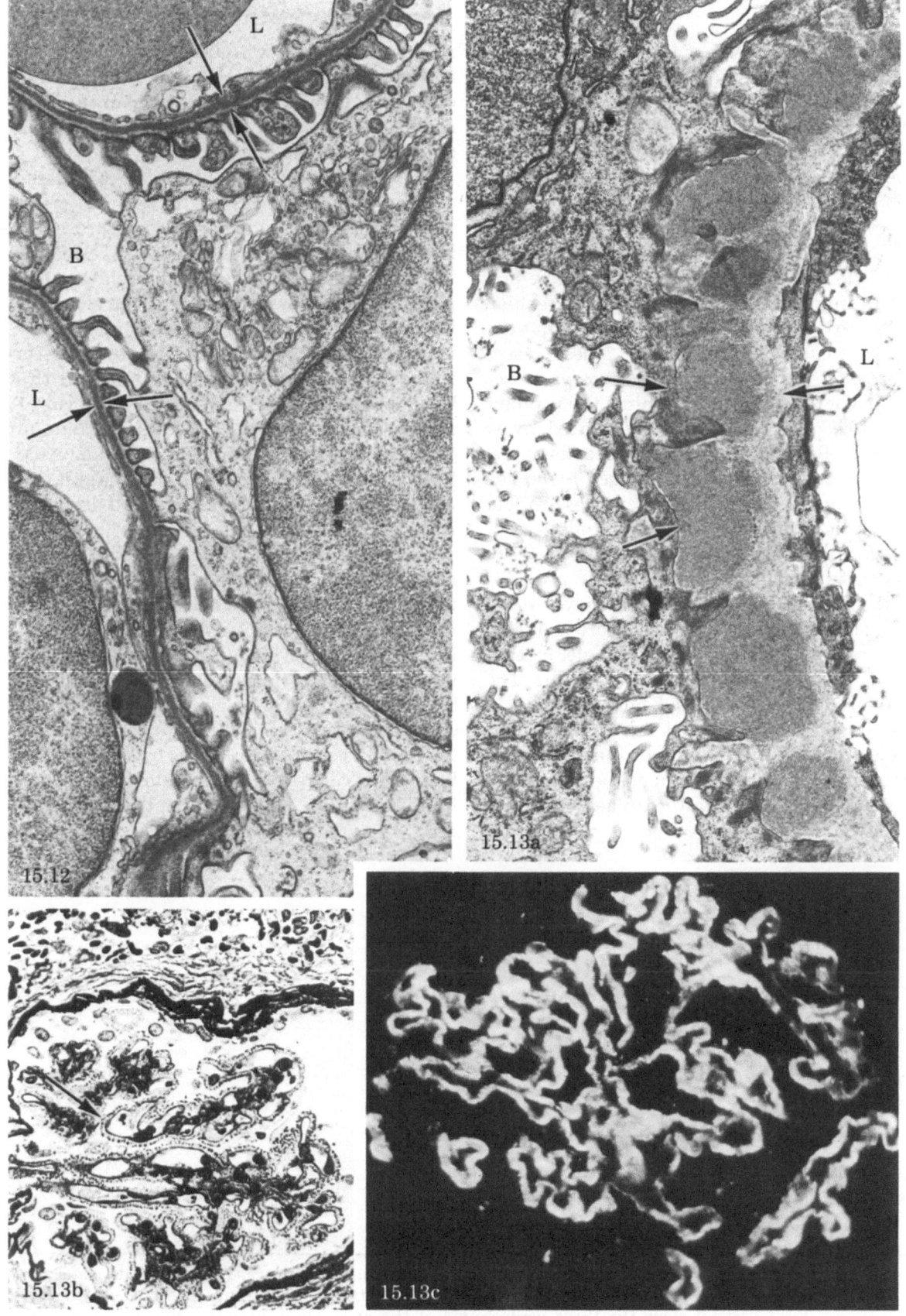

15.12

15.13a

15.13b

15.13c

The epithelial cells of the visceral layer of Bowman's capsule, instead of differentiating into ordinary flat squamous cells, develop into elongated, branched cells termed *podocytes* (Fig. 15.14) applied to the outer surface of the capillaries. There are two orders of branching of podocytes. Each cell has several primary processes. Originating from each primary process numerous parallel *foot processes* extend over the basal lamina. These secondary processes interdigitate in such a precise fashion with those of neighboring podocytes that the interval is always 25 nm wide. These spaces are called *slit pores*. Only the foot processes are in contact with basal lamina; the primary processes and cell bodies are placed away from the basal lamina and the secondary processes, like feet, rest on its surface. Stretched across the slit pore from foot process to foot process is a very thin *slit membrane*.

Approximately 180 liters of filtrate each day pass through the total barrier provided by the combined filters of both kidneys. About 99% of this large volume is reabsorbed during processing by the uriniferous tubule, so that the daily urine production is 1 or 2 liters. The pressure, rate of flow, and filtration rate in the glomerular capillaries are controlled by the sympathetic innervation of afferent and efferent arterioles, by hormones, and, perhaps most important, by autoregulatory mecha-

nisms that are not well understood. The control afforded by these two factors maintains effective glomerular filtration over a wide range of variation of blood pressures, cardiac output, and other factors.

The term glomerulonephritis encompasses a broad group of diseases with various etiologies and clinical and morphologic presentations, all affecting renal glomeruli. Some of the differences within this group relate to the particular layer or component of the glomerulus that is affected. Membranous glomerulonephritis (MGN) is characterized by deposits between the glomerular epithelium and the basement membrane. This is in the form of a diffuse granular layer containing immunoglobulin G (IgG) and complement; it can result from a variety of causes. In some unknown way the glomerular capillary wall is made leaky (Fig. 15.13).

Proximal tubule (Fig. 15.15). At the urinary pole of the renal corpuscle there is a transition from the squamous epithelium of the parietal layer of the capsule to the cuboidal epithelium of the proximal tubule. This tubule is composed of a tortuous portion in the neighborhood of the corpuscle, and a proximal straight portion that courses toward and into the medulla as the *descending limb* of Henle's loop. The cells of the proximal tubule are large and have spherical, centrally located

Fig. 15.14. Drawing of a portion of a *glomerular capillary*. The feet of the *podocytes* are evenly spaced on the outer surface of the basal lamina. The cut ends of the vessel show the three components of the wall which separate the vascular from the urinary space.

Slit pore

Fenestrated endothelium

Basal
lamina

Primary process

Secondary process

Podocyte cell body

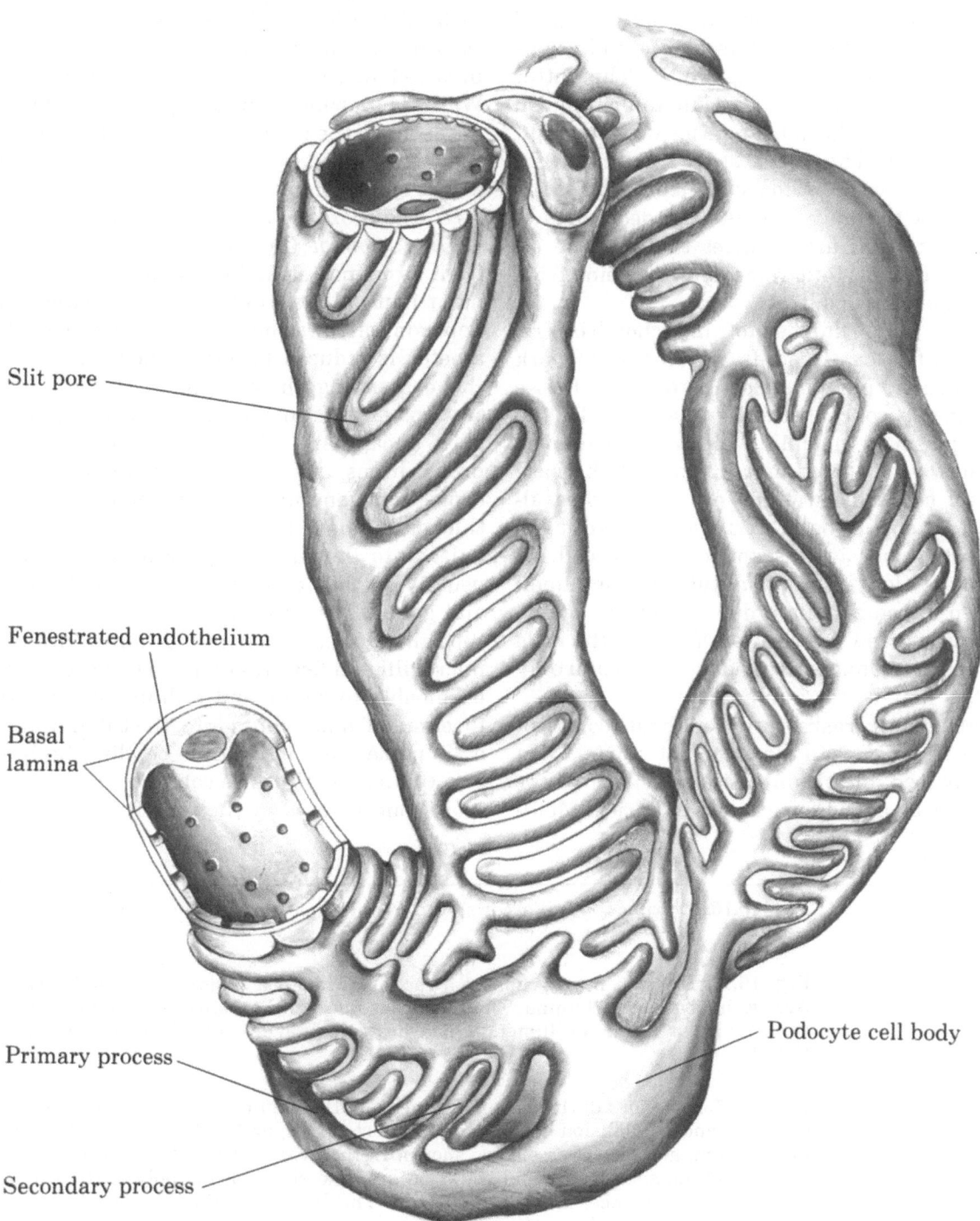

15.14

nuclei. They have a dense *brush border* of long, closely packed microvilli on their apical surfaces and elaborate lateral interdigitations with their neighbors (Fig. 15.16). This latter relationship makes it difficult to distinguish discrete lateral cell boundaries with the light microscope. The cells rest on a distinct basement membrane. Short canaliculi open at the bases of the microvilli. At the deep ends of the canaliculi are vacuoles that are the results of pinocytotic removal of proteins from the glomerular filtrate.

The large number of mitochondria, required for the extraordinary amount of work involved in pumping electrolytes and glucose against a concentration gradient, make the cytoplasm eosinophilic. Mitochondria are particularly elongated and crowded at the base of the cell and, since they are arranged parallel to the apico-basal axis, they appear as basal striations in this portion of the cell. In cross-sections of proximal tubules, the lumen often appears stellate due to collapse of the tubule during preparation. Because the cells are so large, nuclei are widely spaced and only a few may be cut in a cross-section.

Most of the reabsorption of filtrate constituents takes place in the proximal tubule. They are passed into the interstitial connective tissue space and diffuse into capillaries. Meta-bolic wastes, such as creatinine, which are to be discarded in the urine, are not reabsorbed. Specific portions of the tubules are involved in reabsorbing specific substances. Water is probably reabsorbed passively by osmosis along the ionic gradient and the filtrate reaches the descending limb and thin segment at the same osmolality as it had when it entered the proximal tubule (Figs. 15.17, 15.18).

Thin segment (Fig. 15.19). The transition from proximal straight tubule to thin segment is usually abrupt. At this junction the nephron narrows sharply and the outside diameter is reduced to about one-fifth that of the descending thick segment. In ordinary sections anyone may confuse a thin segment with a capillary. However, good histologic preparations and careful examination will show that generally its squamous cells are thicker and have more rounded nuclei, which bulge into the lumen. Endothelial cells are usually so thin as to appear as single lines and generally have dark flat nuclei. Cells of the thin segment are pale with only scattered microvilli and few organelles. They are freely permeable to water and sodium. Water diffuses out of, and sodium into, the tubular fluid as it passes through the descending limb of this tubule and thus the solution has become more concentrated by the time it reaches the

---

Fig. 15.15. *Proximal* (large arrows) and *distal* (small arrows) *convoluted tubules.* ×250.

Fig. 15.16. Electron micrograph of a section through a *distal convoluted tubule.* Arrows indicate basal lamina. The numerous microvilli constituting the brush border (B) appear to fill the lumen, which has collapsed. About ×3300. (Courtesy of R. S. Connell.)

Fig. 15.17. *Functions* of the various segments of the nephron. The basic movements by pump and by diffusion of metabolites, electrolytes, and water between tubules, interstitium, and blood vessels are shown. In the proximal tubule, reabsorption of glucose, amino acids, salts, and water occurs. The rich blood supply of the tubule carries these substances into the circulation. The descending limb lies in an interstitium in which the salt concentration increases toward the papilla. As the fluid passes down the limb, osmotic pressure removes water. In the ascending limb salt is actively pumped out of the tubule into the interstitium, these cells being practically impermeable to water. The fluid in the distal tubule is relatively hypotonic. Here, as in the ascending limb, salt is actively pumped from the tubular lumen and water follows passively. Water is removed passively from the collecting duct by the osmotic pressure provided by the hypertonic medullary interstitium. The permeability of the collecting duct to water is controlled by antidiuretic hormone (ADH). Figures on the right side of the diagram indicate osmolality of the interstitium.

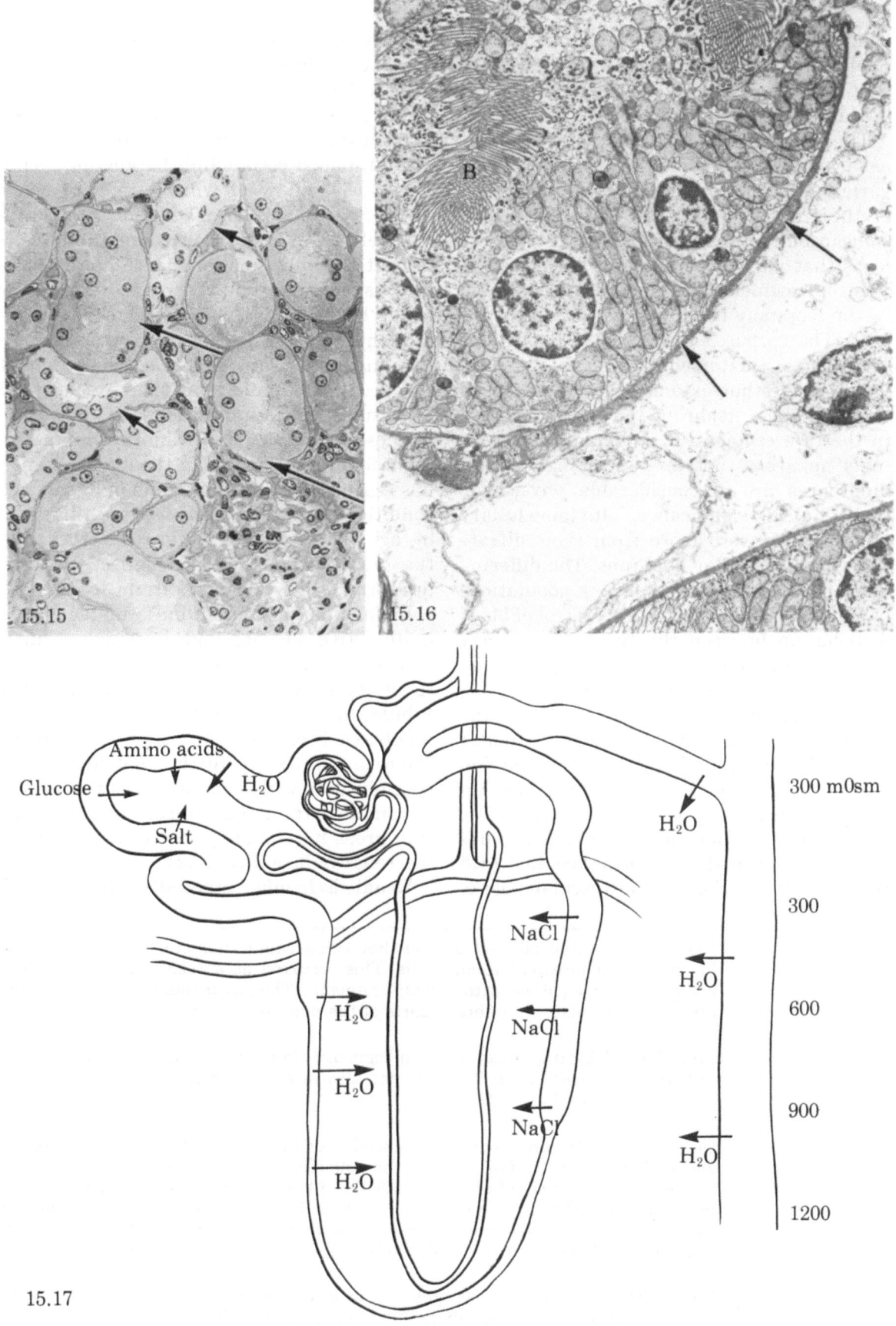

15.15

15.16

Glucose

Amino acids

Salt

H_2O

300 mOsm

H_2O

300

H_2O

NaCl

600

H_2O

NaCl

H_2O

900

NaCl

H_2O

H_2O

H_2O

1200

15.17

bend of Henle's loop. This occurs only in nephrons in the inner portion of the cortex; that is, in those whose loops extend into the medulla.

The length of Henle's loop varies in different populations of nephrons and most of this variation is due to differences in the length of the thin segment. The more peripheral (subcapsular) renal corpuscles have short loops that may not even reach the medulla. The thin segment is very short and the bend in the loop may be in the distal straight tubule. The corpuscles in the deeper portions of the cortex (juxtamedullary nephrons) have longer loops that extend deep into the medulla. In these nephrons the bend is located in the thin segment. It is becoming increasingly apparent that these seemingly minor differences are of considerable physiologic and clinical significance. Juxtamedullary nephrons reabsorb more from their filtrate than do subcapsular nephrons. The differing blood supply to the two differing populations of nephrons, and the sensitive control of blood distribution between the two patterns may permit precise fine tuning of kidney function in balancing body fluid components.

Distal tubule (Figs. 15.15 and 15.20). At the termination of the thin segment, the tubular epithelium abruptly changes again to the simple cuboidal characteristic of the distal tubule. The straight portion of the distal tubule (ascending thick limb of Henle's loop) ascends into the cortex, makes important contact with the afferent arteriole at the vascular pole of its own renal corpuscle, and then becomes the distal convoluted tubule. The distal convoluted tubule joins the collecting tubule (Fig. 15.20) in the medullary ray of its lobule.

The cytoplasm of the cuboidal cells in the distal tubule is eosinophilic because of the mitochondria, many of which are here again aligned to produce basal striations. Distal tubule cells differ from the proximal tubule cells in that they are smaller (hence more nuclei are visible in a tubular cross-section), they lack a brush border, they are shorter (the lumen thus appears larger), their cytoplasm, although eosinophilic, is less so than that of the proximal tubule, and their nuclei tend to be more apical in position.

These cells are effective chloride pumps (sodium follows passively). In the filtrate, which has reached the ascending limb in hypertonic condition, the salt is removed at this level by active transport. Salt is reabsorbed into the medullary interstitial connective tissue fluid, rendering the interstitium hypertonic.

Renal tubular epithelium is metabolically quite active and has high nutritive requirements. Not surprisingly, it is also vulnerable to injury by poisons. As we have seen, the tubule has several distinct anatomic segments, each of which has specific functions. There are probably further subdivisions of specialization within these segments. Depending on the particular chemical agent, only certain areas may undergo necrosis, with ensuing renal failure (Fig. 15.21).

Renal ischemia, especially that due to

Fig. 15.18. A section stained for *iron* shows an accumulation of iron in the glomerular space and proximal tubule cells. This occurred as a result of destruction of erythrocytes in a patient with hemolytic anemia. The picture suggests that different functions take place in different parts of the nephron. ×225.

Fig. 15.19. Collecting ducts (C), thin segments (long arrow), and capillaries (short arrow) in the *renal medulla*. It is not always easy to distinguish between thin segment and capillary. ×225.

Fig. 15.20. Electron micrograph of a section of the junction between *distal tubule* and *collecting tubule*. Two cells of the collecting tubule (C) are seen and one of the distal convoluted tubule (D). Note the difference in complexity between the two cell types. Collecting tubule cells, which have less work to do in pumping, have fewer mitochondria and less folded basal surfaces than does the distal tubule cell. About ×3300. (Courtesy of R. S. Connell.)

Fig. 15.21. *Acute tubular necrosis.* Necrotic tubules (on the left) are contrasted with the normal. Proximal tubule segments are most affected. ×110.

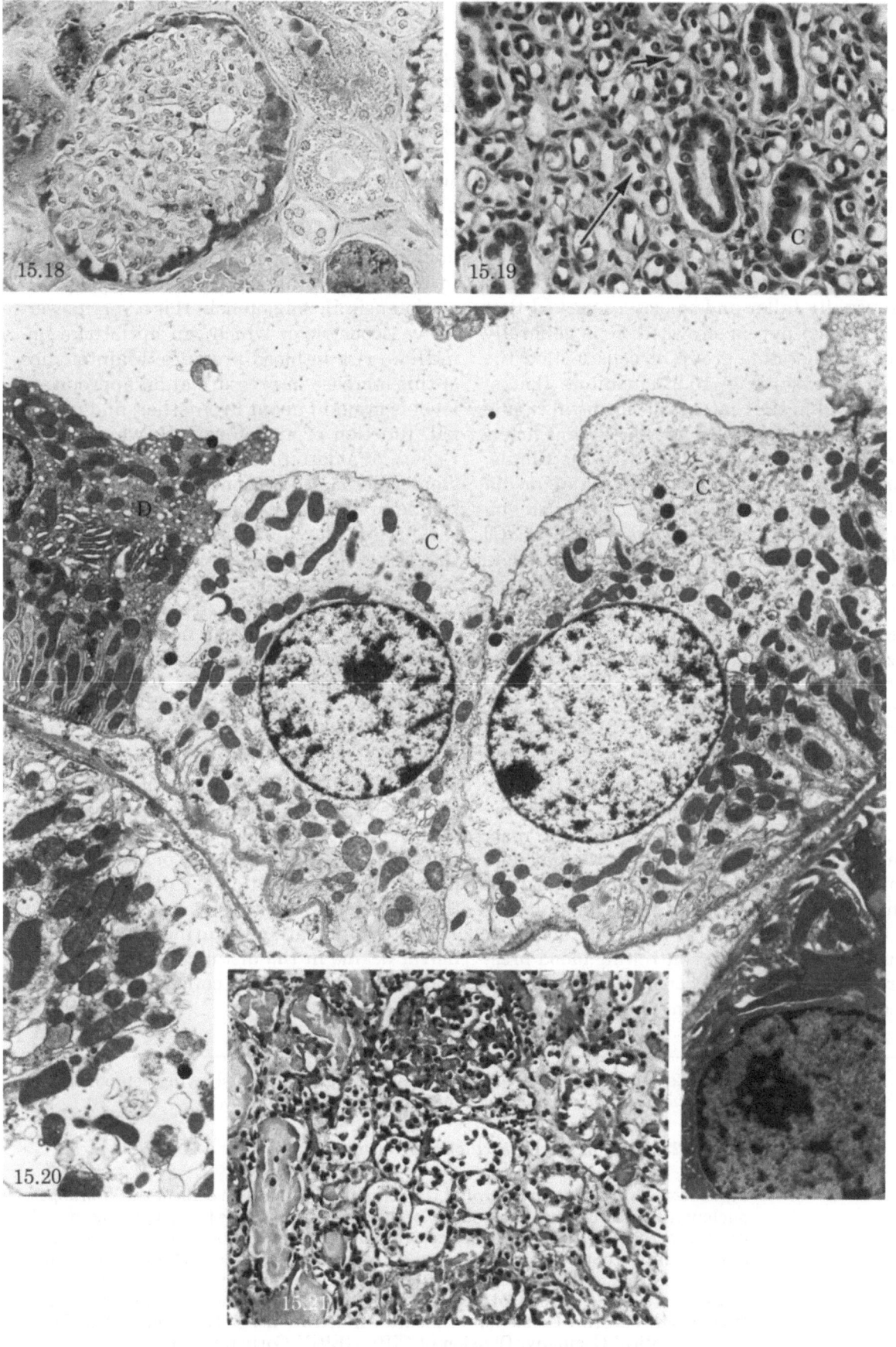

15.18

15.19

15.20

15.21

shock, may also damage tubular epithelium. However, this seldom causes necrosis; usually the tubules in ischemic renal injury are histologically normal and capable of full recovery. These cells do not have to be replaced.

At the point of contact of the distal tubule with the afferent arteriole, both structures show structural modifications (Figs. 15.22). The tubule is somewhat flattened against the arteriole and the cells of this flattened area are usually taller and so closely packed that their nuclei appear crowded. It is generally believed that this group of cells (called the *macula densa*) (Fig. 15.22) monitors the sodium level in the contents of the distal tubule and passes information to the afferent arteriole. In this area of contact with the tubule, the smooth muscle cells of the tunica media of the arteriole are highly modified to an epithelioid form. These *juxtaglomerular (JG) cells* are believed to sense blood pressure levels in the afferent arteriole. They have spherical nuclei and numerous cytoplasmic granules that have been shown to contain an enzyme called *renin*. The segment of the afferent arteriole containing these cells is termed the *JG apparatus* (Fig. 15.23).

Crowded into the triangular space between the vessels and the distal tubule is a cluster of cells (mesangial cells) similar to the pericytes seen outside the endothelium of capillaries. They are probably phagocytic. The macula densa, JG apparatus, and mesangial cells make up the juxtaglomerular complex. The function of this complex is the modulation of the chemical systems that interact with neural mechanisms in controlling blood pressure. There is much controversy over the mechanism. The following is one of several theories. By controlling fluid and electrolyte resorption, it also controls tissue fluid volume. As an example in simplified outline, a lower than normal sodium concentration in the distal tubule sensed by macula densa cells results in the release of renin into the blood by JG cells. Renin converts a blood protein, called angiotensinogen, into a decapeptide, angiotensin I. A converting enzyme present in blood alters this latter to an octapeptide, angiotensin II. Angiotensin II is a very powerful vasoconstrictor which can initiate an immediate rise in blood pressure. Maintenance of this increase in pressure at an appropriate level is brought about by another, and principal, function of angiotensin II, which is the release of aldosterone from the adrenal zona glomerulosa. Aldosterone acts on the distal tubule to increase its sodium absorption from the luminal fluid. The additional sodium in the tissue fluids leads to water retention, which increases blood and interstitial fluid volume and thus increases blood pressure.

If we now return to the first statement in this example in the preceding paragraph and replace the subject clause, ". . . a low sodium level in the distal tubule sensed by macula densa cells . . ." with the words ". . . a low blood pressure in the afferent arteriole sensed by the JG cells . . . ," the rest of the description need not be altered. It follows from this that the response either to low sodium concentration in the distal tubule, or to low blood pressure, is the retention of salt and fluid and the elevation of blood pressure.

The concentration of urine by water removal begins in the distal convoluted tubule and is completed in the collecting tubule.

Fig. 15.22. a: Section of the vascular pole of a glomerulus showing components of the *juxtaglomerular apparatus*. ×480. **b:** Map of **a.**

Fig. 15.23. Drawing of the *juxtaglomerular apparatus*.

Fig. 15.24. *Hypothalamic control* of the tonicity of urine. The cells of the supraoptic nucleus are sensitive to the osmolality of the blood. In response to changes in osmolality, the output of ADH in the pars nervosa varies and thus the permeability of the collecting tubules of the kidneys to water varies. This system assures that appropriate amounts of water are returned from the collecting tubules to the blood and not lost in the urine. (Adapted from an original painting by Frank H. Netter, M.D., from the CIBA Collection of Medical Illustrations. © Copyright 1973, CIBA Pharmaceutical Company, Division of CIBA-GEIGY Corporation.)

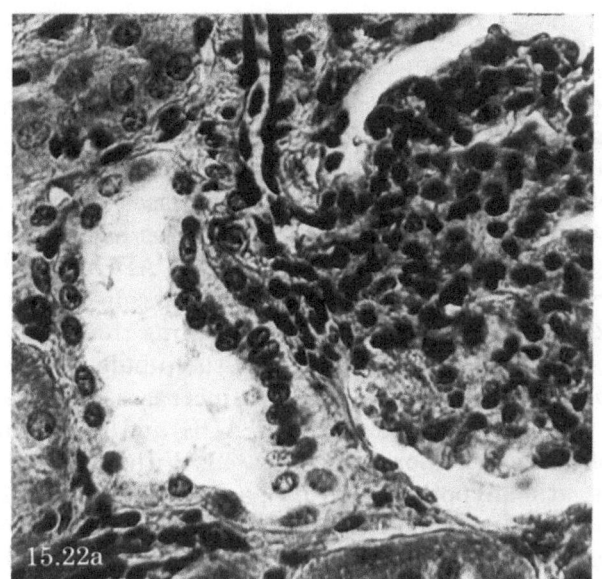

15.22a

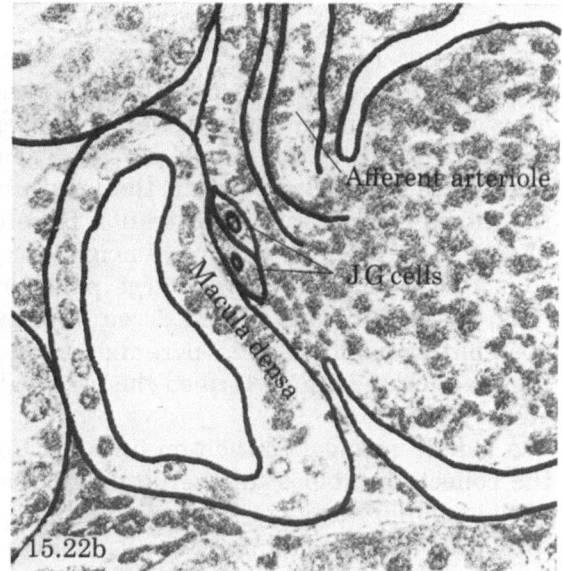

Afferent arteriole

J.G cells

Macula densa

15.22b

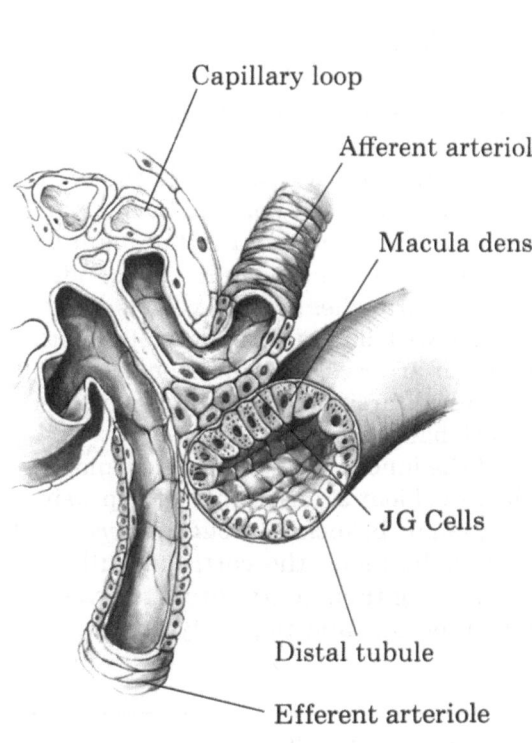

Capillary loop

Afferent arteriole

Macula densa

JG Cells

Distal tubule

Efferent arteriole

15.23

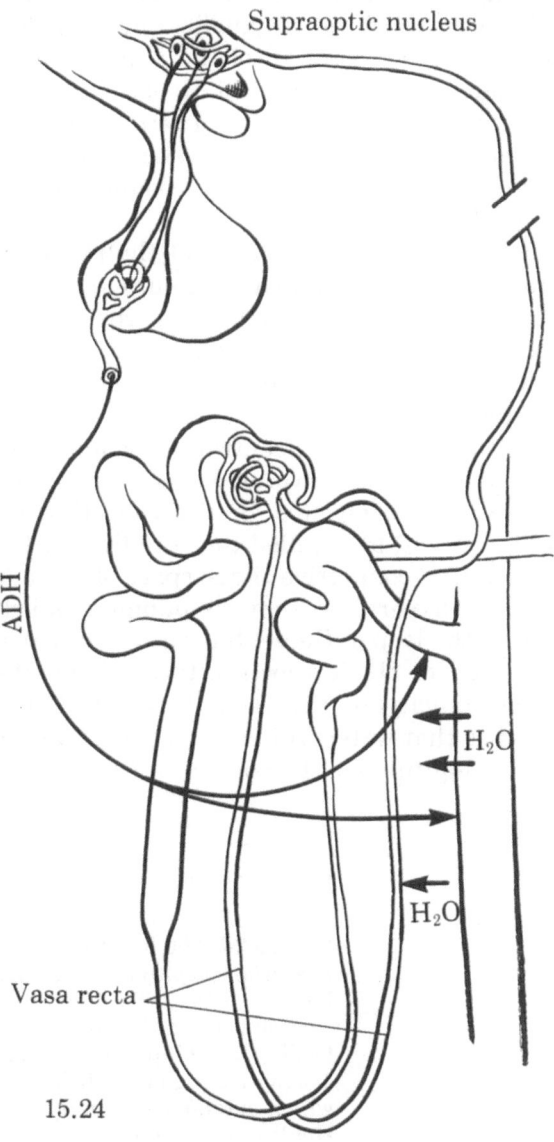

Supraoptic nucleus

ADH

H_2O

H_2O

Vasa recta

15.24

COLLECTING TUBULE. The nephrons of a lobule are connected to collecting tubules in the associated medullary ray by arched collecting tubules. Each collecting tubule pursues a generally straight course through the length of the medullary ray into the medulla. Here it joins, one at a time, with several neighboring collecting tubules to form a large *papillary duct* (of Bellini). One or two dozen of these open on the papilla of each pyramid, producing a perforated region termed the *area cribrosa*.

A simple cuboidal epithelium lines most of the collecting tubules. In the larger tubules of the papillary ducts of the medulla, the epithelium becomes columnar. Their nuclei are darkly staining and spherical, and the cytoplasm has the fewest organelles and the palest staining reaction of all of the regions of the uriniferous tubule; in fact it often appears unstained. These tubules can be readily identified in histologic sections by this light staining and the distinctly evident boundaries between their cells.

The columnar epithelium of the papillary ducts is continuous with a similar epithelium on the surface of the papilla. In the grooves surrounding the papilla, where the calyx is attached, the epithelium becomes transitional.

Although final concentration of urine begins in the distal convoluted tubule, it is accelerated and completed in the collecting tubules. It will be recalled that the fluid of the interstitial connective tissue space of the medulla is hypertonic from the pumping of salt out of the loop of Henle. Indeed the principal function of Henle's loop is to maintain the hypertonicity of the medullary interstitial fluid so that water will be extracted from the collecting tubule. The control of this process lies in the hypothalamus (Fig. 15.24), where a peptide hormone *antidiuretic hormone* (*ADH*), is synthesized in neuroendocrine cells which are sensitive to the osmolality of the blood. When osmolality increases, this hormone is released into capillaries in the pars nervosa of the pituitary gland. ADH renders the distal convoluted tubule and collecting tubules permeable to water. Thus the passive movement of water out of the tubule into the hypertonic interstitium increases with increasing blood levels of ADH and the urine becomes more concentrated. With damage to the hypothalamus or pars nervosa, so that ADH production is reduced or halted, the tubules become impermeable, water is not reabsorbed, and the urine is not concentrated. In this condition, called diabetes insipidus, large amounts (up to 15 or 18 liters per day) of hypotonic urine may be produced.

Blood Vessels (Fig. 15.25)

The renal artery enters the hilus of the kidney and here usually divides into two branches, one to the anterior portion of the organ and one to the posterior portion. Each divides into several *interlobar arteries* that enter the kidney between the medullary pyramids. Since the finer branches of these vessels do not anastomose with similar branches of the other interlobar arteries, these are end arteries. Thus collateral circulation does not exist between interlobar systems.

At the junction between cortex and medulla the interlobar arteries give off approximately right-angle branches (*arcuate arteries*), which at first lie along the corticomedullary junction. Along their course arcuate arteries give off numerous and regularly spaced, roughly

Fig. 15.25. General pattern of the *arterial supply of the kidney*.

Fig. 15.26. The blood supply and tubular pattern of *subcapsular (right) and juxtamedullary nephrons*. The efferent arteriole of the subcapsular glomerulus remains largely cortical. The efferent arteriole of the juxtamedullary glomerulus, although contributing to the vascularity of the convoluted tubules, is largely concerned with feeding blood into the vasa recta which dip down into the medulla. Efferent arterioles arising from glomeruli intermediate in position between these two provide vessels which extend accordingly. The same sort of variation occurs in the depth to which Henle's loop extends into the pyramid.

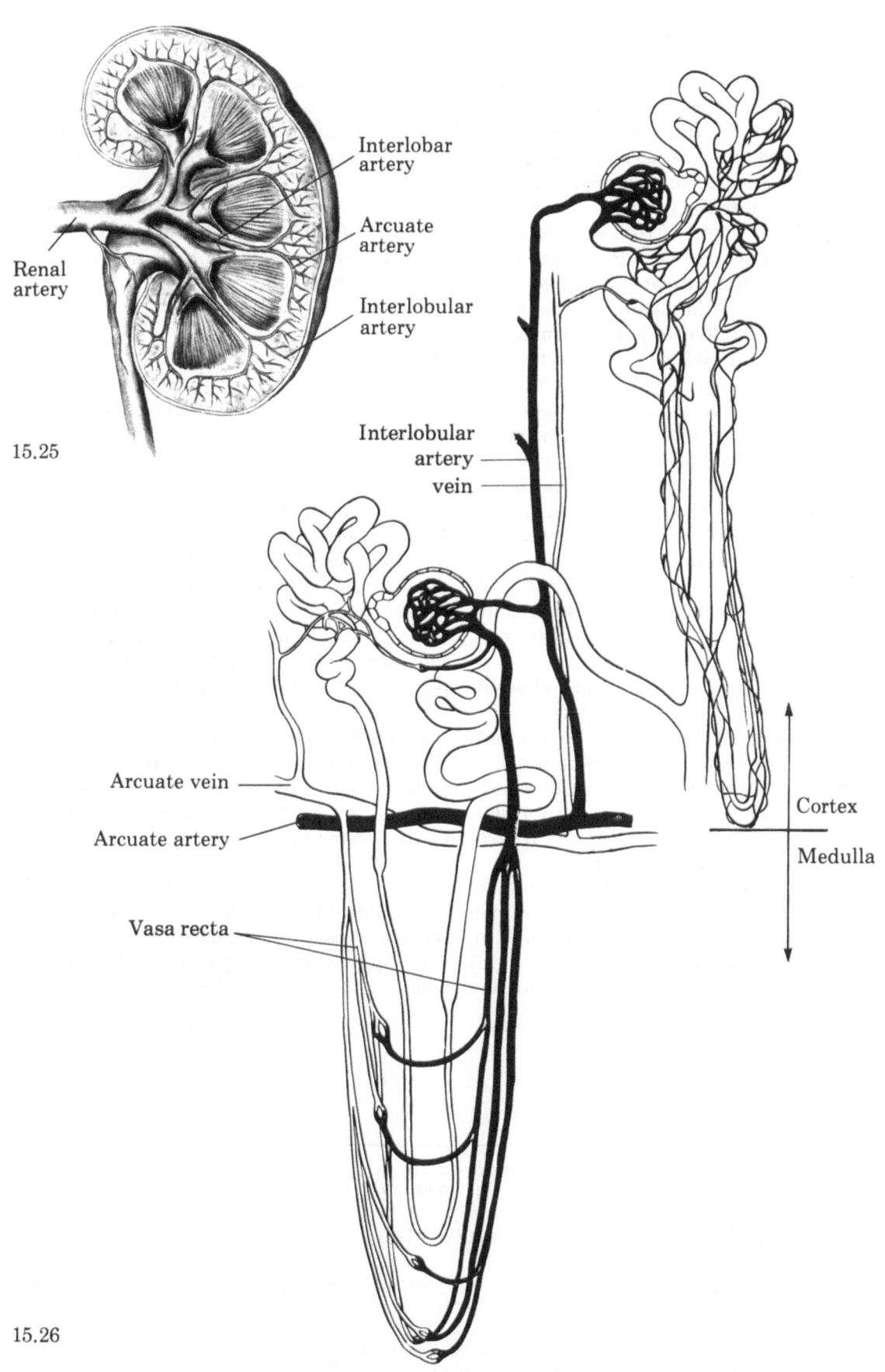

Interlobar
artery

Arcuate
artery

Interlobular
artery

Renal
artery

15.25

Interlobular
artery
vein

Arcuate vein

Arcuate artery

Vasa recta

Cortex

Medulla

15.26

perpendicular branches, which extend into the cortex between the lobules. These are the *interlobular arteries* (Figs. 15.25 and 15.26). Toward the end of its course each arcuate artery, as it branches and becomes smaller, swings upward into the cortex to become the last interlobular vessel of that particular arcuate system. Each interlobular artery gives off numerous radially arranged *afferent arterioles* to the neighboring glomeruli (Fig. 15.26). The glomerular capillaries join to form an *efferent arteriole* draining blood from each glomerulus. From this point the circulation to subcapsular and juxtamedullary nephrons differ. In nephrons of the outer cortex (subcapsular) the efferent arteriole breaks up almost immediately into a network of capillaries around the proximal and distal convoluted tubules. These capillaries drain toward the capsule and empty into the *stellate veins* under the capsule. The sequence of flow is then stellate veins to interlobular veins to arcuate veins to interlobar veins to renal veins to vena cava.

In juxtamedullary nephrons each efferent arteriole provides a capillary plexus for the proximal and distal convoluted tubules, but in addition, provides an arteriole that takes a straight course deep into the medulla parallel to Henle's loop. These are the *arteriolae rectae*, which make hairpin loops and return as the venulae rectae to empty into the arcuate veins. (The arterioles and their venulae together are called *vasa recta*.) From here the path is arcuate veins to interlobar veins to renal veins to vena cava.

The two limbs of the vasa recta and the two limbs of Henle's loop form a complex countercurrent exchange system for manipulation of sodium and water in the conservation of body fluids and the concentration of urine.

Lymph vessels accompany the major blood vessels but their identification and arrangement in the parenchyma have not been completely worked out.

Ureter

The calyx (Fig. 15.27), pelvis of the ureter, and the ureter itself (Fig. 15.28) show the same histologic structure. The mucosa is composed of a sheet of transitional epithelium resting on a thin lamina propria rich in elastic fibers. There is no muscularis mucosae and no submucosa. The muscularis consists of inner longitudinal and outer circular layers of smooth muscle. In the lower third of the ureter, an additional outer layer of longitudinal muscle is present. This outer layer appears to be continuous with the thickest layer of the bladder. The ureter passes obliquely through the wall of the bladder; thus the bladder contents tend to compress this intramural portion of the ureter and prevent reflux of urine. The muscle of the intramural portion of the ureter is all longitudinal, so that its contractions tend to shorten and open the tube.

The adventitia of the ureter contains numerous nerves and blood vessels. These vessels supply a rich plexus in the lamina propria.

Fig. 15.27. *Transitional epithelium* in a calyx. This epithelium lines almost the entire urinary tract below this point. ×110.

Fig. 15.28. *Ureter* in cross-section. ×12.

Fig. 15.29. *Bladder*. The wall is contracted, throwing the inner layers into folds. ×7.5.

Fig. 15.30. *Urethra*. This is a section of the male membranous urethra which at this level is similar to the female urethra. ×16.

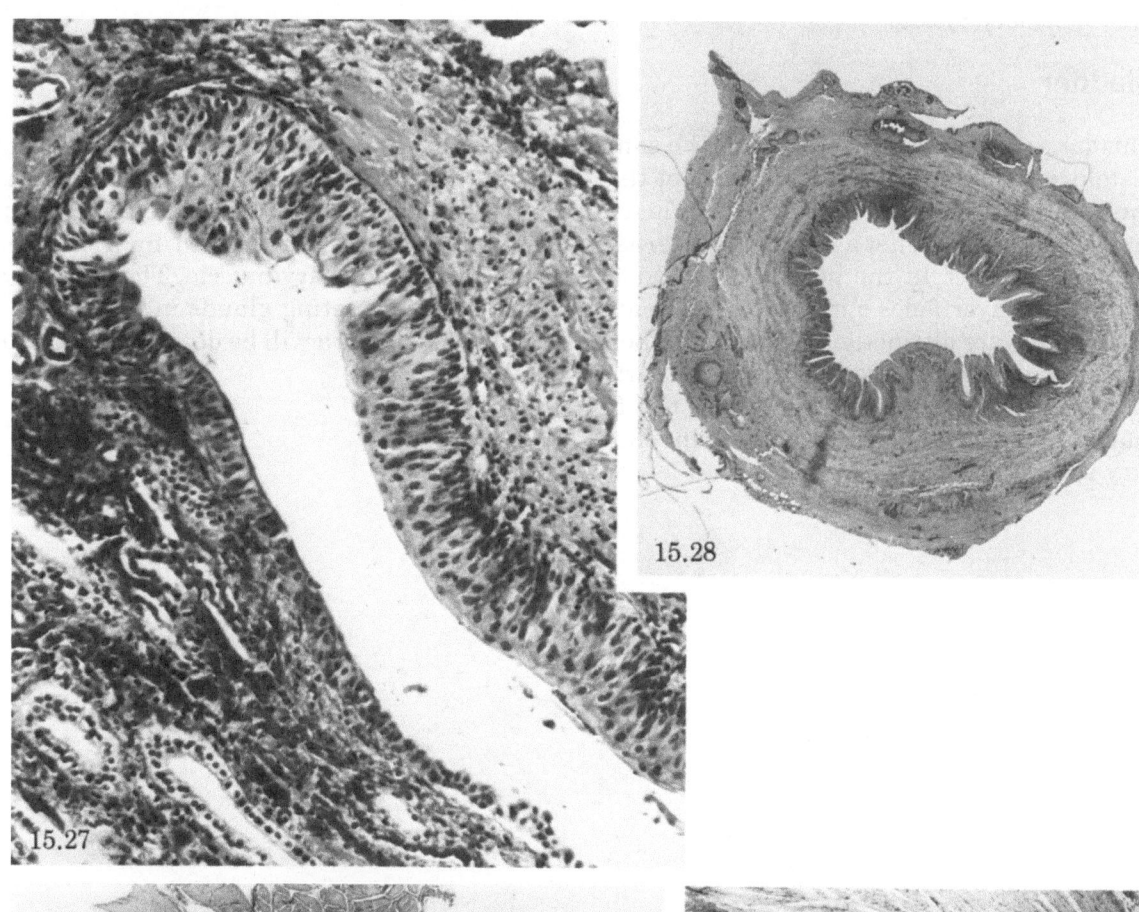

15.27

15.28

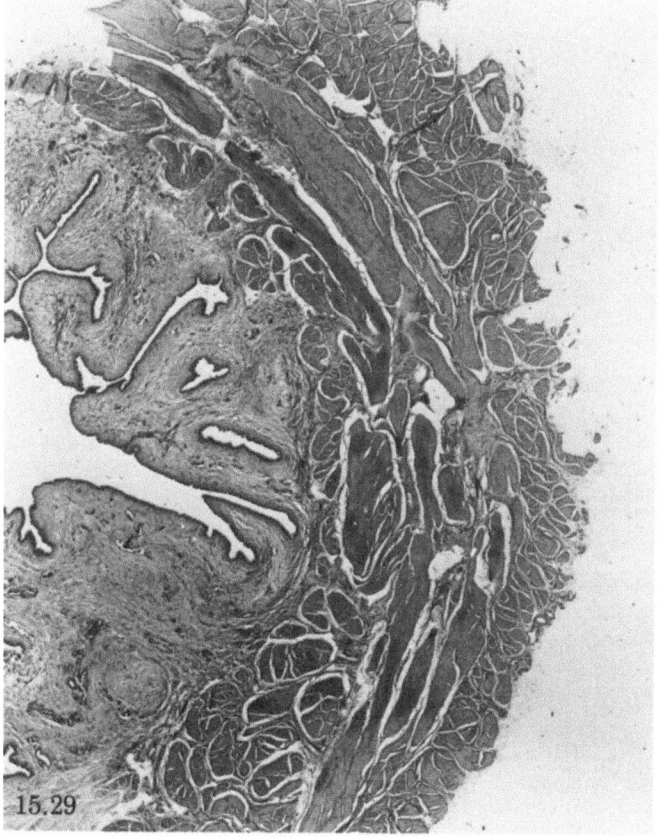

15.29

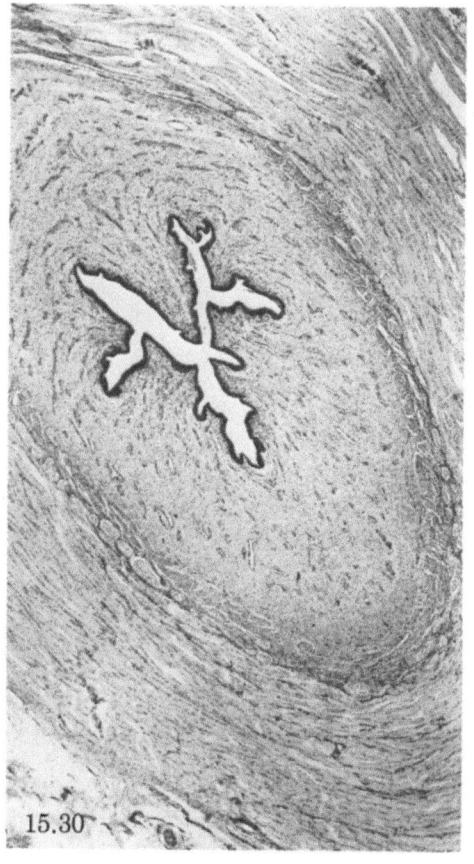

15.30

Bladder

This large reservoir (Fig. 15.29) has the same histologic structure as the ureter except that the muscularis is much thicker and its layers are less discrete and not as distinctly alternating in directions. In the neck of the bladder the middle layer fades out and the inner and outer layers are distinctly longitudinal. These continue into the prostatic urethra in the male and to the urethral meatus in the female. The inner layer constitutes the involuntary sphincter.

Urethra

The female urethra (Fig. 15.30) is 2–3 cm long and 1 cm in external diameter. Its lining is of transitional and stratified squamous epithelium and it is surrounded by a circular sphincter of voluntary muscle. There are few small mucus-secreting glands in the wall.

The male urethra will be described in Chapter 18.

16 Endocrine Glands

General Aspects

Endocrine glands are ductless, and their products are secreted into the interstitial space of their surrounding connective tissue and then pass into blood vessels. Hence the term endocrine, which means secreting internally. Such glands constitute one of two major mechanisms for initiation, integration, and correlation of adjustments to internal and external environmental variations. The other is the nervous system, in which neurons transmit signals as a result of environmental alteration, in the form of waves of depolarization that initiate a distant response. An endocrine gland, in response to a specific stimulus (which may be neural or hormonal), releases into the circulation a chemical messenger that brings about appropriate specific responses in other tissues or organs. The substance is termed a hormone, from the Greek meaning "to set in motion."

On the basis of chemical structure hormones are of three types (Fig. 16.1): tyrosine derivatives; proteins and peptides; and steroids. The first two types do not enter target cells but bind to receptors on the cell membrane and activate an enzyme, adenyl cyclase, that brings about the production of a "second messenger," cyclic adenosine monophosphate (cAMP), which in turn brings about the physiologic response for which the particular cell is programmed. Hormones of the third group, the steroids, enter the target cells, become bound to cytoplasmic receptors, and are carried to the nucleus, where they initiate RNA synthesis.

Hormones generally produce their effects at sites distant from the sites of their secretion. They act on the target tissue by: (1) activating preexisting enzymes; (2) bringing about the release of preformed and stored cell products; or (3) initiating the synthesis of a new protein.

The increased blood level of the product of the target tissue acts, in return, on the endocrine gland to suppress or inhibit the production and/or release of its hormone. This is termed *feedback inhibition* (Fig. 16.2) and is an important mechanism for equilibration of levels of hormones and other substances in the body.

Fig. 16.1. Diagram summarizing the *mechanism of action of hormones*. Three simplified pathways are shown as if occurring in the same cell, one for tyrosine derivatives and protein hormones, one for estradiol, and one for testosterone. In actuality only one mechanism predominates in a given cell. Note that receptors for the tyrosine derivatives and protein are plasmalemmal while those for the steroids are cytoplasmic. Testosterone is converted to dihydrotestosterone (DHT) before it acts on the genome.

Fig. 16.2. The concept of *hormonal feedback control*. The product of a target organ, in addition to performing its basic biologic functions, suppresses the production of its trophic hormone.

Fig. 16.3. Locations of *hypophysis, hypothalamus* and *pineal* gland.

Fig. 16.4. Three stages in the embryonic *development of the pituitary gland*.

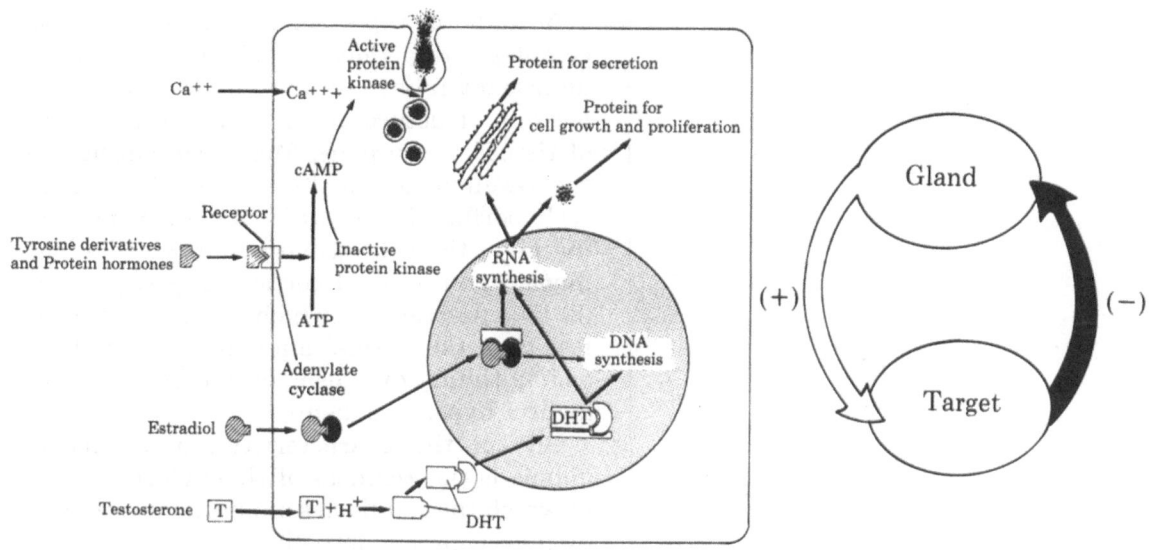

16.1

16.2

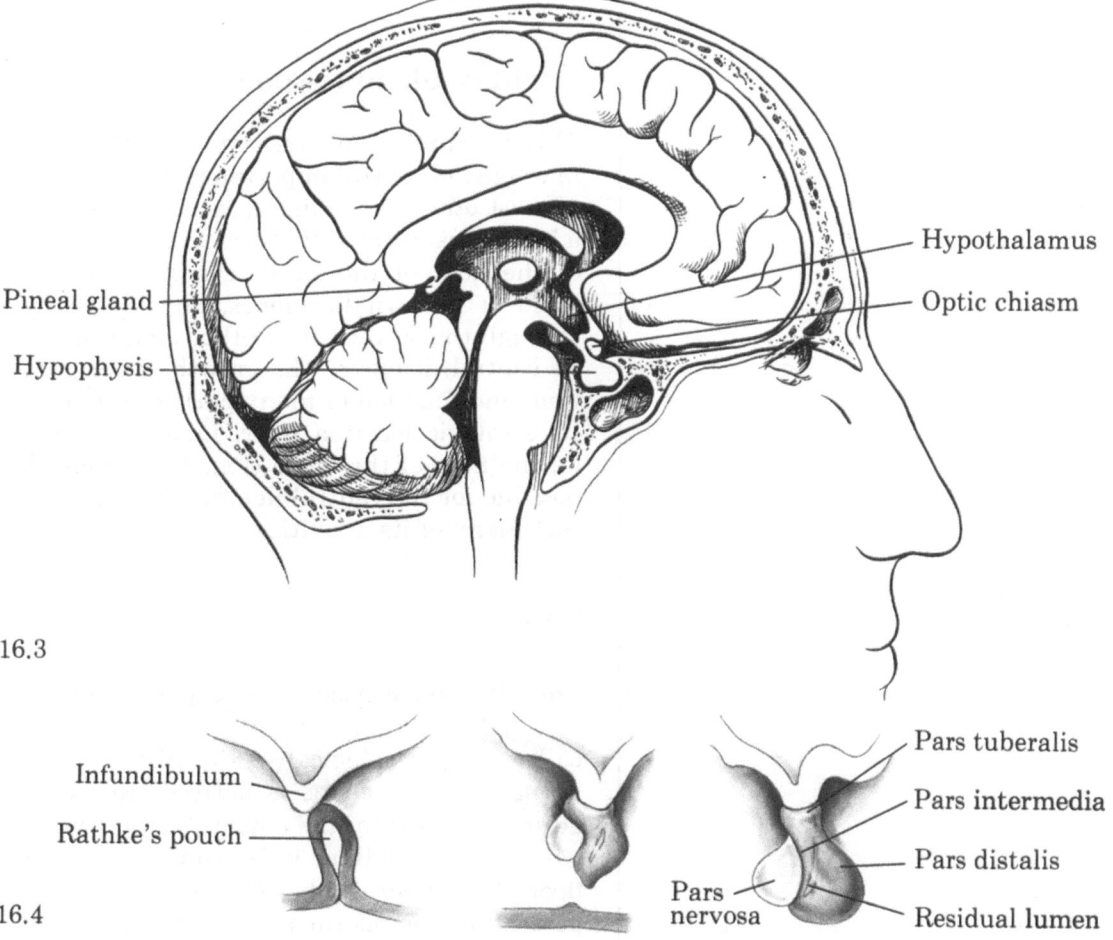

16.3

16.4

As might be expected, disturbances of these complex interactions by genetic errors or by disease often have serious and widespread effects on structure and function of a variety of tissues and organs. Most such effects are the result of one of two states of function: (1) hyperfunction, in which a gland is producing more than the usual quantity of its hormone, as in adrenal cortical hyperplasia, or (2) hypofunction, in which a gland produces less than the normal amount of its product, as in pituitary dwarfism, or in cretinism (congenital hypothyroidism).

One of the characteristics of endocrine glands is the richness of their blood supply, in which the capillaries or sinusoids are lined by fenestrated endothelium.

We have excluded from this chapter brain, liver, lung, kidney, and gonads, because their endocrine functions are secondary in the systems of which they are component organs.

Pituitary Gland (Hypophysis)

This pea-sized organ, averaging about 500 mg in weight, of central importance in the control of most other endocrine organs, is located in a bony pocket (the sella turcica) in the center of the floor of the skull. Directly, through some of its own hormones, and indirectly, through the secretions of other glands under its control, it affects the growth, differentiation, and function of many parts of the body. Its strategic location near, indeed attached to, the floor of the brain (Fig. 16.3) makes it possible for the central nervous system to direct many of its activities.

Parts

The pituitary consists of two parts that are distinctly different embryologically, histologically, and physiologically (Fig. 16.4).

THE ADENOHYPOPHYSIS is derived from ectoderm of the roof of the embryo's stomodeum, where its epithelium is in contact with the floor of the neural tube. This area of contact persists as mesoderm proliferates around it to form the skull and other tissues and to separate the brain from the oral cavity. Thus the area becomes first an epithelial pocket (Rathke's pouch), and then a closed vesicle that loses its connection with the lining of what is now the nasopharynx. The anterior wall of the pouch becomes the pars distalis (Figs. 16.4 and 16.5), the largest hormone-producing part of the gland; the posterior wall remains in intimate contact with neural tissue and is the pars intermedia. The cavity disappears or breaks up into a group of colloid-filled, more or less cystic spaces (follicles). A thin collar of pouch tissue encloses a stalk of neural tissue extending downward from the brain floor, and is termed the pars tuberalis.

THE NEUROHYPOPHYSIS (Figs. 16.4, 16.9, and 16.10), is drawn out from the floor of the brain during development and consists of, from above downwards, a flattened, cone-shaped area (the median eminence of the hypothalamus), an elongated tubular portion (the infundibular stalk), and an expanded end (the infundibular process or pars nervosa).

Cells and Products

PARS DISTALIS. The cells are arranged in the pattern characteristic of endocrine glands, that is, in cords and clumps separated by sheets of tenuous connective tissue with a rich network of capillaries and sinusoids lined by fenestrated endothelium (Fig. 16.7). With the use of sophisticated staining methods and the electron microscope, approximately eight cell types have been demonstrated. Each type probably produces one of the several hormones secreted by this gland. However, with routine stains three cell types are apparent (Figs. 16.7 and 16.8).

Chromophobes are small, lightly stained, or unstained cells with indistinct cell boundaries and few if any demonstrable cytoplasmic granules. They constitute about 50% of the cells in the pars distalis and probably are precursors and/or nonsecreting, resting cells. It may be that some cells of this population secrete adrenocorticotrophic hormone (ACTH). It seems more likely that they represent degranulated cells that have released their secretion.

Acidophils (Fig. 16.8) are cells with acidophilic cytoplasmic granules. This group includes two cell types, one with small and one with large granules.

The *somatotrophs* (acidophils with small granules) produce *growth hormone* (somatotrophin, STH), a simple protein. In its general growth-promoting activity STH affects a number of metabolic processes, but its principal impact is probably through the stimulation of protein synthesis. Its most obvious effect is the stimulation of growth of the epiphyseal plates in bones. This effect is indirect, however, for under the influence of STH, the liver and kidney produce a peptide called somatomedin, which acts on the plates. Acidophil tumors in children and adolescents may result in gigantism. Similar tumors in adults, when epiphyseal plates are no longer present, produce growth of some cartilage and thickening of some bones, particularly those of the extremities, but no growth in height. This condition is known as acromegaly.

The *mammotrophs,* the other group of acidophils, with large granules, produce *prolactin* (lactogenic hormone, luteotrophic hormone, PRL), which also is a simple protein. This hormone's most apparent and first discovered action is the control of milk secretion. However, it also has important behavioral effects; for example, its experimental administration to cocks induces brooding behavior usually characteristic of hens. In addition, receptors for this hormone are present in a number of cell types in both sexes. It seems likely that prolactin will prove to be of far greater significance in a wide variety of body functions than was originally believed.

There appears to be some overlap in function of STH and prolactin, or perhaps each cell type can produce at least some of the other's hormone. These possibilities are indicated by the fact that some female patients with acidophil tumors have not only acromegaly but also galactorrhea (excessive milk secretion).

Basophils (Fig. 16.8). There are at least four and possibly five subgroups in the basophil population of the pars distalis. Three of these subgroups produce glycoprotein hormones and two produce polypeptides.

The *thyrotrophs* are large polyhedral cells with small granules. For the most part they are located in the central portion of the pars distalis. They produce *thyroid-stimulating hormone* (thyrotrophin, *TSH*), a glycoprotein that stimulates both the synthesis and the release of thyroid hormones.

Gonadotrophs. These round basophils produce glycoprotein hormones that control growth and functions of the several tissues making up the ovary and testis. There are two gonadotrophic cell types distributed throughout the pars distalis, each producing a hormone. Because the two hormones were discovered in studies in female laboratory animals, they are named *follicle-stimulating hormone* (*FSH*) and *luteinizing hormone* (*LH*) for the ovarian processes they control. The same hormones are present in males, in whom they have different, but perhaps homologous, functions.

FSH is secreted by large round basophils that have a prominent Golgi apparatus, so large in fact that it may sometimes be seen as a negative, unstained image in routine preparations observed with the light microscope. The hormone is a glycoprotein containing sialic acid as an important functional component. FSH stimulates growth and differentiation of the primordial follicle in the ovary and, via the Sertoli cells, spermatogenesis in the testis.

LH is also referred to as interstitial cell stimulating hormone (ICSH) in the male. It is also a glycoprotein produced by a population of small, round basophils, and it consists of two peptide chains. In the female, LH: (1) stimulates estrogen production by the theca interna; (2) stimulates the final stages in maturation of the follicle; (3) by a sudden increase in its blood level, apparently brings about ovulation; and (4) subsequently controls conversion of the empty follicle to a corpus luteum, thus initiating and maintaining progesterone production by the corpus luteum. In the male LH stimulates the production of androgens by the interstitial cells of the testis. Endocrine relationships of the female and male reproductive systems are further discussed in Chapters 17 and 18.

Hypofunction resulting from disease of the pituitary or of its controlling hypothalamus may lead to greatly decreased output of gonadotrophins and, for example, testicular failure. Such failure includes reduced or absent spermatogenesis (sterility) and reduced secretion of androgens. This is termed secondary testicular failure, since it depends on failure of another organ. In primary testicular failure, the defect lies in the testis; the hypothalamus and pituitary are functioning appropriately. Secondary testicular failure is readily treated by the administration of gonadotrophins. The chorionic trophoblast of the placenta is a good source of these because it produces large quantities of gonadotrophins. Thus human chorionic gonadotrophin (HCG) is readily available and is commonly used to treat this and other clinical problems.

Corticotrophs. Although there is some controversy about this, basophils in the pars intermedia and pars distalis are probably producers of adrenocorticotrophic hormone (ACTH). This is a peptide consisting of only 39 amino acids. It is responsible for control of secretion of steroid hormones by the zonae fasciculata and reticularis of the adrenal cortex. This pituitary-adrenal axis (*also see later*) is a vital part of the body's mechanism for

Fig. 16.5. *Pars distalis* (D) and *pars nervosa* (N) of the pituitary gland, in transverse section. ×6.

Fig. 16.6. *Pars distalis.* ×110.

Fig. 16.7. *Cells* of the *pars distalis.* Acidophils (A), basophils (B) and chromophobes (C). ×560.

Fig. 16.8. Electron micrograph of the *pars distalis* showing portions of two adjacent *chromophils.* Granules of an acidophil (A) and a portion of a basophil (B) are seen. ×20,250. (Courtesy of M. Webb.)

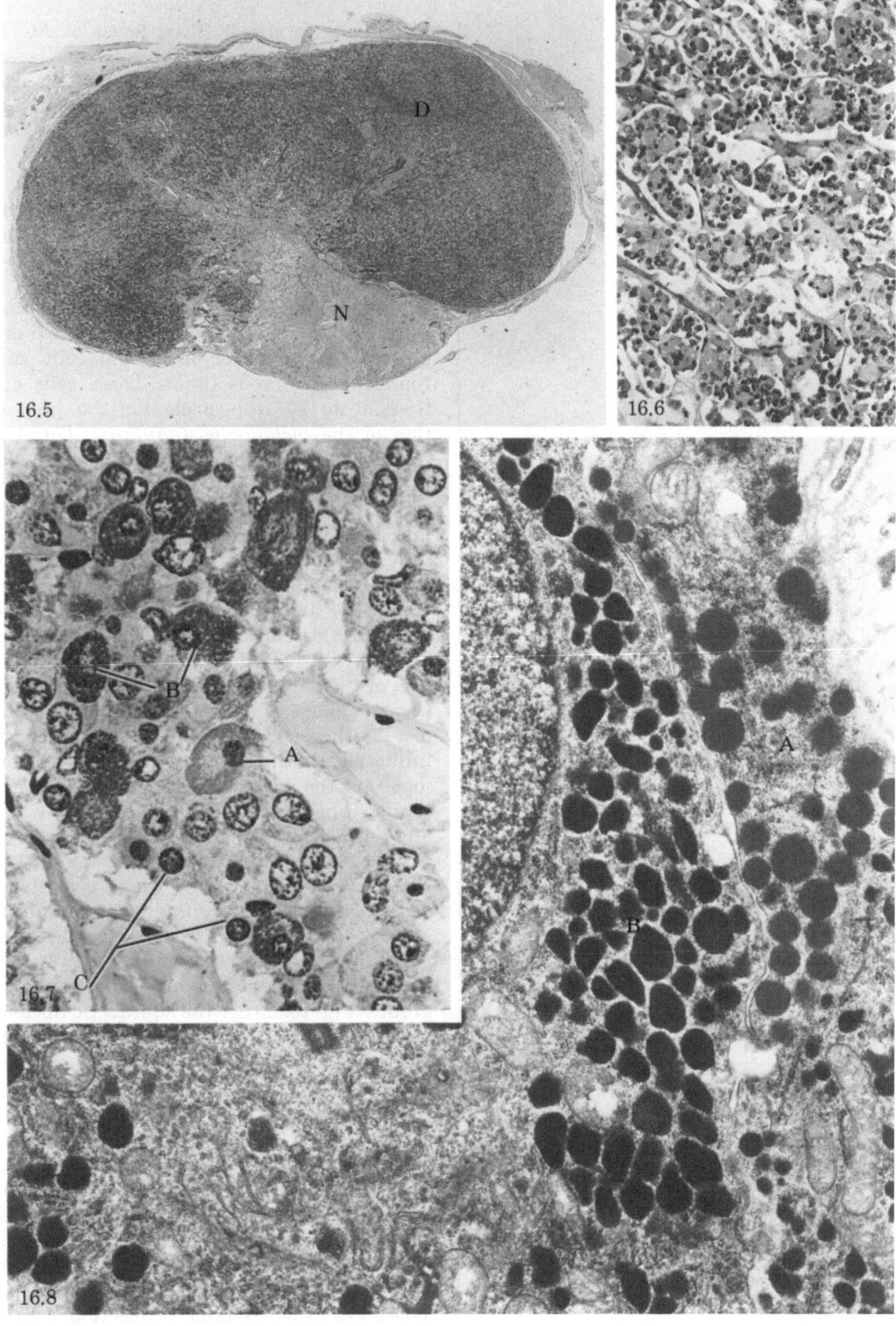

16.5

16.6

16.7

16.8

responding to stress. Blood levels of ACTH show a diurnal rhythm. This system is extremely sensitive to environmental changes and related CNS input, and therefore fluctuations of high frequency and amplitude are superimposed on this rhythm.

PARS INTERMEDIA (Fig. 16.9). The intimate embryologic relations of neural and buccal epithelium are retained in this portion of the pituitary gland. No connective tissue or other barrier separates the pars intermedia from the pars nervosa. Indeed the basophils extend into the pars nervosa and many of them are present as groups or individual cells surrounded by nervous tissue. These cells are thought to be responsible for the production of the *melanocyte-stimulating hormone* (*MSH*, melanotrophin). MSH is a small peptide and occurs in two forms, α-MSH and β-MSH. In some animals MSH produces dramatic changes in melanocytes; in humans its function is more obscure but it probably increases melanin synthesis. The sequence of the first 13 amino acids of ACTH is contained in α-MSH. A relation to ACTH is further suggested by the fact that among signs of destruction of the adrenal cortex (Addison's disease) is an increase of skin pigmentation. In this disease there is an absence of the feedback inhibition that is normally provided by hormones of the adrenal cortex. There is therefore a large increase in the output of ACTH and an associated increase in MSH.

PARS NERVOSA (Figs. 16.10 through 16.12). This part of the pituitary gland consists of modified glial cells (*pituicytes*) and about 100,000 axons that extend into the area through the infundibular stalk from two cell clusters in the hypothalamus. These two cell groups (Fig. 16.12) are the supraoptic nucleus and the paraventricular nucleus (a nucleus in the neurologic sense is a group of nerve cell bodies all concerned with the same function). This mass of nerve fibers (axons) constitutes the hypothalamohypophyseal tract. Each of its fibers conducts secretion manufactured in its cell body in the hypothalamus, down to the fiber's termination near a capillary in the pars nervosa. Here the secretion is stored in the form of droplets in the nerve fiber that are visible in the light microscope. These are called Herring bodies (Fig. 16.11).

The hormone is released from the axon terminal, in response to an impulse coming down the axon in which it is stored, and it passes into the blood vessel to be distributed throughout the body and to bring about the appropriate reactions in its target tissues. The pars nervosa is not like most glands; its products are manufactured elsewhere, it has no epithelial component, and it has no connective tissue stroma supporting cords and clumps of cells. The two hormones of the pars nervosa, *oxytocin* and *antidiuretic hormone* (*ADH*, vasopressin), are both nonapeptides. The same cells synthesize proteins termed neurophysins to which these hormones are bound. Each hormone has its own specific neurophysin, which apparently acts as a carrier.

Oxytocin produced in the paraventricular nucleus has two targets (Fig. 16.12): uterine muscle and myoepithelial cells of the mammary glands. It functions in what are called neuroendocrine reflexes (since both nerve conduction and circulating hormones are involved in the final target response). Distention of the cervix in childbirth and of the vagina in copulation provide afferent impulses to the central nervous system that lead to oxytocin release and thus to uterine contraction. Similarly, nerve impulses initiated in sensory endings in the nipple by nursing are responsible for stimulation of the appropriate hypothalamic neurons, and thus for the release of the hormone in the pars nervosa. The circulating hormone then brings about contraction of myoepithelial cells in the breast and the ejection of milk from the gland.

ADH is mostly derived from cells of the supraoptic nucleus (Fig. 16.12). These cells, closely related anatomically to a "thirst center," are very sensitive to changes in osmolality of the blood of their associated capillaries. In response to an increase in blood osmolality, nerve impulses depolarize axons that release stored ADH. Its targets are the distal tubules and collecting ducts of the kidney, where it increases permeability of the epithelium to water. Water thus leaves the tubule and a concentration of urine occurs. Damage to any portion of the supraopticohypophyseal system may lead to failure of ADH synthesis and/or release and thus to the production of large quantities, sometimes 15 liters per day, of hypotonic urine. This condition is known as diabetes insipidus.

Mechanisms of Control

Integrated normal function of the pituitary gland depends on information from the environment and from many parts of the body via the nervous and vascular systems. Although the pars nervosa is basically a portion of the nervous system, the adenohypophysis has no direct innervation. Therefore all of its input, both from target organ feedback and from the CNS, must come through the vascular system. There are three major components to the system of controls that work together to equilibrate pituitary function: (a) blood supply, (b) hypothalamic neuroendocrine factors, and (c) feedback inhibition.

THE BLOOD SUPPLY is probably best appreciated by a study of the diagram (Fig. 16.13). On each side an inferior hypophyseal artery from the internal carotid provides most of the blood to the pars nervosa, and there is direct venous drainage of its capillary bed. However, some of its capillary vessels anastomose with those of the pars distalis and there are probably direct anastomoses with the superior hypophyseal artery. The latter artery feeds a rich capillary bed in the median eminence and the infundibular stalk. The most important feature of this entire system is that the set of capillaries, which supply neuroendocrine cell groups in the brain floor, are gathered into a series of longitudinal veins that course down the pituitary stalk and break up into another capillary bed, that of the pars distalis. Blood from the pars distalis then returns to the general circulation by way of hypophyseal veins. This arrangement is appropriately termed the hypophyseal portal system. Through this system hormones produced by hypothalamic neuroendocrine cells have relatively quick access to cells of the pars distalis, whose function they at least partially control. Patterns of flow through this system are probably variable, depending upon the behavior of smooth muscle in precapillary arterioles. Blood flow in the portal veins has been seen to temporarily reverse its direction;

Fig. 16.9. *Pars intermedia.* There is a gradual transition from the pars distalis (above) to the pars nervosa (below). ×85.

Fig. 16.10. *Pars nervosa.* ×110.

Fig. 16.11. *Pars nervosa.* The darkly stained nuclei are those of pituicytes. There is a Herring body (H) and a capillary (arrow). ×560.

Fig. 16.12. Functional anatomy of the *neurohypophysis.* Hormones synthesized by cells in various nuclei of the hypothalamus are delivered to the neurohypophysis by the axons. The pathway and target organs for oxytocin from the paraventricular nucleus and for ADH from the supraoptic nucleus are shown.

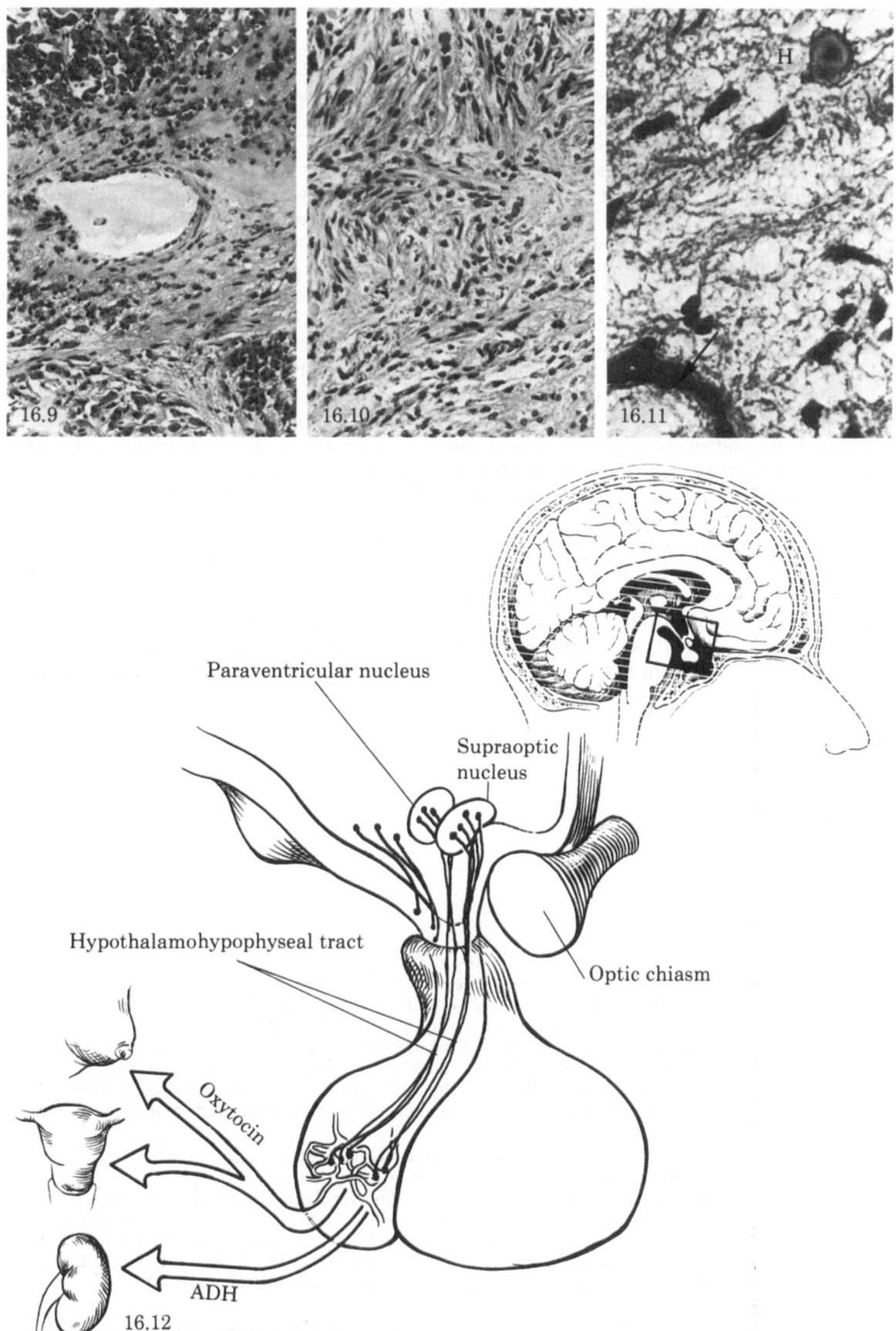

16.9

16.10

16.11   H

Paraventricular nucleus

Supraoptic nucleus

Hypothalamohypophyseal tract

Optic chiasm

Oxytocin

ADH

16.12

such a change might provide quick feedback from the pars distalis to the hypothalamus.

HYPOTHALAMIC NEUROENDOCRINE FACTORS (Fig. 16.14). In response to humoral and neural stimuli, several groups of cells in the hypothalamus produce substances (usually termed factors until they are established as definite compounds, after which they are called hormones) and release them to capillaries in the median eminence and infundibular stalk. These may be releasing factors or inhibiting factors, depending on their action on cells of the pars distalis. There is a thyrotrophin-releasing hormone (TRH), a corticotrophin-releasing factor (CRF), a prolactin-inhibiting factor (PIF), and so on. Each one acts on the appropriate cell type in the pars distalis by stimulating or inhibiting hormone synthesis and/or release.

FEEDBACK INHIBITION (Fig. 16.15). With respect to pituitary function the process of feedback inhibition involves responses of hypothalamus and pituitary to blood levels of target tissue products. It includes the following four interactions or feedback loops.

(1) Target organ-pituitary gland inhibition. For example, thyroxin may act directly on pituitary thyrotrophs to inhibit TSH production.

(2) Target organ-hypothalamus inhibition. For example, cortisol from the adrenal gland acts on hypothalamic cells to reduce the production of CRF.

(3) Adenopyhophysis-hypothalamus inhibition (short loop). For example, ACTH inhibits hypothalamic CRF production.

(4) Pituitary-pituitary inhibition (ultra short loop). For example, local levels of ACTH in pars distalis inhibit the production of ACTH by corticotrophs.

In some instances it is likely that feedback control is brought about by varying the activity of lysosomes in digesting cell products before they are released. Thus the net amount available for secretion into the circulation would be the difference between the rate of synthesis and the rate of lysosomal digestion. Interestingly, although positive feedback is a theoretical possibility, only the existence of negative feedback systems has been proved.

Fig. 16.13. *Blood vessels of the pituitary gland.* Capillaries in the median eminence at the top of the pituitary stalk and in the stalk itself are fed by the superior hypophyseal artery. Blood from these beds passes through the portal veins to the sinusoids of the pars distalis and then into the general circulation through hypophyseal veins. The capillaries of the pars nervosa are supplied by the inferior hypophyseal arteries and lead into the general circulation through hypophyseal veins.

Fig. 16.14. Endocrine *output and feedback* of the pars distalis. On the right are shown products of the basophils, their target organs and the products of the target organs that exert feedback control. This feedback affects the production of hypothalamic releasing hormones or of pituitary production of trophic hormones. On the left are shown the products of acidophils and their targets. Direct feedback loops are not known to occur in this group. (Based on Fig. 21.7 in Junqueira L., Carneiro J. Basic Histology, Los Altos, Lange Medical Publications, 1980.)

Fig. 16.15. Diagram of *releasing and trophic hormones* (stippled) and the various feedback loops that control them (black).

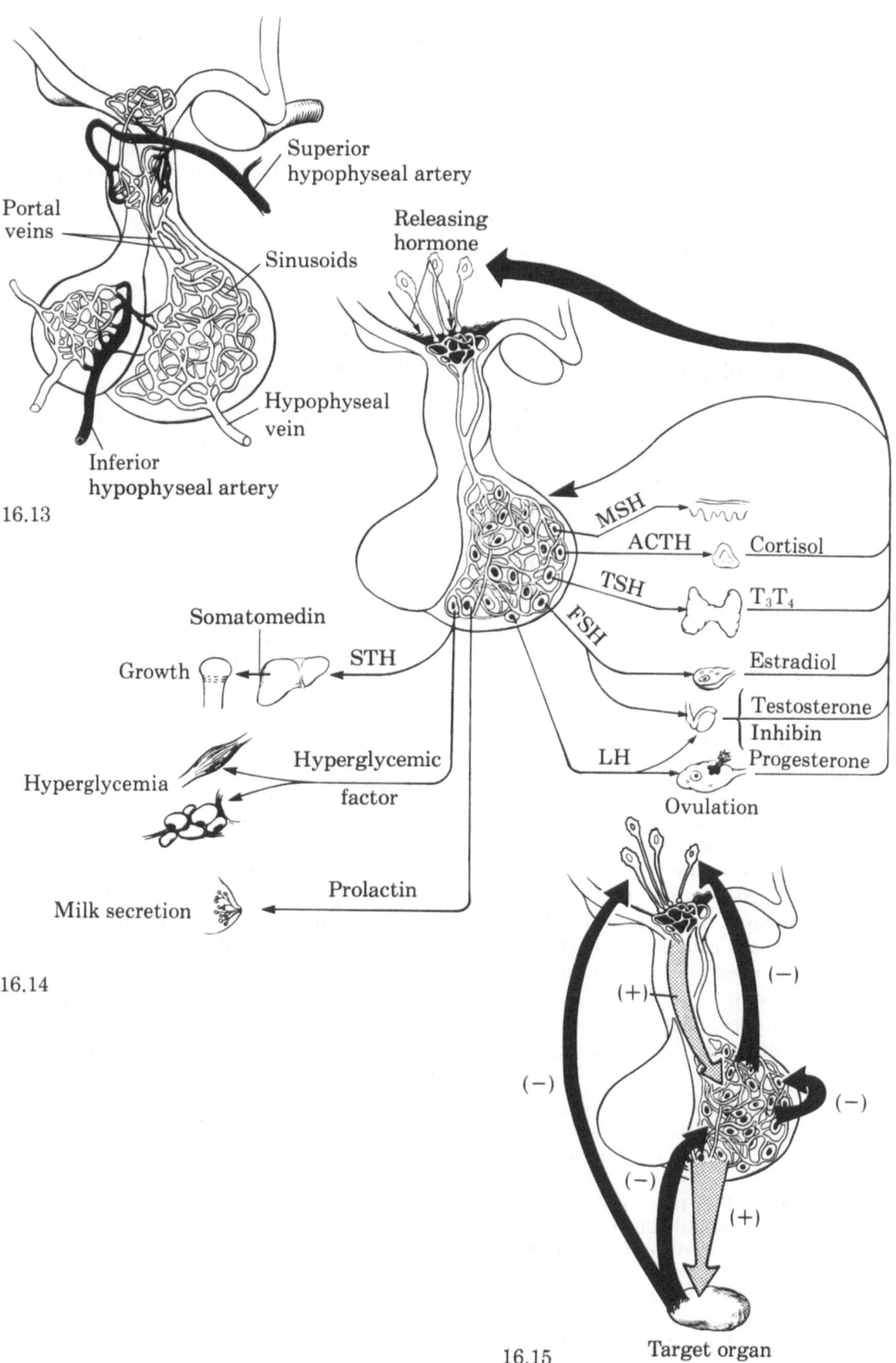

Superior hypophyseal artery

Portal veins

Sinusoids

Hypophyseal vein

Inferior hypophyseal artery

16.13

Releasing hormone

MSH

ACTH   Cortisol

TSH   T₃T₄

FSH

Estradiol

Testosterone
Inhibin
Progesterone

LH

Ovulation

Somatomedin

Growth   STH

Hyperglycemia   Hyperglycemic factor

Milk secretion   Prolactin

16.14

(+)   (−)

(−)   (−)

(−)   (+)

Target organ

16.15

Thyroid Gland

The thyroid gland is a 30–35 g, encapsulated mass (Fig. 16.16) of small epithelial *follicles* (*see later*) that contain stored, inactive secretion called *colloid*. Although the gland is of fairly simple structure, it releases two iodinated amino acid derivatives of major importance in the development of many tissues, and in the control of their oxidative metabolism.

Control of Development

Although other hormones are also involved in development, the thyroid secretion is a necessity for development and functional differentiation, particularly of nervous, reproductive, and musculoskeletal systems. Without it these systems are inadequately formed and infantile. It is particularly important for adequate CNS function.

Control of Metabolism

Metabolic effects of thyroid hormone are complex and not thoroughly understood.

OXIDATIVE METABOLISM, and thus metabolic rates, in many tissues are controlled by thyroid hormone (particularly in liver, skeletal muscle, and cardiac muscle). Unexpectedly, although the CNS requires thyroxin for adequate development and continuing function, its basal metabolic rate is not affected by this hormone. Other less well-known mechanisms are involved here.

THERMOREGULATION. Although it does not act alone in this function, thyroid hormone is important for the mobilization of heat-producing substrates such as fats.

Hypo- and hyperfunction of this gland may have dramatic clinical effects. Thyroid disease presents the physician with a large range of diagnostic and therapeutic problems.

Embryonic Development (Fig. 16.17)

The thyroid rudiment first appears as a pit in the floor of the pharynx in the region destined to become the tongue. This pit deepens and elongates to become the thyroglossal duct. The duct grows downward into the neck and the gland develops from its deep end. Normally the duct degenerates and the original pit is represented on the adult tongue by the foramen cecum. Accessory thyroid tissue may be found along the migration route and remnants of the duct may persist and dilate with accumulated fluid to form thyroglossal duct cysts.

Structural and Functional Organization

The units of structure and function are the follicles (Fig. 16.18). These spheroids range from 50 to 900 μm or sometimes more in diameter. In some forms of goiter (thyroid enlargement), they may reach a centimeter.

FOLLICULAR CELLS. The follicle wall is composed of simple cuboidal epithelium (Fig. 16.19), but this also may vary. The cells may become columnar or the follicles may sometimes become distended with colloid so that the epithelium becomes squamous. The apices of the cells, provided with scattered microvilli, are directed toward the cavity of the follicle and the bases rest on a thin basement mem-

---

Fig. 16.16. Anterior view of the *thyroid gland* in place.

Fig. 16.17. The path of *migration of the thyroid* rudiment during development is indicated by the dotted line. Two possible locations for thyroglossal duct cysts are shown, but they may develop at any position along this route.

Fig. 16.18. *Thyroid* (T) and *parathyroid* (P) glands. ×35.

Fig. 16.19. *Thyroid gland.* Note the characteristic preparation artifact, "chatter," in the colloid. ×250.

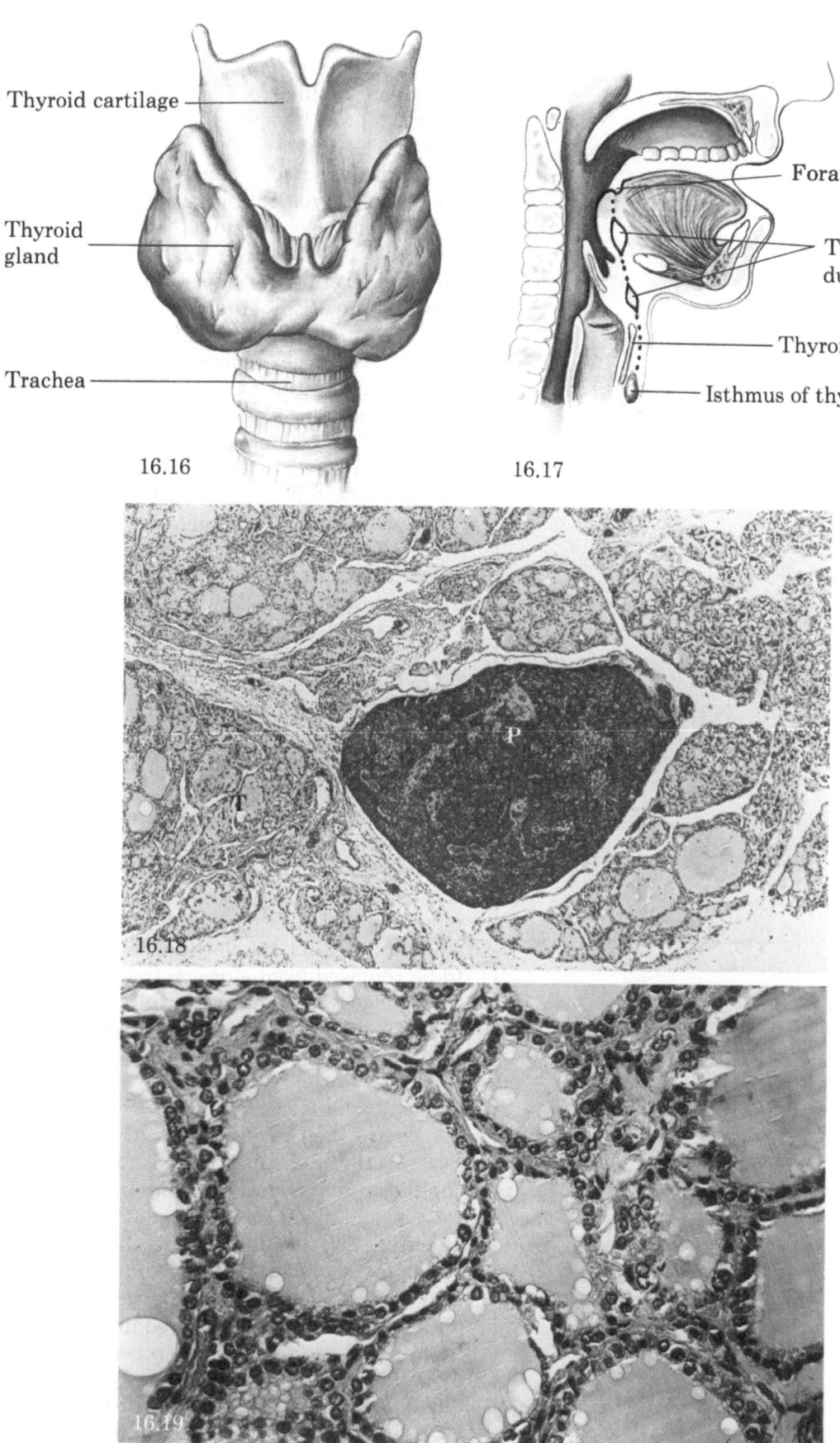

Thyroid cartilage

Thyroid gland

Trachea

16.16

Foramen cecum

Thyroglossal duct cysts

Thyroid cartilage

Isthmus of thyroid gland

16.17

16.18

16.19

brane. They are joined near their apices by junctional complexes. Gap junctions are present and probably provide for synchrony of function.

The initial secretory product of the follicular cell is thyroglobulin, a very large (about 670,000 daltons), hormonally inactive, iodinated glycoprotein (Fig. 16.20). As is usual in protein-secreting cells, peptides are synthesized in the RER. Mannose is incorporated into the peptide in the RER. The product is carried by transfer vesicles to the Golgi apparatus, which is on the colloid-facing side of the nucleus. Here galactose is added and polymerization is completed. Secretory vesicles from the Golgi carry the product to the apical surface, where it is released into the lumen.

The basal and apical membranes act as iodine pumps, transferring iodide from the blood, first into the cell, where it is oxidized, and then into the follicular lumen. Here the tyrosyl radicles are iodinated to complete the thyroglobulin. The pump is sufficiently powerful to maintain an iodine concentration differential of 25 to 1 between thyroid and blood. The pump is controlled by TSH from the pars distalis. Increased TSH levels stimulate rapid increase in iodine uptake.

Thyroglobulin is strictly a storage product. The active substances are tetraiodothyronine (thyroxine, T4) and triiodothyronine (T3). T4 is the principal circulating hormone; T3 is the more potent substance and is produced in smaller amounts. When these compounds are to be removed from storage, thyroglobulin is first phagocytosed from the follicular lumen by the follicle cells. The phagosomes so formed then fuse with primary lysosomes. Proteases in the lysosomes cleave the macromolecule and free the T3 and T4. These hormones are then released from the basal surface of the follicular cells and enter the capillaries for general circulation. The phagocytosis and lysosomal breakdown of thyroglobulin (Fig. 16.20) are controlled by TSH.

The metabolic activity of iodine in the thyroid is a useful clinical diagnostic tool. When a palpable nodule is discovered in the thyroid by physical examination, a tracer dose of radioiodine is injected intravenously and subsequent scanning of the thyroid area with a counter is likely to show that the nodule is either "hot" (has taken up an excessive amount of iodine) (Fig. 16.21) or "cold." Cold nodules are more likely to be neoplastic and they therefore require surgical removal and histologic diagnosis. Hot nodules are usually hyperplastic, but occasionally may be neoplastic, so that one cannot confidently leave them in place. Removal is usually recommended.

Other uses of radioactive iodine are: (1) location of distant metastases of thyroid carcinoma, and; (2) suppression of thyroid function with radioactivity when the gland is overactive (hyperthyroidism).

Presumably, fluctuations occur in the activity of different parts of the thyroid. This is consistent with the histologic appearance—follicles, colloid, and epithelium all vary. The variation is perhaps effected by special arrangements in the branches of the thyroid arteries, which may act to shunt blood.

PARAFOLLICULAR CELLS (C CELLS) are scattered, small, lightly staining cells lying just within the basal laminae of the follicles. They are responsible for the production of a hormone termed *calcitonin*. C cells are difficult to find with the light microscope, but the electron microscope (Fig. 16.22) shows small, membrane-bound granules characteristic of peptide-producing endocrine cells. These cells can also be localized by their selective binding of fluorescent antibody against calcitonin. They may be of neural crest origin and may migrate into the last pair of pharyngeal pouches early in development. From here they apparently are carried into the thyroid when those pouches join the developing thyroid gland by the 7th week of embryonic life.

Calcitonin is a substance that lowers the blood concentration of calcium by supressing the activity of osteoclasts. An appropriate balance between this hormone and parathyroid hormone, which stimulates osteoclast activity, is necessary for the maintenance of serum calcium levels within the remarkably narrow range of normalcy (8.5–10.5 mg/100 ml). Very small departures from this range produce serious and sometimes fatal consequences (*see below under* Parathyroid Gland).

The C cells are directly responsive to changes in levels of calcium in the blood. Increased calcium levels produce rapid release of calcitonin. Although these cells are not under continuing hypophyseal control, growth hormone may bring about some of its effects on bone in growing individuals by stimulating release of calcitonin, which in turn may stimulate an increase in the population of osteoblasts.

STROMA. The thyroid gland is enclosed by a thin capsule of connective tissue from which tenuous internal extensions or trabeculae divide the gland into irregular and incomplete lobules. A delicate mesh of connective tissue, largely of fine reticular fibers, surrounds each follicle.

The gland is richly vascularized; a network of blood and lymphatic capillaries lies in the sparse interfollicular connective tissue around each follicle. The capillary endothelium, as in other endocrine glands, is of the fenestrated variety. Thyroid hormone is primarily passed into blood capillaries but can also leave the gland via the lymphatic channels.

Small nerves found in the stroma are primarily vasomotor. However, sympathetic fibers have been found to terminate in very close relationship to the basal lamina of each follicle. Although control of thyroid function is certainly dominated by the hypothalamus and hypophysis, it is possible that some degree of neural control also exists.

Functional Disorders

Goiter is a nonspecific term for chronic enlargement of the thyroid gland and may occur in a number of diseases of this organ. Until the development of general awareness of the need for dietary iodine, deficiency of this element was the major cause of goiter. A minimum daily intake of 10 μg is necessary to maintain effective hormone function. At lower levels the braking effect of thyroxine on the pituitary gland is reduced and TSH output rises. This results in proliferation of follicular epithelium and enlargement of the thyroid (*hyperplastic goiter*).

If iodine is now added to the diet, thyroglobulin is synthesized, TSH production is suppressed, and normal colloid storage occurs. However, the increased parenchyma derived from the previous hyperplasia provides increased follicular storage space for colloid, and the gland enlarges still further. This is termed *colloid goiter*. Commonly both stages are seen together.

Hyperthyroidism occurs in a number of thyroid diseases. Probably the most common is *exophthalmic goiter* (Graves' disease). In this disorder there is a γ-globulin in the circulation that imitates TSH. This stimulates thyroid secretion and suppresses pituitary production of TSH. The mechanism of exophthalmia (protrusion of the eyes) is not fully understood.

Hypothyroidism has varying impact depending on the time of life at which it occurs. But whenever it occurs, its clinical manifestations involve all organ systems.

If hypothyroidism begins prenatally or during infancy, it produces a condition of mental and physical retardation termed *cretinism*. Failure of the gland to develop is the most

common cause of this serious disorder, but there are numerous other causes such as production of an abnormal thyroglobulin, failure of the proteolytic enzymes in the phagolysosomes, failure of the iodine pump, defective hormone receptor function in the target tissues, failure of the hypothalamus to produce TRH, accidental accumulation of radioiodine, and so on. With early diagnosis most thyroid deficiencies can be effectively treated with the hormone. But if this is delayed, receptors are not maintained, treatment is ineffective and the change becomes irreversible.

Hypothyroidism in the adult is less devastating because normal development of tissues and organs has been completed. This disorder, *myxedema*, (Fig. 16.23), is characterized by a slowing of most metabolic processes and results in cold intolerance, lethargy, slowness of thought and speech, and alterations in probably every body function, as well as characteristic changes in physical appearance.

Fig. 16.20. Diagram summarizing the functional anatomy of a *thyroid follicular cell*. At the left of the nucleus are shown the routes for iodine accumulation and thyroglobulin synthesis. At the right is shown the removal of thyroglobulin from the follicular lumen, its degradation by lysosomal digestion and the delivery of T3 and T4 to the circulation through the fenestrated endothelium of thyroid capillaries.

Fig. 16.21. Scintiscan of *thyroid gland with "hot" nodule*. The radioactivity due to the uptake of ^{131}I is greatest in the nodule. Arrow indicates midline marker. (Courtesy of J. Haines.)

Fig. 16.22. Electron micrograph of a portion of thyroid *parafollicular* cell. The hormone is apparently released soon after synthesis since very few secretory granules (arrows) are seen. ×10,000. (Courtesy of R. Brooks.)

Fig. 16.23. Nearly complete *atrophy of thyroid*. The patient, age 44, had been markedly hypothyroid for most of her life. The only remaining thyroid tissue consists of a few small gland nests in loose connective tissue. ×100.

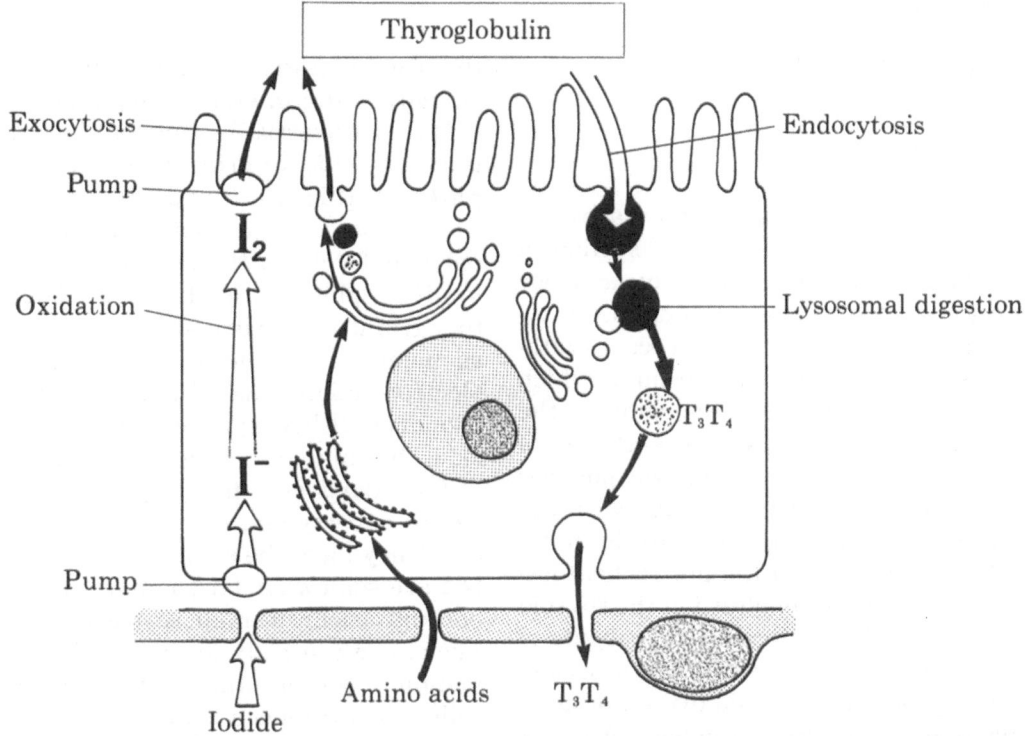

Thyroglobulin

Exocytosis

Pump

I₂

Oxidation

I⁻

Pump

Iodide

Amino acids

T₃T₄

Endocytosis

Lysosomal digestion

T₃T₄

16.20

16.21

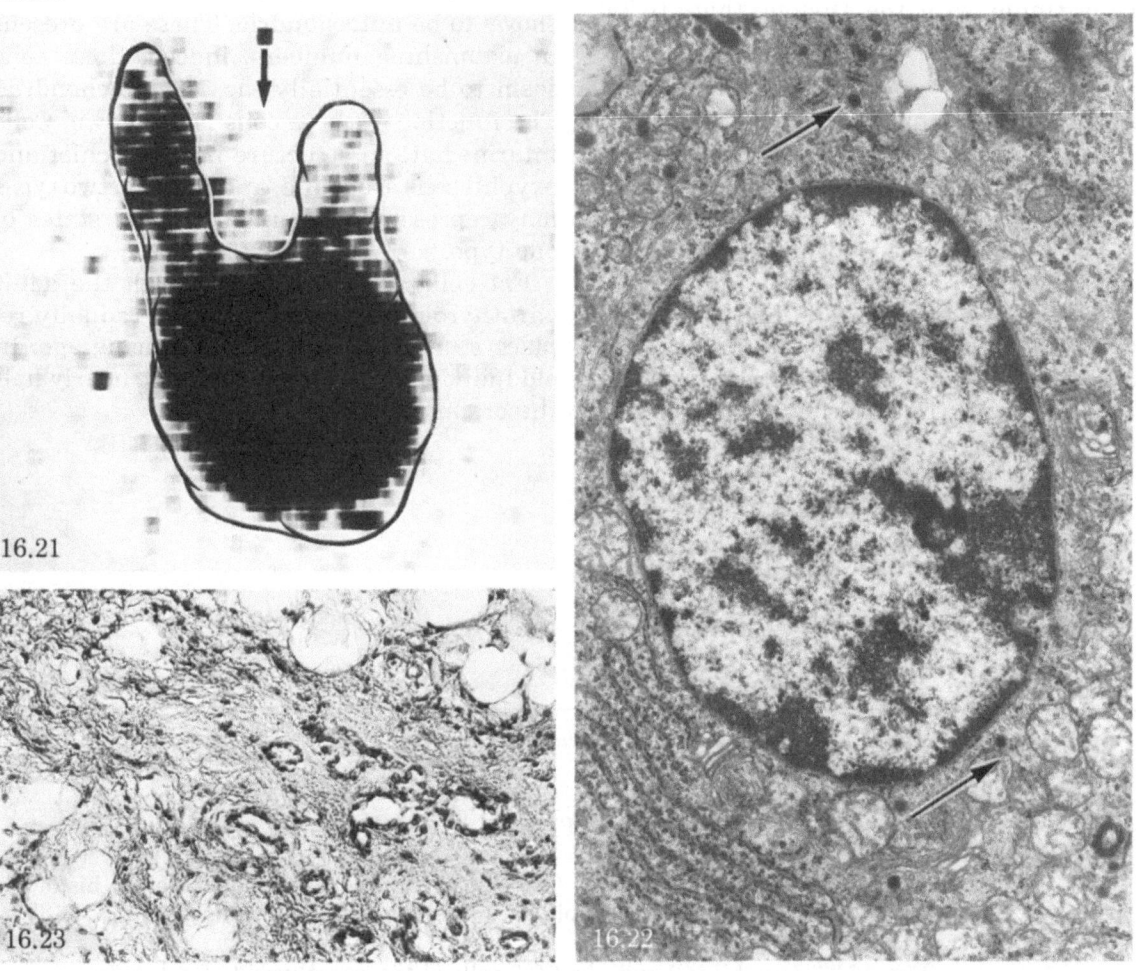

16.22

16.23

Parathyroid Gland

General Features

There are normally four tiny parathyroid glands, one bound to the posterior surface of each of the upper and lower poles of each lobe of the thyroid (Fig. 16.24). Although their total weight is less than 0.2 g, death occurs without adequate supply of their hormone, which maintains normal levels of calcium in the blood. One gland develops from each one of each pair of embryonic pharyngeal pouches III and IV, and becomes associated with the thyroid as the latter migrates into the neck. With the development of the pretracheal fascia, the glands become enclosed in the thyroid capsule, and each develops a thin capsule of its own. They may, however, fail to associate with the thyroid, and occasionally one or more may be found elsewhere in the neck or in the mediastinum with the thymus (Fig. 16.25), which is also a pharyngeal pouch derivative.

Histologic Organization (Fig. 16.26)

The parathyroids exhibit a typical endocrine histology; that is, the cells are arranged in clumps and cords with delicate connective tissue and many small blood vessels intervening.

STROMA. The thin capsule has inward extensions (trabeculae) that divide the parenchyma into irregular and incomplete lobules. The rich vascularization is by capillaries with the usual fenestrated endothelium characteristically found in endocrine glands.

THE PARENCHYMA is composed of two cell types, the *chief* or principal cells, and the *oxyphil* cells (Fig. 16.27 and 16.28).

The chief cells are small, lightly staining, polygonal cells with more or less centrally located, spherical, dark nuclei. Their secretory granules are very small and are apparent as membrane-bound vesicles only with the electron microscope. There are few mitochondria. RER, Golgi, free ribosomes, and considerable amounts of glycogen are present.

The oxyphil cells first appear about 2 years before puberty and increase in number with age. They have the same shape as chief cells, but are somewhat larger and fewer in number; they occur in small, scattered groups. The nuclei are centrally located and are smaller and more densely staining than those of chief cells. The cytoplasm is filled with fine eosinophilic granules which the electron microscope shows to be mitochondria. These are present in astonishing numbers; indeed, these cells seem to be essentially sacs of mitochondria. The function of these cells is unknown. Cells intermediate in structure between chief and oxyphil cells are found, and thus the two types may represent different functional states of one type.

Fat cells are scattered through the adult parathyroid gland and seem to gradually replace secretory cells with advancing age. In old individuals they may make up nearly half the organ.

Fig. 16.24. Posterior view of *pharynx* and thyroid gland to show the location of the *parathyroid glands*.

Fig. 16.25. *Parathyroid gland* (P) found in the *thymus* (T). ×35.

Fig. 16.26. *Parathyroid gland*. The photograph repeats the universal histologic pattern of endocrine glands; capillaries are plentiful and regularly spaced. ×35.

Fig. 16.27. *Oxyphil* (O) and *chief* (C) cells of the parathyroid gland. ×200.

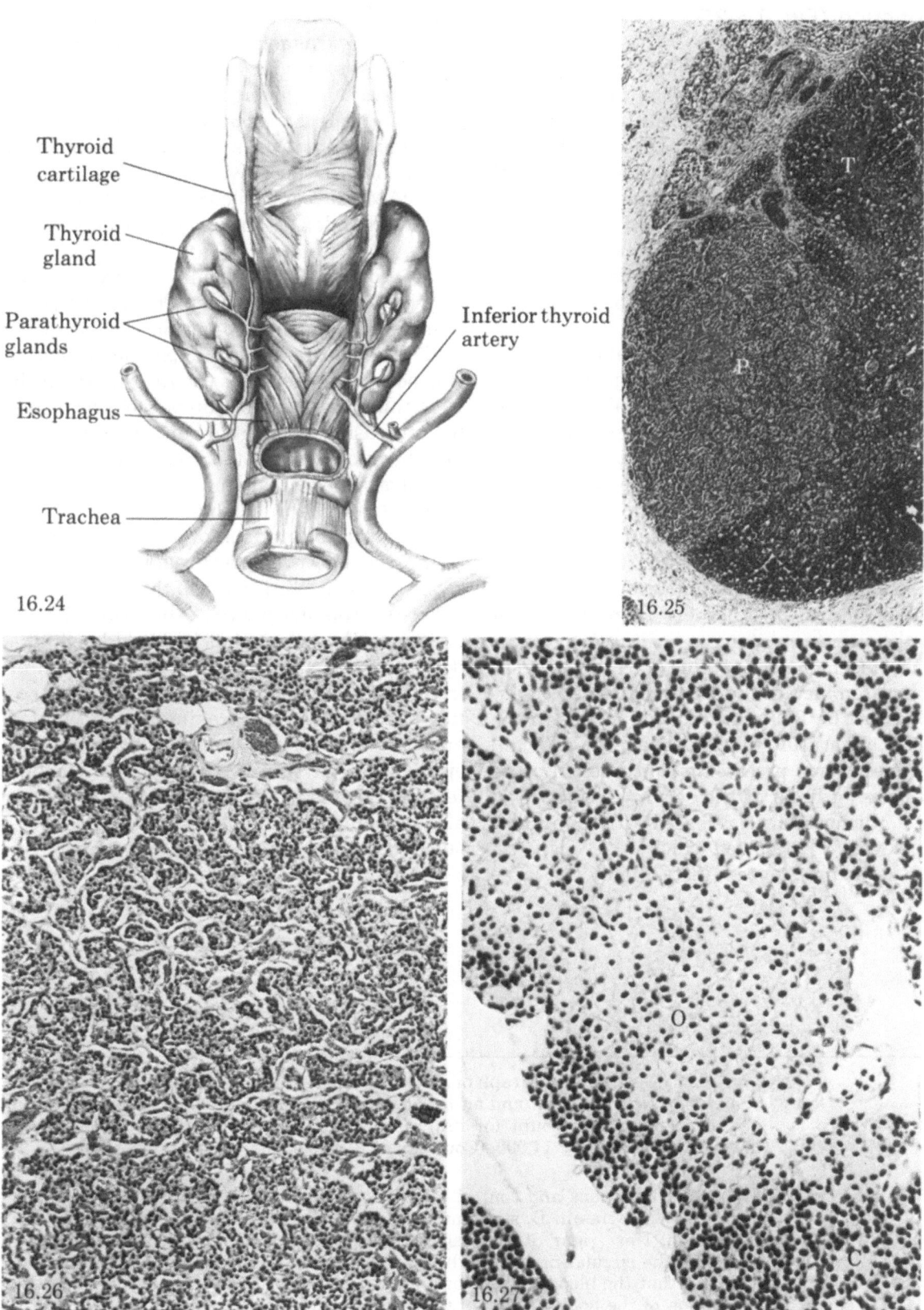

Thyroid
cartilage

Thyroid
gland

Parathyroid
glands

Esophagus

Trachea

Inferior thyroid
artery

16.24

16.25

16.26

16.27

Function (Fig. 16.29)

As indicated in the section on thyroid parafollicular cells, precise control of the level of calcium in the blood is essential to provide for the needs of many cells and tissues throughout the body. Calcium plays a vital role in membrane structure and permeability and in secretory mechanisms. It controls ionic gradients across plasmalemmas in the nervous and muscular systems where depolarization of cell membranes is basic to their function. Although many factors, such as renal function, dietary intake, vitamin D, and intestinal absorption are important for general long-term maintenance of blood calcium, some mechanism must be present to provide rapid fine tuning of these levels because the range of tolerance is so narrow. The parathyroid glands constitute the primary regulator of acute changes in blood calcium. The output of parathyroid hormone (PTH) is directly responsive to blood calcium levels, and is not under control of other endocrine glands or of the nervous system.

The hormone is a peptide of 84 amino acids. It is assembled in the form of a large prohormone in the RER and reduced in size in the Golgi apparatus, which packages it in small vesicles. Some processing continues to occur in these vesicles. If the serum calcium level falls, the hormone is released within minutes. However, when blood calcium is high, secretion is not stopped; instead only the large C-terminal fragment of the molecule is released. This fragment is biologically inert. A balance is maintained between the secretion of this inert fragment and the active entire molecule. The hormone acts by way of the receptor-adenyl cyclase-cAMP system. This system is so responsive in so many tissues that cAMP levels in blood and urine provide a clinical index of the biological activity of PTH.

The body pool of calcium is 1000–1200 g, of which 99% is in bone. The parathyroid glands (perhaps in cooperation with the thyroid C cells) are the principal managers of this pool. PTH increases the rate of osteolysis by stimulating the function of osteoclasts and by increasing their numbers (and perhaps also by increasing osteolysis by osteocytes). Osteolysis makes calcium available for general distribution in the blood.

Along with calcium, phosphate is also freed from bone. However, PTH reduces phosphate reabsorption in the kidney. If the level of PTH increases, the phosphate in the urine also increases to the extent that its blood level falls below normal. In addition to freeing calcium from bone, PTH also stimulates the reabsorption of calcium by the proximal renal tubules and the absorption of calcium by intestinal epithelium. Vitamin D is required for the latter function. The effects of PTH on bone are also partially dependent on vitamin D; without it PTH does not cause osteolysis.

Fig. 16.28. Electron micrograph of a section of parathyroid gland showing a portion of a *chief cell* at the right and an *oxyphil cell*. The large numbers of mitochondria in the oxyphil cell account for its granular acidophilia in sections viewed with the light microscope. ×14,000. (Courtesy of R. Brooks.)

Fig. 16.29. Functions and control of *parathyroid hormone* (PTH). At the left the hormone, with vitamin D, stimulates absorption of calcium from the gut into the circulation. Next right, it acts, again with vitamin D, to release calcium from bone into the circulating blood. The dashed arrow ascending to the gland (center) indicates that the blood concentration of calcium exerts negative feedback on the production of the hormone. The two arrows to the kidney indicate that PTH promotes reabsorption of calcium into the blood and loss of phosphate into the urine. In each case the dashed arrow represents calcium.

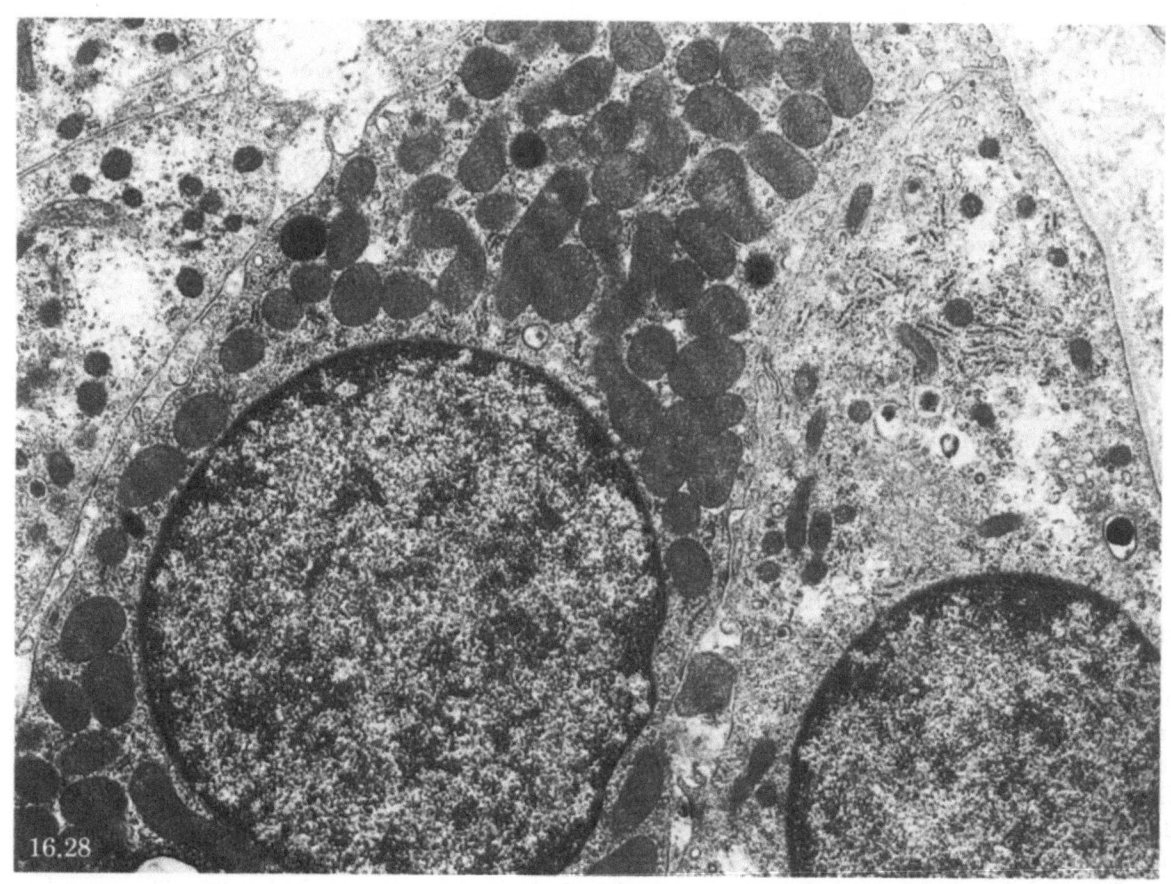

16.28

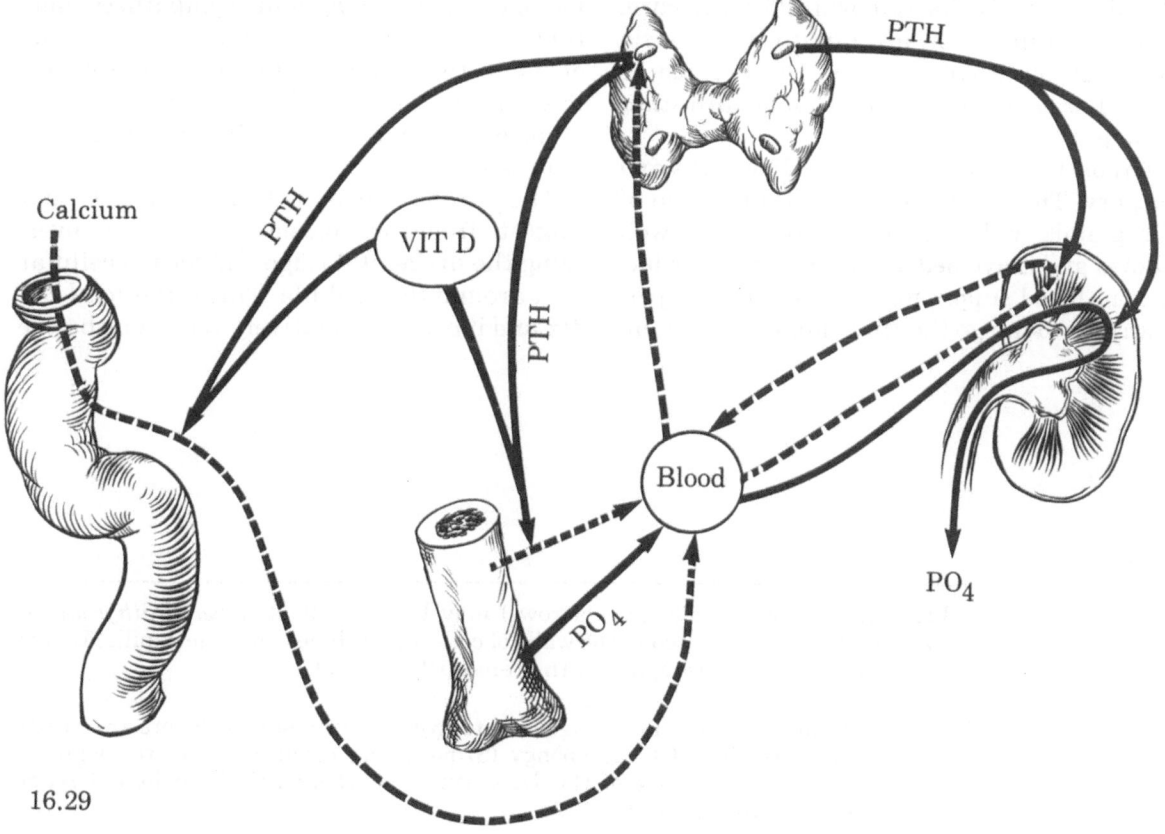

Calcium

VIT D

PTH

PTH

PTH

Blood

PO₄

PO₄

16.29

Functional Disorders

As with most endocrine glands, pathologic processes may produce either increased output of the hormone or its reduction to lower than normal levels.

IN HYPERPARATHYROIDISM greater than normal amounts of calcium are removed from bone, recovered by the kidney and absorbed from the gut. Thus the blood calcium level increases (hypercalcemia) and the phosphate level decreases (hypophosphatemia). The calcium equilibrium between blood and tissue is unbalanced and calcium, even while it is being removed from bone, may be deposited in a variety of abnormal locations such as arterial walls (Fig. 16.31) and kidneys (renal stones) (Fig. 16.30). Over a period of time continued decalcification of bone results in weakening of its structure to the extent that spontaneous fractures may occur, sometimes following even minimal normal movements. Decalcification is irregular and produces radiolucent patches in radiographs. In 85% of instances of hyperparathyroidism the cause is a functioning tumor (adenoma) of one of the four glands; its removal effects a cure. The remaining 15% are due to hyperplasia of all four parathyroid glands. However, there are other causes of hypercalcemia, all rather serious.

HYPOPARATHYROIDISM often follows thyroid surgery. The impact of accidental removal of the glands with thyroidectomy is now well known and is avoided, but scarring or a reduction in blood supply may temporarily or permanently damage the tiny glands. In such instances the blood level of calcium falls and phosphate increases. Bone density increases. Neuromuscular excitation threshold is reduced; tetany occurs, which, unless exogenous PTH is provided, progresses to generalized convulsions and death.

Adrenal (Suprarenal) Glands

General Features

The adrenal glands are paired, flattened organs, one capping the upper pole of each kidney. Their combined weight is about 8–12 g, but size and weight vary with age and with physiologic status of the individual. Each gland is an association of two morphologically and functionally discrete glands, the adrenal *cortex* and adrenal *medulla* (Fig. 16.32), which are enclosed in one capsule and share a common blood supply.

The two components have different embryonic origin (Fig. 16.33). The medulla is derived from a group of neural crest cells which migrate into the urogenital ridge. They are homologues of postganglionic sympathetic neurons but they do not develop axons. Instead of using their epinephrine as a neurotransmitter, they secrete it into the circulation in response to stimulation by their preganglionic neurons.

The adrenal cortex is formed by cells that migrate from the adjacent mesothelium overlying the urogenital ridge and form a cellular coat around the medulla. This is the *fetal cortex* and it becomes relatively very thick before

Fig. 16.30. Renal calcification (arrows) may be a result of *hyperparathyroidism.* Excess calcium is deposited in the walls of collecting tubules near the papilla. Larger stones may form and slough into the renal pelvis. ×200.

Fig. 16.31. Bony and arterial changes due to *hyperparathyroidism.* There are irregular fraying of cortical (C) and spongy (S) bone and calcification in the walls of arteries (arrows). (Courtesy of the Department of Diagnostic Radiology, Oregon Health Sciences University.)

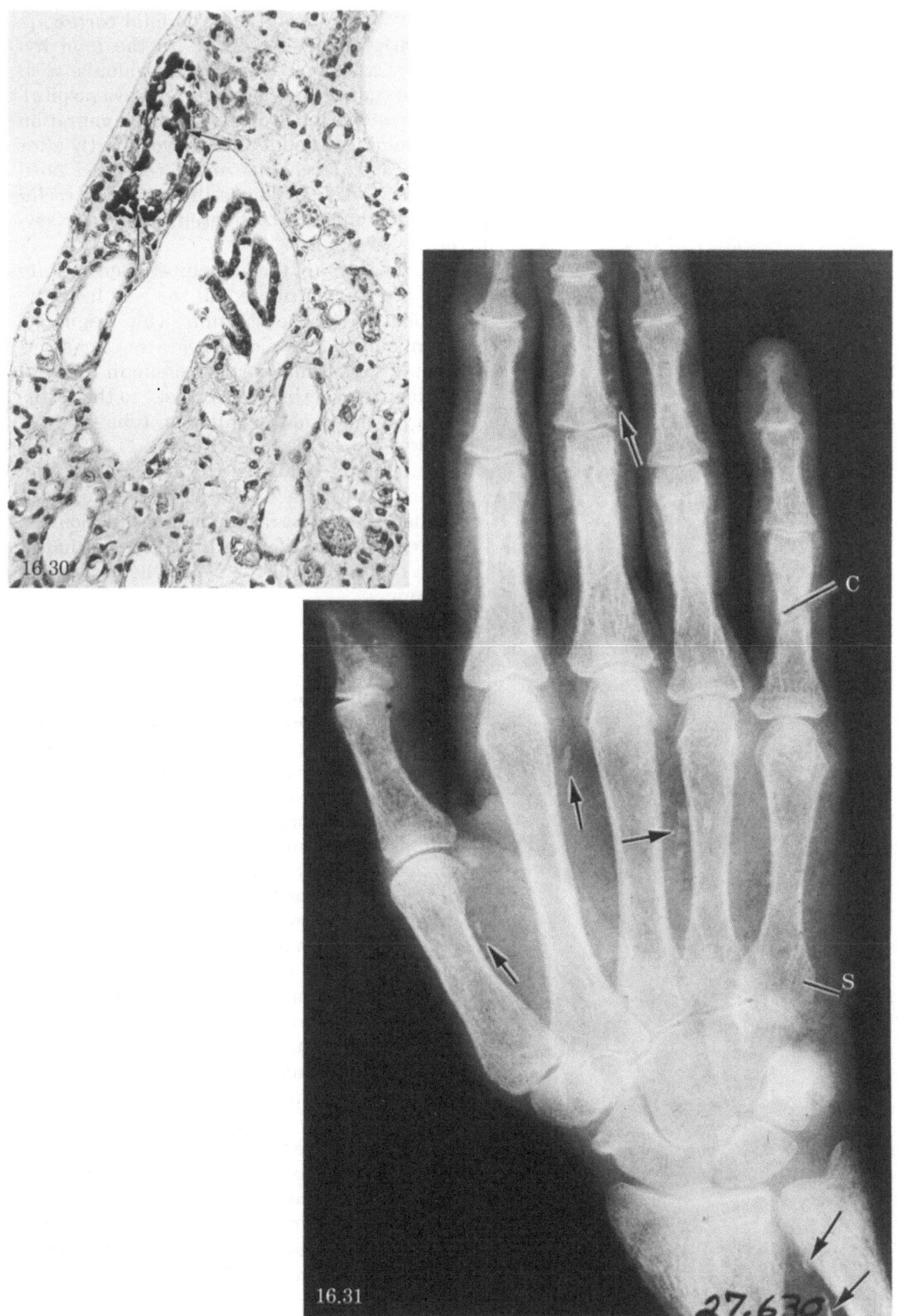

16.30

16.31   27.630

its postnatal involution. The fetal cortex apparently owes its presence to the fetal hypophysis. (Anencephalics, individuals with only a rudimentary or no brain, have no pituitaries and no fetal cortex). A second migration of celomic epithelial cells arrives shortly after the first but remains undifferentiated until late in fetal life. This is the *definitive cortex* and it completes its differentiation over several years.

Components of the urogenital ridge migrate and become distributed all the way from the diaphragm to the scrotum. This origin accounts for the occasional appearance of small nodules of adrenal cortical tissue in the wall of the ureter or bladder, or next to the testis, ovary, epididymis, or fallopian tube (see Fig. 16.34).

Functional failure of the cortex, or its destruction by disease, is fatal. The medulla, although it has several important functions, is not essential to life; its functions are shared with other units of the sympathetic nervous system.

Stroma

Each adrenal gland is embedded in the perirenal fat and is provided with a thin capsule of connective tissue. Very delicate, parallel sleeves of connective tissue, mostly reticular fibers, extend from the capsule through the cortex, surrounding and supporting the clumps and columns of cortical cells. At the corticomedullary junction they blend to form a fine fibrillar meshwork around the interwoven and anastomosing cords of medullary cells. Although a few scattered, thick, incomplete trabeculae extend inwards, there is no distinct lobulation. However, variations in the histologic regularity, or evenness, of the cortex are common, and large (up to 2 cm in diameter) and small nodules of cortical tissue may often be found in the adrenal gland itself and occasionally in any of the other tissues which are derived from the urogenital ridge (Fig. 16.34). This complicates surgical decisions about the need for their removal in the treatment of hyperadrenocorticism. Not every adenoma is functional; not every adenoma should be removed.

Blood Vessels (Fig. 16.35)

Arterial supply to the adrenal gland is usually through branches of three arteries: aorta, inferior phrenic artery, and renal artery. These provide numerous small vessels that ramify and anastomose over the surface of the gland. A plexus of arterioles from these lies in the capsule and feeds a rich network of parallel and interconnected capillaries in the cortex between the columns of cortical cells. These capillaries drain into vessels of the medulla. Additional vessels, the medullary arterioles, arise from the capsular arterioles and follow trabeculae through the cortex directly to the medullary capillaries. All of the capillaries in the adrenal gland are lined by fenestrated endothelium.

Each gland is drained by a single medullary vein that is peculiar in having an irregularly arranged and unusually thick coat of smooth muscle, presumably involved in controlling the volume of blood leaving the organ.

Adrenal Cortex

FETAL (PROVISIONAL) CORTEX (Fig. 16.36). The adrenal gland of the newborn is relatively larger than that of the adult as a result of the presence of the thick fetal cortex lying between the thin, undifferentiated, definitive cortex and the medulla. Its cells are arranged in cords similar to, but less distinct than, those of the adult or definitive cortex. The principal function of this zone apparently is the production of sulfated steroid precursors which are converted to estrogens in the syncytiotrophoblast of the placenta, which lacks the capacity to make these precursors. After birth, involution of the fetal cortex occurs during the first few postnatal months, and the definitive cortex gradually differentiates into its characteristic three layers.

ADULT (DEFINITIVE) CORTEX. The adrenal cortex is usually divided into three zones on the basis of both morphology and function (Fig. 16.37). In the ideal section one may see these three zones. More often the boundaries are indistinct; the nodules and/or adenomas mentioned before may distort or obliterate them,

and it is seldom clear as to which zone these belong.

Structure and function. The three zones are the (outer) zona glomerulosa, (intermediate) zona fasciculata and (inner) zona reticularis. The cells of all three zones are structurally somewhat similar (Fig. 16.38). They have acidophilic cytoplasm and spherical central nuclei. As in other steroid-producing cells, the mitochondria have tubular cristae and there is a large amount of SER. With the light microscope their cytoplasm appears vacuolated, an artifact since the vacuoles represent lipid droplets from which the contents have been dissolved in preparing the section. These droplets contain cholesterol esters for use in synthesizing the steroid hormones produced by the cortex.

The cortex is probably entirely under humoral control (Fig. 16.39). There are no nerve fibers here.

Zona glomerulosa. This thin, outer zone is composed of more or less columnar cells arranged in spherical or ovoid groups. They produce steroids that regulate the levels of sodium and potassium in the body and thus are known as the *mineralocorticoids.* Aldosterone is the most important and most potent of them. It acts on renal tubules (primarily the distal), salivary glands, sweat glands and gastric mucosa to promote the reabsorption of sodium and the equivalent loss of potassium. The zona glomerulosa is not under control of the hypothalamohypophyseal system. Its secretion of aldosterone is stimulated by angiotensin II. (At this point the student may wish to review the renin-angiotensin system in Chapter 15.) A decline in the level of potassium also stimulates aldosterone secretion.

Zona fasciculata. This, the largest zone of the cortex, is composed of parallel columns of cells separated by capillaries. Cytoplasmic vacuoles are particularly noticeable in this layer, sometimes giving the cells a foamy appearance. The cells are polyhedral and have spherical, central nuclei. SER is more abundant than in the other zones and considerable amounts of RER make the cytoplasm slightly basophilic under the light microscope. Cell surfaces facing the endothelium are provided with microvilli.

Fig. 16.32. *Adrenal gland.* Medulla (M) and cortex (C). ×4.

Fig. 16.33. *Embryonic origins of the adrenal gland.* **a:** Diagrammatic cross sections of portions of two embryos at different stages of development. Above, the *neural crest cells* are shown leaving the ectoderm and migrating into the mesenchyme; these become the medulla. The lower figure shows migration of *celomic epithelial cells* to meet, and form a cortex over, the medulla. **b:** Diagrams of four stages in the *further development of the adrenal gland* after assembly of neural crest and celomic epithelial cells. In the fetal stage the second wave of migrating cells is shown forming the definitive cortex.

Fig. 16.34. Locations of *ectopic adrenal tissue.*

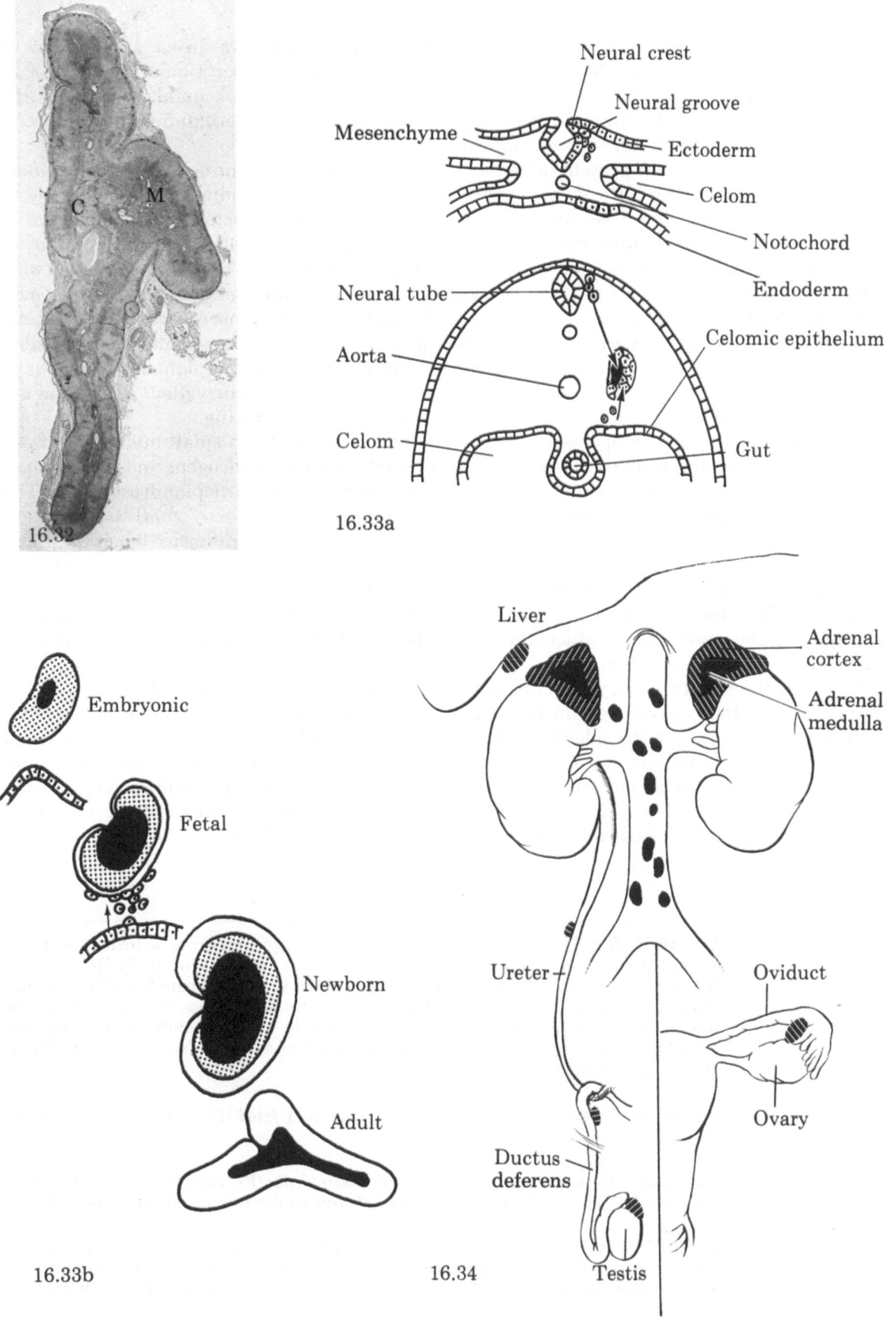

16.32

16.33a

Neural crest

Neural groove

Mesenchyme

Ectoderm

Celom

Notochord

Endoderm

Neural tube

Aorta

Celomic epithelium

Celom

Gut

16.33b

Embryonic

Fetal

Newborn

Adult

16.34

Liver

Adrenal cortex

Adrenal medulla

Ureter

Oviduct

Ovary

Ductus deferens

Testis

This zone produces a group of steroid hormones termed *glucocorticoids* because of their action in the production and mobilization of glucose. The principal steroid is cortisol. Glucocorticoids act on the liver, stimulating the formation of glucose from protein (gluconeogenesis), converting some of the glucose to glycogen (glycogenesis), and releasing the remainder into the blood. Raw materials for these processes are provided from other tissues, notably skin, muscle, lymphoid tissue, and adipose tissue, where cortisol suppresses synthetic activities and stimulates the breakdown of protein and lipids. The resulting amino acids and fatty acids are utilized in the liver for gluconeogenesis.

Cortisol also strongly suppresses the immune response by inhibiting mitosis in lymphoid tissue, accelerating lymphocyte destruction and sequestering eosinophils in the lungs and spleen. Because of this action, glucocorticoids are given to patients receiving organ transplants to help prevent graft rejection. They are also prescribed in treatment of innumerable conditions in which there is an excessive immune reaction.

The zona fasciculata is very responsive to ACTH, which binds to receptors in the plasmalemma and acts, via the adenyl cyclase-cAMP system, to stimulate steroid synthesis and release. Under continued excessive stimulation hypertrophy of the zone occurs. Cortisol provides negative feedback control of ACTH production by direct suppression of adenohypophyseal secretion of the corticotrophin. Whether cortisol can also suppress CRF secretion in the hypothalamus has not been clearly established.

Zona reticularis. The cells of this, the innermost cortical zone, adjacent to the medulla, are arranged in branching and anastomosing cords with a complementary, interwoven mesh of capillaries. The cells are smaller with more darkly staining cytoplasm; fewer vacuoles; and smaller, denser nuclei than the cells of the other zones. They contain considerable amounts of lipofuscin pigment. Some have pyknotic (dark and shrivelled) nuclei and appear to be degenerating.

This zone produces small quantities of sex steroids. Most are androgens and the predominant one is dehydroepiandrosterone. The amounts produced are so small that they are not of physiologic significance when the gland is functioning normally. This zone, although structurally different from the zona fasciculata, has some functional similarities. It probably produces some glucocorticoids in addition to the sex steroids; its production of both substances is stimulated by ACTH.

The principal overall function of the adrenal cortex (Fig. 16.39) is the maintenance of the chemical constitution of the intra- and extracellular fluids in equilibria appropriate for the metabolic activities of the cells that depend on these fluids. The hypothalamic-pi-

Fig. 16.35. *Blood supply of the adrenal.* **a:** Although numerous arteries enter the gland through the capsule, there is but a single vein draining it. **b:** Branches of the *adrenal arteries* ramify over the surface of the gland and penetrate the capsule. Blood is fed into the sinusoids of the cortex and from these to the sinusoids of the medulla. Alternately, blood may pass directly to the medullary sinusoids via medullary arterioles (arrows). The adrenal vein has several large longitudinal bundles of smooth muscle.

Fig. 16.36. *Adrenal cortex* with *definitive* (D) and *fetal* (F) zones in the newborn. ×35.

Fig. 16.37. *Zona glomerulosa* (G), *zona fasciculata* (F), *zona reticularis* (R), and *medulla* (M). The cortical zones are not always as distinct as shown here. ×35.

Fig. 16.38. Portions of two *adrenal cortical cells*. Although cells of the three zones differ in detail, they all contain the abundant SER (arrows) and mitochondria (M) with tubular cristae which characterize steroid-producing cells. ×13,000. (Courtesy of J. Thliveris.)

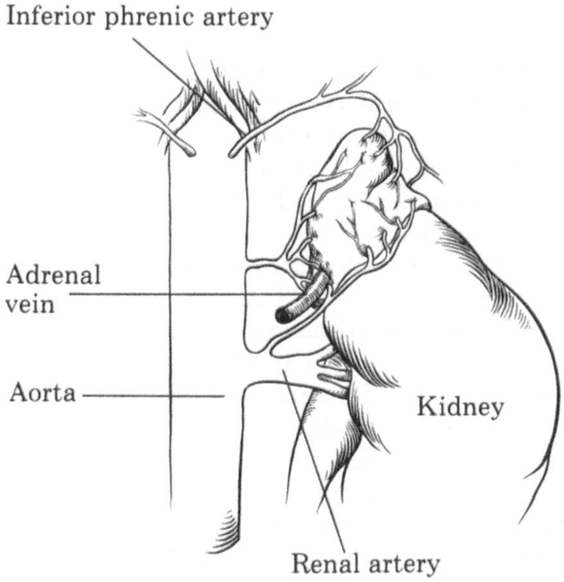

Inferior phrenic artery

Adrenal vein

Aorta

Kidney

Renal artery

16.35a

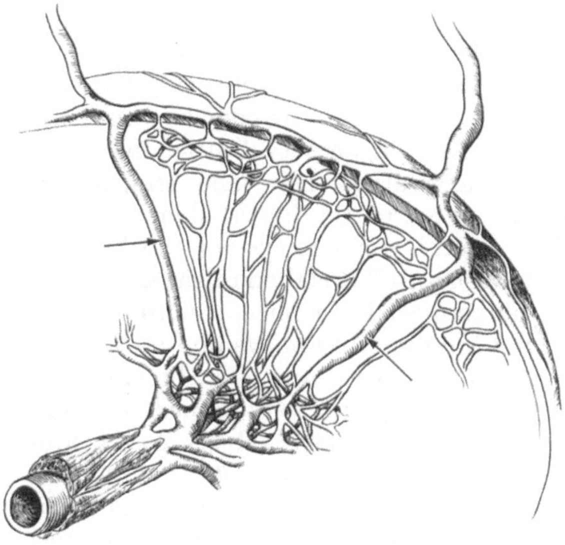

16.35b

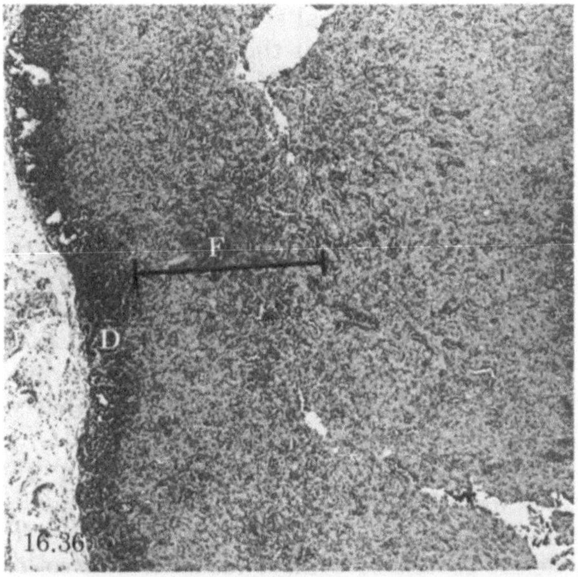

F

D

16.36

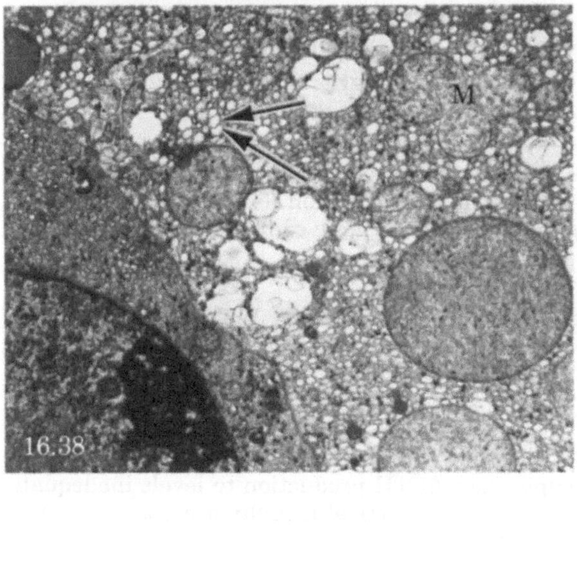

M

16.38

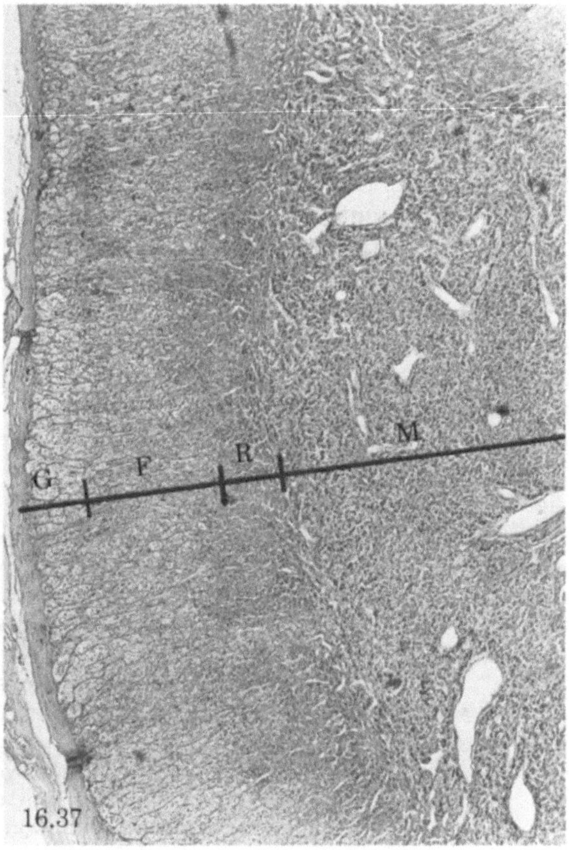

G   F   R   M

16.37

tuitary-adrenal axis (HPA) responds rapidly to adjust these equilibria to altered needs. Many external factors affect this system, and the needs imposed on the body by stress take precedence. Pain, anxiety, fasting, infections, hemorrhage, drugs, fear, and temperature change all act on the hypothalamus by way of the central nervous system and humoral mechanisms. ACTH is then released to stimulate adrenal cortical response. Acting via the mechanism described above and others, vascular, renal, hepatic, and other functions are modified and adjusted to fit immediate needs. The body is continuously subject to such stimuli at various levels of intensity, and the HPA acts continuously with other systems, in an integrated manner, to maintain an appropriate internal environment.

Functional disorders. Hypofunctional disorders. Primary adrenal cortical insufficiency (Addison's disease) may result from destruction of the cortex by disease, such as tuberculosis, metastatic tumor, or autoimmune process, or from surgical removal of the glands. In the absence of cortisol ACTH levels are high. Pigmentation increases in the skin, probably because of increased production of MSH parallel to the increase in ACTH (MSH may be a fragment of the ACTH precursor; see section on Pituitary Gland). Lymphocytes and eosinophils leave tissues and accumulate in the blood. Sodium is lost and potassium is retained. Hypotension results from the absence of aldosterone (see Chapter 15). Treatment with gluco- and mineralocorticoids reverses these changes.

Secondary adrenal cortical insufficiency (Fig. 16.40) is the result of reduced ACTH production from hypothalamic or hypophyseal disorders. Glucocorticoid production is absent, but mineralocorticoids are still present, since the zona glomerulosa is independent of pituitary control. In the USA the commonest cause of cortical atrophy is the therapeutic use of cortisol.

Hyperfunctional disorders. These may be primary or secondary. The former are due to high levels of corticosteroids from adenomas or hyperplasias of one or all zones of the cortex (Fig. 16.41). Secondary hyperfunction results from overproduction of ACTH due to, for example, a functioning pituitary tumor. (An adenoma may or may not produce excessive amounts of hormones.)

Excessive amounts of any or all of the adrenal steroids may be secreted, producing a complex array of possible physiologic effects and corresponding clinical syndromes.

Hypercortisolism, if the result of overproduction of CRF or ACTH, accompanies cortical hypertrophy of both adrenal glands. If it is the result of a functioning cortical adenoma in one gland, the increased cortisol level suppresses ACTH production and the contralateral adrenal is atrophic. (Figs. 16.40 and 16.41). In both instances protein wasting, due to the catabolic effect of glucocorticoids on proteins, occurs with thinning of the skin, muscle weakness, and poor wound healing. Because of the high rate of gluconeogenesis, diabetes mellitus may become apparent.

In a disorder termed *congenital adrenal cortical hyperplasia* (Fig. 16.42), an enzyme deficiency occurs that results in inability to synthesize cortisol. Negative feedback control is reduced and the resulting increase of ACTH produces marked enlargement of the adrenal cortices up to eight times normal weight at

---

Fig. 16.39. *Adrenal gland functions.* Note the hypothalamo-pituitary-adrenal axis, which is responsible for cortisol and androgen production. Note also renal control of the zona glomerulosa and preganglionic sympathetic control of the adrenal medulla.

Fig. 16.40. *Adrenal cortical atrophy* due to cortisol therapy. Withdrawal of cortisol treatment after establishment of such atrophy causes a crisis because the gland cannot resume normal function. Compare with Fig. 16.32. ×4.

Fig. 16.41. *Effects of feedback.* Above are shown *ACTH and cortisol production* in normal equilibrium. Below, a functioning tumor in one adrenal cortex produces large amounts of cortisol, which suppresses ACTH production to levels inadequate for maintenance of normal adrenal structure. Cortical atrophy occurs.

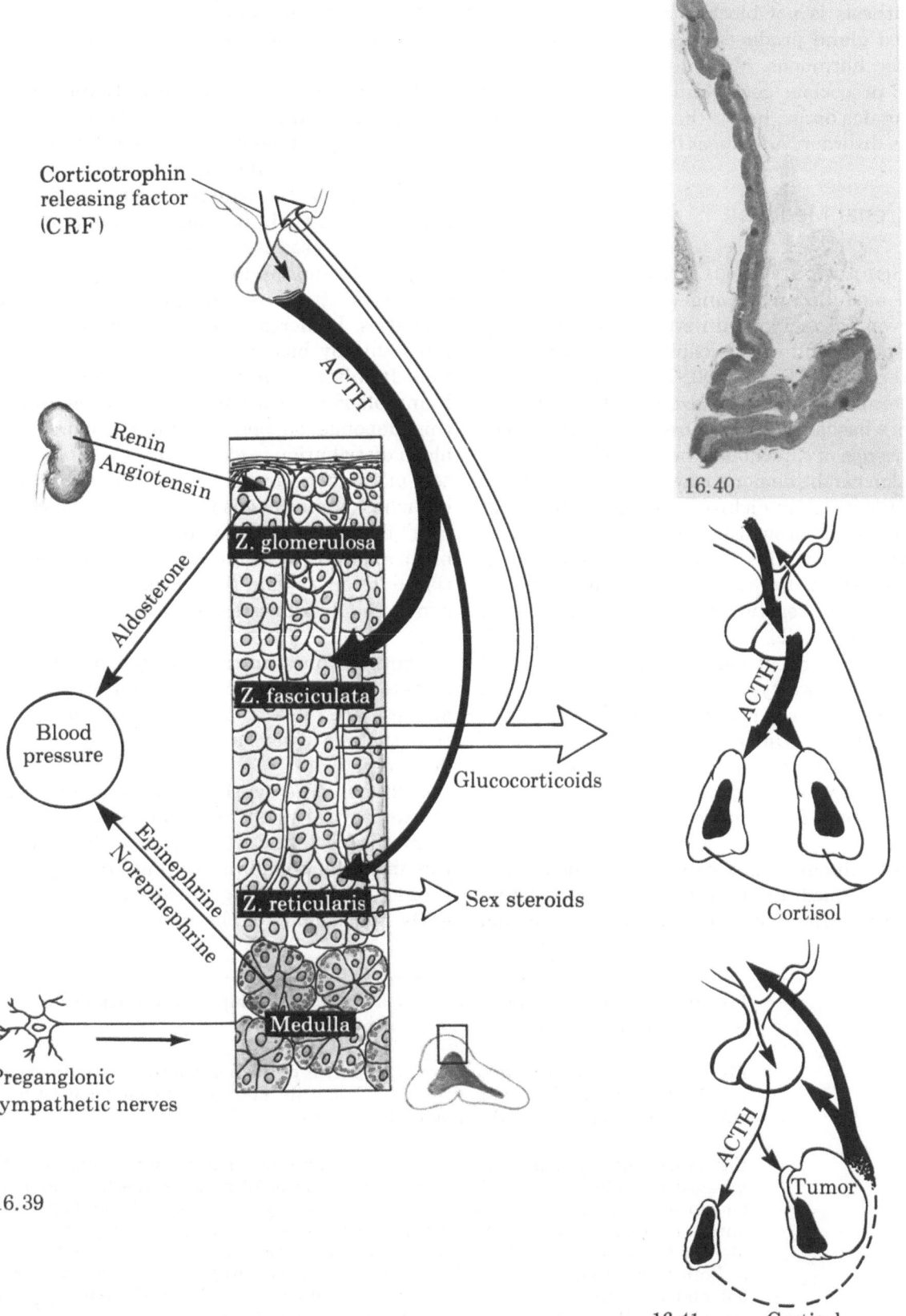

Corticotrophin
releasing factor
(CRF)

ACTH

Renin
Angiotensin

Z. glomerulosa

Aldosterone

Blood
pressure

Z. fasciculata

Glucocorticoids

Epinephrine
Norepinephrine

Z. reticularis

Sex steroids

Medulla

Preganglonic
sympathetic nerves

16.39

16.40

ACTH

Cortisol

ACTH

Tumor

16.41   Cortisol

birth. Usually in these instances, androgen synthesis is not blocked and the overstimulated gland produces excessive quantities of these hormones. Masculinization of females and precocious genital and hair development in males occur; hence the alternate name for this disorder, *adrenogenital syndrome*.

Adrenal Medulla

HISTOLOGIC STRUCTURE. The cells of the adrenal medulla are arranged in tortuous, interwoven cords with thin strands of connective tissue and numerous capillaries and venules intervening (Fig. 16.43). The cells show considerable variation in size and shape and are more basophilic than those of the cortex. The presence of catecholamines stored in the cytoplasm can be demonstrated by oxidizing them with potassium dichromate, a procedure that produces a brownish yellow, granular reaction product. This is known as the chromaffin reaction. Catecholamine-storing cells, in which this reaction takes place, are called chromaffin cells. With additional histochemical procedures it can be demonstrated that there are two types of chromaffin cells, one producing norepinephrine and one producing epinephrine. Differences in the granules of the two cell types are visible with the electron microscope. About 80% of the chromaffin cell population is of the epinephrine-producing type.

Not all chromaffin cells are confined to the adrenal medulla. Groups of them are found in association with some of the thoracic and abdominal sympathetic ganglia. These are called *paraganglia* and, together with the adrenal medulla, they constitute the *chromaffin system*.

HORMONES AND THEIR FUNCTIONS. Epinephrine is synthesized from tyrosine via DOPA, dopamine, and norepinephrine. About 20% of the cells in the medulla carry the reaction sequence only as far as norepinephrine and release this as their product. Norepinephrine is a potent vasoconstrictor.

Epinephrine, the major product, has widespread effects on physiologic and metabolic activities. It increases respiration and facilitates this by bringing about bronchial dilation. It raises cardiac output and heart rate. Many blood vessels constrict but some dilate; this depends on specific innervation. Thus blood distribution is altered; for example, vessels of the skin are constricted and the skin blanches, while vessels to skeletal muscles dilate. Epinephrine activates enzymes which bring about the breakdown of lipids in adipose tissue (lipolysis) and the breakdown of glycogen in the liver to release glucose (glycogenolysis).

The hormones are synthesized and stored in the cytoplasmic granules and only some of these are released during normal activity; thus there is always a reserve supply for sudden needs.

CONTROL. The synthesis of epinephrine is at least partially dependent on glucocorticoids from the cortex. Cortisol passes directly to the medullary capillaries (Fig. 16.43) from those of the cortex (Fig. 16.35B) and is apparently responsible for the induction of the en-

---

Fig. 16.42. *Congenital adrenal cortical hyperplasia.* Compare the thickness of the cortex with that shown in Figs. 16.32 and 16.40. ×4.

Fig. 16.43. *Adrenal medulla* (upper three-fourths of the field) here apparently composed completely of chromaffin cells. Ganglion cells, known as a component of medulla, are not apparent in this photograph. ×110.

Fig. 16.44. *Pheochromocytoma,* a functioning tumor of the adrenal medulla. A middle-aged man died in 1952, 2 years after the onset of severe hypertension. The diagnosis of pheochromocytoma was considered because of the severity and episodic nature of the hypertension, but it was never established during the patient's life. Modern techniques now permit this diagnosis to be made more easily and certainly. **a:** Both adrenal glands bivalved, in cross section, at autopsy. The medulla of the left gland is enlarged by the tumor. **b:** The tumor cells (above) simulate normal medullary cells. Note compression of the cortex (C). ×110.

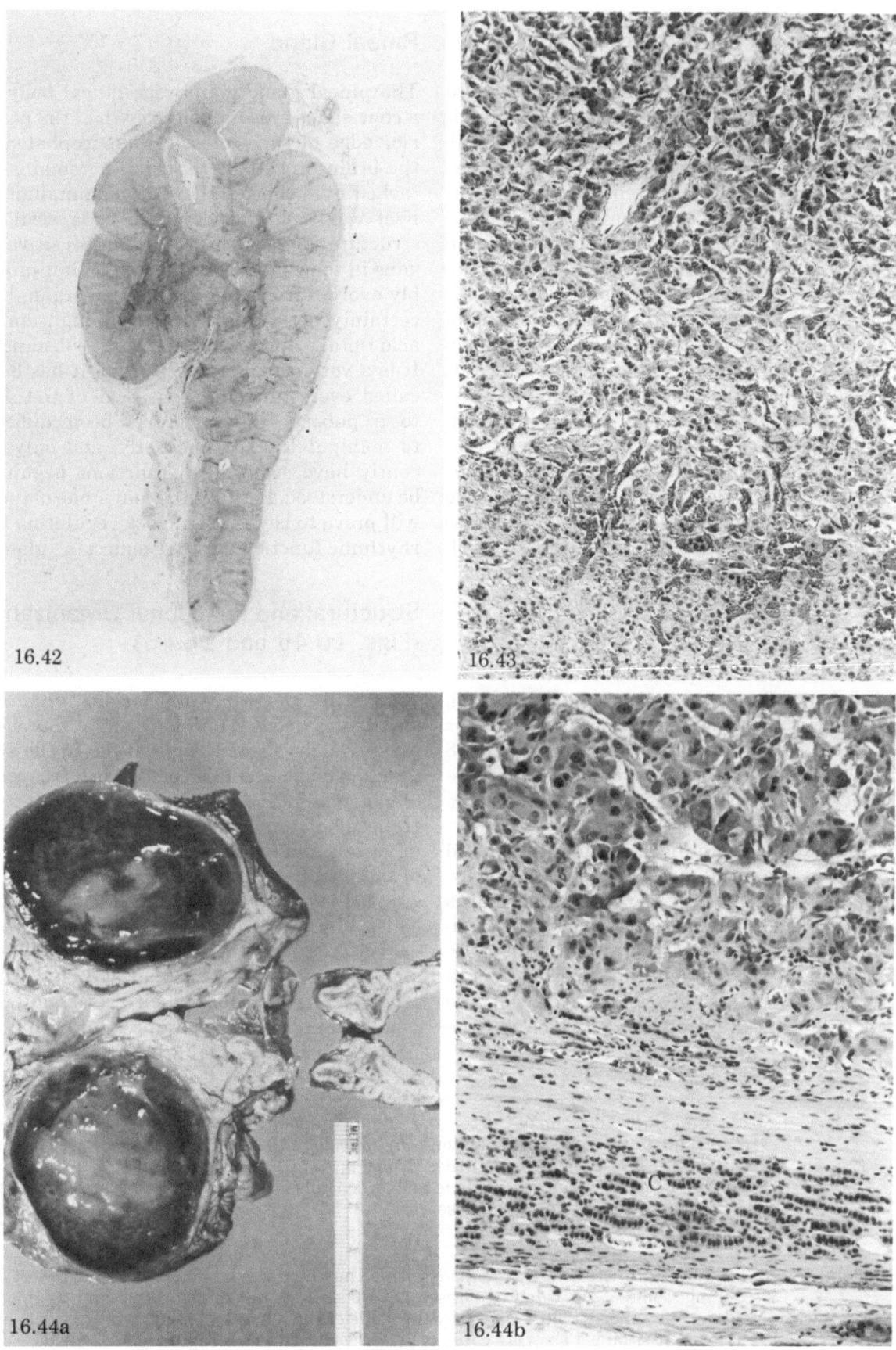

16.42

16.43

16.44a

16.44b

zyme which converts norepinephrine to epinephrine in the last step of its synthesis.

Release of medullary hormones is brought about by acetylcholine from the preganglionic sympathetic neurons which end on the medullary cells. The physiologic effects described above occur rapidly in response to increased blood levels of the hormones.

Although the ordinary small oscillations in medullary function are subliminal, when unusual physical or emotional stress occurs, the physiologic impact of the sudden release of either epinephrine or norepinephrine is obvious to the individual. The changes one feels in heart and breathing rates, blood pressure, and skin temperature, together with the unnoticeable metabolic and other changes, constitute the "fight or flight" response, preparing the body to deal with an emergency. The release of epinephrine and norepinephrine is mediated by preganglionic fibers that reach the chromaffin cells. Hence these effects demonstrate that the autonomic nervous system is intimately related to the CNS and not entirely autonomic.

DISORDERS. The adrenal medulla is the usual site of an important tumor of childhood, the neuroblastoma. Sometimes this tumor presents at birth but it rarely occurs after 8 or 10 years of age. Occasionally it may be functional and secrete either norepinephrine or epinephrine, or both.

In adults a more highly differentiated and usually benign tumor, the pheochromocytoma (Fig. 16.44), may secrete both hormones or sometimes only norepinephrine. The clinical signs related to high blood levels of these substances are as would be expected from a knowledge of their physiologic effects. These include arterial hypertension, which may be paroxysmal, and its sequelae.

Pineal Gland

The pineal gland (epiphysis; pineal body) is a cone-shaped median outgrowth of the posterior edge of the roof of the diencephalon of the brain (Fig. 16.3), to which it remains attached by a short stalk. The mammalian pineal was long considered to be a vestigial structure related to median, light-sensitive organs in some other animals. Though it probably evolved from a light-sensitive organ, it is certainly not vestigial. It has a high amino acid uptake and produces several substances. It is a very active organ. In man it has been called everything from the seat of the soul to a puberty timer. It has been difficult to manipulate experimentally, and only recently have some of its functions begun to be understood. Perhaps the major one of these will prove to be that of a clock regulating the rhythmic function of other endocrine glands.

Structural and Functional Organization (Figs. 16.45 and 16.46)

This still somewhat mysterious organ is small; it is about 7 mm long and 4 mm wide and it weighs about 120 mg. It lies in the subarachnoid space and is coated with a capsule of pia mater. It is irregularly lobulated by trabeculae from the capsule. A rich supply of vessels and nerves enter the organ by way of these trabeculae. There are two organ-specific cell types, pinealocytes and interstitial cells.

PINEALOCYTES (Figs. 16.5 and 16.46b) have slightly basophilic cytoplasm and characteristically large nuclei, which are irregularly lobulated and folded. Not apparent with ordinary stains are the long branched cytoplas-

Fig. 16.45. Diagram of the cellular *organization of the pineal gland.* Neural stimuli result in the release of melatonin by pinealocytes into the perivascular space and thence into the capillaries. (Based on Fig. 3 in Kappers J, Smith A and DeVries R. The mammalian pineal gland and its control of hypothalamic activity. In Kappers J. (ed): Progress in Brain Research, Vol. 52. Amsterdam, Elsevier North-Holland Biomedical Press, 1979.)

Fig. 16.46. a: *Partially calcified pineal.* The tissue was not decalcified before sectioning; some of the calcified masses have been torn out of the tissue and fragments have been distributed over it by the blade of the microtome. ×11.5. b: High magnification of pineal showing cords of *pinealocytes* and rich capillary bed. ×250.

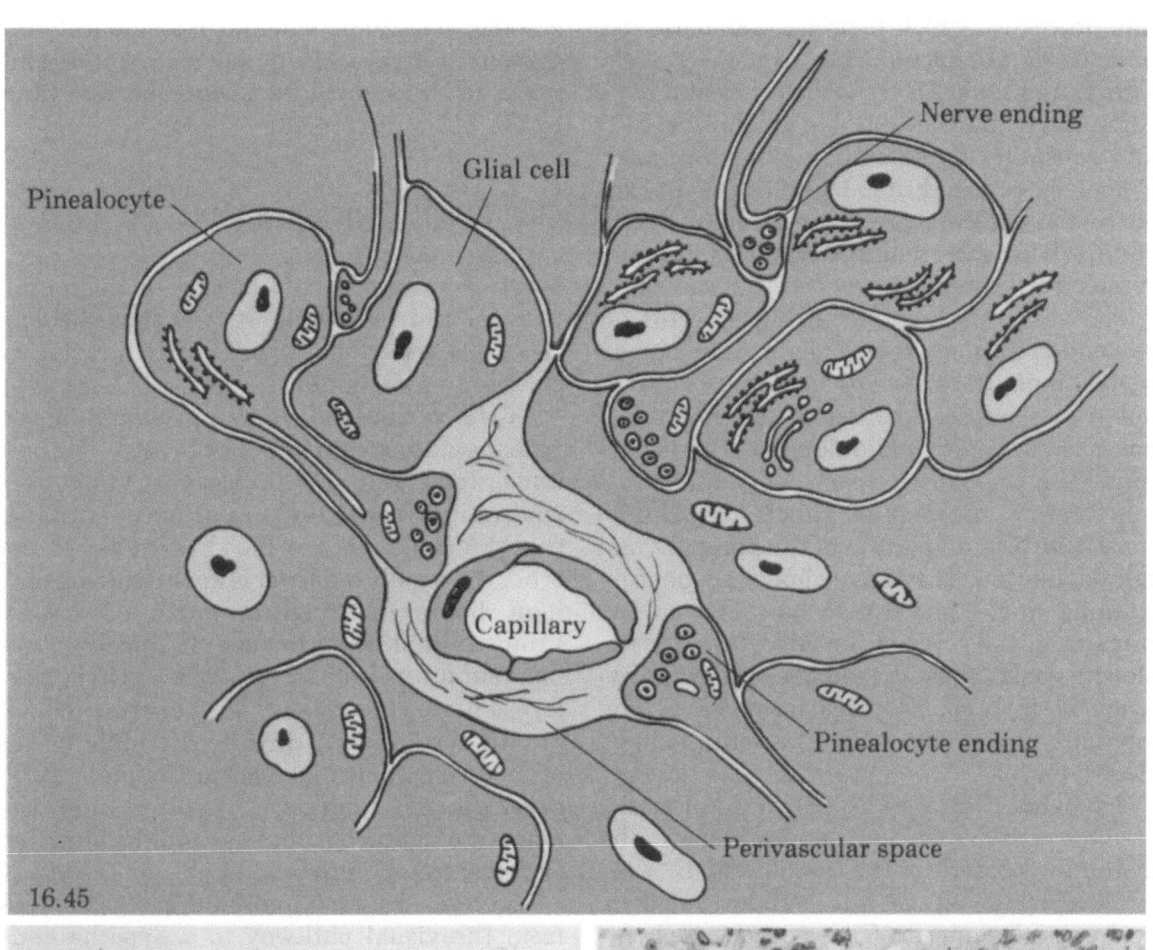

Pinealocyte

Glial cell

Nerve ending

Capillary

Pinealocyte ending

Perivascular space

16.45

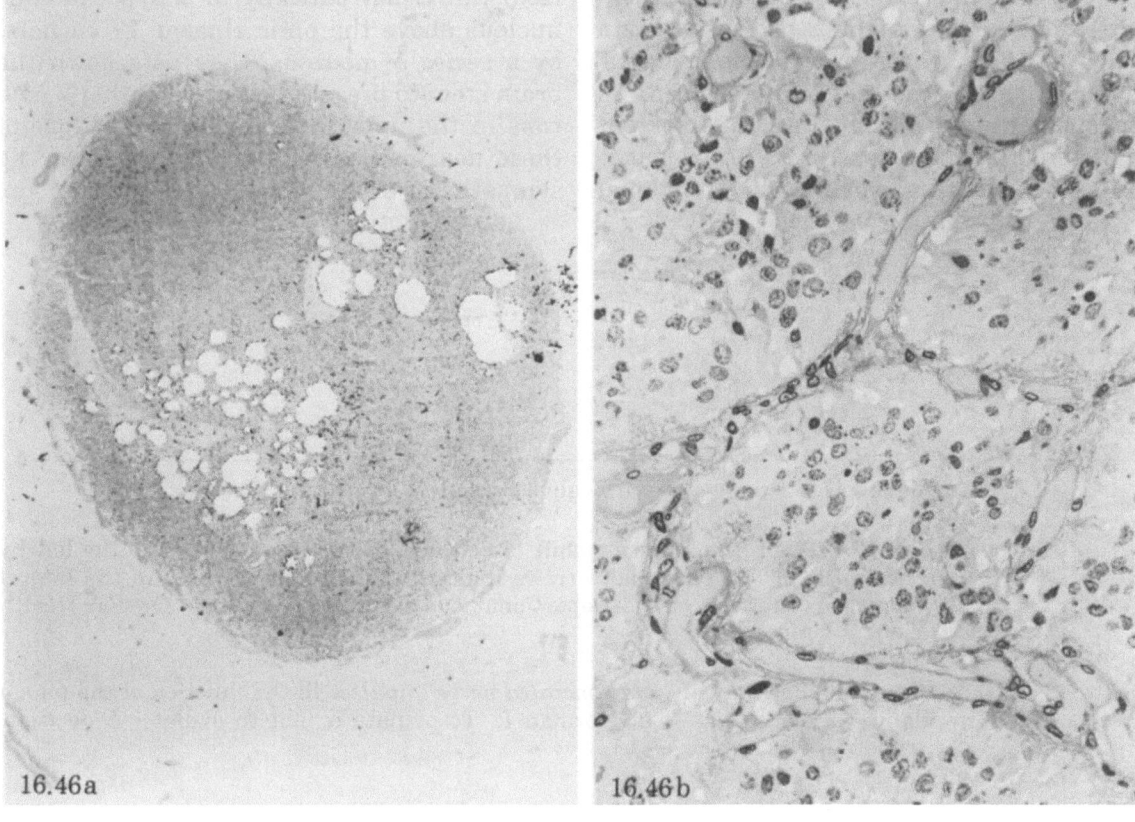

16.46a

16.46b

mic processes, which terminate as flattened, bulbous enlargements close to blood vessels. There are numerous free ribosomes and little RER. There are considerable amounts of SER and unusually large numbers of microtubules. Pinealocytes constitute about 95% of the parenchymal cells, and are arranged in cords and clumps with intervening capillaries and pial connective tissue.

The numerous nerve fibers entering the organ end in intimate relationship to the pinealocytes, many forming contacts, but probably not true synapses with these cells. Many, if not most, are postganglionic sympathetic neurons from the superior cervical ganglion.

INTERSTITIAL CELLS (Figs. 16.45 and 16.46b) constitute a small portion of the parenchymal cell population. They have elongated, densely staining nuclei and are to be found on the surfaces of the cords of pinealocytes near the blood vessels. They have long cytoplasmic extensions with considerable numbers of fine microfilaments. They may represent modified astrocytes.

True glial cells are also present. Mast cells are frequently seen and, appropriately, the histamine content of the gland is high.

With increasing age, intercellular, calcified, oval granules appear. These are termed corpora arenacea, psammoma bodies or brain sand (Fig. 16.47). These are variable in diameter and tend to occur in groups, not only in and about the pineal, but to a lesser extent in the subarachnoid space and brain generally. Nothing is known of their functional

significance. Since calcium is comparatively opaque to X-rays, the gland is a helpful landmark to the radiologist in interpreting films of the head (Fig. 16.48).

Functional Considerations

Much concerning the function of this organ remains to be worked out, and thus the concepts presented here will almost certainly change to some extent.

Of the various substances produced by the pineal gland, *melatonin* is at present the best understood. It is an indole that undergoes rhythmic, diurnal fluctuation in quantity in the gland and in the blood of humans and other mammals. Its level is lowest during daylight hours and highest during darkness. From animal experiments, it appears that light suppresses the activity of a methyl transferase that is the rate-limiting enzyme in melatonin synthesis. Although rhythmic cycles of secretion continue even in complete darkness, diurnal light-dark rhythms alter the amount of material released and the duration of the secretory process.

Light-generated impulses (Fig. 16.49) pass from the visual pathway to a hypothalamic nucleus above the optic chiasm. From here, by a series of neurons, they pass down the brain stem to preganglionic sympathetic neurons in the upper spinal cord. The axons of these neurons leave the cord and enter the sympathetic trunk, in which they pass up-

Fig. 16.47. *Pineal gland* with calcific granules (brain sand) (arrows). ×35.

Fig. 16.48. CAT scan showing shift of calcified *pineal* (large arrow) to the left by a brain tumor (T). The small arrows indicate the choroid plexuses in the lateral ventricles. (Courtesy of the Department of Diagnostic Radiology, Oregon Health Sciences University.)

Fig. 16.49. Pathway of *light-generated nerve impulses* in the function of the pineal gland. (Based on Fig. 3 in Norman R. To ovulate or not to ovulate. A decision. Primate News 19:2–7, 1981.)

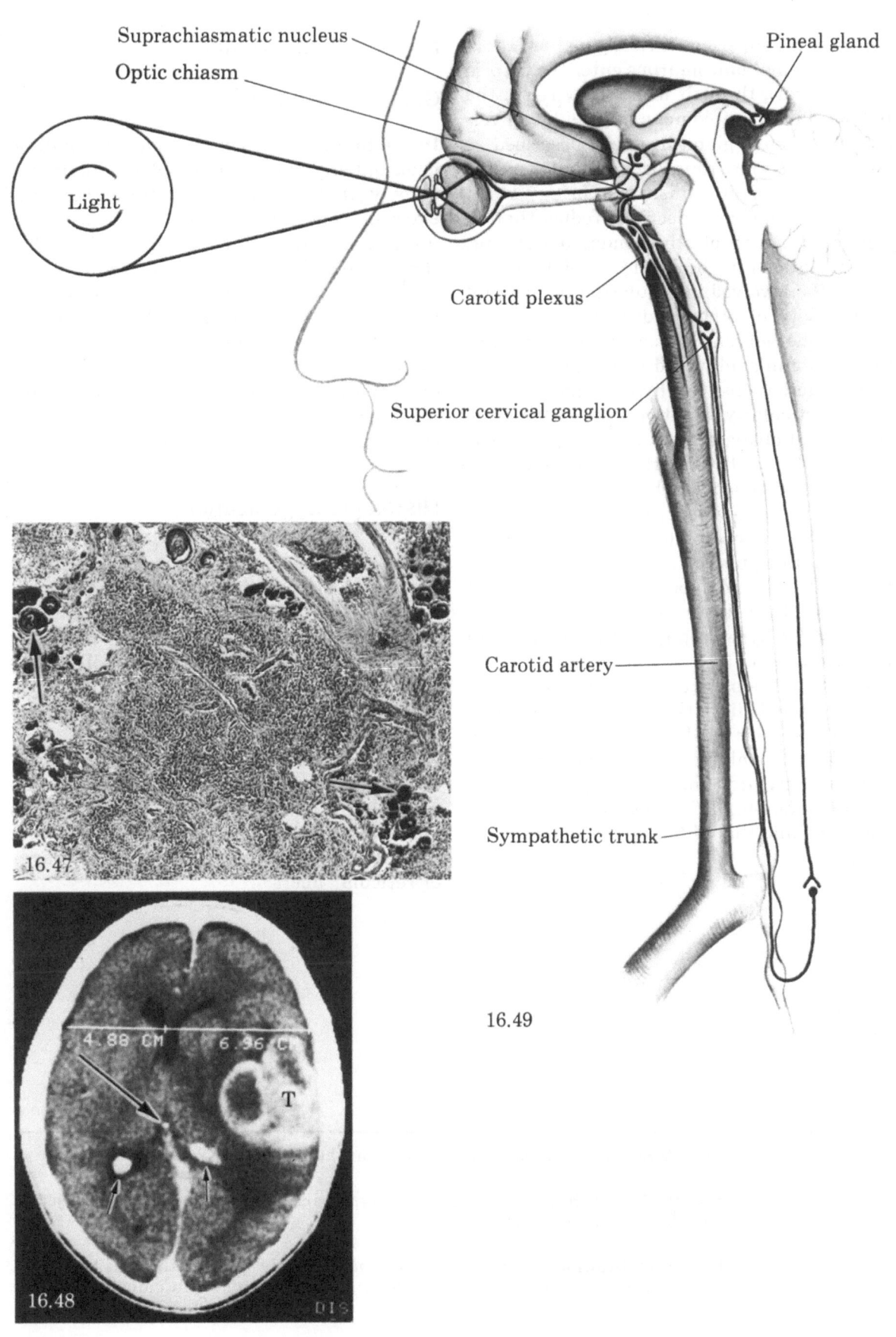

Suprachiasmatic nucleus

Optic chiasm

Pineal gland

Light

Carotid plexus

Superior cervical ganglion

Carotid artery

Sympathetic trunk

16.47

16.48

T

4.88 CM   6.96 CM

DIS

16.49

wards to the superior cervical ganglion. From here postganglionic neurons enter the carotid nerve plexus, through which they reach the pineal gland by accompanying its blood vessels. The pineal gland has been described as a neuroendocrine transducer, in that synaptic release of a neurotransmitter brings about the secretion of an endocrine product that alters the function of other endocrine organs.

Fluctuations in the level of melatonin appear to be involved in regulating the diurnal rhythmicity of other endocrine glands. Although the nervous system in general takes up melatonin avidly, and is therefore subject to its fluctuations, the hypothalamus seems to be particularly sensitive to the substance. By diurnal changes produced here, it apparently rhythmically suppresses the release of hypophyseal gonadotrophins.

There is some evidence that in children the pineal may suppress the development of the gonads before puberty, again probably via the hypothalamus and hypophysis. Destruction of the pineal by a tumor in childhood has been followed by hypertrophy of the gonads and precocious puberty.

Again on the basis of animal studies, some investigators believe that the gland produces a peptide similar to ADH that has very strong antigonadotrophic effects, but this peptide is effective only in young individuals.

Understanding of pineal function has lagged behind that of the other endocrine organs.

Islets of Langerhans

General Features

In the human pancreas there are 1–2 million islets of Langerhans, small, spheroidal masses of polygonal cells scattered throughout the exocrine pancreas (Fig. 16.50). They are most numerous in the tail of this organ. Together they weigh about 1 g and constitute about 1.5% of the pancreas. In aggregate they make up the *endocrine pancreas*. They have long been thought to develop from the same embryonic diverticula of the foregut that produce the exocrine pancreas. However, some investigators believe they arise from neural crest rather than from endoderm.

Histologic Organization

As in other endocrine organs, the parenchymal cells are arranged in anastomosing cords with a delicate investment of reticular fibers. There are intercellular junctions, including gap junctions, binding adjacent cells. It is likely that every islet cell has at least one face in contact with a capillary. The islets are richly vascularized by capillaries (Figs. 16.51 and 16.52) lined with fenestrated endothelium. Autonomic nerve fibers, both sympathetic and parasympathetic, enter the islets and terminate in close association with islet cells. Each islet is coated with a thin layer of reticular fibers.

Fig. 16.50. *Islets of Langerhans* (arrows) in the pancreas. ×24.

Fig. 16.51. Islets have a richer *capillary bed* than the rest of the pancreas. Injected and cleared specimen. ×100.

Fig. 16.52. Drawing of pancreas showing *blood supply*. Some of the cells have been omitted from the islet to demonstrate its greater vascularity. Compare with Fig. 16.51.

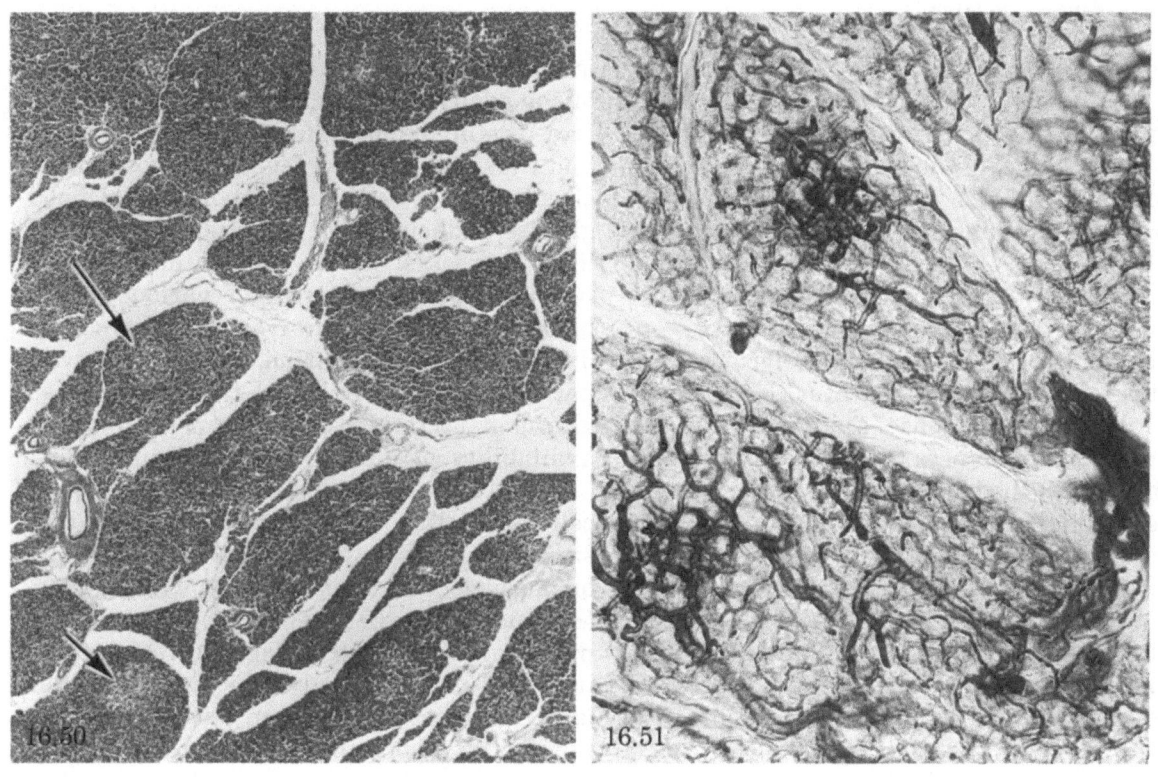

16.50

16.51

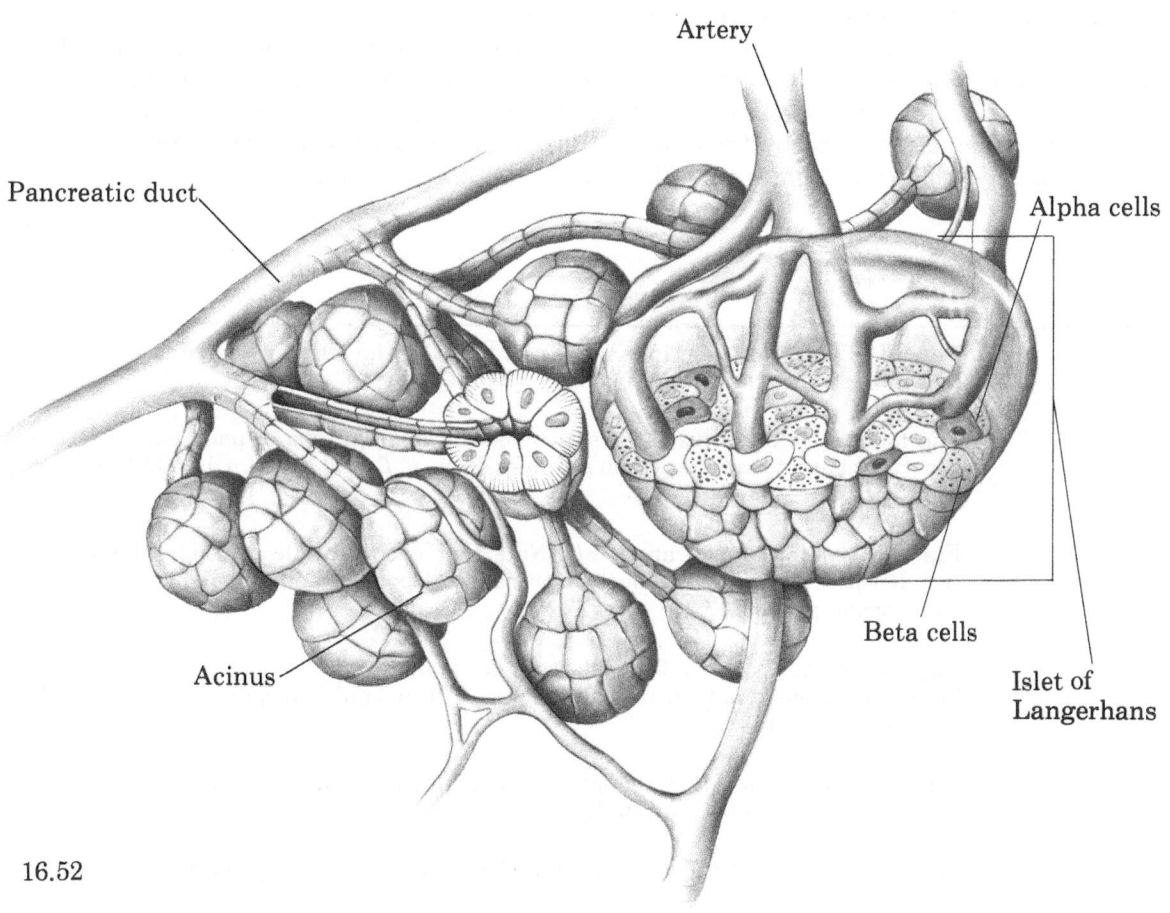

Artery

Pancreatic duct

Alpha cells

Acinus

Beta cells

Islet of
Langerhans

16.52

354   Endocrine Glands

Cells and Hormones

Although in sections stained with hematoxylin and eosin all of the cells appear alike, special stains help to differentiate among the three cell types termed α, β, and δ cells (Fig. 16.53).

With the electron microscope, all types have features of cells synthesizing polypeptides for export; that is, free polyribosomes, diffuse RER, Golgi apparatus, and small, membrane-bound, dense, secretory granules. The visible differences between cell types are primarily in the electron microscopic appearance (Figs. 16.54 through 16.56) and the light microscopic staining properties of these granules. Nerve fibers can be seen terminating on all three cell types, and physiologic studies indicate that some may stimulate and others inhibit secretion. However, the principal control is probably exerted by the levels of glucose brought to the islets in the blood.

α CELLS are generally located at the periphery of the islet and make up about 20% of the cells. They are slightly larger than the other cell types. Their granules have dense, spherical, central cores with a zone of low density between core and membrane (Fig. 16.54). The hormone produced by the α cell is a small polypeptide called *glucagon*. This

is a glycogenolytic substance; that is, by way of the adenyl cyclase-cAMP system, it stimulates the breakdown of glycogen in the liver, and thus increases the level of glucose in the circulation. α Cells are responsive to blood glucose, reducing their secretion as the blood level increases. In physiologic emergencies produced by acute stress of various kinds, blood-borne epinephrine from the adrenal medulla and norepinephrine, released by sympathetic nerves to the islets, also increase glucagon secretion, thereby increasing the availability of glucose for metabolic needs.

β CELLS constitute about 75% of the islet cell population. Their secretory granules, smaller than those of alpha cells, contain one or more electron-dense crystals with an electron-lucent zone between the crystals and the membrane (Fig. 16.55). Their secretion product is *insulin,* a hypoglycemic hormone (that is, it reduces blood glucose level). It accomplishes this by promoting the transport of glucose across cell membranes and by stimulating glycogen formation, particularly in liver and muscle.

The hormone is synthesized in the RER, passed by transfer vesicles to the Golgi where it is packaged in crystalline form in storage vesicles. In response to elevated blood glucose, the crystals are extruded by exocytosis, dis-

Fig. 16.53. An *islet*. The individual cell types in the islet are not much different by routine light microscopy. ×300.

The following three illustrations are electron micrographs of pancreatic islets to show the characteristic secretion granules of the α, β, and δ cells. ×14,600. (Courtesy of R. Brooks.)

Fig. 16.54. A portion of an α *cell*. Note that each granule contains material of two densities, a peripheral electron-translucent portion and a central nearly electron-opaque portion.

Fig. 16.55. The β *cell* contains electron-dense material of variable shape in membrane-bound electron-transparent vesicles. The irregular fragments probably are crystals of insulin.

Fig. 16.56. In the δ *cell*, although granules may differ in density, each granule is itself of uniform density throughout.

Fig. 16.57. *Islet cell tumor*. This caused recurrent hypoglycemia and is a tumor of β cells. ×35.

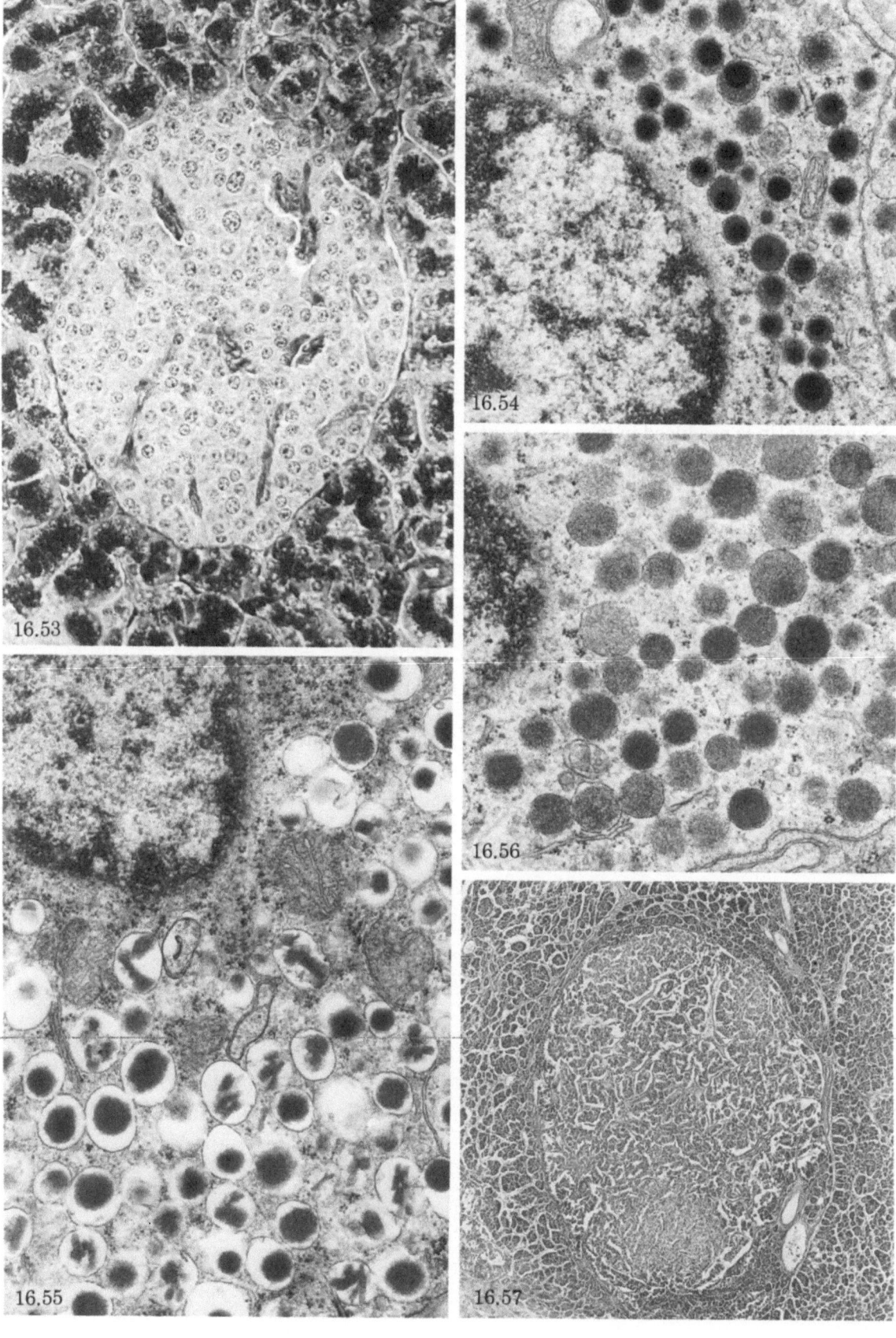

16.53

16.54

16.56

16.55

16.57

solved in the extracellular fluid, and passed into the capillaries. The total population of β cells in all of the islets produces about 2 mg of insulin per day.

Increased epinephrine from the adrenal gland in the circulation suppresses insulin secretion, as probably also does norepinephrine from sympathetic nerve terminals in the islets.

δ CELLS have secretory vesicles with dense granules, but with contents of uniform moderate density, and no electron-lucent halos (Fig. 16.56). They are similar in many respects to some of the enteroendocrine cells found in the stomach. They produce *somatostatin* and perhaps *gastrin*.

Somatostatin is produced in greater quantities in the hypothalamus, where it is the somatotrophin-release inhibiting factor for the hypophysis. Here in the islets, it is produced in too small a quantity to have systemic effects, but probably functions locally on neighboring cells to suppress the secretion of insulin and glucagon.

Gastrin is a hormone that stimulates release of acid by the parietal cells of the stomach. Its function in the islets of Langerhans is unknown.

Functional Disorders

Any pathologic process that destroys the islets, or genetic effect that makes the function of β cells inadequate, produces the disease *diabetes mellitus*. This is a common disorder and often presents serious clinical problems. In the absence of insulin, blood glucose rises to a high level. It comes to exceed the ability of the kidney to reabsorb it from the glomerular filtrate, and hence glucose appears in the urine. A consideration of the complex ramifications of this disease is beyond the scope of this book.

Islet cell hyperplasia and tumors of one or another of the cell types occur (Fig. 16.57). Increased amounts of insulin result in hypoglycemia with serious consequences, such as severe neurologic and mental damage. Functioning tumors of α or β cells have results predictable from knowledge of their hormones' actions.

The endocrine pancreas, composed of the islets of Langerhans, is a complex group of interacting and antagonistic cells with widespread important functions in controlling metabolic activity in many tissues and organs. Only a small sample of its numerous disorders have been introduced here.

17 Female Reproductive System

Introduction

The female reproductive system consists of two groups of structures, the *internal genitalia* (Figs. 17.1 through 17.3) located in the pelvic cavity, and the *external genitalia* (Figs. 17.3 and 17.38) located in the perineum. The former include the ovaries, oviducts (fallopian tubes), uterus, and vagina; the latter include the labia minora, labia majora, and clitoris. Although the breasts are glands of the integument and have been described in Chapter 11, they are importantly related to reproductive function and these aspects will be included here.

Normally the development and differentiation of the organs of this system are not complete until the pituitary gonadotrophic hormones begin to appear at about age 10. Under the influence of these hormones, maturation of the system is completed and the first reproductive cycle occurs at 12 to 14 years of age. Although this complex cycle involves primarily the hypothalamus, pituitary gland, ovaries, and uterus, cyclic changes also occur in breasts, libido, basal body temperature, psyche, and other structures and functions. Since these changes occur on an average of every 28 days, or every lunar month, they are said to compose the *menstrual cycle (mensis,* month). In healthy women the length of the cycle varies from 21 to 35 days. If pregnancy ensues, the cycle ceases until nursing is terminated, at which time it begins again. Menstrual cycles continue fairly regularly throughout the 30–35 years of reproductive life and cease between the ages 45–55. This, the end of the reproductive period, is termed the *menopause,* and is accompanied by a variety of sometimes profound morphologic, physiologic, and psychologic changes.

Ovaries

General Features

Each of the two ovaries is an almond-shaped body measuring about $4 \times 2 \times 1$ cm, lying near the lateral wall of the pelvis (Figs. 17.2 through 17.4). Each is attached to the posterior surface of the broad ligament by a fold of peritoneum (the *mesovarium*). Vessels and nerves gain access to the hilus of the ovary between the layers of the mesovarium.

Fig. 17.1. *Internal genitalia,* posterior view. Arrow indicates a small leiomyoma (a common benign tumor of uterine smooth muscle).

Fig. 17.2. *Internal genitalia* drawn as if removed from the pelvis and viewed from behind, as is the specimen photographed in Fig. 17.1. The posterior wall of the vagina has been removed so that the vaginal portion of the cervix is visible.

Fig. 17.3. Right half of the *female pelvis.* Sagittal section.

Fig. 17.4. Cut surface of *ovary* with corpus hemorrhagicum (C) at lower left and follicles (arrows).

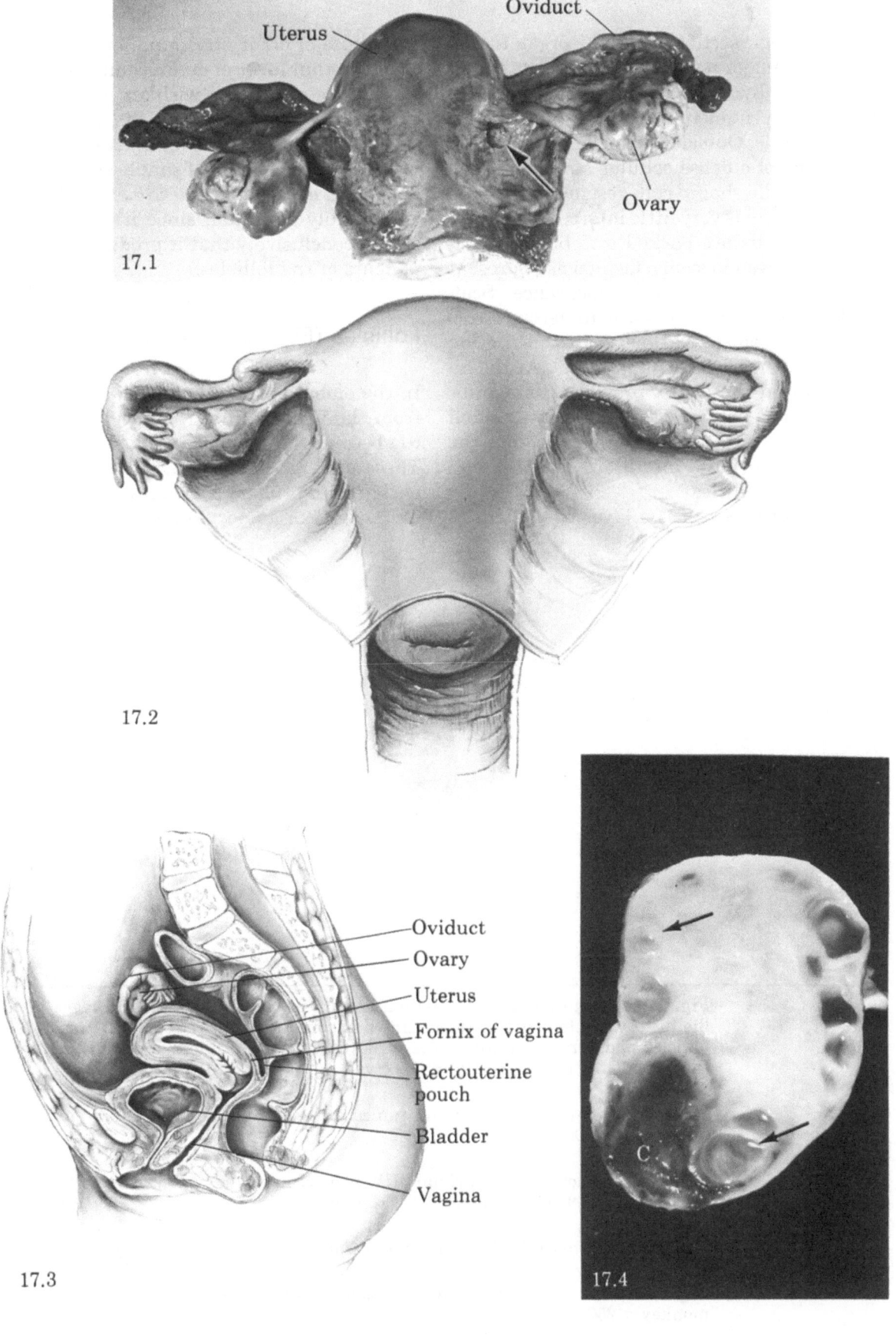

Uterus

Oviduct

Ovary

17.1

17.2

Oviduct
Ovary
Uterus
Fornix of vagina
Rectouterine pouch
Bladder
Vagina

17.3

17.4

A histologic section shows the organ to consist of two major portions (Fig. 17.5). Its center is occupied by a *medulla* of loose connective tissue with numerous tortuous and coiled blood vessels. Outside the medulla is a *cortex* consisting of a dense cellular *stroma* of elongated, spindle-shaped cells resembling smooth muscle. There is very little intercellular material. The cells are packed into bundles that are interwoven in such a fashion as to present a characteristic whorled appearance. Scattered through the cortex are numerous structures representing various stages in the life history of the egg-bearing *follicles*. At the hilus a gap in the cortex provides passage for blood and lymph vessels, whose small branches radiate from the medulla into the cortex to provide a meshwork between and around the follicles.

Outside the cortex is a layer equivalent to the serosa of other abdominal organs. It consists of a thin layer of dense connective tissue (the *tunica albuginea*) with an epithelial covering (Fig. 17.6). Instead of the simple squamous epithelium that characterizes other viscera, it is composed of simple cuboidal cells and is termed the *germinal epithelium*. (It is not truly germinal, since it has not been shown conclusively that it produces any components of the follicles.)

Follicles (Figs. 17.6 through 17.8)

In the embryo primordial germ cells migrate from the yolk sac into the developing gonad to become oogonia (singular, oogonium). These undergo mitosis and eventually differentiate into *primary oocytes*. An ovarian follicle consists of an oocyte and its surrounding

Fig. 17.5. Diagrammatic longitudinal section of *ovary*. The various stages in the life history of a follicle have been drawn in counterclockwise sequence. In actuality follicles and corpora in all stages of development are found randomly scattered throughout the ovary, mostly in the cortex.

Fig. 17.6. *Ovarian cortex* (C) and tunica albuginea (T) with germinal epithelium on surface. ×300.

Fig. 17.7. Primordial (Po), primary (P), and secondary (S) *follicles* from the ovary of a monkey. ×300. (Courtesy of R. Brenner.)

Fig. 17.8. *Tertiary follicle* with antrum from the ovary of a monkey. ×85.

Fig. 17.9. *Cumulus oophorus* (C) and *zona pellucida* (arrow) from the ovary of a monkey. ×250.

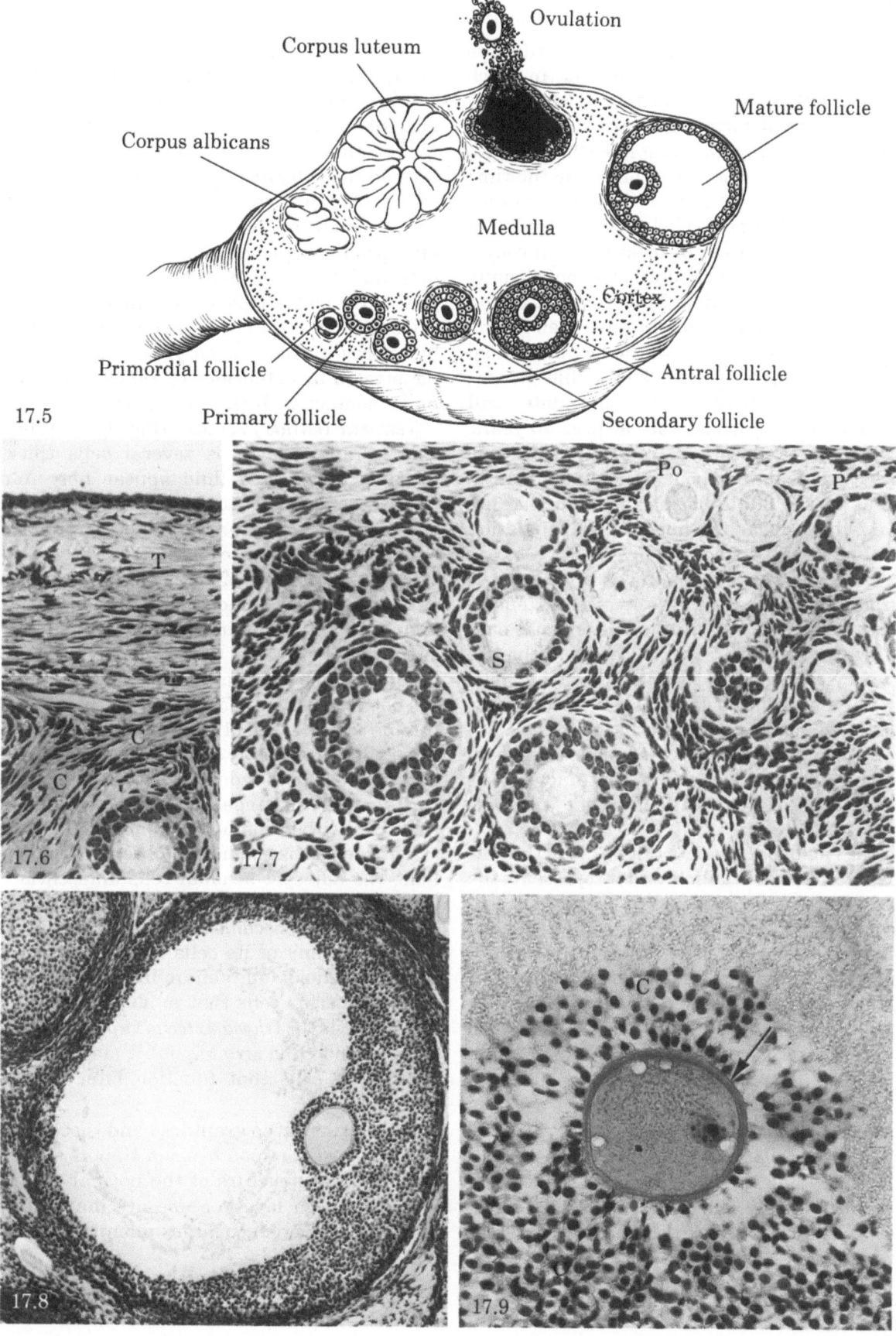

Ovulation

Corpus luteum

Corpus albicans

Mature follicle

Medulla

Cortex

Primordial follicle

Antral follicle

Primary follicle

Secondary follicle

17.5

T

C

C

17.6

Po

P

S

17.7

17.8

C

17.9

cellular wrappings. During intrauterine life 150,000–200,000 follicles develop in each ovary. Although even during fetal life many degenerate, at birth there are still perhaps 100,000 or more remaining in each ovary. No new ones are formed after birth. By the time of birth all oogonia have become primary oocytes and have proceeded to the prophase of the first cell division of meiosis. Each oocyte remains in this phase until it is hormonally called up for ovulation. Thus the first oocyte to ovulate at puberty might have been in prophase for 12 years, and in the last menstrual cycle of a woman's reproductive life at, say, age 45, the particular egg to be ovulated will have been in prophase I for at least 45 years. Except in producers of fraternal twins, one oocyte is ovulated about every lunar month. Thus in the 30- to 35-year reproductive life only about 400 of the huge oocyte population will be released from the ovary.

Over the years the number of follicles is gradually reduced by a process of degeneration termed *atresia,* until at menopause only a few remain. There are increases in the frequency of atresia at times of marked change in the endocrine balance, such as just after birth, at puberty, and during pregnancy.

Although the changes the follicle undergoes during its maturation are continuous, it is possible to distinguish four stages with specific characteristics.

THE PRIMORDIAL FOLLICLE (Fig. 17.7) is the earliest recognizable follicle and it represents the only stage to be seen before puberty. It consists of an oocyte and a layer of flat cells applied to its surface. The follicle cells are not clearly differentiated from stromal cells, which in fact they may be at this stage. The oocyte is a large cell, 30–40 μm in diameter, with a large, clear nucleus and a distinct nucleolus.

PRIMARY FOLLICLE (Fig. 17.7). At this stage the oocyte has enlarged and begins to develop numerous Golgi apparatuses and small vesicles in the cytoplasm. The distinctive feature is the beginning of differentiation of the follicle cells. The single layer of flat cells now becomes a single layer of cuboidal or low columnar cells and these divide to keep pace with the enlargement of the oocyte.

SECONDARY FOLLICLE (Figs. 17.6 and 17.7). Under the influence of hypophyseal FSH, follicle cells proliferate rapidly. The resulting presence of several layers of follicle cells characterizes this stage. This thickening layer is termed the *follicular epithelium.* Its cells are called granulosa cells and are separated from the stroma by a basement membrane. A thick glycoprotein layer develops between the oocyte and the immediately adjacent coat of granulosa cells. This is the *zona pellucida* (Figs. 17.8 and 17.9). It is partially penetrated by microvilli from the oocyte and completely penetrated by extensions of follicle cells that make contact with the surface of the oocyte.

TERTIARY (ANTRAL) FOLLICLE (Fig. 17.8). When the granulosa layer is several cells thick, droplets of secreted fluid appear here and there among the cells. As fluid accumulates, these droplets enlarge and coalesce to form a single cavity or *antrum,* eccentrically splitting the granulosa layer about midway between the zona pellucida and the basement membrane. The antrum does not completely surround the oocyte; it allows the latter to occupy a hillock of granulosa cells (the *cumulus oophorus*) (Figs. 17.8 and 17.9), projecting into it from the wall of the follicle. The granulosa cells immediately surrounding the oocyte and attached to the zona constitute the *corona radiata.* At this stage the oocyte reaches its full size, with a diameter of about 100 μm.

Outside the basement membrane of the follicle, the adjacent stromal cells differentiate into two layers (Fig. 17.10). The inner layer (*theca interna*) becomes noticeably vascularized, and many of its cells become enlarged and epithelioid (epithelium-like). These become endocrine cells that produce estrogens. The outer layer (*theca externa*) appears to be simply condensed stroma, but it may contain contractile cells that function later during ovulation.

Neoplasms of the granulosa and theca cells are the most common ovarian tumors. These simulate the structure of the normal granulosa and theca layers. Some are malignant, and they may produce large amounts of estrogen (Fig. 17.14).

Up to this point in follicular development, the changes have been largely under the control of FSH. The increasing amount of estrogens from the growing follicle applies a brake to the production of FSH-releasing hormone and a stimulus to the production of LH-releasing hormone.

MATURE FOLLICLE. By the midpoint of the menstrual cycle, about 12–14 days after its growth begins, the follicle is mature. This, the *Graafian follicle,* is nearly a centimeter in diameter, greater than the thickness of the cortex; it projects as a visible blister on the surface of the ovary. Growth ceases because of the reduction in FSH, and a brief period of inactivity ensues, preceding the critical surge in LH production.

Ovulation (Figs. 17.4 and 17.11)

About midway in the menstrual cycle there is a sudden sharp increase in secretion of LH. This is a key factor in initiating the several important correlated events that comprise the process of ovulation.

A fundamental response to this LH surge is the completion of the first division of meiosis, which reduces the chromosome number to haploid. The division produces a large *secondary oocyte* and a small cell, the *polar body,* whose only function apparently is to contain the discarded chromosomes. The secondary oocyte then begins the next division. The process proceeds as far as metaphase and stops. Division proceeds to anaphase and telophase only when, and if, fertilization occurs.

Another response to the surge of LH is a sudden increase in the amount of fluid in the follicle. The raised intrafollicular pressure stretches the surface blister and an ischemic spot (the *stigma*) develops where the overlying tunica albuginea is compressed. The stigma finally breaks open, probably as a result of this pressure. This is also probably assisted by an enzymatic weakening of the overlying connective tissue and, at least in some species, by the contraction of smooth muscle-like cells in the theca externa of the follicle. The follicle collapses (Figs. 17.5 and 17.11) and the oocyte, with its corona radiata and variable numbers of granulosa cells, is flushed into the peritoneal cavity. From here it normally is swept into the oviduct by the movement of cilia, which line this organ and which are particularly numerous and active in its funnel-shaped mouth at this stage in the cycle.

Corpus Luteum (Figs. 17.5 and 17.12)

After ovulation, the rupture point heals over and the remaining cavity is filled with a serous fluid and some clotted blood. Macrophages and fibroblasts from the ovarian stroma invade the area, the debris is removed, and the serous fluid is gradually replaced by connective tissue. The basement membrane of the follicular epithelium disappears and blood vessels invade the folded, collapsed wall of the follicle. The structure is converted to a short-lived endocrine gland, the *corpus luteum,* which produces estrogen and progesterone to prepare the uterus for the ovum, which is descending through the oviduct. The cells of the follicle wall do not undergo mitosis but enlarge to become *lutein cells* (Fig. 17.12) by the action of LH. The previously small granulosa cells become much enlarged *granulosa lutein cells* and develop cytoplasmic lipid droplets, abundant SER, and numerous mitochondria with tubular cristae. The large amounts of lipid give a yellow color to the gross specimen. The smaller cells of the theca interna become the *theca lutein cells.*

The corpus luteum functions during the last half of the menstrual cycle. Its secretory activity ceases with the reduction of hypophyseal LH production. This decrease results from feedback inhibition by progesterone. The lutein cells lose their lipid and their yellow color, and the corpus luteum becomes a lobular, acellular scar, the *corpus albicans* (Fig. 17.13). This scar gradually disappears over several months or years.

If pregnancy occurs, the placenta produces LH and the corpus luteum does not regress, but enlarges and becomes known as a *corpus luteum of pregnancy* (Figs. 17.15 and 17.16). It continues to produce estrogen and progesterone under the influence of placental gonadotrophin.

Preovulatory Follicular Degeneration (Atresia)

Since only about 1 in 1000 of the follicles present at birth will progress to ovulation, and since the number is gradually reduced until very few are present in the postmenopausal ovary, follicular degeneration is a prominent activity in the ovary. For a given follicle, this may appear at any stage in its development from primordial to mature. In atresia of young follicles the oocyte shows an irregular outline and a shrunken nucleus. The cells separate and undergo autolysis. As they disappear, they are replaced by ovarian stroma and no trace remains. In antral stages, granulosa cell nuclei become pyknotic, and the cells become small and separate from each other and from the basement membrane. Many become loose in the follicular fluid. The basement membrane breaks down, blood vessels invade the follicle, and the cell debris is removed by macrophages. Stromal fibroblasts also invade the area and a scar of connective tissue (corpus atreticum) replaces the follicle. In histologic sections, a collapsed and folded zona pellucida or basement membrane may sometimes be seen in the scar as the only recognizable follicular components. Eventually the scar is completely replaced by ovarian stroma.

Oviducts (Uterine Tubes; Fallopian Tubes)

General Features

The oviducts are narrow, muscular tubes lined by a folded mucous membrane. They are 7–14 cm long and vary in external diameter at different levels. They are enclosed in the free margin of the broad ligament. Each is horizontally placed, with its lateral end curved posteriorly so that the opening faces more or less medially toward the lateral portion of the ovary. It is shaped like the capital letter J lying on its side, with the ovary in the bend. Its narrow medial end (the top of the J) opens into the upper lateral angle of the uterine cavity (Fig. 17.17). As in the gallbladder, with which it is sometimes confused, a muscularis mucosae and submucosa are lacking and its layers are three: mucosa, muscularis, and serosa.

MUCOSA (Figs. 17.18 and 17.19). The lining epithelium is one of the simple columnar variety and contains two types of cells, one ciliated and the other probably secretory. Estrogens control ciliogenesis and the rate of ciliary movement in this organ. Thus the number of ciliated cells and their activity, as would be expected, reach a peak at about the

---

Fig. 17.10. *Granulosa layer* (G), *theca interna* (I), and *theca externa* (E) in the wall of a follicle. ×300. (Courtesy of R. Brenner.)

Fig. 17.11. *Rupturing follicle* with oocyte. ×85.

Fig. 17.12. Wall of *corpus luteum* with theca lutein (T) and granulosa lutein (G) cells. ×250.

Fig. 17.13. *Corpus albicans.* ×35.

Fig. 17.14. *Granulosa cell tumor.* This ovarian tumor simulates normal granulosa cells in appearance and by its excessive secretion of estrogens. The small spaces are rudimentary antra. ×100. (Courtesy of F. Vellios, K. Ireland, and the American Society of Clinical Pathologists.)

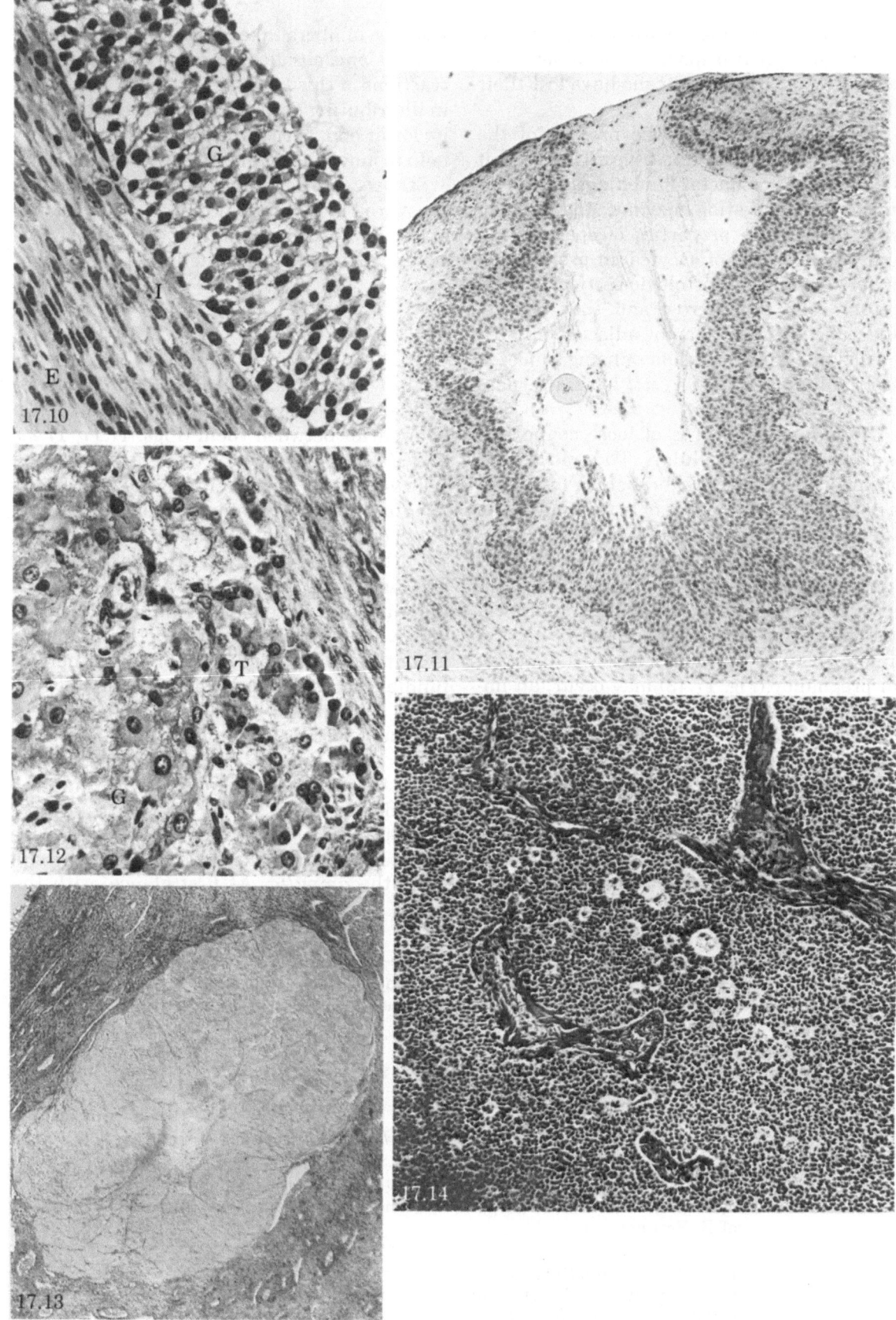

time of ovulation (Fig. 17.18), when they are most needed for transport of the gametes. By the end of the cycle most cells have lost their cilia (Fig. 17.19).

The precise nature of the product of the secretory cell type is uncertain. However, it is known that oviductal fluid plays an important part in activating enzymes, and in modifying the surface properties of spermatozoa (and probably also of oocytes) in preparation for fertilization. In histologic sections the secretory cells are narrow and they usually bulge above the surface of adjacent ciliated cells, giving the impression of being squeezed into the lumen. Thus *peg cell* is an alternate name for this type.

The lamina propria is of loose connective tissue and quite cellular. The mucosa is formed into longitudinal branching folds that vary in height and degree of branching in the different segments.

If the zygote is delayed in the tube until it loses its zona pellucida, it may implant in the oviductal mucosa, and the lamina propria will respond to its presence in somewhat the same fashion as does endometrium. Thus tubal pregnancy (Fig. 17.43) may occur, an important clinical problem because of the limited space for fetal and placental growth, which may result in rupture of the oviduct and sudden, copious intraperitoneal hemorrhage.

MUSCULARIS. Although the muscle is roughly divided into inner circular and outer longitudinal layers, these are not sharply defined.

Bundles of fibers take spiral, as well as longitudinal and circular, courses. Ring-like contractions of this layer are probably important in distributing sperm through the tube. Near its lower end, peristaltic movements probably help to move the ovum into the uterine cavity.

SEROSA. The outer surface of the oviduct is covered by a thin, but quite vascular, layer of loose connective tissue and the usual simple squamous cells of mesothelium.

Segments

Each oviduct is divided into four regions or segments of varying length, without sharp boundaries between them (Figs. 17.17, 17.20, and 17.21).

INFUNDIBULUM. Nearest the ovary is the *infundibulum*, shaped like a funnel, with its large open end (*ostium*) facing medially toward the upper lateral portion of the ovary. The rim of this funnel is provided with finger-like mucosal extensions (*fimbriae*), one of which is attached to the ovary. Each fimbria is continued into the lumen of the funnel (infundibulum) as a tall, branching fold of mucosa.

About the time of ovulation the movements of this segment increase dramatically, gliding over the surface of the ovary with fimbriae extended.

AMPULLA (Fig. 17.20). The infundibular funnel leads to the next widest portion of the tube, the *ampulla*. At first glance, with the

---

Fig. 17.15. Diagram correlating sequential events and functions in *hypophyseal*, *ovarian*, and *uterine cycles*. At the right the regular cycle is interrupted by pregnancy.

Fig. 17.16. A single, lobulated *corpus luteum of pregnancy* occupies almost the entire ovary. ×2.

Fig. 17.17. Dorsal view of the right *oviduct* and associated structures.

Fig. 17.18. *Epithelium of oviduct* during the proliferative phase of the endometrial cycle. Note the ciliated (large arrow) and peg (small arrow) cells. ×560. (Courtesy of R. Brenner.)

Fig. 17.19. *Epithelium of oviduct* near the time of menstruation. The cells are shrunken, more darkly staining and less distinct than during the proliferative phase. Ciliation is drastically reduced. ×560. (Courtesy of R. Brenner.)

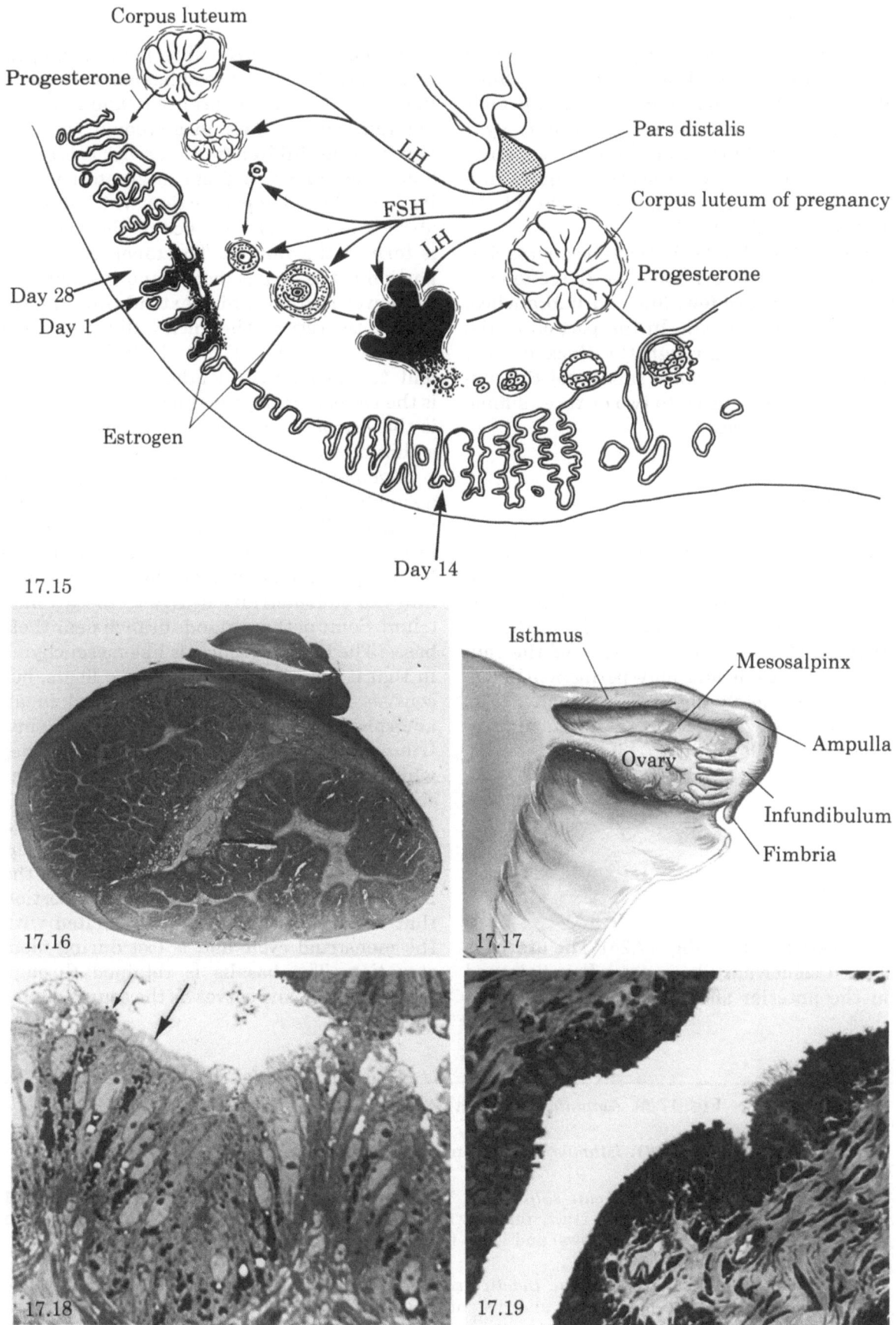

Corpus luteum

Progesterone

LH

Pars distalis

FSH

Corpus luteum of pregnancy

LH

Progesterone

Day 28

Day 1

Estrogen

Day 14

17.15

17.16

Isthmus

Mesosalpinx

Ovary

Ampulla

Infundibulum

Fimbria

17.17

17.18

17.19

low power of the microscope, a cross-section appears to show no lumen, since it is filled with thin, branching and rebranching folds of cilia-covered mucosa separated only by a small layer of fluid. It appears like a tightly constructed maze, with spaces of quite uniform width. This is the segment in which fertilization most frequently occurs.

ISTHMUS (Fig. 17.21). As the tube approaches the uterus, the lumen narrows. In section the mucosal folds are few, low and unbranched.

INTRAMURAL SEGMENT. In the portion of the tube that passes through the thick uterine wall, the lumen becomes small and the mucosal folds are reduced to two or three simple longitudinal ridges.

Salpingitis

Gonorrhea causes acute inflammation of the reproductive system, particularly the oviducts. In early stages there is a thick purulent exudate in the lumen and involving the epithelium (Fig. 17.22). Adhesions of the mucosal folds result and may permanently distort or completely obstruct the lumen (Fig. 17.23). If fertilization occurs at all, tubal pregnancy may follow (Fig. 17.43).

Uterus

Corpus

GENERAL FEATURES (Fig. 17.24). The uterus is shaped somewhat like a pear. It is flattened on the anterior and posterior surfaces, and suspended between the anterior and the posterior sheaths of the broad ligament. It varies in size at different stages in life and in different functional states. In a woman who has never borne children (nulliparous), it is about 8 cm long, and 4 or 5 cm in greatest width. Its dome-shaped upper portion, which projects above the level of entrance of the oviducts, is termed the *fundus*. The tapering, largest portion is the *corpus* (body), and the cylindrical, lower portion, which extends into the vagina, is the *cervix*. The thick wall is composed of three layers (Fig. 17.24): the lining, equivalent to the mucosa of other hollow organs, is the *endometrium;* the thick, muscular layer is the *myometrium,* and this is covered with a thin *serosa.*

Endometrium. This layer is composed of a simple columnar epithelium with scattered ciliated cells and a thick, cellular lamina propria. The latter contains numerous parallel, simple tubular glands that extend deep into the endometrium nearly to the myometrium. Some of these glands branch near their bases. The lamina propria is like mesenchyme in that it has no connective tissue fibers, but consists of numerous cells contained in an amorphous ground substance. The endometrium is divided indistinctly into two zones which, although they are structurally rather similar, have different functions (Fig. 17.26). The thicker, more superficial zone is termed the *zona functionalis* and the thinner layer, applied to the myometrium, is termed the *zona basalis.* The functionalis is the portion that undergoes the changes associated with the menstrual cycle and is lost during menstruation. The basalis is retained through menstruation, and serves as the source of new

Fig. 17.20. *Ampulla* of oviduct. ×23. (Courtesy of R. Brenner.)

Fig. 17.21. *Isthmus.* ×42. (Courtesy of R. Brenner.)

Fig. 17.22. *Acute salpingitis.* The infectious disease gonorrhea, having traveled up the genital tract, remains mainly within the lumen. However, it does injure epithelium (arrows) and leads to deformities, as seen in Fig. 17.23. ×110.

Fig. 17.23. *Chronic inactive salpingitis.* Adhesions between mucosal folds have caused obstruction and distention of the lumen. ×7. (Courtesy of F. Vellios, K. Ireland, and the American Society of Clinical Pathologists.)

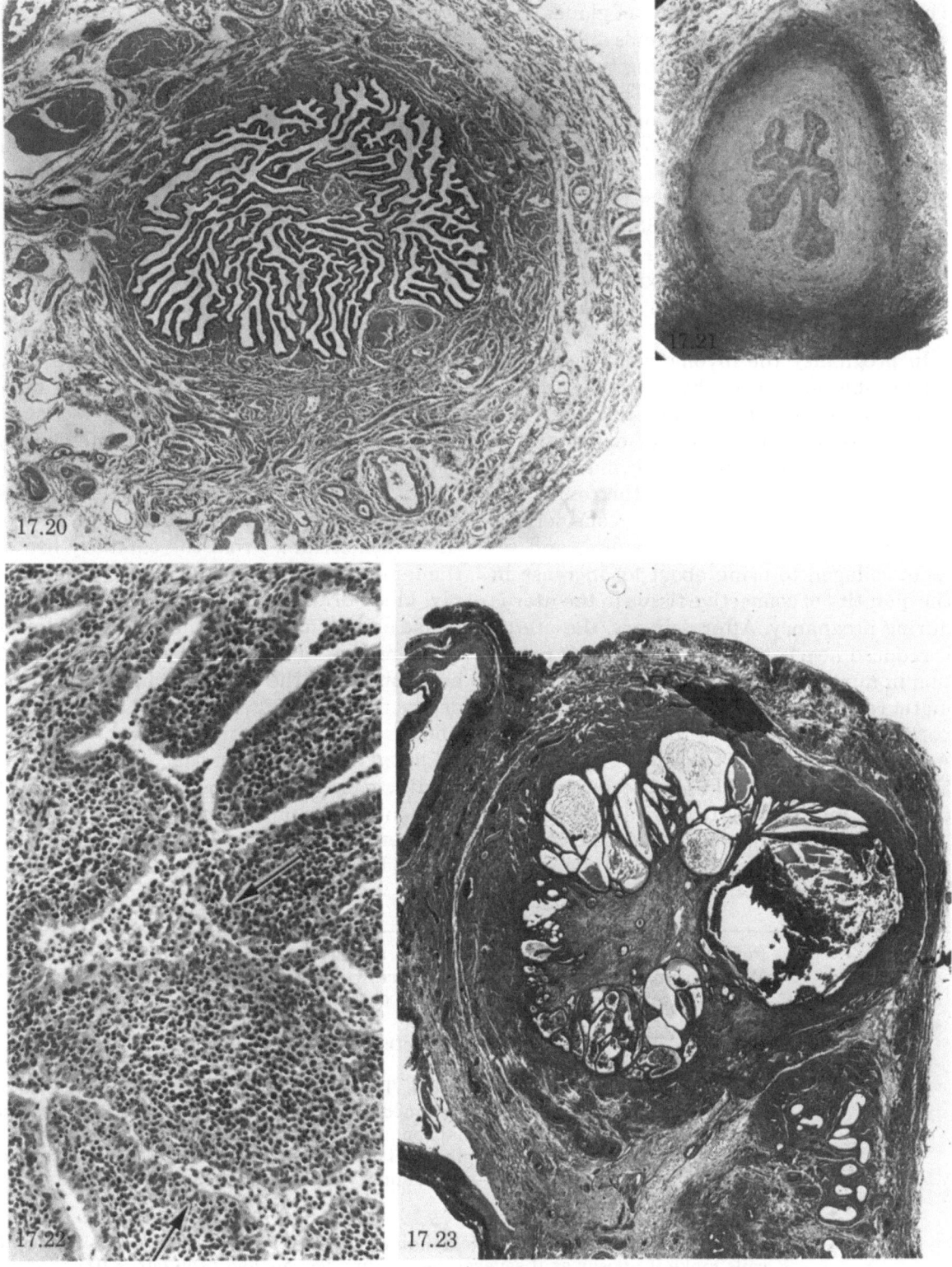

tissue to replace that lost at menstruation. The basalis, with its remnants of glands, provides new lamina propria, glands and surface epithelium for the regenerating functionalis.

Myometrium (Fig. 17.25). This muscular layer is 12 mm or more thick and is subdivided into three components. The outer and inner layers are longitudinally oriented, hence useful in expulsion of the fetus at birth. The intermediate layer contains bundles running in all directions. Also located in this layer is a rich venous and arterial plexus; accordingly this layer is often termed the stratum vasculare.

In pregnancy the myometrium undergoes remarkable growth by hypertrophy and increase in the number of muscle cells. This increase is both by mitosis of existing cells and by differentiation of new muscle cells from undifferentiated cells in the connective tissue. Muscle cells develop considerable amounts of endoplasmic reticulum, and secrete collagen to bring about an increase in the quantity of connective tissue in the uterus during pregnancy. After delivery, the uterus is reduced nearly to its original size by reduction in number of smooth muscle fibers, enzymatic removal of collagen, and return of hypertrophic muscle fibers to their usual size. A cell that originally may have been about 50 μm in length, but that has become 10 times that long, may then return to its original size.

The serosa is composed of the usual connective tissue and overlying simple squamous mesothelium. It covers the corpus and the posterior portion of the cervix.

Blood vessels (Figs. 17.27 and 17.28). Although the pattern of blood supply within the uterus is difficult to determine from routine histologic preparations, it is of great significance to the function of the organ, and to the cyclic changes that occur during menstruation. One needs a concept of this pattern before discussing these functional activities.

The branches of the uterine arteries within the myometrium follow a course parallel to the surface, forming a basket of arching vessels in the shape of the uterus and buried in the myometrium. From some of these arcuate arteries, radial arteries pass to the endometrium. These radial branches give rise to two types of vessels. The *basal arteries* supply blood to the basal zone of the endometrium. *Spiral arteries* (Fig. 17.27) are coiled and tortuous and extend into the functional zone of the endometrium. From the capillary bed of the lamina propria, which these arteries supply, blood drains into dilated, thin-walled lacunae and then into veins. The spiral arteries are sensitive to changes in endocrine status and constitute the basic mechanism for the degenerative processes that lead to menstruation.

ENDOMETRIAL (MENSTRUAL) CYCLE. Every month, more or less, the functional zone of the endometrium undergoes degenerative changes and is shed. The resulting mixture of blood, cellular debris, and tissue fluid con-

Fig. 17.24. *Uterus,* opened. Half of the uterus has been separated and removed. Myometrium (M), endometrium (large arrow), cervical canal (small arrow), vaginal portion of cervix (V). (Courtesy of E. Jacobson.)

Fig. 17.25. *Wall of the uterus.* Endometrium (E), myometrium (M). ×5.

Fig. 17.26. *Zones of the endometrium.* The basal zone, next to the myometrium, has a more compact and darkly stained stroma with simple and smooth-walled glandular elements. The functional zone has a lightly stained, less packed cellular stroma and the portions of the glands at this level have a less regular lumen and more folded epithelial lining. The boundary between the two zones is indicated. ×28.

Fig. 17.27. *Endometrial artery* (extending from lower right to upper left). Its tight coils make it appear as if several neighboring vessels had been cut. ×100.

Fig. 17.28. *Blood supply* of the uterus. **Left:** Overall pattern of arterial distribution. Rectangle indicates area enlarged. **Right:** Diagram of arteries and veins of the endometrium.

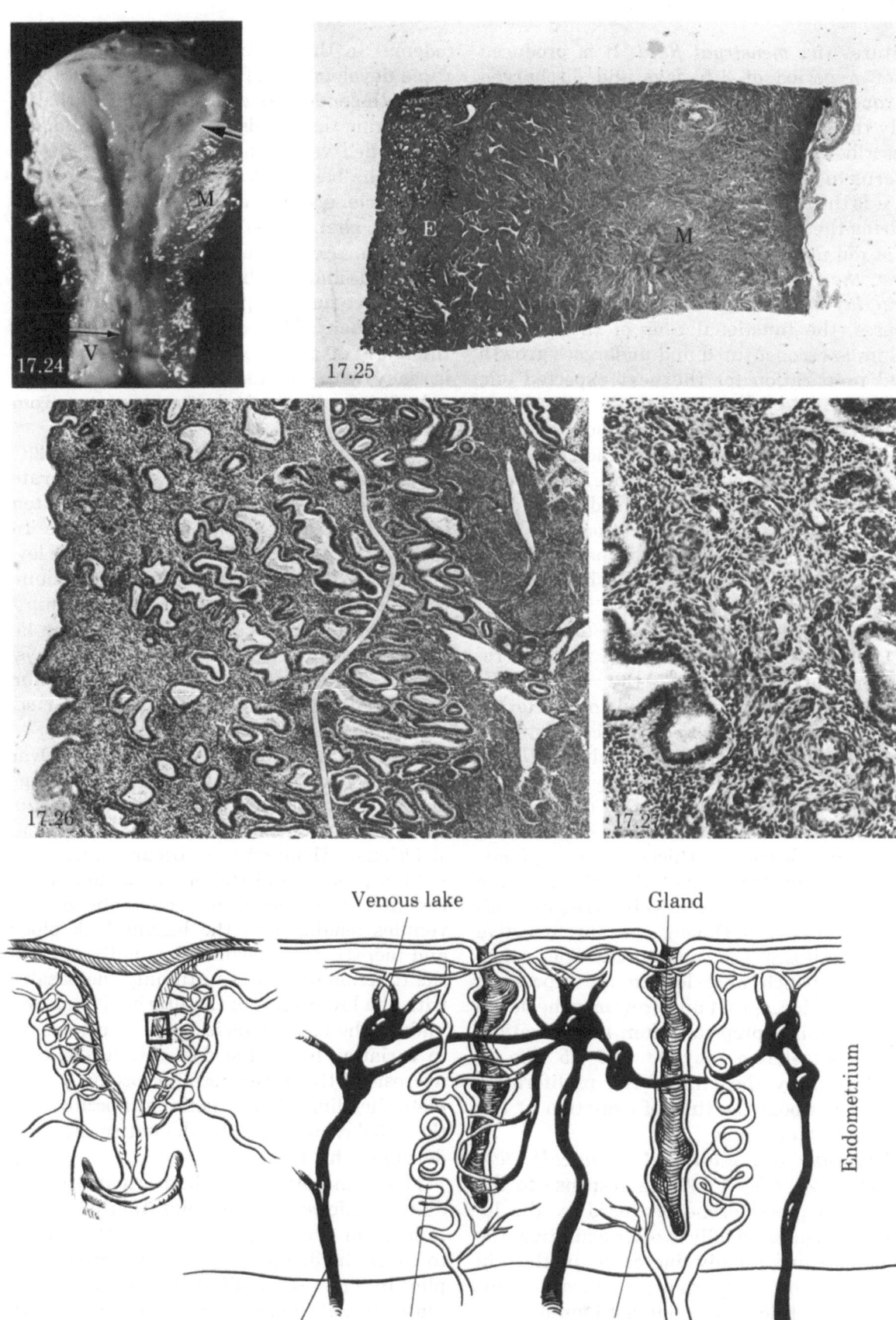

17.24

17.25

17.26

17.27

17.28

Venous lake   Gland

Vein   Spiral artery   Basal artery

Endometrium

stitutes the *menstrual fluid*. It is produced over a period of 3–5 days and discharged through the vagina. Menstruation is functionally the termination of the cycle. It has been described as the response of a disappointed uterus to failure to receive a fertile egg; that is, it is the shedding of endometrium prepared during the preceding 3½ weeks for an embryo that did not arrive. *In clinical practice, however, the cycle is timed as beginning with the first day of menstruation*. After menstruation ceases, the functional zone of the endometrium is reconstituted and undergoes growth and preparation for the next expected embryo. As these changes occur in response to the changing levels of ovarian hormone, the histologic picture of the endometrium goes through a series of stages. Since, in biologic terms, the cycle begins with the development of the endometrium in preparation for an embryo, and then is terminated by menstruation, the stages and the processes will be described in that sequence.

Proliferative (estrogenic) stage (days 5–14), (Fig. 17.29). After menstruation the only remaining uterine mucosa is the zona basalis. The epithelial cells now begin to proliferate and to cover the exposed surface of stroma to reconstitute a surface epithelium. Under the influence of the gradually increasing amount of estrogen from the ovaries, the stroma proliferates and the endometrium gradually becomes thicker. The glands lengthen and throughout this phase of the cycle they remain relatively straight with narrow lumens. During the proliferative phase mitoses are numerous. The spiral arteries, which were lost in the process of menstruation, sprout and grow into the developing lamina propria. After menstruation, the endometrium may be 0.25–0.5 mm in thickness. By the end of the proliferative phase, at about the time of ovulation, it has grown to 2 or 3 mm.

Secretory (progestational or luteal) stage (days 15–27) (Fig. 17.30). In response to the increased progesterone produced by the luteinized, ruptured follicle after ovulation, the endometrium rapidly increases further in thickness and its glands begin secreting. This increase in thickness is due not to mitotic activity, but to an increase in tissue fluid (edema) in the lamina propria, and to the rapid development of intense secretory activity by the endometrial glands. The epithelial cells lining the glands become taller, and glycogen-filled vacuoles appear in the cells between the basement membrane and the nuclei. Nuclei are thus displaced from the basal position characteristic of the preovulatory condition. Accumulated secretion distends the glands and they become tortuous, appearing to have tufts of epithelium projecting into their lumens. The endometrium attains a thickness of about 5 mm at this stage and is ready, with secreted nutrients and rich vascularity, for the arrival of a blastocyst from the oviduct.

Premenstrual (ischemic) stage (days 27–28). Instead of being given the status of a separate stage, this brief but important phase is often included as a part of the secretory stage. In response to the reduction in progesterone levels with early regression of the corpus luteum, the spiral arterioles undergo repeated, temporary contractions. Water is lost from the lamina propria to the lacunae and venous system, so that edema is reduced and the functionalis becomes thinner. Glandular secretion ceases.

Menstrual stage (days 1–5) (Fig. 17.31). Over a day or two, the repeated ischemia brings about necrosis of the endothelium and rupture of the vessels distal to the vascular constrictions. Hemorrhage occurs into the lamina propria and the outer portion of the functionalis becomes detached. The deeper venules leading into the basalis leak blood and menstruation begins. Gradually more of the functionalis is lost until only the basalis, with the lower ends of the uterine glands, remains. The basal arteries are not responsive to variation in the blood steroid levels; thus necrosis of this layer does not occur. A complete shedding of the functionalis occurs over the 3–5-day period, until the entire uterus is devoid of this layer.

The termination of menstruation is immediately followed by the migration of epithelium from the basal portions of the glands to cover the denuded surface. Estrogen, supplied by a new wave of follicular growth, stimulates these changes and initiates the proliferative stage.

Typical endometrial tissue is not always restricted to the lining of the uterine cavity. In the condition called ectopic endometriosis (Fig. 17.32), islands of this tissue (both stroma and glands) are found in a variety of sites, most of which are in the pelvis. Any pelvic organ, particularly on its peritoneal surface, is likely to be affected. Sometimes this lesion may occur in other, even distant, sites such as mediastinum or lung. This condition is of interest here because its manner of clinical presentation is entirely predictable from the facts already presented. The disease is characterized clinically by periodic episodes of pain, corresponding to whatever sites are involved. The pain is caused by the hemorrhage, which occurs on a cyclic schedule along with that of the normal endometrium. There is no possibility of excretion of the blood and shed mucosa through the normal route. Consequently there is a local tissue reaction. This includes scarring and the appearance of macrophages laden with hemosiderin (a breakdown product of blood).

Cervix

The cervix (neck) (Figs. 17.2, 17.3, and 17.33) of the uterus is as much an organ distinct from the uterine corpus and vagina as is the duodenum from the stomach and jejunum. It is a firm, fibromuscular tube, barrel-shaped overall, with a mucosal lining and a very narrow lumen about 3 cm long. This lumen is continuous above with the uterine cavity at the *internal os,* and opens below into the vagina through its *vaginal* or *external os.* The lower end of the cervix projects into the vagina, as the *vaginal portion.* This portion is accessible for direct examination and for the acquisition of biopsies or smears of exfoliated cells, an important attribute since cervical cancer is a common occurrence (Fig. 17.36).

Most of the wall of the cervix is composed of dense irregular connective tissue with small but varying amounts of smooth muscle. It is nearly ligamentous in its firmness; indeed, the upper end may be thought of as the insertion of the uterine musculature that must expel the fetus through the canal at birth.

The cervical lamina propria is more dense and fibrous than that of the corpus. The mucosa of the cervical canal has a mucus-secreting, simple columnar epithelium, longitudinal furrows and numerous long, branched mucous glands (Figs. 17.33 and 17.34). These glands are obliquely placed, with their mouths slanting toward the vagina. Cysts, sometimes 1 or 2 cm diameter, are common in normal cervix and represent obstructed and dilated glands (nabothian cysts).

The mucosa of the vaginal portion of the cervix is without glands and is covered by a nonkeratinized stratified squamous epithelium like that of the vagina. The level of the squamocolumnar junction (Fig. 17.35) varies in different individuals and may vary with age in the same individual. In a condition known as eversion, the junction may be on the exterior of the cervix and columnar epithelium may thus be exposed to the vaginal environment.

Although during the menstrual cycle there are only minor changes in the cervical mucosa, the properties of the cervical mucus vary significantly. At the time of ovulation there is a marked reduction in viscosity. This is an important change for the advancing sperm because the thick, viscid, mucous plug presents a formidable barrier at other times in the cycle. After ovulation, under the influence of progesterone, the mucus again becomes viscous and resumes its important function of preventing germs, whether human or microbial, from entering the reproductive tract and thence the peritoneal cavity. The relative viscosity of the mucus is a helpful indicator of ovulation time.

Vagina

The vagina (Figs. 17.37 and 17.38) is a fibromuscular tube whose upper end is fitted, as the circular *fornix,* around the vaginal portion of the cervix. Below the cervix the vagina is flattened anteroposteriorly and folded along its lateral margins so that the collapsed lumen is shaped like a broad, short H in cross section. It has three layers: mucosa, muscularis, and adventitia. A portion of the fornix is also provided with a serosa in place of the adventitia, where it borders directly on the pelvic cavity.

Phases of the endometrium. In each case the lower magnification is at the top. The myometrial–endometrial junctions are aligned. **a:** ×17. **b:** ×100.

Fig. 17.29. *Endometrium, proliferative phase.* Glands are relatively straight, epithelium is smooth and even, and the stroma is compact.

Fig. 17.30. The endometrium in the *secretory phase* is much thicker. Glands are tortuous, epithelium is convoluted and the stroma is more loose and more variable.

Fig. 17.31. Endometrium, *menstrual phase.* Some endometrium has sloughed off; the surface is ragged and without epithelium. Some glands contain blood. Basal glands remain unchanged.

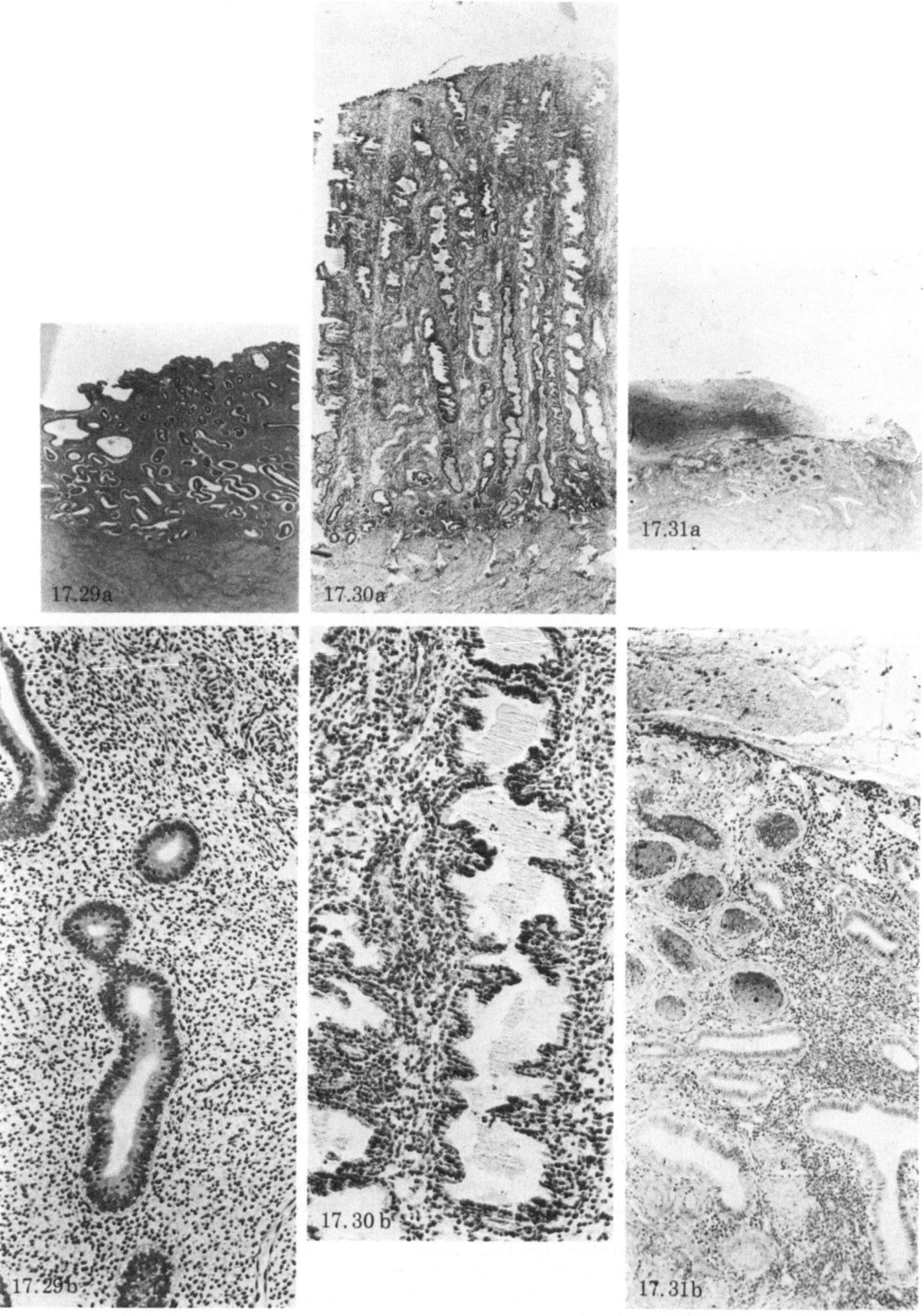

Fig. 17.32. *Ectopic endometriosis.* The presence of endometrium in abnormal sites, where it may function as in its normal position and cause periodic bleeding into local tissue. This specimen is from the abdominal wall in the region of the umbilicus. **A:** ×24. **B:** ×110.

Fig. 17.33. *Cervix* of the uterus with cervical glands (G), one cystic gland (C), and squamocolumnar junction (arrow). ×5.5.

Fig. 17.34. *Cervical gland.* ×100.

Fig. 17.35. *Cervical squamocolumnar* junction. Stratified squamous epithelium mixes irregularly with columnar both on the surface and in glands. ×120. (Courtesy of F. Vellios, K. Ireland, and the American Society of Clinical Pathologists.)

Fig. 17.36. *Early carcinoma* of stratified squamous epithelium of *cervix*. Clues to the diagnosis in this view are: glands lined with squamous epithelium (S); areas of excessive density of cell population (hypercellularity) (Ce); and the markedly irregular interface between epithelium and connective tissue, more significant on the left side of the photograph. There is only minimal invasion across basement membrane (arrow) but the findings necessary for the diagnosis of malignancy exist at higher magnification, in the cells and their arrangement. Compare with Figs. 3.9 through 3.12. ×17. (Courtesy of F. Vellios, K. Ireland, and the American Society of Clinical Pathologists.)

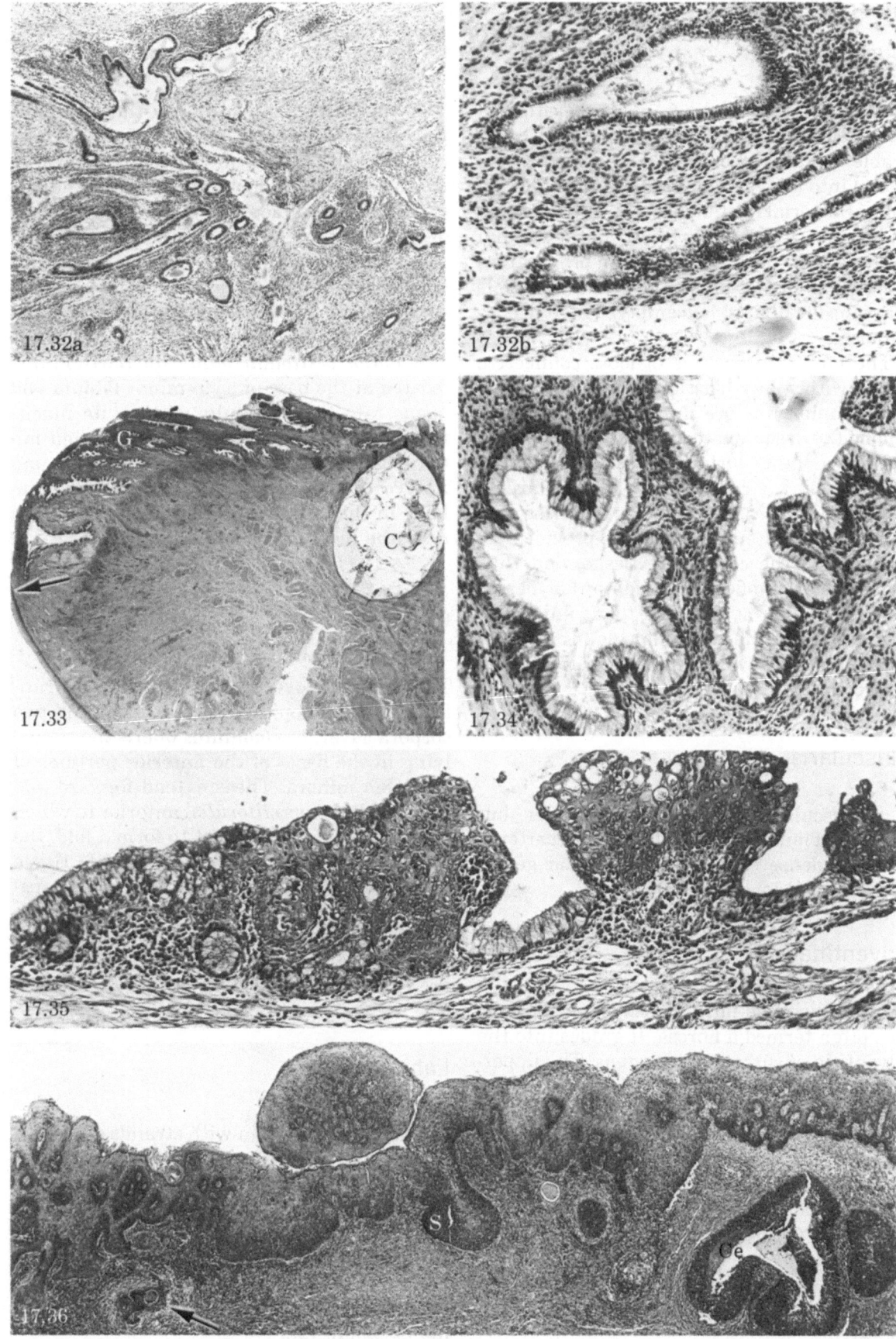

17.32a

17.32b

17.33

17.34

17.35

17.36

Mucosa

The mucosal epithelium is nonkeratinized stratified squamous. The cells contain considerable quantities of glycogen, which is released into the vaginal lumen from exfoliated cells. Bacterial metabolism of this glycogen accounts for the normal acidity of the vaginal contents. Glycogen is dissolved in preparation of routine histologic sections and the cells may appear dilated but empty. There are no glands.

The lamina propria is of loose connective tissue with many elastic fibers. Neutrophils and lymphocytes are numerous and appear among the desquamated epithelial cells in the vaginal contents during part of the menstrual cycle. There is a rich vascular plexus, largely of venous sinuses. Engorgement of these during sexual excitement probably provides extra fluid to the connective tissue, and thus accounts for the fluid transudate that passes into the vagina at this time. This fluid, plus secretion from the vestibular glands and cervical glands, provides lubrication for sexual intercourse.

Muscularis

The muscularis is not a distinct layer, but consists of bundles of smooth muscle scattered through dense connective tissue and generally oriented longitudinally.

Adventitia

The adventitia is fairly dense connective tissue, often termed a fibrosa. It grades into the adventitia of surrounding organs. The uppermost portion of the vagina, the posterior fornix, is covered by a serosa consisting of the peritoneum of the rectouterine pouch (of Douglas).

External Genitalia

The external genitalia include the *labia minora*, the *clitoris*, and the *labia majora* (Fig. 17.38).

Labia Minora

The vagina opens below into the vestibule, the space between the labia minora. These are folds of skin with an epidermis of keratinized stratified squamous epithelium. There is usually a large amount of melanin in the cells of the stratum germinativum. The dermal core of the labia minora is of loose connective tissue rich in elastic fibers. Sebaceous and sweat glands are present, but hairs are absent.

A *major vestibular gland* (of Bartholin) is located at the base of each minor labium and opens into the vestibule, so that its mucus moistens the inner surfaces of the labia minora. Numerous small, scattered, mucous, *minor vestibular glands* are present, particularly in the anterior portion of the vestibule, near the urethral opening and clitoris.

Clitoris

The clitoris is covered with keratinized stratified squamous epithelium and contains two corpora cavernosa (columns of erectile tissue) lying in the bases of the anterior portions of the labia minora. These extend forward and meet in the *glans clitoridis*, anterior to which the two labia minora meet to form a fold, the *prepuce*, over the glans. The erectile tissue consists of a plexus of venous channels capable of distention by blood during sexual excitement. This is more fully developed in the penis of the male and the details of structure are considered in Chapter 18.

Labia Majora

These are folds of skin with strands of smooth muscle (dartos) in the dermis. They are homologous to the scrotum. Their subcutaneous cores contain quantities of fat. Their outer surfaces are provided with hair, sebaceous glands, and sweat glands. The inner surfaces are similar to those of the labia minora in having sebaceous and sweat glands and in being devoid of hair.

Pregnancy

In the establishment and maintenance of pregnancy, and during the complex postpartum period, many parts of the female organism undergo modification of function and/or structure. Changes must occur to allow a number of processes ranging from the transport of spermatozoa and the maturation and protection of the fetus to the maintenance of lactation.

Gamete Transport

The female reproductive tract must provide mechanisms for transporting the spermatozoa and oocytes to the portion of the oviduct most appropriate for fertilization, and for moving the zygote into the uterus, where it will develop (Fig. 17.39).

SPERM TRANSPORT. Sperm that have been ejaculated into the upper vagina must almost immediately escape this damaging environment and enter the alkaline cervical mucus if they are to retain their fertilizing capabilities. Sperm have been found in cervical mucus within 90 seconds after ejaculation (hence the ineffectiveness of the postcoital douche as a method of contraception). At the time of ovulation, as an effect of stimulation by estrogens, the micelles of cervical mucus are arranged linearly. These are aligned parallel to the cervical canal and are suspended in a watery medium. This arrangement provides channels through which sperm swim easily and are guided toward their target. The estrogens also reduce the membrane potential of uterine muscle and lower the threshold for depolarization. The uterus thus increases its contractile activity. Sperm arriving through the cervix are rapidly distributed throughout the organ by these movements. A process of aspiration of sperm into the uterine cavity from the vagina by these movements has also been suggested as playing a part in their transportation.

The uterotubal junction presents an obstacle to passage of sperm. Those that reach the oviduct are soon distributed throughout its length by a combination of swimming, contractions of tubal muscle, and epithelial cili-ary motion. Swimming becomes of critical importance to the few that arrive in the neighborhood of the oocyte. This movement increases the chance of colliding with a corona, and is necessary for penetration of the corona and zona.

Substances in oviductal fluid destabilize the sperm membrane, complete the preparation of the penetrating enzymes, and greatly increase their fertilizing abilities. These activities constitute the process known as *capacitation.*

OOCYTE TRANSPORT. Under the influence of estrogen, oviductal cilia are fully developed and most active at, and for a few days after, ovulation. The ciliary activity on the fimbriae, together with the accelerated movements of the infundibulum over the ovary, almost always succeeds in immediately sweeping the freshly ovulated oocyte into the oviductal lumen. Most of the cilia beat toward the uterus and are probably the principal factor in the passage of the oocyte through the ampulla. There is some evidence that the cilia may have electrically charged areas at their tips, and that these assist in grasping the oocyte in the process of moving it. Fertilization normally occurs in the ampulla; by the time the oocyte has proceeded to lower segments it is too old to be fertilized.

FERTILIZATION (Figs. 17.39 and 17.40). When random swimming movements bring a spermatozoon in contact with a corona, it is probably trapped, and its direction is now guided toward the oocyte by the radial arrangement of the corona cells. It carries corona-penetrating enzymes, one of which is hyaluronidase, which aid in penetration through intercellular materials. It also contains a proteinase (acrosin) in its head cap (acrosome) that is released on contact. This *acrosome reaction* makes possible the digestion of a tunnel through the zona pellucida. The components of the sperm which recognize and bind with complementary substances on the oocyte plasmalemma are located on the flat surfaces of the sperm head. One of these surfaces is now applied to the oocyte surface. Both membranes in the area of contact break down and the contents of the sperm are injected into the oocyte. The sperm membrane is left behind as a mosaic patch in the oocyte membrane. Microtubules of the tail are disassembled, mitochondria are dispersed, and the sperm nucleus enlarges to produce the male pronucleus. The oocyte completes the second meiotic division to produce a second polar body and the female pronucleus. The two pronuclei approach and fuse in the process known as syngamy. Fertilization is now complete.

Cleavage to Blastocyst

About 24 hrs later the zygote undergoes its first mitosis to produce the two-cell stage. These are equivalent, totipotent cells; one type of identical twinning results from the separate development of each of the two blastomeres within the same zona pellucida. Cleavage continues to partition the cytoplasm into smaller and smaller cells without changing the overall dimensions. The cluster of cells so produced is termed morula (i.e., mulberry).

On the 5th day cavities containing fluid appear among the cells. Thus the conceptus (product of conception) enters the uterus as a hollow ball, the *blastocyst*. The cavity of the blastocyst is eccentric. The group of cells bulging into the cavity from one side is the inner cell mass (or embryoblast), and the single, outer layer of cells in contact with the zona pellucida is the *trophoblast*. After about a day in the uterine lumen, nourished by the glycogen-rich secretion of uterine glands, the blastocyst loses its zona pellucida and *implantation (nidation)* begins.

Implantation and Decidual Relations

As soon as the zona is shed, the area of trophoblast overlying the inner cell mass (the polar trophoblast) attaches to the uterine epithelium (Fig. 17.39). Attachment and implantation will occur on any epithelial surface available when the zona is lost (ovarian germinal epithelium, peritoneal mesothelium, tubal epithelium). This allows the development of ectopic pregnancy (Fig. 17.43). At the area of contact the trophoblast undergoes mitosis. Membranes of cells fuse and a multinucleate syncytium forms a new, outer layer in contact with, and invading, the uterine mucosa. From this time on, the trophoblast has two layers, an inner layer of discrete cells, the *cytotrophoblast,* and a peripheral layer of syncytium, the *syncytiotrophoblast* (Fig. 17.41). An increase in syncytiotrophoblast keeps pace with the insertion of the blastocyst into the endometrium, so that during inplantation syncytiotrophoblast is the only embryonic tissue in contact with maternal tissue (Fig. 17.44). With very little destruction of uterine tissue, the syncytiotrophoblast separates the endometrial epithelial cells, and the blastocyst gradually moves into the lamina propria. The endometrial epithelium and stroma close over the conceptus. Implantation is now complete (Fig. 17.42).

As soon as it begins forming, syncytiotrophoblast produces a gonadotrophic hormone similar to hypophyseal LH. The latter is being turned off at about this time by the high progesterone levels from the corpus luteum. This

---

Fig. 17.37. *Vaginal wall.* The vascularity and the muscle bundles (arrows) are characteristic. ×35.

Fig. 17.38. Female *external genitalia.* External view of the female perineum (left). Frontal section through the external genitalia in the plane of the vagina (right).

Fig. 17.39. Diagram illustrating the major morphologic *stages of development* during the first week after ovulation, with the approximate location of the conceptus at each stage.

Fig. 17.40. *Fertilization.* Ovum just after penetration by sperm (arrow). Nucleus of the ovum is in late anaphase or telophase of the second meiotic division. ×560.

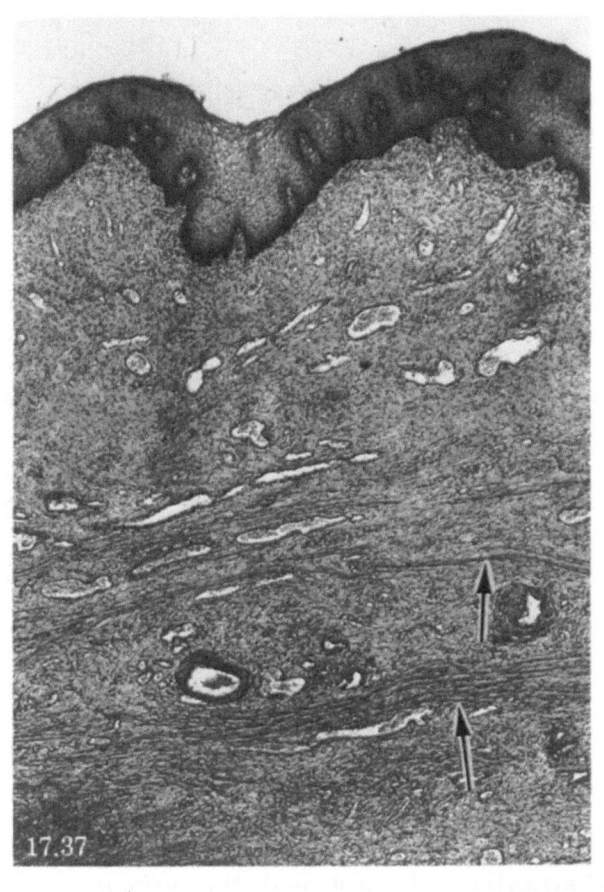

17.37

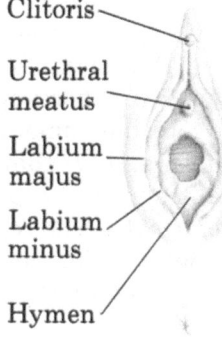

Clitoris

Urethral meatus

Labium majus

Labium minus

Hymen

Cervix

Vagina

Hymen

Labium minus

Labium majus

17.38

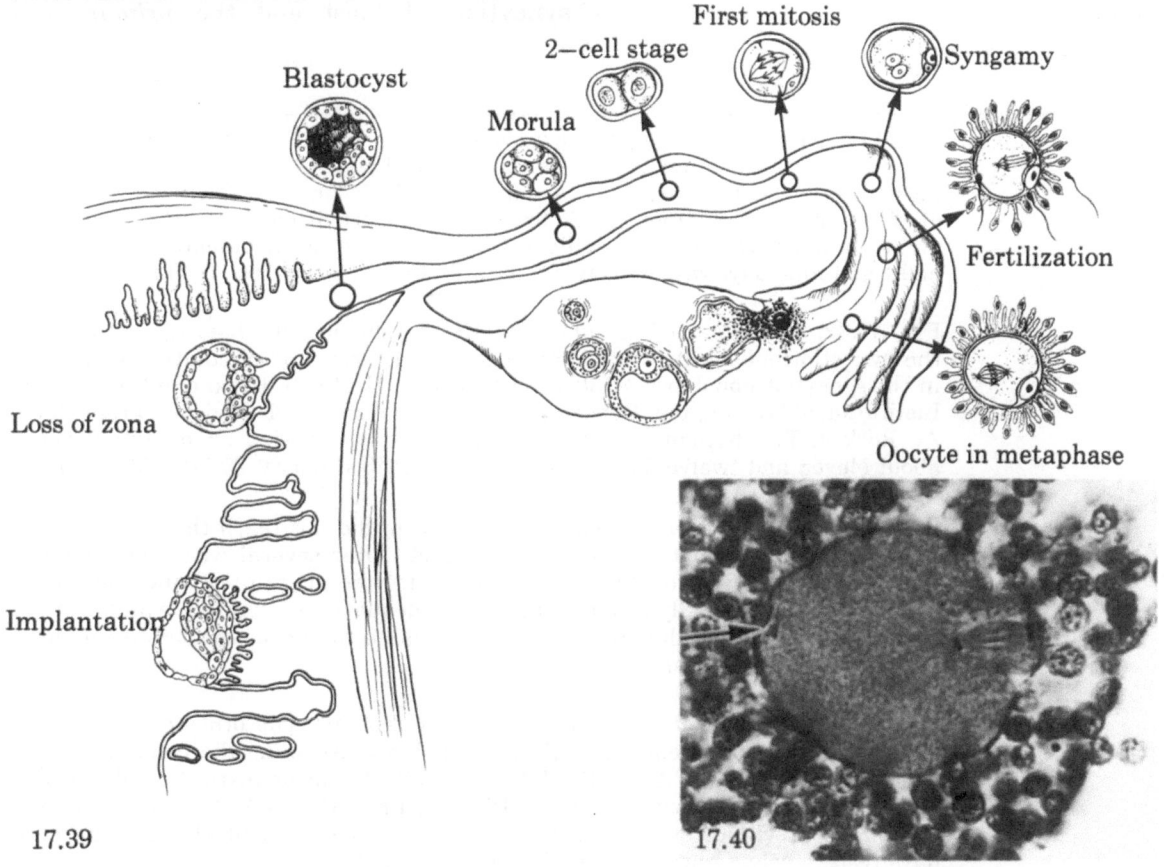

Blastocyst

Morula

2—cell stage

First mitosis

Syngamy

Fertilization

Loss of zona

Implantation

Oocyte in metaphase

17.39

17.40

new hormone is termed *human chorionic go-nadotrophin* (HCG) and, since it is not subject to negative feedback, it keeps the corpus luteum functioning. Indeed it stimulates the further growth of the corpus, which increases its progesterone production. Progesterone inhibits uterine contractility (hyperpolarizes the muscle membrane) and maintains the endometrium for the enlarging conceptus.

The presence of the conceptus splits the endometrial zona functionalis at the implantation site into two components: (1) that portion between the conceptus and uterine lumen, termed the *decidua capsularis,* and (2) that portion between the conceptus and the myometrium, termed the *decidua basalis.* The remainder of the zona functionalis, lining the rest of the uterus, is *decidua parietalis* (Fig. 17.45).

The term decidua refers to something that is (to be) shed. At birth the entire decidua is delivered after the fetus in the last stage of labor. It cleaves from the zona basalis as in menstruation, but all at once, leaving the basalis behind to regenerate a new endometrium.

Placenta

The completed placenta has two components, fetal and maternal. The fetal component consists of the trophoblast-coated *villi (see below).* The maternal component consists of a modified uterine stroma (decidua basalis), and the vessels that deliver and remove blood from the intervillous spaces. The two components interact in some as yet unknown fashion to prevent rejection of this foreign tissue graft, the conceptus.

FETAL COMPONENT. The trophoblast undergoes active cell division and produces on its outer surface a thick coat of syncytiotrophoblast, in which develop irregular channels and spaces (lacunae). During its invasion of the stroma, the syncytiotrophoblast meets and opens endometrial capillaries and venules (Fig. 17.44). These openings allow blood to percolate through the lacunae of the now sponge-like tissue, providing nutrients and gas exchange for the conceptus (Fig. 17.46A). Soon columns of cytotrophoblast cells grow outwards into the extending projections of syncytiotrophoblast and the *primary villi*

Fig. 17.41. *Implantation* of fertilized ovum in endometrium. Syncytiotrophoblast (S) is invading maternal tissue. The cytotrophoblast (C) is still a single layer in most places. ×400. (Courtesy of A. Hertig, J. Rock, and the Carnegie Institution of Washington, Department of Embryology, Davis Division. From Hertig A., Rock J. Two human ova of the previllous stage having a developmental age of about eight and nine days respectively. Contrib Embryol 33:169–186, 1949.)

Fig. 17.42. *Formation of the placenta.* Cytotrophoblast (C) has begun to invade the syncytiotrophoblast (S) and maternal blood (arrow) is circulating in lacunae in the syncytiotrophoblast. ×130. (Courtesy of A. Hertig, J. Rock, and the Carnegie Institution of Washington, Department of Embryology, Davis Division. From Hertig A., Rock J. Two human ova of the previllous stage, having an ovulation age of about eleven and twelve days respectively. Contrib Embryol 29:129–156, 1941.)

Fig. 17.43. *Tubal pregnancy.* The fertilized ovum did not reach the uterine cavity but was implanted in the wall of the oviduct. After several weeks of growth of the conceptus the wall of the oviduct ruptured. Note placenta (P) and embryo (E). Such pregnancies usually lack the support of adequate decidual tissue and, whether because of this or another reason, they are liable to end in serious hemorrhage. ×5. (Courtesy of A. Stier.)

Fig. 17.44. *Trophoblast* (T) eroding a blood vessel (V). The other cells bordering the vessel are stromal endometrial cells which are assuming the form of decidual cells. ×330. (Courtesy of A. Hertig, J. Rock, and the Carnegie Institution of Washington, Department of Embryology, Davis Division. From Hertig A., Rock J. Two human ova of the previllous stage, having an ovulation age of about eleven and twelve days respectively. Contrib Embryol 29:129–156, 1941.)

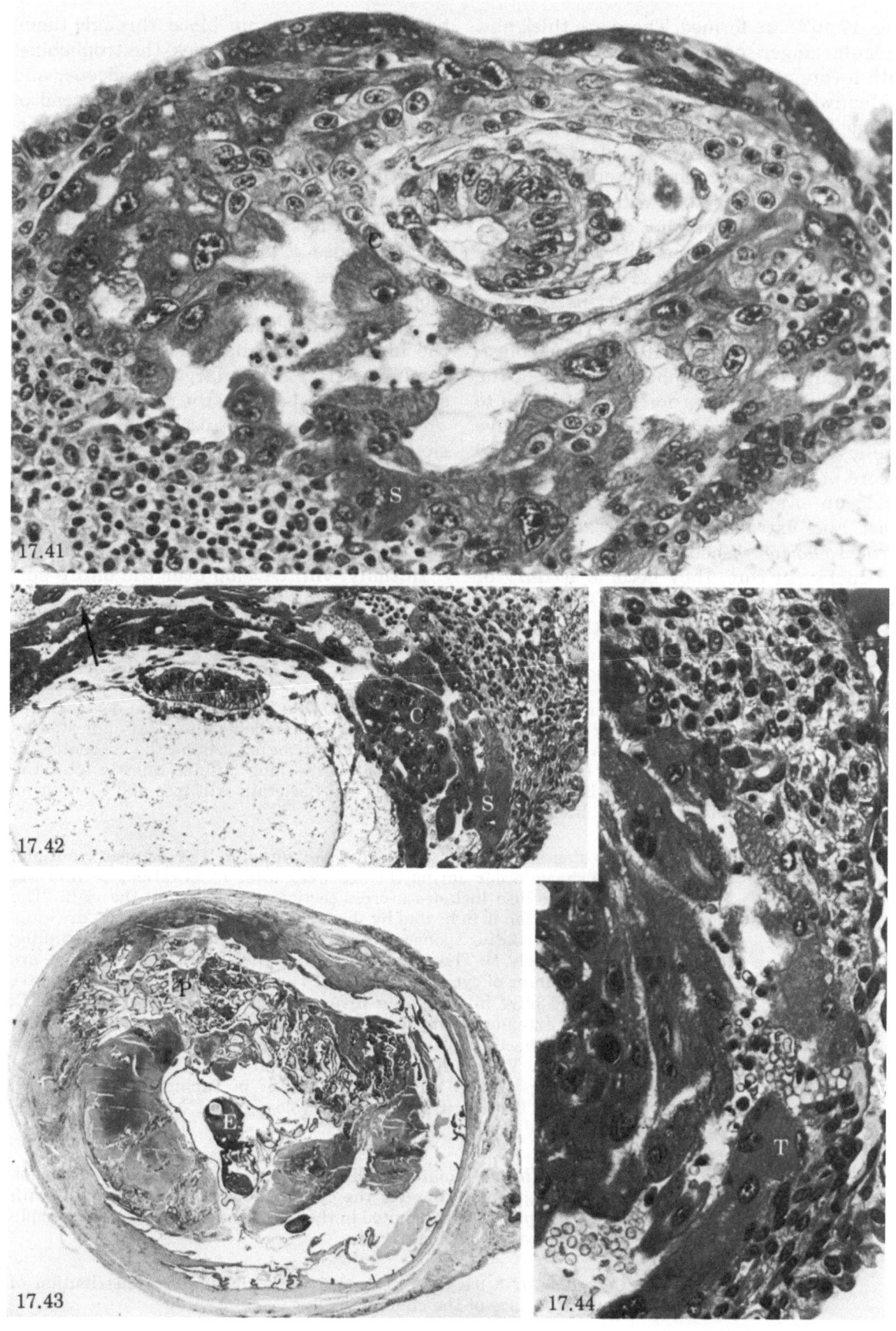

17.41

17.42

17.43

17.44

(Fig. 17.46B) are formed. These are thick and irregular fingers of syncytiotrophoblast, each with a core of cytotrophoblast.

Meanwhile, on its inner surface, the cytotrophoblast has been producing another population of cells to line the blastocyst cavity. This is the extraembryonic mesenchyme. This layer contains cells that will soon arrange themselves into endothelial channels to connect with each other and with blood vessels developing in the embryo. They will in this way provide vascular connections between embryo and villi. The mesenchyme, visibly different from its parent cytotrophoblast, pushes into the cytotrophoblast cores of the primary villi. This invasion converts them to secondary villi (Fig. 17.46C), which now have two layers of trophoblast on the surface and a core of mesenchyme. The composite layer, made up of syncytiotrophoblast, cytotrophoblast and extraembryonic mesenchyme, is termed chorion. When vessels appear in the mesenchymal core, they become tertiary or definitive villi (Fig. 17.46D, 17.47, and 17.49). At about the time this occurs, the embryo's heart begins to pump blood through them.

As the conceptus enlarges, the trophoblast facing the decidua basalis pushes deeper and taps some of the spiral arterioles instead of the capillaries and lacunae encountered earlier. Blood is now delivered forcefully and in pulsating spurts into the syncytiotrophoblast-lined spaces among villi. The chorionic plate, the more or less flat surface from which villi are suspended, is pushed away and the intervillous spaces are enlarged by the increased blood flow. Anchoring villi, firmly attached by syncytiotrophoblast to the decidua, keep the fetal and maternal compartments from coming apart. Each enlarged space fed by a spiral arteriole becomes the cavity of a cotyledon. A cotyledon is a grossly visible subdivision of the placenta containing, in addition to the anchoring villi, numerous floating villi suspended in maternal blood. These floating villi arise from the chorionic plate and from the sides of the anchoring villi (Fig. 17.49).

Initially, villi develop over the entire surface of the conceptus (Fig. 17.48). However, the opportunity for the trophoblast to contact

---

Fig. 17.45. Diagrams of the pregnant uterus to illustrate the general development of deciduae and placenta. Deciduae, derived from endometrium, are indicated by hatched lines. A: At first villi are uniformly distributed around the conceptus. B: Later they are limited to the side facing the decidua basalis. Shortly after the stage shown in B, the deciduae capsularis and parietalis will fuse and the uterine lumen will be obliterated.

Fig. 17.46. Four stages in the development of the placenta. The changes are rapid; all of the stages shown occur during the 3rd week after fertilization. Each of the 4 stages of this figure also includes a cross section of a villus on the right. The plane of each cross section is indicated by the transverse line in the main drawing. A: The conceptus has a coating spongework of syncytiotrophoblast that is beginning to erode maternal vessels. B: The partitions in the syncytiotrophoblast sponge are being invaded by columns of cytotrophoblast. C: The cytotrophoblast columns have reached decidua and have in turn been invaded by columns of mesenchyme. D: Cytotrophoblast has extended along decidua-syncytiotrophoblast boundary to make a complete cytotrophoblastic shell around the conceptus. Syncytiotrophoblast lines maternal blood spaces. Vessels have differentiated in the mesenchymal cores of the villi. (Based on Figs. 1, 2, 3, and 4, pp. 66 and 67 in Tuchmann-Duplessis H., David Y., and Haegel P. Illustrated Human Embryology, Vol. 1. New York, Springer-Verlag, 1972.)

Fig. 17.47. Placental villi. a: Immature villi with a peripheral double row of nuclei, one for the syncytiotrophoblast, one for the cytotrophoblast. b: Mature villi with more blood vessels peripherally distributed in the villus and clumping of the peripheral nuclei in the syncytiotrophoblast. ×250.

Fig. 17.48. Conceptus at 5 weeks of gestation. Note the uniform distribution of villi over the entire surface of the chorion.

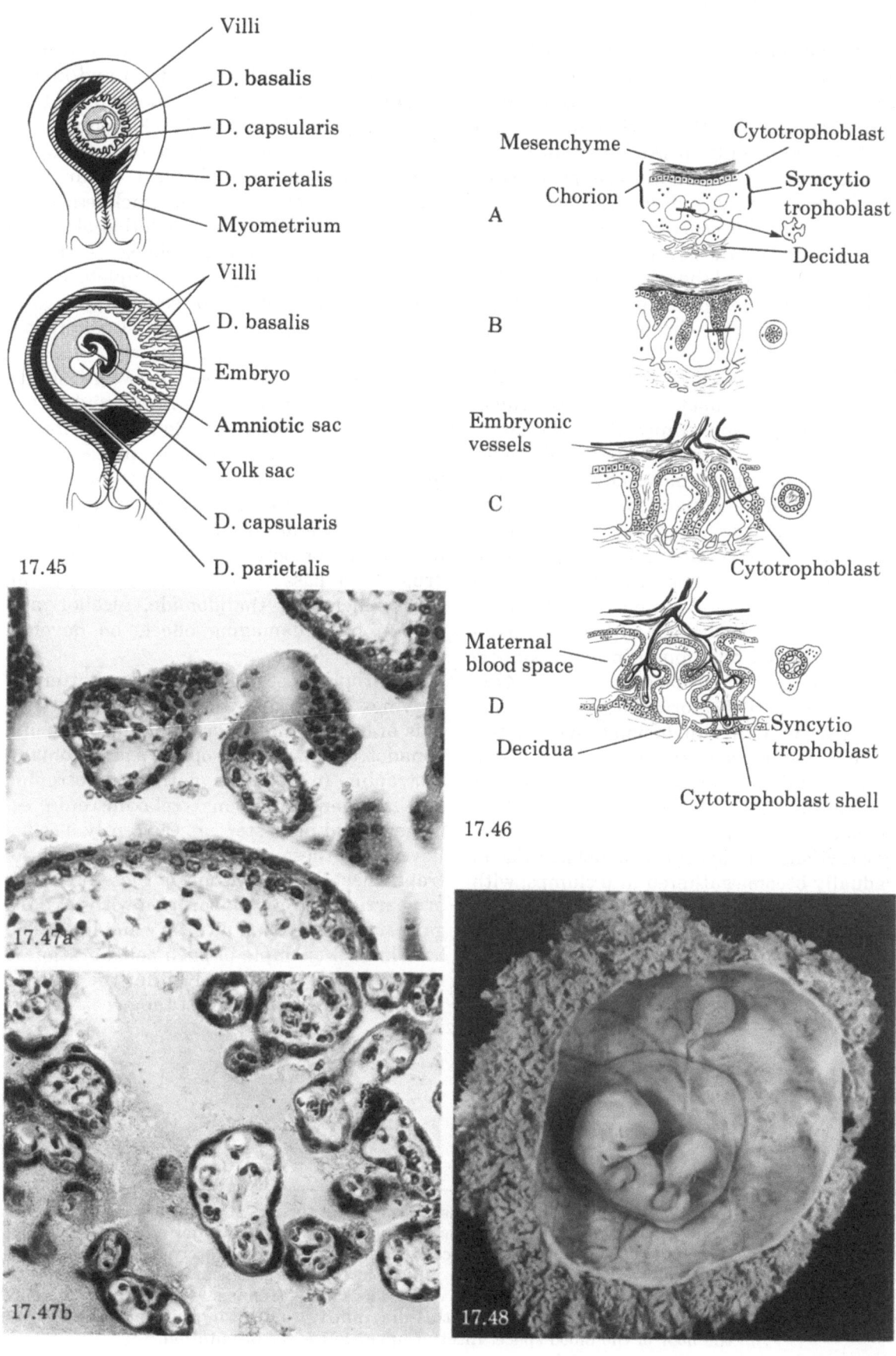

Villi
D. basalis
D. capsularis
D. parietalis
Myometrium

Villi
D. basalis
Embryo
Amniotic sac
Yolk sac
D. capsularis
D. parietalis

17.45

Mesenchyme
Chorion
Cytotrophoblast
Syncytio trophoblast
A
Decidua

B

Embryonic vessels
C
Cytotrophoblast

Maternal blood space
D
Decidua
Syncytio trophoblast
Cytotrophoblast shell

17.46

17.47a

17.47b

17.48

spiral arterioles is of course limited to the area of the decidua basalis. The decidua capsularis is stretched thin as the enlarging conceptus balloons into the uterine lumen. Villi develop further only in the direction of the decidua basalis; the others disappear. Thus the chorion is bald and smooth over much of its surface (the *chorion laeve*), and thick and bushy toward the decidua basalis (*chorion frondosum*). Around the periphery of this disc of chorion frondosum the decidua basalis is firmly attached to the chorion, forming a continuous ring known as the marginal zone. When fully developed the placenta is a disc about 18 cm in diameter and 2.5 cm thick.

The histologic appearance of the definitive villi changes during the life history of the organ (Fig. 17.47). In the mesenchymal core the vessels, initially simple loops, sprout new branches, thus increasing blood supply to the villi. The vessels become more peripheral in each villus and therefore closer to the maternal blood. The original mesenchyme becomes loose connective tissue, but without the array of differentiated cells found in adult connective tissue. In a young placenta (Fig. 17.47a), the proliferation of cytotrophoblast for a time keeps pace with the conversion to syncytiotrophoblast. Later, proliferation lags behind and, by the middle of pregnancy, cytotrophoblast is becoming scarce. In the last trimester of pregnancy it is difficult to find any in histologic sections. The syncytiotrophoblast nuclei gradually become gathered into clumps, with long stretches of attenuated cytoplasm between them (Fig. 17.47b). These clumps may occasionally fuse with those of neighboring villi, forming trophoblastic bridges across the intervillous space.

In summary, during the first half of pregnancy, the barrier between fetal and maternal blood consists of endothelium of fetal capillaries, basal lamina of endothelium, connective tissue, basal lamina of cytotrophoblast, and syncytiotrophoblast. Near *term* (the end of pregnancy), the thickness is reduced to endothelium, endothelial basal lamina and syncytiotrophoblast. Although the barrier always appears complete in sections, there is evidence of some exchange of blood cells between mother and fetus, particularly toward the end of pregnancy.

All materials exchanged between mother and fetus must cross these layers and a very large array of substances do so. All three of the basic physiologic transfer processes are utilized: diffusion, facilitated diffusion, and active transport. Respiratory gases, metabolic wastes, nutrients, hormones, and antibodies pass in one or both directions. A number of drugs also pass into the fetal circulation; many, including thalidomide, alcohol, and heroin, have damaging effects on development.

The trophoblast contains a large battery of enzymes appropriate to its many functions. It is of course an endocrine organ producing gonadotrophins, thyrotrophin, a somatomammotrophin (a hormone with somatotrophic and lactogenic functions), relaxin, renin, estrogens, and progesterone. Currently it is believed that these are all products of syncytiotrophoblast. Probably some of these functions are carried out in collaboration with fetal organs such as adrenal, pituitary and liver. The best known example of such collaboration is that of estriol synthesis. Neither the fetus or the placenta contains all of the necessary en-

Fig. 17.49. Diagrammatic reconstruction of a portion of a *mature placenta*. One simplified cotyledon with villous tree is shown. The decidual surface, including the septa between cotyledons, is coated with trophoblast. Maternal blood is injected into the blood space around the villi from more or less centrally located arteries and drained away in peripheral veins. The villous tree is suspended from the chorionic plate by its "trunk." In this diagram two anchoring villi are attached to the floor of the blood space. Inset at upper left is for orientation.

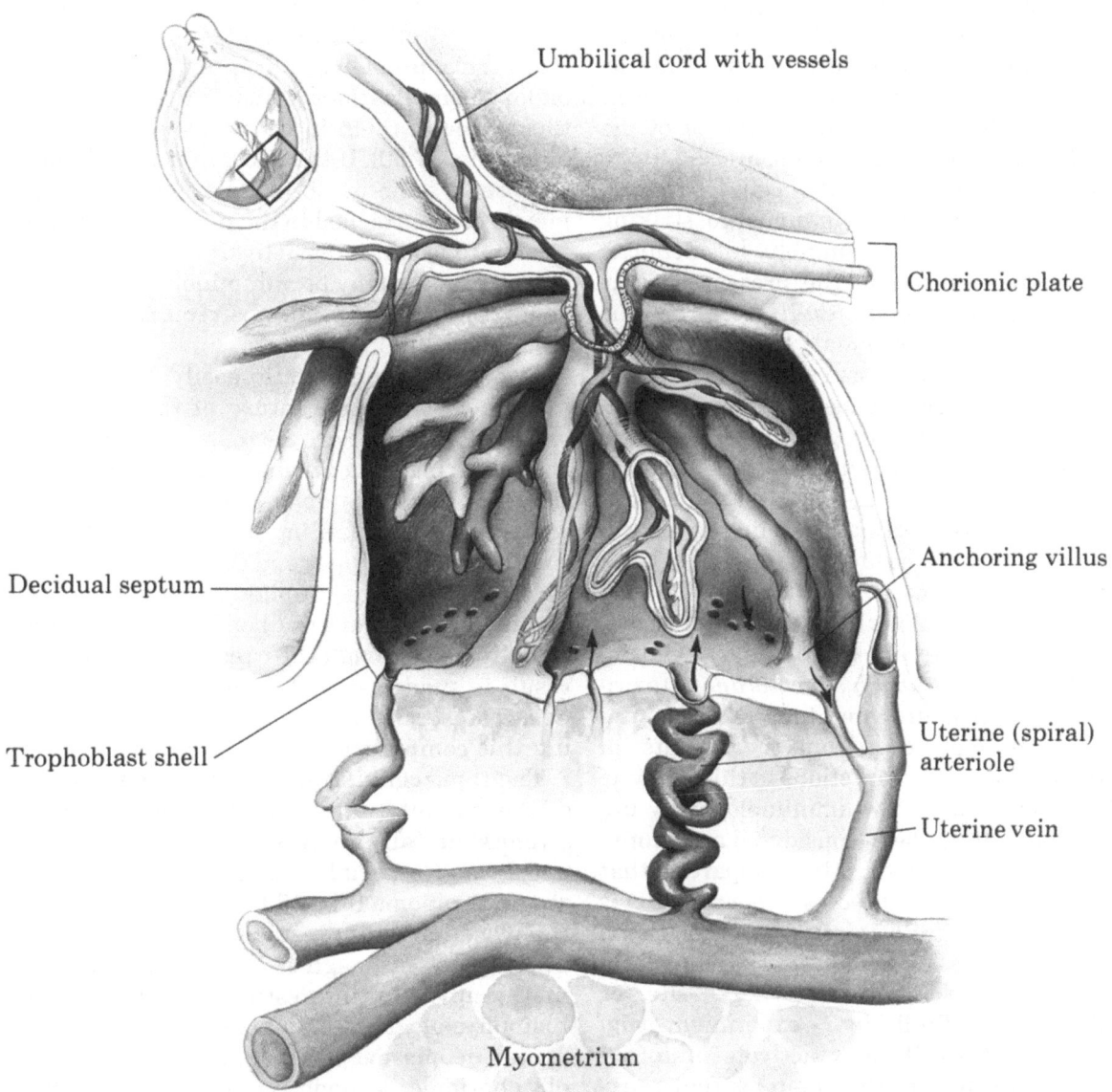

Umbilical cord with vessels

Chorionic plate

Decidual septum

Anchoring villus

Trophoblast shell

Uterine (spiral) arteriole

Uterine vein

Myometrium

17.49

388   Female Reproductive System

zymes for synthesis of this estrogen. The fetal adrenal produces a steroid precursor in the form of a sulfate, and the placenta contains the sulfatase necessary for the final step in producing the estriol. Thus a concept of the *fetoplacental unit* has developed.

MATERNAL COMPONENT. The cells of the endometrial lamina propria undergo striking morphologic, and presumably biochemical, changes in response to the presence of trophoblast. They, as *decidual cells,* become much enlarged, polygonal, epithelioid cells with vacuolated cytoplasm and a vesicular nucleus with a large nucleolus. They contain large quantities of glycogen and lipids. It is possible that they participate in collaborative activities with the fetal-placental unit. However, at this time almost nothing is known of the function of this large population of cells.

FETAL-MATERNAL TISSUE JUNCTION. At the zone of contact between fetal and maternal tissues, there gradually develops a thin layer of fibrin-like material (*Nitabuch's membrane*). Its origin, basic structure and functions are unknown. It may represent the results of antigen–antibody interactions in this the zone of contact between two immunologically unlike tissues. It has been considered an "immunologic no man's land." It is apparent that the allograft represented by the conceptus is not immunologically rejected as other tissue grafts would be. Ectopic pregnancy indicates that the uterus is not a privileged site for such a "graft." Preliminary experiments suggest that fetal cells may activate maternal suppressor cells and thus help prevent rejection.

It is remarkable that this hastily constructed system works as reliably as it does and yet that it can be discarded so easily when its job is done. Of course it does not always work this well. There are several potential mechanical problems and quite a range of secondary complications which may arise from these. One of them is known as placenta accreta (Fig. 17.50). If the decidua is incomplete or absent, some or all of the anchoring villi may become attached to the myometrium and unable to separate at delivery. Hemorrhage, due to tearing, may be voluminous and emergency hysterectomy may be required to control this.

Two other dangers, also easily understood in concept from the nature of the placenta and its formation, are retroplacental hemorrhage and placenta previa. In the latter condition the blastocyst implants low in the uterine cavity and the enlarging placenta may eventually cover the upper end (internal os) of the cervical canal. This implies that a tear must be made in the placenta before the fetus can be delivered through the canal. This also may result in sudden large loss of maternal blood. Cesarean section is the usual means of avoiding this complication.

The rapid cellular proliferation and growth of the placenta, its vascularity and its invasiveness are all prominent characteristics of neoplasms, especially malignant ones. The choriocarcinoma (Fig. 17.51), a malignancy of the placenta, is a devastatingly rapidly growing cancer—although it is amenable to chemotherapy. An interesting and important histophysiologic relationship is that placental neoplasms secrete excessive amounts of chorionic gonadotrophin (HCG). This fact affords a relatively simple and reliable test by which to clinically follow the progress, or the response to treatment, of such tumors.

Fig. 17.50. *Placenta accreta.* a: ×33. b: There is no decidua and villi (arrows) are degenerated and embedded in solid amorphous mass of old blood clot (B) lying directly on the myometrium (M). ×110. (Courtesy of F. Vellios, K. Ireland, and the American Society of Clinical Pathologists.)

Fig. 17.51. *Choriocarcinoma,* a rapidly progressive cancer originating in germ cells. Like its normal counterpart, this tumor is always extremely vascular and therefore hemorrhagic. a: Multiple hemorrhagic metastases in the liver. b: Cytologic criteria of malignancy (nuclear enlargement, hyperchromatism, variability) are obvious. Note the appearance of syncytio- (S) and cyto- (C) trophoblast and adjoining blood-filled spaces (B). ×250. (Courtesy of F. Vellios, K. Ireland, and the American Society of Clinical Pathologists.)

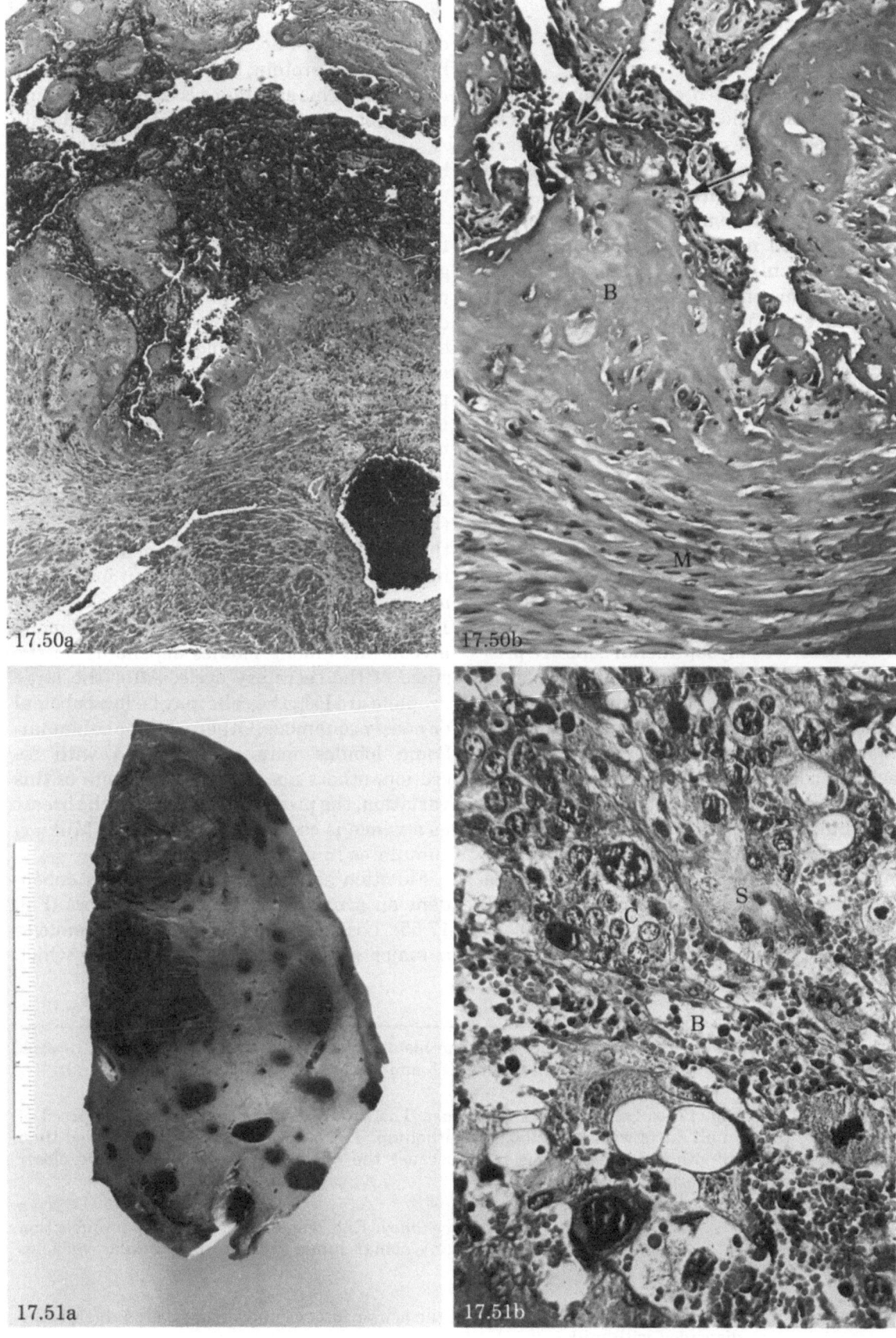

17.50a

17.50b

17.51a

17.51b

Breast

The breast, as pointed out in Chapter 11, is composed of modified sweat glands and its basic histology is described there. Changes in the breast that occur during pregnancy and lactation, however, are described here.

The glandular components of the breasts in the mature nonpregnant woman consist largely of ducts (Fig. 17.52). The tiny lobules containing their terminal ducts are separated by variable amounts of interlobular connective tissue and fat.

ACTIVE MAMMARY GLAND (Fig. 17.53). As the blood level of estrogen rises during pregnancy, further growth, proliferation and budding of ducts take place; with the added influence of progesterone, acini develop. Somatotrophin, prolactin, some adrenal steroids, thyroxin, and insulin are also necessary for complete development and function of the mammary gland. By the middle of pregnancy, the lobules are expanded with closely packed, small, empty acini. Their epithelium is cuboidal and scattered myoepithelial cells are present. Different lobules in the same gland show rather striking differences. Some may be well developed and packed with alveoli, while others may still appear inactive. Intervening stages of course may also be present in the same section. As development proceeds, the interlobular connective tissue and fat are reduced and compressed to septa between adjacent lobules. By the end of the second trimester of pregnancy, although some alveoli will be added, epithelial growth is nearly complete. Most breast enlargement after this is due to scattered accumulations, not of milk, but of a high-protein, low-fat secretion termed *colostrum*. This substance contains type A immunoglobulin (IgA), antibodies and vitamin A, and is an effective laxative. It is the newborn "starter" food for 2–3 days after birth, until milk production begins.

LACTATING MAMMARY GLAND (Fig. 17.54). In lactation the secretory activity is intense. One gram of mammary tissue may produce 1–2 ml of milk per day. The cells have features characteristic of protein-secreting cells, i.e., extensive RER, large Golgi, and apical, membrane-bound, secretory vesicles containing protein, along with lactose added by the Golgi. In addition to proteins, sugars and minerals, milk contains large amounts of fat. The fat appears in the cytoplasm in the form of lipid droplets. When these reach the cell surface, they acquire a coating of plasmalemma as they are extruded into the lumen. The large lipid droplets in the cells are seen in sections as apically located, empty vacuoles (Fig. 17.54b). The epithelium varies greatly among alveoli and among lobules depending on the stage of the secretory cycle. After the large droplets are lost, the cells may be low cuboidal or nearly squamous. Others may be columnar. Some lobules may be distended with secretion, others nearly empty. In spite of this variation, the production of milk by the breast as a whole is essentially continuous. Milk accumulates in alveoli and ducts.

Function as well as development is dependent on a number of endocrine factors (Fig. 17.55). Loss of the placenta at birth removes a major source of several hormones which

---

The figures on this plate show the histology of the breast at three stages. In each case the figure on the left is at ×85 and that on the right at ×250.

Fig. 17.52. Section of *resting breast*. The small scattered lobules are composed of small ducts with low cuboidal epithelium. This appears more deeply stained than the other figures on this plate because the nuclei are more compact and closer together.

Fig. 17.53. The *breast during pregnancy*. Enlargement and cellular proliferation in the lobules have produced many acinar lumens. Some intracellular vacuoles are present.

Fig. 17.54. *Lactating breast*. Both the acinar lumens and vacuoles are larger, being distended with milk.

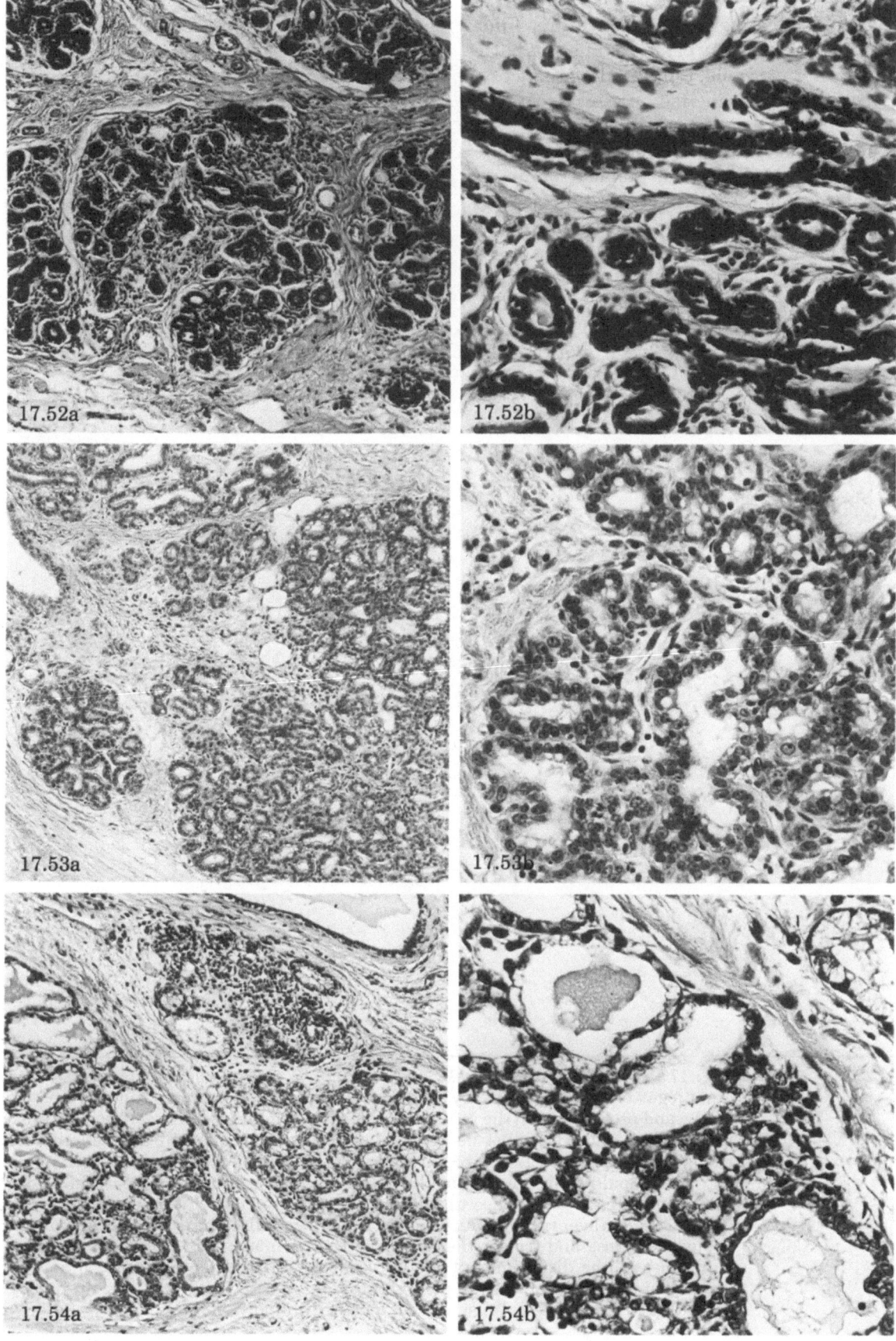

have been affecting maternal pituitary function. Suckling, by way of afferent neural pathways from the nipple, inhibits the production of prolactin inhibiting factor (PIF) by the hypothalamus. Therefore pars distalis increases its output of prolactin. Suckling also suppresses the production of gonadotrophin-releasing hormone (GRH) so that ordinarily ovulation and menstruation are inhibited as long as breast feeding continues. However, occasionally ovulation, and sometimes an unexpected pregnancy, may occur.

Suckling is also responsible for the movement of milk out of the alveoli and through the ducts to the nipple. Sensory endings in the nipple give rise to afferent impulses which ascend through spinal cord pathways to the hypothalamus. Here they synapse with cells of the paraventricular nuclei. Impulses pass down the hypothalamohypophyseal tract to the pars nervosa, to initiate release of oxytocin stored there as Herring bodies. In response to oxytocin in the circulation, myoepithelial cells around the alveoli and ducts contract. Milk is thus delivered to the dilated portion (*lactiferous sinuses*) of the large ducts near the nipple from which it is drawn by the suckling infant.

Fig. 17.55. The *control of growth and function* of the mammary gland. Estrogen and progesterone from the ovary stimulate the growth of the ducts and acini respectively, and prolactin from the pituitary acidophils stimulates milk secretion. Thyroxine, cortisol, and STH must be present for normal development and function although their specific actions are not clear. The release of oxytocin is brought about by nerve impulses initiated by suckling. These impulses pass through spinal nerves to the spinal cord and thence up the cord to increase the synthesis of oxytocin by cells of the paraventricular nucleus. From here impulses pass down the axons to the pars nervosa and trigger the release of the hormone from Herring bodies into capillaries at the distal ends of the nerve fibers. Milk is moved to the nipple by the action of oxytocin from the pars nervosa on myoepithelial and smooth muscle cells. The major hormonal factors are indicated in heavier lines.

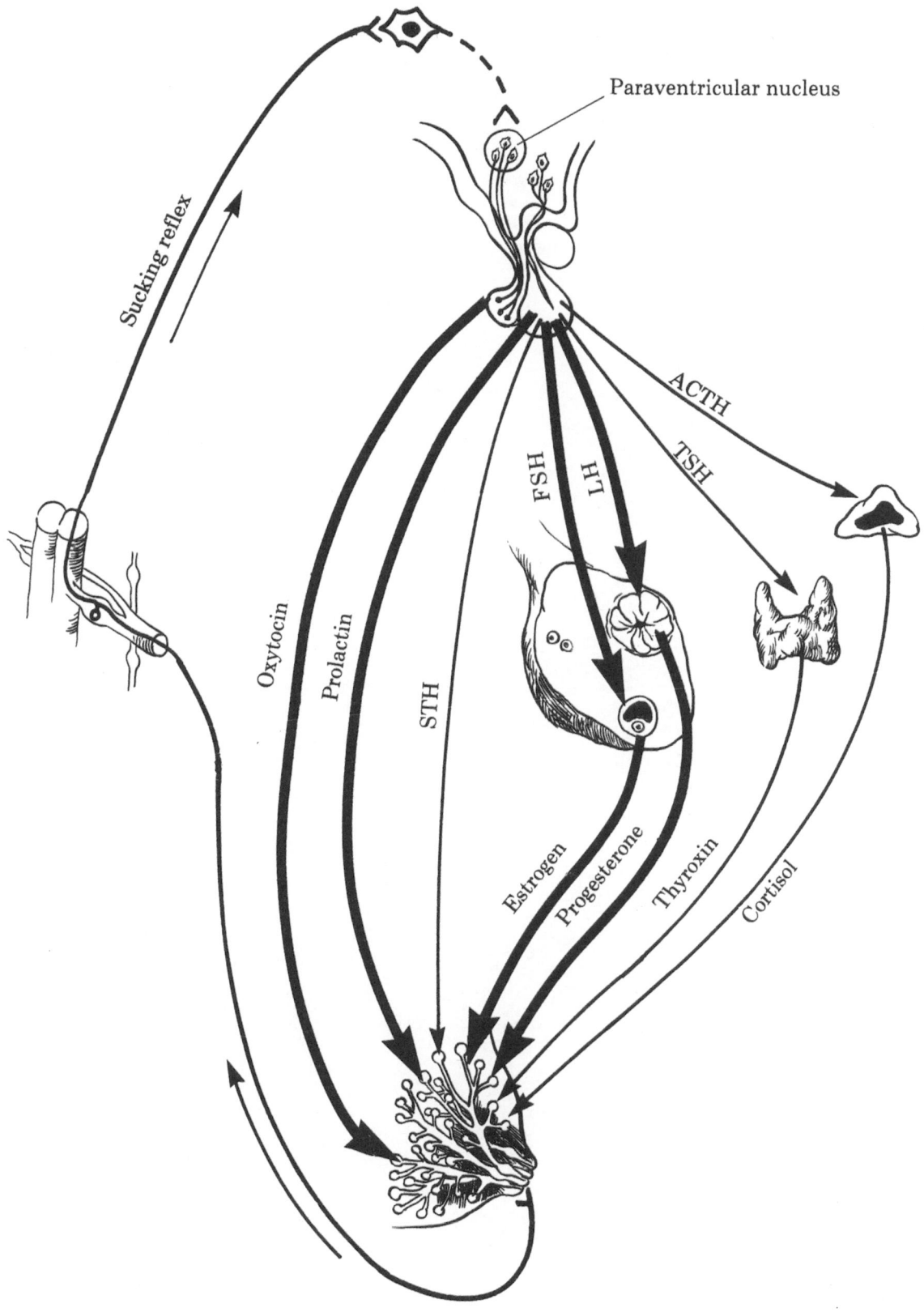

Paraventricular nucleus

Sucking reflex

ACTH

TSH

FSH

LH

Oxytocin

Prolactin

STH

Estrogen

Progesterone

Thyroxin

Cortisol

17.55

18 Male Reproductive System

Introduction

The male reproductive system (Fig. 18.1) consists of paired primary sex organs, the *testes*, and a series of secondary sex organs. The secondary organs are the (paired) *rete testis*, the *ductuli efferentes, vas deferens, seminal vesicle* and *bulbourethral gland*, the (single) *prostate gland*, and *penis*. The secondary organs are so called because they are dependent on a hormone (*testosterone*) from the testes for development and maintenance of their structure and function. In addition, there are secondary sex characters, such as hair and fat distribution, form of the laryngeal cartilages and of the pelvis, and sexual behavior patterns, which are also dependent on testosterone.

The various components of the male reproductive system develop from diverse embryonic tissues in widely separate areas, and, by differential growth and migration, make structural and functional contact with each other. This developmental complexity predisposes to a variety of congenital malformations. The differentiation of the system during intrauterine life is dependent on interaction between the component tissues and on the maternal and fetal hormones. This differentiation is completed only after puberty with the development of hypothalamohypophyseal function. Maturation of the male reproductive system must be coordinated with that of the nervous system. The nervous system is an important target of fetal androgens in order that behavior, years later, will be appropriate for function of the system.

Testis

The testis is a paired, firmly encapsulated, compound tubular gland whose parenchyma is incompletely subdivided by tenuous connective tissue septa into about 250 lobules. It is both an endocrine gland, producing testosterone and possibly other steroids, and an exocrine gland, producing sperm cells (spermatozoa).

Gross Relations

Although the testis originates in the urogenital ridge on the dorsal body wall high in the embryo's abdomen, before birth it has ordinarily shifted into a small outpouching of the peritoneal cavity that has extended into a pouch of skin, the *scrotum*. Each pocket of peritoneum projecting from the abdominal cavity is a processus vaginalis (Fig. 18.2a). Its connecting channel normally closes to isolate it from the abdominal cavity (Fig. 18.2b). The lining is the *tunica vaginalis*. Each testis is suspended in its serous cavity in the same fashion as an abdominal organ is suspended in the peritoneal cavity, that is, in a fold of the wall. Thus there is a visceral tunica vaginalis and a parietal tunica vaginalis.

During development the processus vaginalis has carried with it the layers of the abdominal wall that lay in front of it. Therefore, outside of the parietal tunica vaginalis, among other layers, is a thin sheet of striated muscle derived from the internal oblique muscle of the abdominal wall. This sheet is the *cremaster muscle* (Fig. 18.1 and 18.3). In addition to coating the parietal tunica vaginalis, it forms a muscular investment of the group of testicular blood vessels, lymphatics, nerves, and the ductus deferens, all of which have been carried along by the descending gonad. The cremaster muscles, by lowering the testes or lifting them closer to the abdomen, help to regulate the temperature of the gonads, which is an important determinant of sperm development. Testing of the cremasteric reflex (lifting of the testis on stimulation of the medial surface of the thigh) is a routine part of the physical examination. The cremaster will be seen in histologic sections of the *spermatic cord*, which includes all of the structures passing to the scrotum through the inguinal canal. In addition to the ductus deferens, the cord contains the testicular artery, which is surrounded by an anastomosing network of testicular veins, the *pampiniform plexus*. The artery and veins form a countercurrent exchange system that helps to keep the testicular temperature about 2 degrees lower than that of the rest of the body, and also helps to maintain a higher concentration of testosterone in the testis than in the rest of the body.

Stroma

The stroma of the testis consists of a capsule of dense connective tissue (*tunica albuginea*) underlying the visceral tunica vaginalis. The capsule has a thickened portion (the *mediastinum*) on the posterior surface of the organ.

Fig. 18.1. Drawing of a portion of the *male reproductive system* seen from the ventral aspect.

Fig. 18.2. Diagram of development of *processus and tunica vaginalis*. **a:** Extension of the peritoneal cavity through the inguinal canal into the scrotum. **b:** Closure of the upper portion of the processus vaginalis isolates the lower portion from the parent peritoneal cavity.

Fig. 18.3. Cross-section of *spermatic cord* with ductus deferens (D), spermatic artery (A) in the midst of a group of veins, the pampiniform plexus, and cremaster muscle bundles (C). ×11.

Fig. 18.4. *Testis and epididymis.* Capsule (C), rete (R), head (H) and body (B) of epididymis, ductus deferens (D) and trabeculae (arrows). ×35.

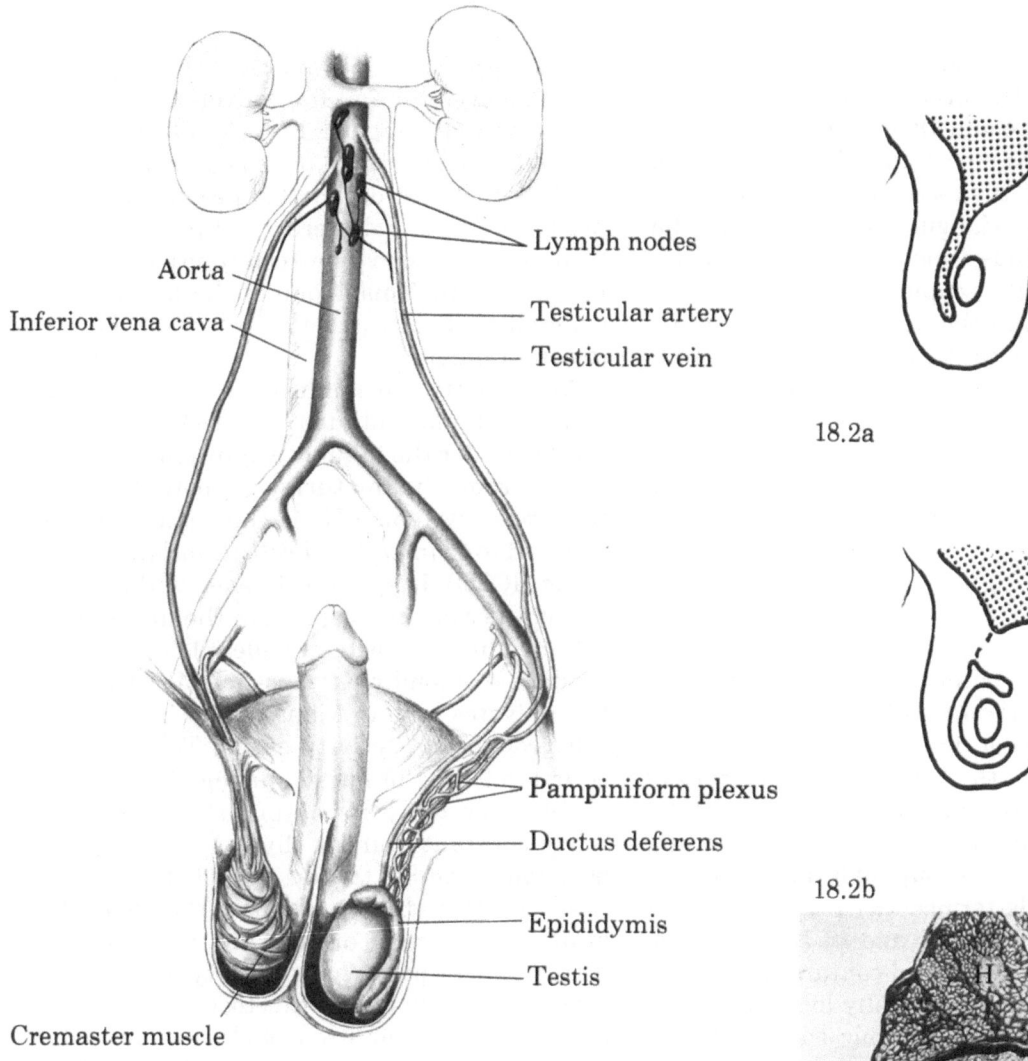

Aorta

Inferior vena cava

Lymph nodes

Testicular artery

Testicular vein

Pampiniform plexus

Ductus deferens

Epididymis

Testis

Cremaster muscle

18.1

18.2a

18.2b

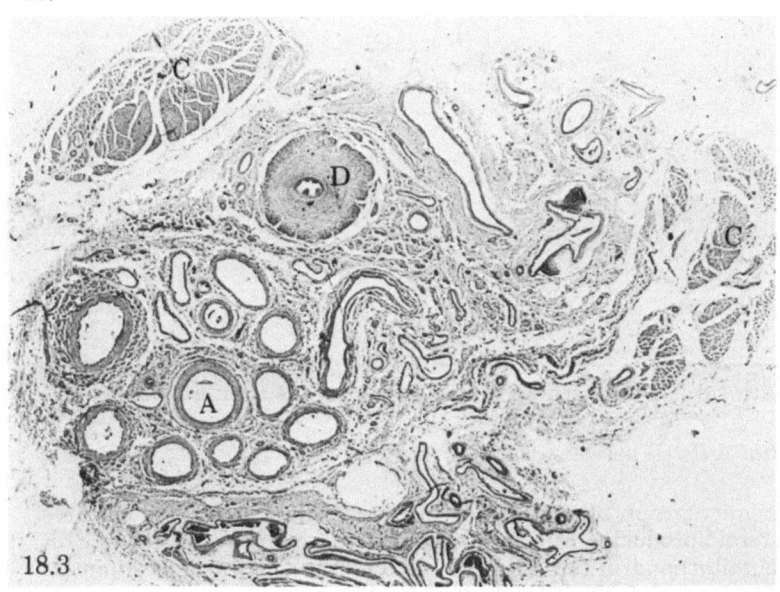

18.3

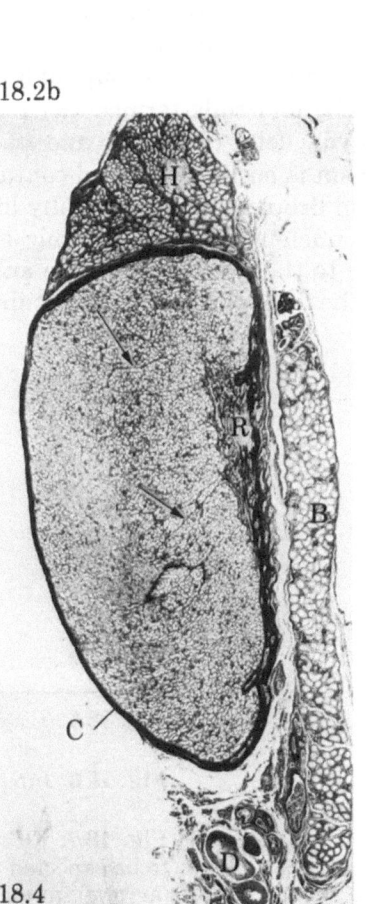

18.4

Numerous *septa* radiate from the mediastinum through the organ to the tunica albuginea (Figs. 18.4 and 18.5). They are thin and incomplete, only partially dividing the parenchyma into the testicular lobules.

The roughly triangular areas among adjacent seminiferous tubules (*see below*) of the parenchyma are occupied by richly vascularized, loose connective tissue, which contains the testosterone-secreting cells, in addition to the usual array of connective tissue cells. This is the endocrine portion of the testis. The vessels of the capillary network are lined with fenestrated endothelium and there is also an unusually rich supply of lymphatic vessels.

Parenchyma

The testicular parenchyma includes endocrine *interstitial cells* (of Leydig) and *seminiferous tubules* (Fig. 18.5).

INTERSTITIAL CELLS. From about 10 weeks of fetal life until the end of gestation, and then again after puberty, the interstitial connective tissue contains groups of large, polygonal, epithelioid cells termed the *interstitial cells* (Leydig cells) (Figs. 18.6 and 18.7). Their cytoplasm is eosinophilic and contains numerous lipid droplets and a centrally located, spherical nucleus. The cytoplasmic eosinophilia is due to the presence of large amounts of SER in the form of anastomosing tubules. The SER contains the enzymatic machinery for synthesis of cholesterol and for conversion of pregnenolone to androgens. Mitochondria are numerous and have tubular, instead of lamellar, cristae. In these organelles pregnenolone is produced from cholesterol, and passed to the SER for conversion to testosterone (the principal androgen). This is one of the best-known examples of intracellular cooperation between organelles.

At puberty this hormone synthesizing equipment differentiates and produces testosterone, under the influence of luteinizing hormone from the maturing hypothalamohypophyseal system. LH in the male is often referred to as *interstitial-cell-stimulating-hormone* (ICSH). It apparently acts, without entering the cell, on receptors in the interstitial cell membrane to activate adenyl cyclase and produce a second messenger, cAMP. The latter activates protein kinases, and interstitial cell growth and activity ensue. Testosterone is first released in bursts during sleep at puberty. Eventually its output stabilizes to a fairly constant diurnal rhythm with a peak between 6 and 8 A.M. and a low between late evening and midnight. Either early differentiation of this system, or interstitial cell tumors may result in precocious puberty, due to the premature production of testosterone. Variations in number and morphology of interstitial cells are associated with endocrine dysfunctions.

Fig. 18.5. *Testis* with tunica albunginea (T) and seminiferous tubules. ×250.

Fig. 18.6. *Interstitial cells* (I) between tubules. ×250.

Fig. 18.7. Electron micrograph of portions of two *interstitial cells*. The features to be expected in steroid-producing cells are present; that is, large amounts of SER (arrows), numerous mitochondria (M) with tubular cristae, and variable numbers of lipid droplets (L). About ×10,000. (Courtesy of N. Alexander.)

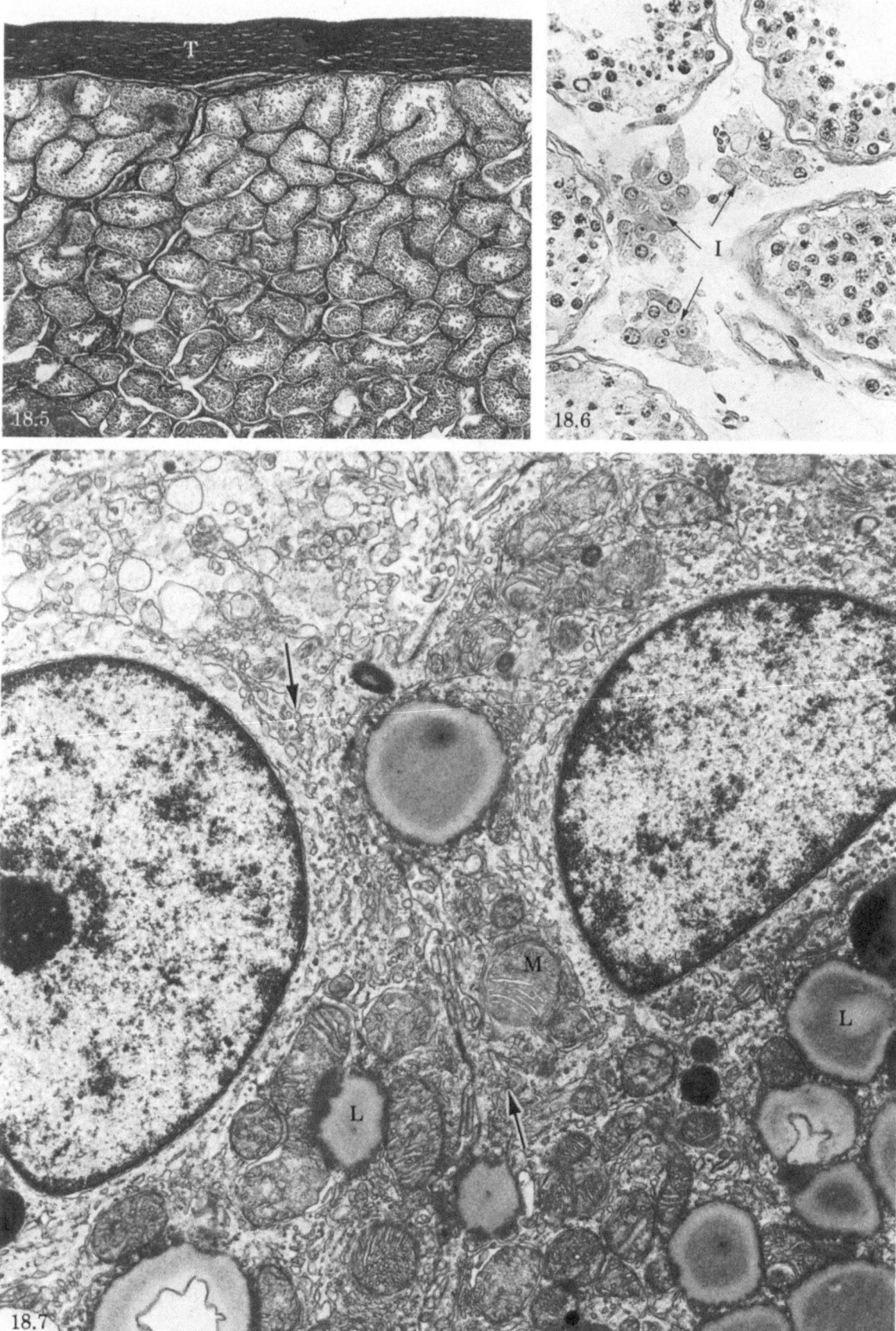

SEMINIFEROUS TUBULES. Each seminiferous tubule is about 30–70 cm in length; the caliber varies from about 150 to 300 μm, though it is fairly constant in each individual. Each of the (about) 250 lobules contain approximately 1.2 m of tubule. Thus each testis contains about 300 m of tubule, enough to assure the production of the 100 million or so spermatozoa in each of the 3 or 4 ml of the average ejaculate. This astonishing number is required for fertilization, even though only one sperm is successful. If this number falls markedly, the individual is usually, but not always, sterile. There are few if any blind-ending tubules; loops and terminal connections with the terminations of neighboring tubules are common. Each tubule has a *spermatogenic epithelium* resting on a complex *basement membrane,* and is modified at its downstream end to form a straight tubule. The spermatozoa pass through the straight tubules (tubuli recti) into a meshwork of epithelium-lined spaces (the *rete testis*) in the dense connective tissue of the mediastinum to reach the extra-testicular ducts. We will describe the tubules from the outside toward the lumen to follow the sequence of sperm cell differentiation from basal to luminal surfaces.

Basement membrane. This structure is termed the *boundary layer* because it differs somewhat from the usual organization of a basement membrane. A well-developed basal lamina is present. External to this is a tenuous reticular lamina with numerous scattered flat cells, the innermost of which are contractile and termed *myoid cells.* The thickness of the basement membrane increases with age and often in systemic illness.

Spermatogenic epithelium. The epithelial lining of tubules consist of: (1) tall, irregular, columnar or pyramidal cells (*Sertoli cells*) that extend from the basement membrane to the lumen, and; (2) several layers of cells in various stages of spermatogenesis (*see later*). In sections examined with the light microscope, cytoplasm and all cell outlines are obscure. However, the nuclei are clear and distinctive and make the identification of the various cells reasonably simple.

Sertoli cells (Figs. 18.8 and 18.9). These

large cells are adherent to the basement membrane. In spermatozoa that have reached the last stages of development, the heads are buried in deep indentations of the apical (luminal) surface of the Sertoli cells, and the tails extend into the lumen. The lateral surfaces of Sertoli cells are deeply pockmarked with indentations into which are fitted the earlier forms of developing spermatozoa. As these earlier spermatogenic stages mature, they are moved toward the lumen; thus the plasmalemmal pockets in which each developing germ cell is contained moves apically with its contained cell. The Sertoli cell transports nutrients imported from the interstitial space through its cytoplasm to nourish the developing germ cells. Materials discarded from the germ cells are phagocytosed and disposed of by Sertoli cell lysosomes.

In ordinary sections of testis, Sertoli cells are easily identified by their large, clear, oval nuclei with dark nuclear envelopes and sharply stained nucleoli. The electron microscope shows extensive SER, abundant mitochondria and lysosomes, and large Golgi apparatus. These are obviously busy cells.

Just internal to the basal lamina, each Sertoli cell is joined to its neighboring Sertoli cells by a zonula occludens and gap junctions. Thus, in effect, this zone of occluding junctions forms a continuous barrier all around the tubule (Fig. 18.8). This divides the tubule into a *basal compartment* below the zone of junctions, and an *adluminal compartment* above the zone of junctions. This barrier accounts for the fact that many substances present in blood and tissue fluids are not present in fluid sampled from testicular tubular lumens. Only substances that Sertoli cells will absorb and pass around this barrier are transmitted between basal and adluminal compartments. This block to free passage to and from the lumen of the tubule is the *blood–testis barrier.* As germ cells differentiate into spermatozoa, they develop specific surface antigens. If these were to have free access to the general circulation, the immune system would produce antibodies that would be returned to the testes and react with the developing germ cells (Fig. 18.10). Even if sperm

antigens do get into the circulation (and some individuals have antisperm substances in their serum), antibodies cannot ordinarily enter the tubules to impair fertility by destroying spermatozoa or their precursors.

An additional Sertoli cell function is to secrete a fluid that is absorbed in the extratesticular ducts. This absorption produces a current in the tubules that carries the nonmotile sperm out of the testes. In addition, Sertoli cells, in response to FSH, synthesize and secrete *androgen-binding protein.* This protein is secreted into the lumens of the tubules and binds testosterone, thus assuring a high concentration of the androgen in the seminiferous tubule. High levels of testosterone are required here for adequate spermatogenesis.

Spermatogenic cells. The cells of the spermatogenic epithelium, which are eventually to give rise to the spermatozoa, are crowded together between Sertoli cells. The earliest stages are applied to the basement membrane in the basal compartment of the tubule, while more mature stages are arranged in developmental sequence toward the lumen. Studies with tritiated thymidine have shown that, in the human testis, the entire process from spermatogonium to mature spermatozoa takes just about 64 days.

Spermatogenesis (Fig. 18.11 and 18.12) is the process by which spermatozoa are produced from undifferentiated germ cells. The stem cells in this sequence are the *spermatogonia.* As in most epithelia, they are located close to the basement membrane. They consist of two types. The A spermatogonia divide by mitosis and serve as a continuing source of germ cells. Eventually some A spermatogonia produce somewhat different appearing cells, the B spermatogonia, which enlarge greatly and become *primary spermatocytes.* All of the daughter cells of a given spermatogonium remain connected by thin, intercellular bridges until they are shed into the lumen as spermatozoa. This probably helps to account for the high degree of synchrony in the stages of cells grouped together in the epithelium. It will be noticed that, in a tubule section, all the cells in a cluster of, say, primary

Fig. 18.8. *Sertoli cells and the blood–testis barrier.* Drawing shows two complete and two incomplete Sertoli cells and their relations to each other and to the stages of spermatogenesis. A short distance above the basal lamina, the Sertoli cells are joined by tight junctions, thus creating the blood–testis barrier. Spermatogenic cells occupy deep pockets in the plasmalemma of the Sertoli cells. All cells derived from a single spermatogonium remain connected by intercellular bridges until they are mature spermatozoa. Three stages in spermiogenesis are also shown, progressing from left to right.

Fig. 18.9. *Sertoli cells,* made more apparent because of severe atrophy of the spermatogenic cells. ×250.

Fig. 18.10. *Sperm granuloma,* a reaction of macrophages and lymphocytes to the "foreign" antigen in sperm (the small dark cells in the photograph), which have escaped from the lumen of the genital tract into the surrounding tissue due to some defect or rupture in the wall. ×250.

Fig. 18.11. Tubules with normal *spermatogenesis.* Spermatogonia (Sg), primary spermatocytes (P), spermatids (Sd) and Sertoli cells (Se). ×300.

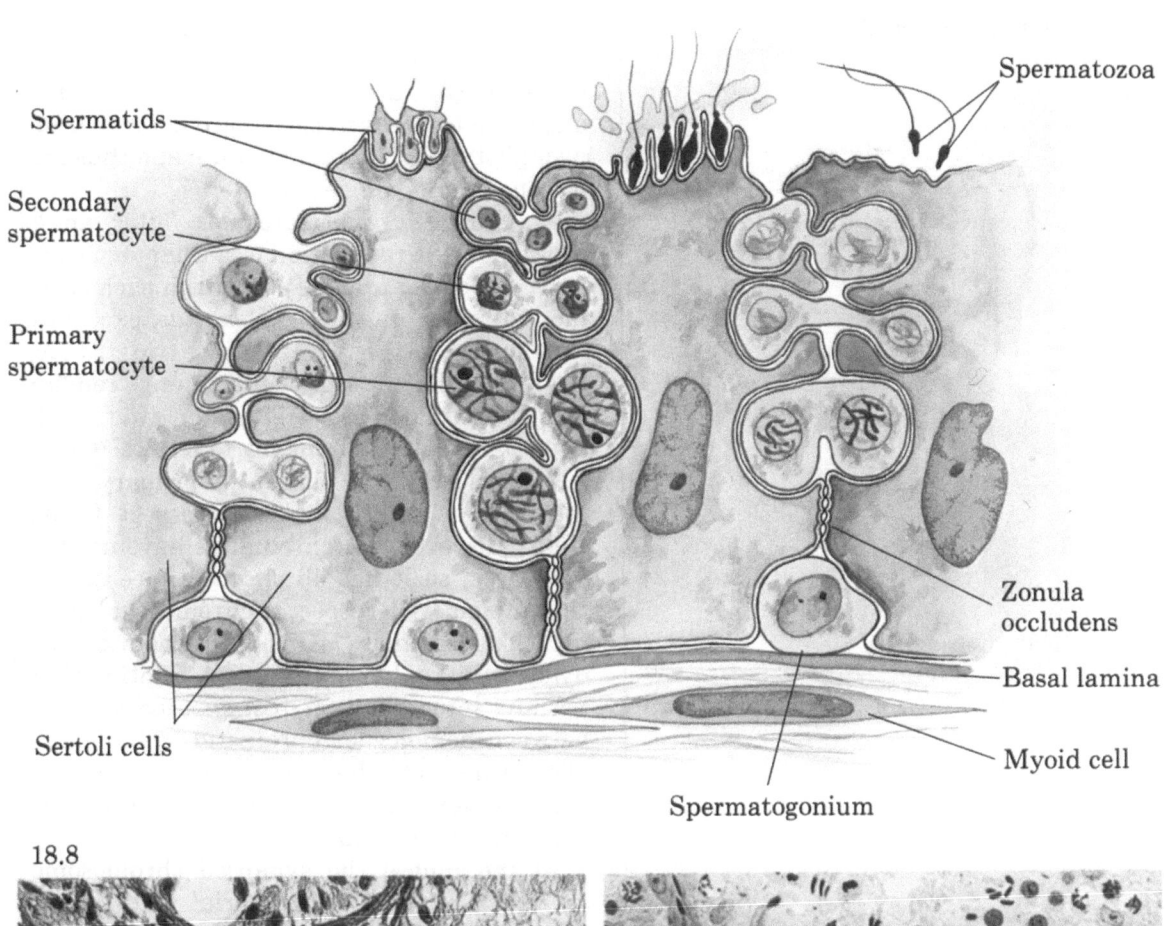

Spermatids

Secondary
spermatocyte

Primary
spermatocyte

Spermatozoa

Zonula
occludens

Basal lamina

Sertoli cells

Myoid cell

Spermatogonium

18.8

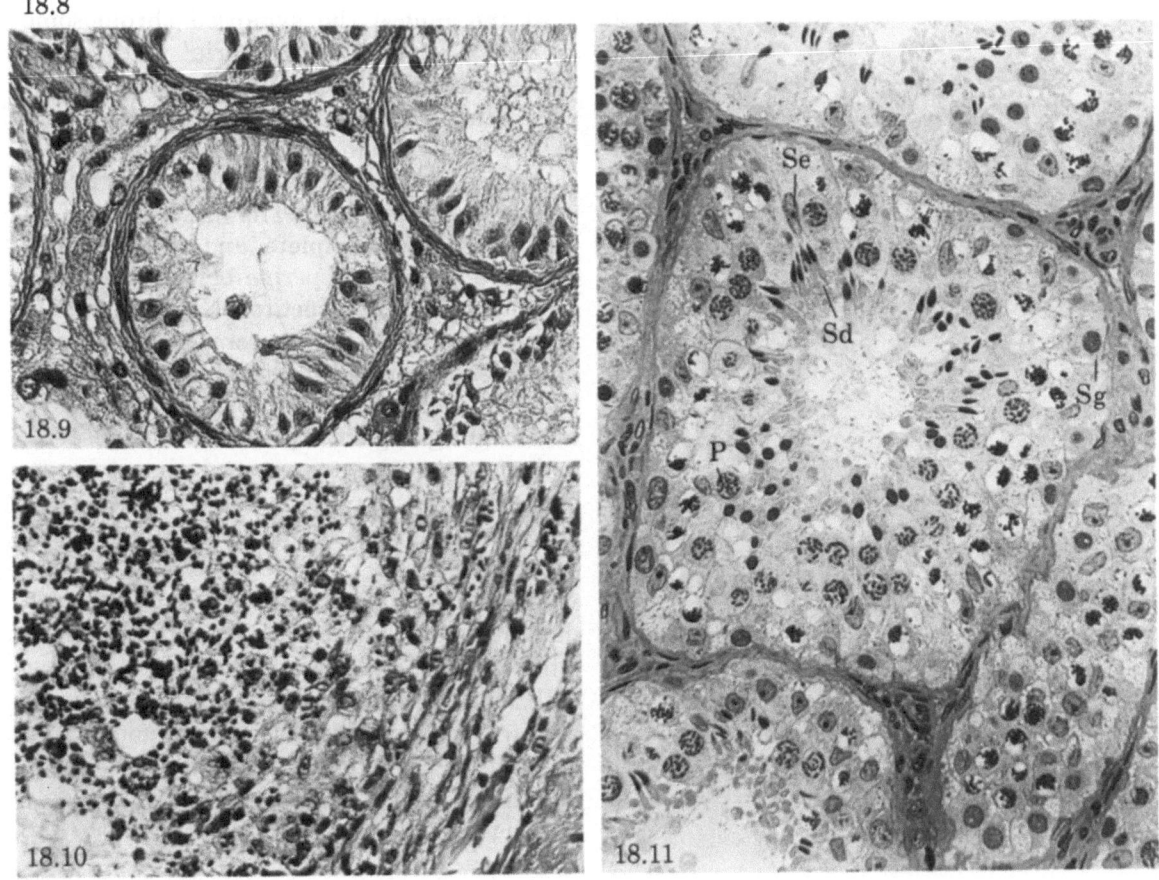

18.9

18.10

18.11

spermatocytes are in almost exactly the same stage. All the cells in such a group arose from a single type A spermatogonium and thus are a clone from a single ancestor.

The primary spermatocytes, after an S phase of DNA replication (see Chapter 2), enter a prolonged prophase in which each chromosome splits into two *chromatids*, except at the *centromere* (Fig. 18.12). These two strands, held together at the centromere, remain tightly associated as a *bivalent* or *dyad*. Each dyad pairs with its homolog to form a *tetrad*. At the end of the S phase, the primary spermatocyte is tetraploid with respect to its DNA. However, the chromatids have not yet separated, so it has 46 chromosomes and is thus diploid with respect to chromosome number. The intimate pairing of homologous dyads is termed *synapsis*, an association that permits interchange (*crossing-over*) of genes between homologous chromatids. The points of crossing-over, where chromatids are temporarily innerconnected during the exchange, are termed *chiasmata*.

At metaphase the synapsed chromosome pairs line up on the equatorial plate of the division spindle. Microtubules of the spindle attach to the centromere of each dyad. In anaphase, the two homologous centromeres separate from each other and each dyad is pulled into a daughter cell. The first division of meiosis is now complete and the daughter cells are *secondary spermatocytes*. These are diploid ($2n$) with respect to DNA, and haploid (n) with respect to chromosome number, since daughter chromatids are still united by their centromeres.

Without going through G_1 or S stages, secondary spermatocytes proceed almost immediately to the second meiotic division. The chromosomes line up at the equator and the spindle develops. The centromeres now divide, as in mitosis, and in anaphase each daughter centromere and the chromosome of which it is a part are pulled into a daughter cell. These daughter cells are the *spermatids*, and are haploid (n) in both chromosome number and DNA content. Now they begin the astounding series of morphologic changes by which they are converted to spermatozoa (Fig. 18.13).

Spermiogenesis is the term applied to this transformation. Its goal is to provide each cell with the biochemical and structural equipment required for sustained swimming and for penetration of an egg. Spermiogenesis also allows these cells to discard all components not needed for these or later functions. For this purpose, a sequence of five steps takes place.

(1) The Golgi apparatus becomes closely applied to the nucleus. One of its vesicles enlarges, develops a dense internal granule, and assumes the shape of a cup fitted over one pole of the nucleus. This, the *acrosome*, is a specialized lysosome. It contains the proenzymes to be activated at fertilization, and then released from the sperm. These enzymes bring about separation of corona cells and digest a path through the zona pellucida about the ovum.

(2) The paired centrioles migrate to the pole opposite the developing acrosome to control the development of the flagellum (tail). Here one of the pair is involved in the assembly of tubulin subunits into the usual arrangement of pairs of microtubules; thus it becomes the basal body of the flagellum. The microtubules grow out from the caudal end of the cell, carrying a plasmalemmal investment with them. The fate of the other centriole is not clear.

(3) As the flagellar microtubules stretch the cell, mitochondria shift position so as to lie alongside these tubules, and then finally become wound around them in a spiral pattern. This region, containing the mitochondria, becomes the *middle piece* of the completed spermatozoon. The mitochondria provide the energy for flagellar movement. Substrates for their enzymes are provided by the components of reproductive tract fluids, since in the mature spermatozoon there is no storage space for such materials. Ordinarily sperm do not swim until after storage and maturation in the epididymis.

(4) The chromatin in the nucleus becomes so densely packed into its characteristic flattened, oval form that no internal structure can be seen. It is so reduced in size that it is finally not much larger than the nucleolus of some cells.

(5) The final step is the shedding of all cytoplasm and of all of the Golgi except the acrosome. These components are not absolutely required by the spermatozoon. This material is pinched off as the unfortunately called residual body* which is phagocytosed by the Sertoli cell. The mature spermatozoon is now free, and is swept down the tubule and out of the testis by movement of fluid. It will come to a halt in the epididymis, where biochemical maturation will be completed and where it will remain until ejaculated. The structure of the mature spermatozoon is best presented graphically (Fig. 18.13D).

Identifying features other than position, of the spermatogenic cell types observed with the light microscope are seen in their nuclei. The spermatogonial nuclei lie next to the basement membrane, and are generally similar to nuclei of other epithelia. The next nuclei above are those of the primary spermatocytes, which are the largest nuclei in the spermatogenic series. The chromosomes in different cell clusters may be seen in the various stages of condensation that occur during the long prophase. Because of the approximately 22-day length of this prophase, large numbers of the cells seen in the tubule are primary spermatocytes. Secondary spermatocytes are rarely seen since they proceed so rapidly through the next division. When found, their nuclei are about two-thirds the diameter of those of primary spermatocytes and are darkly stained. Spermatids show a great range in nuclear appearance, as would be expected from the morphologic changes that occur in spermiogenesis. When first formed, the nuclear diameter is about half that of primary spermatocyte nuclei and less than that of most nuclei seen in other tissues. Reduction in size and increase in staining density continue. Their form changes from spherical to oval to wedge-shaped. Form also varies depending on their orientation in the section. Fully mature sperm, unattached to Sertoli cells or to other sperm of their clone, are rarely seen in sections of human testes. They have already moved on to the epididymis.

_____
* This term also applies to the retained remnants of lysosomal digestion (see Chapter 2).

Fig. 18.12. Simplified diagram of stages of *meiosis*. Instead of attempting to follow all 23 pairs, only a single pair of homologous chromosomes (one derived from each parent) is followed through the process. See text for description.

Fig. 18.13. *Spermiogenesis.* **A:** Young spermatid with an early stage of development of the acrosome from a single Golgi vesicle. **B:** Development of flagellum and further differentiation of acrosome. Beginning of nuclear condensation. **C:** Acrosome has capped the nucleus. Mitochondria are spiraled around the proximal portion of the flagellum. Residual body has been shed. **D:** Mature spermatozoon. (Based on Fig. 23.4 in Junqueira L, and Carneiro, J. Basic Histology. Los Altos, Lange Medical Publications 1980.)

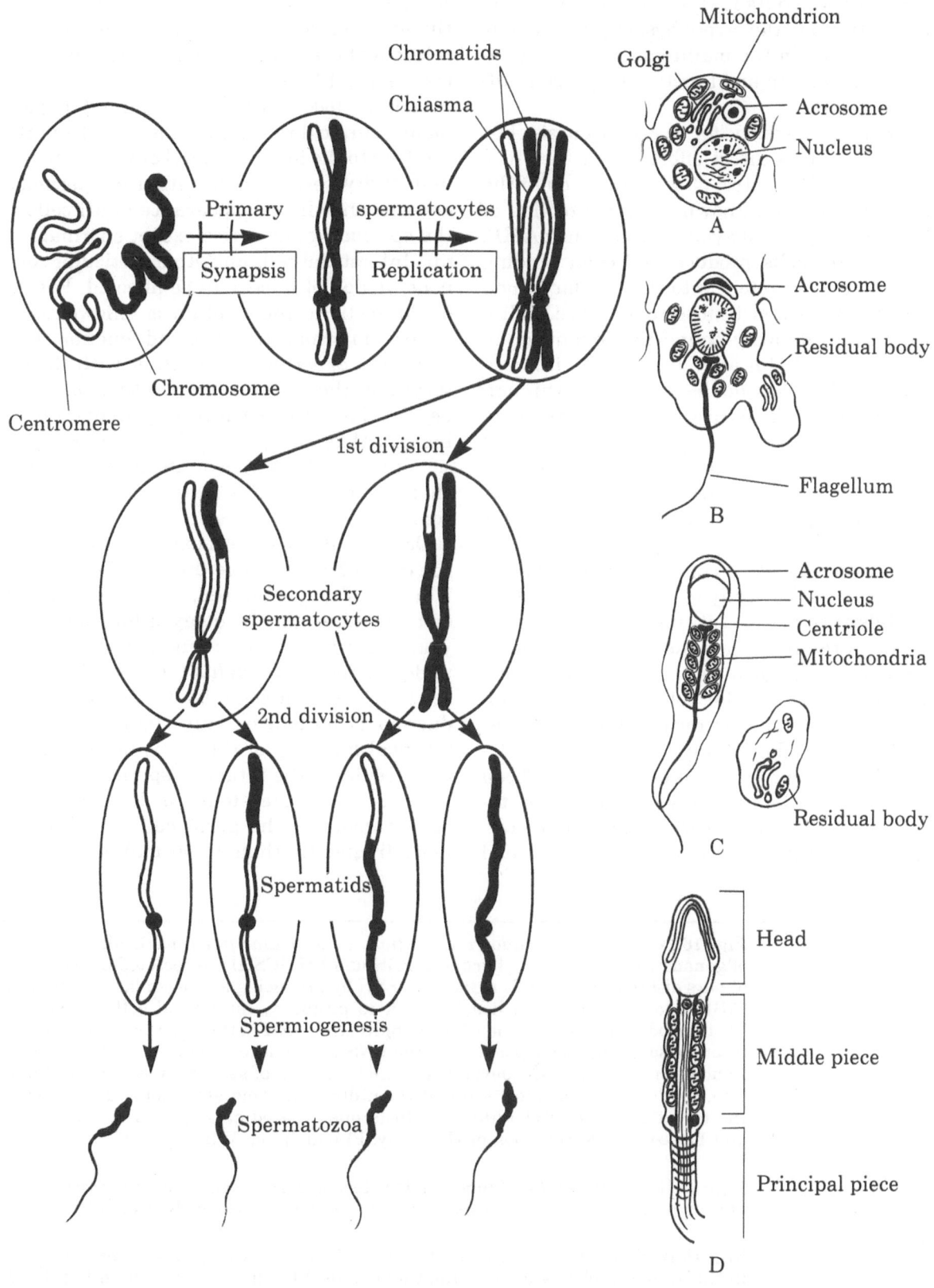

18.12   18.13

ENDOCRINE CONTROL (Fig. 18.14). Both FSH and LH from the hypophyseal pars distalis are involved in the maintenance and regulation of structure and function in the seminiferous tubules.

FSH is necessary for spermiogenesis, but whether this is direct effect or whether it is indirect by its control of some function of the Sertoli cell is not known. Under direction of FSH, by way of adenylate cyclase and cAMP, the Sertoli cells produce androgen binding protein and secrete it into the tubular lumen along with bound testosterone. Since androgens are ordinarily bound to albumin or to a specific globulin after leaving the interstitial cell, they may not be able to pass through the blood–testis barrier without this help from Sertoli cells. Testosterone is needed in the adluminal compartment for maintenance of spermatogenesis, and is carried into the extratesticular ducts in the testicular fluid.

Negative feedback control of FSH is probably channeled directly to the hypophyseal basophils that produce it, instead of indirectly through the hypothalamus. The feedback, or controlling, hormone is thought to be a product from some tubular cells, probably Sertoli cells. This product is termed inhibin. Other actions of inhibin, if any, are obscure.

LH, the other functions of which have been discussed earlier, is involved indirectly in tubular function since testosterone from its target (interstitial cells) is required for normal spermatogenesis. Feedback control of hypothalamic production of LH(gonadotrophin)-releasing hormone is brought about by testosterone (see Fig. 18.4).

TEMPERATURE CONTROL. In animal experiments, surgical relocation of a testis from the scrotum to the inguinal canal or to the abdominal cavity results in cessation of spermatogenesis, and the disappearance of all cells of the spermatogenic series except spermatogonia. Interstitial cells and other testicular components do not appear to be affected. Return of the testis to the scrotum is followed by a return of normal structure and function. This and other experiments, together with the observation that scrotal temperature is 1 or 2 degrees lower than basal body temperature, indicate that male germ cells are temperature sensitive. Little is known about the physicochemical basis for this need for a lower environmental temperature.

Occasionally a natural experiment imitates the one described above (Fig. 18.15). In about 1 or 2% of male children, the descent of one or both testes may be delayed for months or years, or it may never occur. Biopsies of such undescended (*cryptorchid*) testes show absence of spermatogenesis. Testosterone production is normal or only slightly reduced. Surgical lowering of the testis into the scrotum results in the return of spermatogenesis. Undescended testes tend to develop malignant tumors of the germ cells (Fig. 18.16), more frequently than do normal ones.

Fig. 18.14. *Neural and endocrine relations in testicular function.* Under direction of gonadotrophin-releasing hormone, FSH and LH (ICSH) are secreted by basophils of pars distalis. Sertoli cells respond to FSH by producing androgen-binding protein (ABP) and inhibin, which has feedback to pituitary. Interstitial cells respond to LH by producing testosterone which suppresses LHRH in the hypothalamus. Testosterone also affects other portions of the CNS in the development of male behavior. In addition it controls the development and function of secondary sex organs (prostate, seminal vesicles, etc.), some of them directly, some after being converted in the target tissue to DHT (dihydrotestosterone). (Based on Fig. 32.37 in Bloom W. and Fawcett, D. A Textbook of Histology. Philadelphia, WB Saunders, 1975.)

Fig. 18.15. A *cryptorchid* (undescended) testis. Sertoli cells and interstitial cells appear normal; spermatogenesis is absent. ×130. (Courtesy of K. Ireland.)

Fig. 18.16 *Seminoma* (a germ cell tumor of the testis). Lymphocytes are abundant in this tumor, probably because the tumor cells, like the spermatozoa in Fig. 18.11, are "foreign" antigens outside of the normal boundaries. ×130. (Courtesy of K. Ireland.)

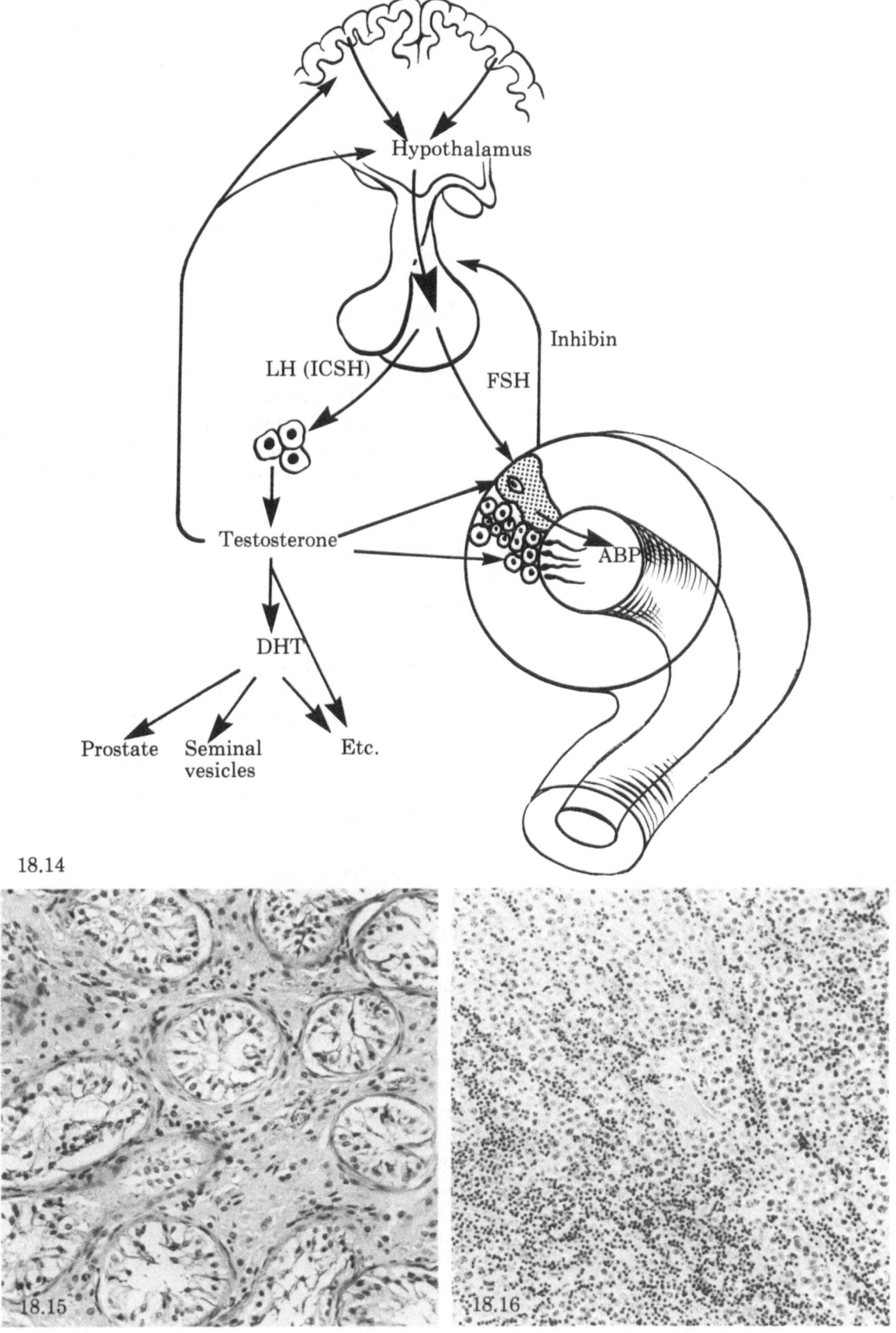

Hypothalamus

LH (ICSH)

FSH

Inhibin

Testosterone

ABP

DHT

Prostate   Seminal   Etc.
           vesicles

18.14

18.15

18.16

Ducts

The duct system can be divided into intratesticular and extratesticular portions (Fig. 18.17). The former include the *tubuli recti* and *rete testis;* the latter include *ductuli efferentes, epididymis,* and *ductus (vas) deferens.* Each of these structures has a different embryologic origin; it is remarkable that during development they make such constant and dependable connections to complete this complex passageway.

Tubuli recti (Straight Tubules)

Rather suddenly, as a seminiferous tubule approaches the mediastinum of the testis, its germinal cells disappear and only Sertoli cells remain. These give way after another short distance to low columnar or cuboidal cells. The tubule then enters the mediastinum where its epithelium become continuous with that of the rete.

Rete Testis

This structure (Fig. 18.18) is rather like a flattened sponge. It consists of numerous, flat, roughly parallel, interconnected spaces in the dense mediastinal connective tissue. The epithelial lining varies from simple cuboidal to simple squamous. Some of these cells may be equipped with a single flagellum.

Ductuli Efferentes

These channels (Fig. 18.19), of which there are about a dozen, lead obliquely upward from the rete, beginning at the outer surface of the mediastinum. Each is derived from an embryonic mesonephric nephron, from which the renal corpuscle has been removed. They conduct sperm superiorly and posteriorly around the curvature of the testis. At the posterior-superior portion of the testis, each becomes very tortuous and is packed into a cone-shaped package whose apex is pointed toward the testis. These are the coni vasculosi. The total assembly of these 12–15 coni is held together by connective tissue and is covered by visceral tunica vaginalis. This constitutes the *head* (caput) of the epididymis. The epithelium of these tubules is variable in height. Areas of low columnar or cuboidal cells alternate with groups of tall columnar cells. This arrangement gives the characteristic appearance in sections of a folded lining. Many but not all of the cells are ciliated. There is a very thin layer of smooth muscle outside the basement membrane. The ductuli merge, like ramps onto a freeway, to form the ductus epididymis.

Ductus Epididymis

This is a single tube 5 or 6 m in length, folded and packed into a small 2.5 × 0.5 cm *body* (corpus) and *tail* (cauda) of the epididymis (Fig. 18.20). This structure lies along the posterior border of each testis. It is held together by loose connective tissue and covered by visceral tunica vaginalis. In histologic sections it is characterized by a tall pseudostratified epithelium of uniform thickness, whose luminal surface is covered by *stereocilia* (see Chapter 2). Although the stereocilia make occasional shortening and lengthening movements, they have no basal body and no organized internal system of microtubules. They are not considered motile, and play no part in moving the spermatozoa. Their principal function appears to increase the surface area of the epithelium.

The epididymal epithelium shows evidence of secretion, pinocytosis and phagocytosis. The cytoplasm contains numerous granules, vesicles, phagosomes, and lysosomes. There are many Golgi bodies. The complex, mixed epididymal secretions are present in seminal fluid, but little is known about their function. Considerable amounts of glycerylphosphorylcholine have been found. Metabolism of this substance requires an enzyme not found in the epididymis, but present in the uterus and oviductal secretions. This enzyme splits the molecule to release glycerophosphate, which can then be metabolized by sperm for their swimming energy.

The epididymis is the major storage compartment for maturing sperm. The changes they undergo here are not understood, but passage through the epididymis is required for full development of motility and fertility. For example, the motion which can be experimentally elicited in sperm obtained from the ductuli efferentes, is an uncoordinated thrashing without forward progression. The epididymal fluid contains a protein that converts this to an effective swimming motion, resulting in forward movement.

The ductus epididymis is provided with a layer of smooth muscle, which is thin in its upper portion. This becomes gradually thicker in the cauda. Here the tube is less tortuous. It finally bends sharply upward, acquires a thick muscular coat, and becomes the ductus deferens.

Ductus (Vas) Deferens, Ampulla, and Ejaculatory Duct

This long, straight, thick-walled tube (Fig. 18.21) ascends along the posterior border of each testis and enters the spermatic cord. As one of several components of the cord, it traverses the inguinal canal and enters the abdomen. Then it curves caudally and medially around the urinary bladder, passes through the prostate gland, and opens into the urethra on the *urethral crest*. Just before piercing the prostate gland, each duct becomes dilated and is called the *ampulla;* it then receives the duct of the seminal vesicle, and passes through the prostate as the much narrowed *ejaculatory duct.*

Except at the ampulla the vas has a narrow lumen and a very thick wall largely composed of tightly spiralled bundles of smooth muscle. There are three layers of muscle: a nearly circular and very thick middle layer, and nearly longitudinal, somewhat thinner, outer and inner layers. The lumen is usually nearly stellate because of the contraction of the muscle. In the dilated ampulla, the lining is much folded into a complex system of spaces, giving a lacy appearance in section. The epithelium is similar to that of the epididymis, that is, pseudostratified columnar with stereocilia. It is underlaid by a fibroelastic lamina propria.

The function of the ductus is obviously the transport of spermatozoa. During sexual excitement, some epididymal contents are moved to the ampulla for temporary storage.

Fig. 18.17. The *duct system* traversed by spermatozoa from seminiferous tubule to ductus deferens.

Fig. 18.18. *Seminiferous tubules, rete testis* (large arrow) and *efferent ductules* (small arrow). ×10.

Fig. 18.19. *Efferent ductules.* ×150.

Fig. 18.20. *Epididymis* with stereocilia (arrow) and spermatozoa (S). ×250.

Fig. 18.21. *Ductus (vas) deferens.* ×36.

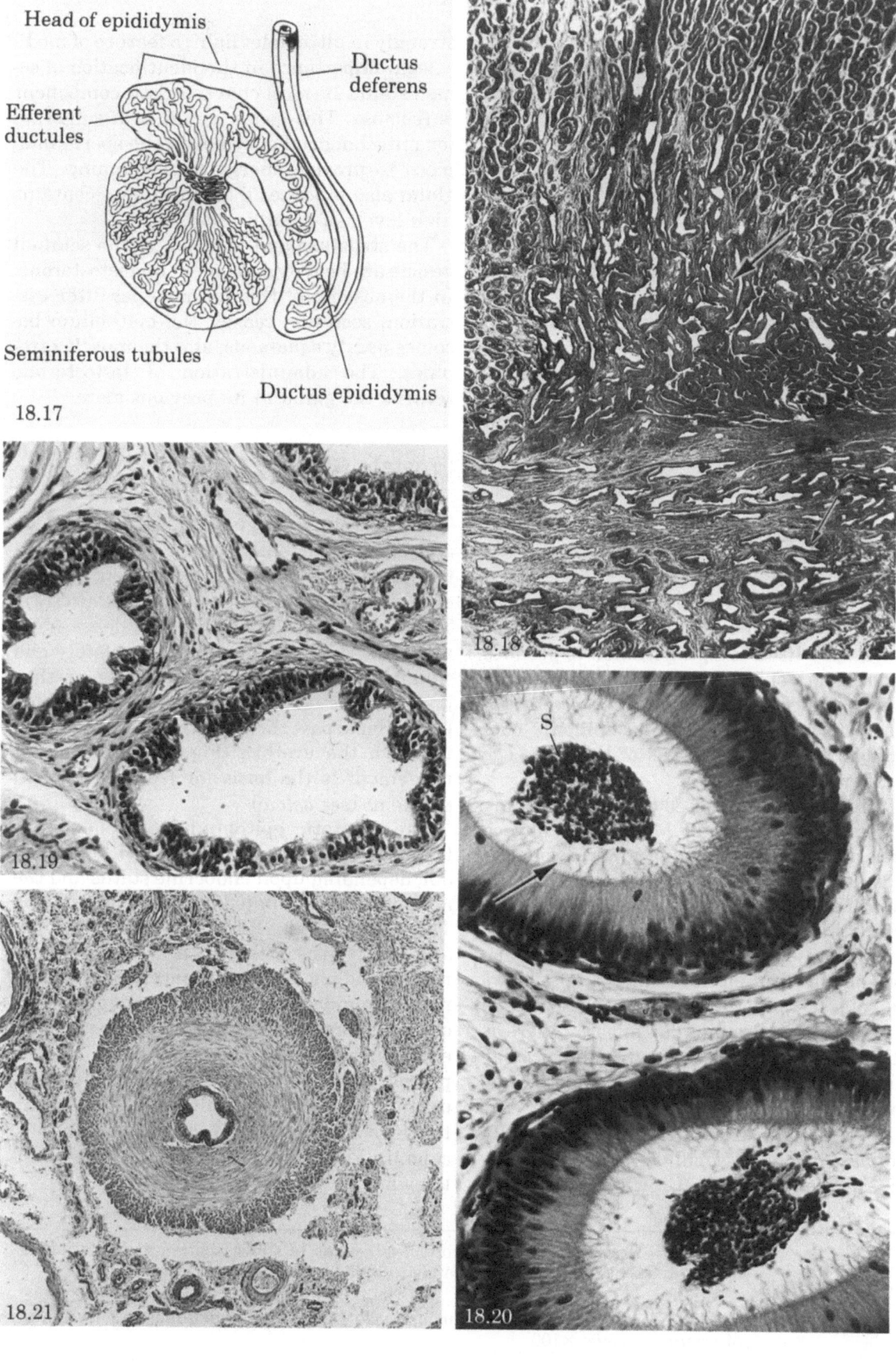

Head of epididymis

Ductus
deferens

Efferent
ductules

Seminiferous tubules

Ductus epididymis

18.17

18.18

18.19

18.20

S

18.21

At ejaculation, more sperm are moved rapidly to the ampulla, and all are ejected into the urethra along with secretions of the seminal vesicle and prostate.

Glands

The principal glands of the male reproductive system are paired *seminal vesicles,* a median *prostate gland,* paired *bulbourethral glands* (of Cowper) (Fig. 18.22) and numerous, small *urethral glands* (of Littré). The first two supply most of the volume of the seminal fluid. Each gland has its own special products which it contributes to the seminal plasma, the buffered vehicle or "culture medium" in which the sperm become suspended.

Seminal Vesicles

These glands (Fig. 18.23) are paired, narrow sacs about 15 cm in length. Each vesicle is folded upon itself in zigzag fashion to produce a final length of 5–7 cm. The folds are adhered by the connective tissue of their adventitia. A section of the organ thus commonly cuts through two or three levels of the same sac in different planes.

The mucosa is composed of thin, branching and anastomosing folds. Major folds have a thick, fibromuscular lamina propria; smaller folds have a very thin, inconspicuous lamina propria of loose connective tissue. The epithelium, which at first glance appears simple, is in fact pseudostratified columnar of variable height. The electron microscope shows the cells to have the usual features of cells manufacturing proteins for export. There is a thick coat of poorly defined inner circular and outer longitudinal layers of smooth muscle.

The secretion of this gland is chemically complex. It contains small amounts of yellowish pigments (flavins), which fluoresce strongly in ultraviolet light, a feature of medicolegal importance in the identification of semen stains. Its most characteristic component is fructose. This sugar serves as a substrate for mitochondrial enzymes in the sperm midpiece to provide energy for swimming. The gland also produces a globulin, and contains high levels of ascorbic acid.

The structure and function of the seminal vesicle are heavily dependent on testosterone. In the absence of this hormone, as after castration, secretion ceases, the epithelium becomes nearly squamous, and the muscle atrophies. The administration of testosterone returns the gland to its previous state.

Prostate Gland

This chestnut-sized gland (Figs. 18.22, 18.24, and 18.27) is actually an aggregate of about two dozen branched, tubuloacinar glands, each of whose ducts opens into the urethra. These glands are imbedded in a dense fibromuscular stroma. The organ completely and snugly surrounds about an inch of the urethra just below its exit from the bladder. The ejaculatory ducts pass through its posterior portion to reach the urethra (Fig. 18.27c). This arrangement is the basis for frequent clinical problems (*see below*).

The prostatic epithelium is pseudostratified, and varies from columnar to low cuboidal, depending upon endocrine status and the amount of accumulated secretion (Fig. 18.25). The cells contain RER, secretion granules, and many lysosomes, which are particularly rich in acid phosphatase. Concentrically laminated, rounded granules of varying size are often seen in the lumens of acini. They apparently are accumulated precipitates of a glycoprotein component of the secretion, and range up to about 0.2 μm in diameter. These are the *corpora amylacea* (prostatic concretions; calculi) (Fig. 18.26). Their significance is unknown.

Fig. 18.22. Drawing of male *reproductive organs* to show location and relations of ductus deferens and accessory glands to bladder, urethra and penis.

Fig. 18.23. a: *Seminal vesicle* and *ampulla* (A) of ductus deferens. ×2. **b:** Lining of *seminal vesicle.* ×100.

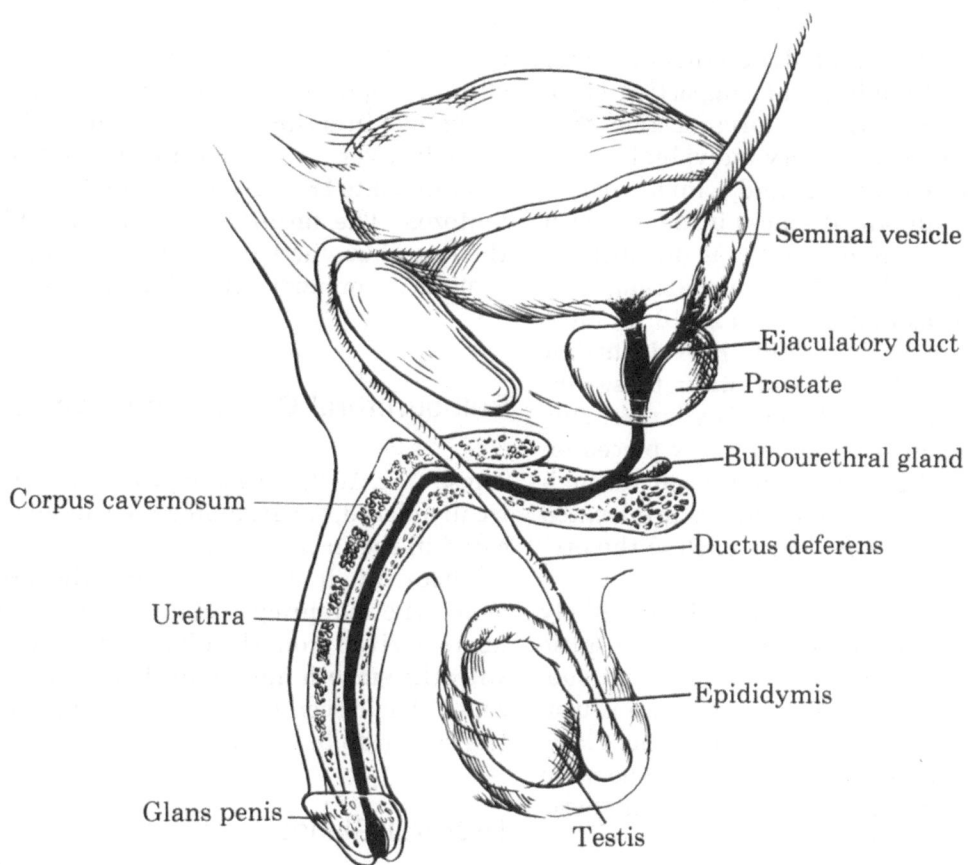

Seminal vesicle

Ejaculatory duct

Prostate

Bulbourethral gland

Corpus cavernosum

Ductus deferens

Urethra

Epididymis

Glans penis

Testis

18.22

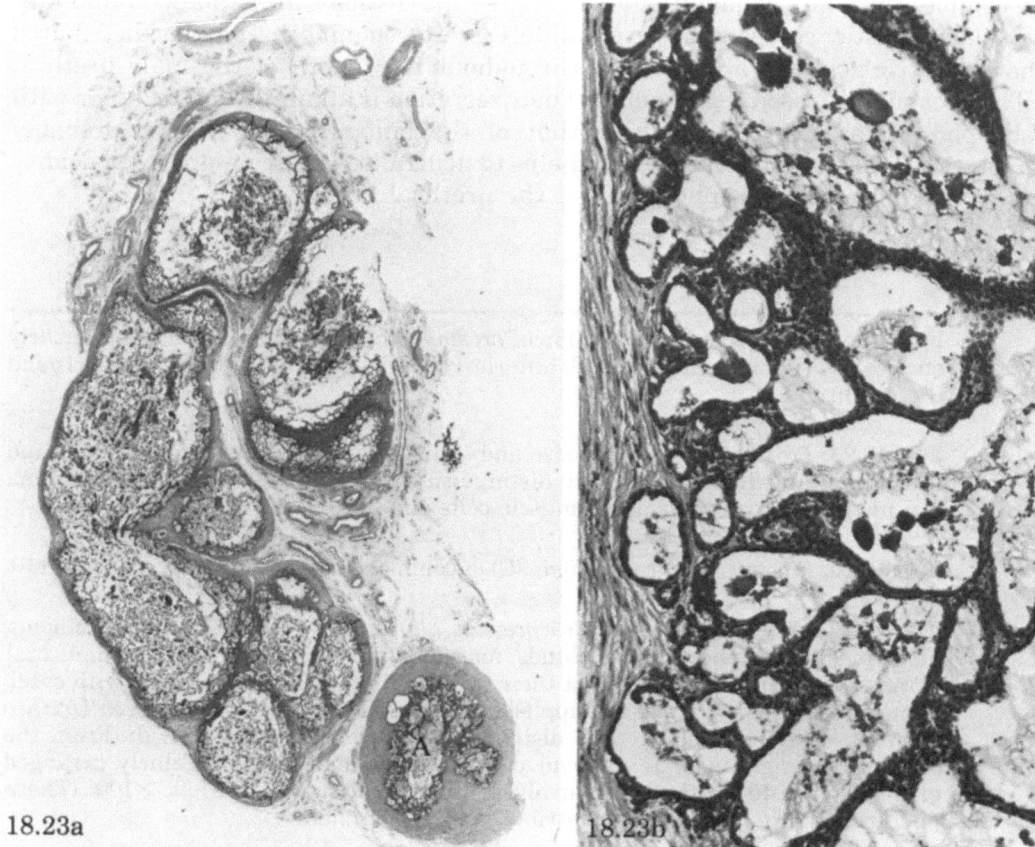

18.23a

18.23b

Just outside the glandular epithelium there is a thin basal lamina. The supporting fibromuscular tissue, without organization into layers, invests nearly every individual acinus in the organ. The tubules and acini are essentially epithelium-lined spaces in the uniform fibromuscular stroma; there is no distinct lamina propria. The glands are arranged in three groups as indicated in Fig. 18.24. Most of the glands near the urethra have ducts that open through the anterior wall; these are termed the mucosal glands. The larger, submucosal glands are symmetrically placed on each side of the urethra, and open through its lateral wall. The main glands are located peripherally and completely enclose the others.

The different groups of glands are likely to be affected by different diseases. Prostatic hypertrophy involves the mucosal and submucosal glands; thus its first evidence is usually urethral obstruction. Prostatic carcinoma, on the other hand, develops in the main glands in the periphery. Obstruction is therefore a late result (Fig. 18.27).

The slightly acidic (pH 6.5) prostatic secretion is a complex mixture of many substances. Its characteristic components are acid phosphatase, citric acid and a potent fibrinolysin. The prostate also secretes a small amount of acid phosphatase into the circulating blood. Prostatic cancers often cause elevations of this content. The serum acid phosphatase level has therefore become a common clinical laboratory test and the determination of changes in serum levels assist in evaluating the effectiveness of therapy. The citric acid is assumed to be of use in metabolism of spermatozoa. The fibrinolysin is responsible for the later liquefaction of semen that normally coagulates immediately after ejaculation.

Bulbourethral Glands (of Cowper)

These (Fig. 18.22) are two pea-sized, symmetrically placed, encapsulated mucous glands located in the urogenital diaphragm of the pelvic floor. Their ducts open into the urethra below the diaphragm. Some skeletal muscle fibers derived from the diaphragm are mixed with the smooth muscle in their interlobular septa. Their secretion is the first material of the semen to be ejaculated.

Urethral Glands (of Littré)

These (Fig. 18.28b) are small, numerous, widely scattered mucous glands distributed throughout the length of the male urethra. Their secretion is alkaline and, together with that of the bulbourethral glands, probably helps to neutralize the urine-produced acidity of the urethral lumen.

Fig. 18.24. Basic organizational plan of *prostate gland*. The main glands (Ma) nearly enclose the submucosal glands (S) anteriorly (below). Mucosal glands (M) surround the urethra (U).

Fig. 18.25. *Prostate gland*. Note size and shape of acini, columnar epithelium and absence of fat (which may help to distinguish this from breast tissue). The stroma is a uniform mixture of smooth muscle cells and fibroblasts. ×85.

Fig. 18.26. *Prostate* with *concretions* (C), a common finding in elderly males. ×110.

Fig. 18.27. a: Section of an entire *prostate gland*, showing two foci of carcinoma involving the peripheral main glands, and nodular hyperplasia of the submucosal glands, which are bulging against their surroundings. ×2.5. **b:** *Map of* **a** with carcinoma (black) and hyperplasia (stippled). **c:** (From the larger rectangle in **a**) *Urethra* compressed by hyperplastic and distended submucosal glands. ×11. **d:** (From the smaller rectangle in **a**) *Carcinoma* consisting of small and irregularly arranged glands, contrasted with the uninvolved prostatic tissue at the left. ×100. (These photographs are from a slide contributed by D. Kircheim).

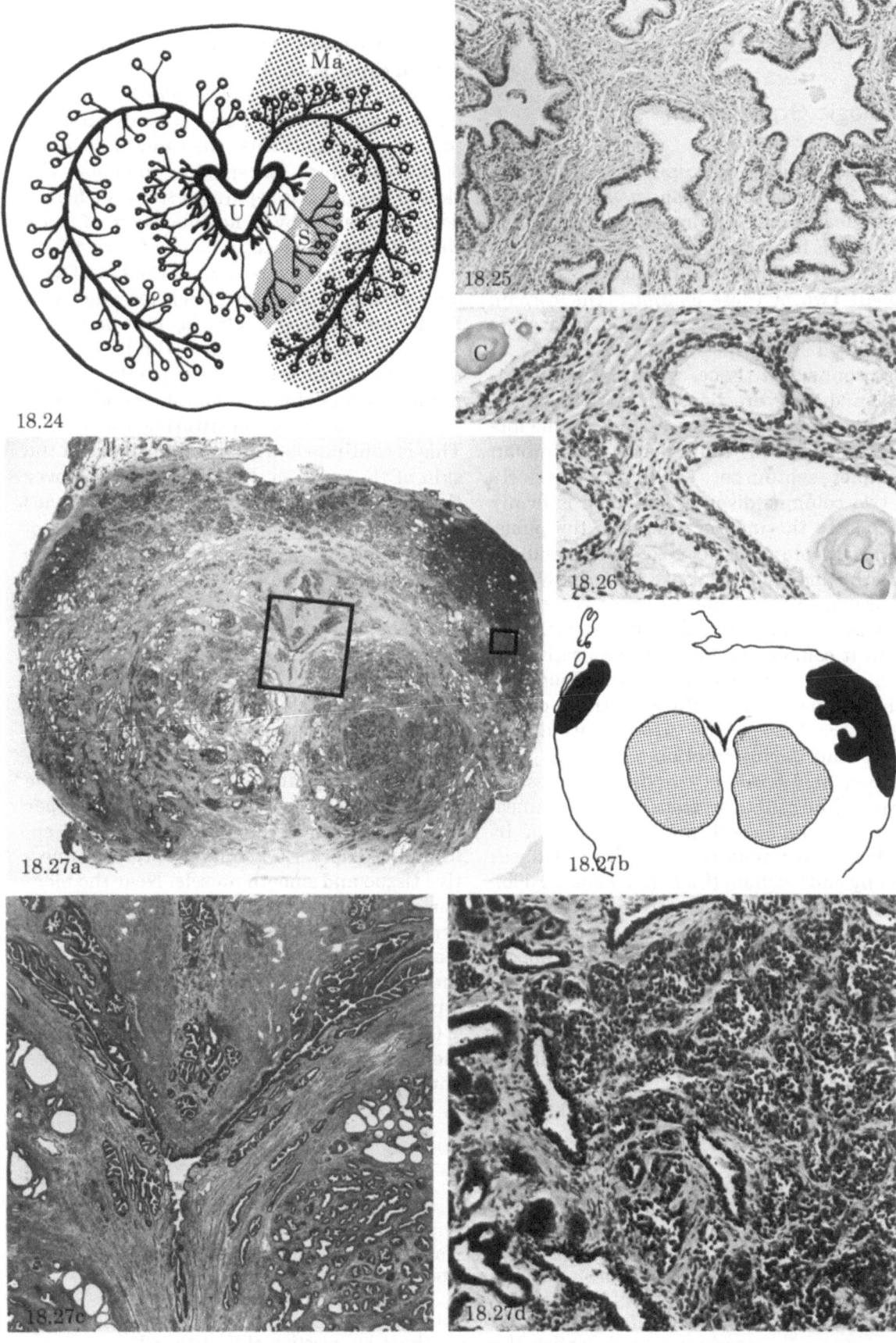

18.24

18.25

18.26

18.27a

18.27b

18.27c

18.27d

Penis

Histologic Organization

Since the penis is the copulatory organ, its largest component is a spongy, vascular erectile tissue arranged in three parallel, cylindrical columns bound together by connective tissue and covered with skin (Figs. 18.28a and 18.30a). Two of these columns, the *corpora cavernosa,* are dorsally placed, and each is surrounded by a thick *tunica albuginea* of dense connective tissue, which limits its expansion during erection. Through much of their length they are in contact along the median plane, and the tunicas are fused into an incomplete septum between them. Posteriorly the two columns diverge, and each is firmly attached to the inferior ramus of the pubis. The third column is located in the midline beneath, and in the groove formed by, the corpora cavernosa. This is termed the *corpus spongiosum* (Fig. 18.28b). Throughout its length it completely encloses the urethra. It has a thin and distensible tunica albuginea. If this tunica were as thick as those of the corpora cavernosa, the urethra would be tightly shut during erection.

The spongy tissue of corpora cavernosa is composed of countless trabeculae of connective tissue and smooth muscle separating irregular, interconnected, vascular sinuses lined by endothelium (Figs. 18.29 and 18.30b). Blood supply to all of the tissues of the penis is provided by branches from the paired dorsal artery. Blood from capillaries of the trabeculae in the erectile tissue passes into the cavernous spaces, then into peripherally placed veins which leave the corpora through the tunica albuginea, and drains into the superficial veins of the penis.

At the free end of the penis the corpus spongiosum is expanded and forms a more or less conical cap over the distal ends of the corpora cavernosa. This cap is the *glans.* Over the glans, the dermis of the skin is firmly attached to, and continuous with, the tunica albuginea of that structure. Except over the glans, the skin of the penis is separated from the firmer deep structures by a flexible layer of loose connective tissue rich in elastic fibers, which permits the relatively free movement of skin over the organ. The thin skin is provided with numerous sebaceous glands, but hairs are scarce or absent except near the base of the organ. In deeper layers of the penile skin are numerous small bundles and sheets of smooth muscle, collectively constituting the *dartos.* This is continuous with a similar layer in the skin of the scrotum. Extending forward over the glans from just behind its rim (*corona*) is a thin, retractable, cylindrical fold of skin, the foreskin or *prepuce.* Circumcision is the removal of this fold.

The male urethra consists of three regions:

(1) The *prostatic urethra* traverses the prostate gland. From the posterior wall of this portion of the urethra, the longitudinal urethral crest projects anteriorly into the lumen, and makes it V-shaped in cross-section. At the apex of the crest opens the *prostatic utricle,* a blind median pocket lying between the openings of the ejaculatory ducts. The upper prostatic urethra is lined by transitional epithelium. There is a lamina propria of connective tissue and smooth muscle. Near the bladder this muscle is thick and circularly arranged, and it contributes to the sphincter. Near the lower margin of the prostate gland the epithelium becomes pseudostratified or stratified columnar.

(2) The *membranous urethra* is a short segment, about 1 cm in length, which passes downward through the urogenital diaphragm to leave the pelvis. Here striated muscle of

---

Fig. 18.28. a: *Penis,* in cross-section, from an infant. ×12. **b:** *Urethra* and periurethral glands from **a.** ×85.

Fig. 18.29. *Erectile tissue* composed of collapsed vascular spaces separated by fibrous columns. Note tortuous helicine artery (arrows). ×35.

Fig. 18.30. *Adult penis.* **a:** Distended vascular spaces. ×35. **b:** Cross section of whole specimen after distention of erectile tissue by injection of fixative. ×2.

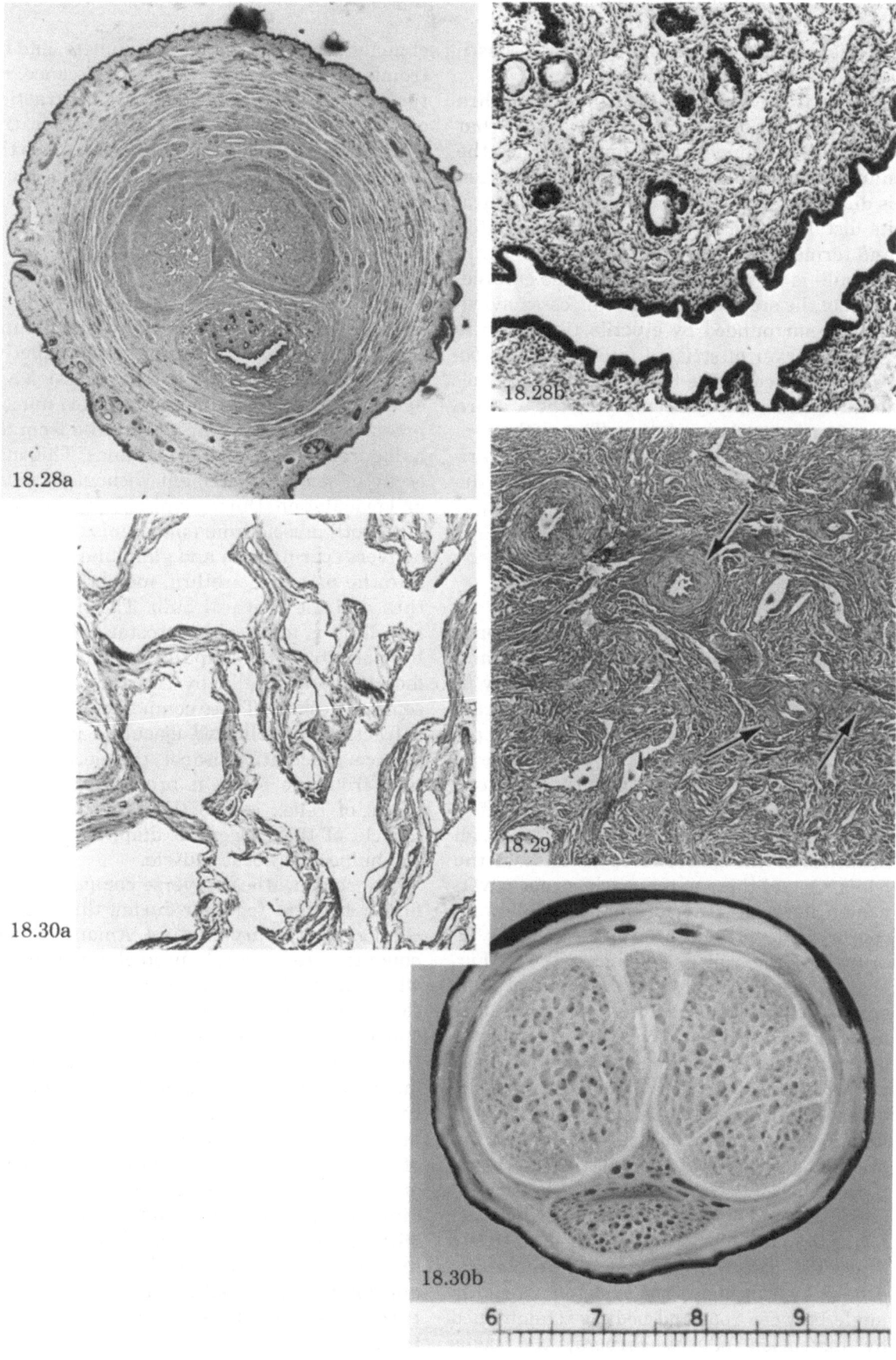

18.28a

18.28b

18.30a

18.29

18.30b

the diaphragm surrounds the tube and constitutes the *sphincter urethrae.*

(3) As it leaves the diaphragm, the urethra becomes surrounded by erectile tissue that coats the remainder of its length; hence the name *cavernous urethra.* Its posterior portion is dilated and termed the bulb of the urethra; its distal portion in the glans is also dilated and termed the *fossa navicularis.* The urethral bulb is surrounded by a bulbous enlargement of the erectile tissue, as the fossa navicularis is surrounded by erectile tissue of the glans. A layer of striated muscle (the *bulbocavernosus*) coats the bulb and functions voluntarily and reflexly in emptying the urethra in urination and ejaculation. The epithelium is generally stratified columnar, but is variable and becomes stratified squamous in the distal part of the fossa navicularis.

Erection

The process of erection requires an additional mechanism for by-passing capillary beds and delivering large amounts of blood rapidly to the spaces near the center of each corpus cavernosum. This is needed to compress the peripheral spaces against the inner surface of the tunica, thus reducing the outflow of blood to a rate less than that of the inflow. The increased inflow is accomplished through branches of the paired deep arteries of the penis. One of these enters each corpus cavernosum near its posterior end, and follows a course through the center of the column. Its branches, the coiled *helicine arteries* (Fig. 18.29), open directly into the cavernous spaces. The helicine arteries are unusually muscular for such small vessels, and have additional longitudinal ridges of muscle in the tunica intima. This vascular smooth muscle, and that of the trabeculae, remain contracted under sympathetic control except during erection. In response to sexual stimulation via parasympathetic innervation, the muscle fibers relax and blood enters the erectile tissue faster than it can be drained away (Fig. 18.30). Since the posterior portions of the corpora are firmly attached to the skeleton, when the angle between root and body is straightened by distension of the corpora, the penis

changes position, erection is complete, and intromission can take place. Detumescence, return to the flaccid state, follows contraction of the smooth muscle in arteries and in trabeculae. The drainage rate then overtakes the arterial inflow rate and the amount of blood in the corpora is gradually reduced.

Ejaculation

This process involves the coordinated function of several parts of the male reproductive system. It consists of two phases, emission and ejaculation. A small amount of clear, mucoid preejaculatory fluid is first expressed from the bulbourethral and urethral glands. This may occur in sexual excitement without emission and ejaculation. During emission, contraction of smooth muscle from epididymis to prostate delivers spermatozoa and glandular secretion into the prostatic urethra, membranous urethra and the urethral bulb. The preejaculatory fluid is followed by prostatic fluid, then by sperm from the ampulla and from the epididymis, and finally by secretion from the seminal vesicles. These components appear in a fractionally collected ejaculate in this sequence. Ejaculation proper, the ejection of semen from the penis, is brought about by a series of reflex contractions of the skeletal muscle of the urogenital diaphragm and of the bulbocavernosus muscle.

The semen, whose diverse components are finally brought together during this process, is an extraordinary mixture. Among its components are several proteolytic enzymes which break down some of its larger proteins to peptides and amino acids, numerous carbohydrates in free and bound forms, more than a dozen prostaglandins, ascorbic, citric, lactic and other organic acids and numerous hydrolytic and oxidative enzymes. All of these are contained in a complex buffered solution of electrolytes. Each of them presumably has one or more functions in constituting a medium for spermatozoa, and for interaction with substances in the secretions of the female reproductive tract. The seminal plasma appears to provide optimal conditions for fertilization by healthy well nourished spermatozoa.

19 Organs of Special Sense

Eye

The eye is a fluid-filled sphere with a transparent opening through which light enters and is focused on an epithelium whose highly modified cilia are sensitive to the impact of photons. The membrane depolarization initiated by such impact is then passed through a chain of neurons to the CNS, where it is interpreted as light. In the visual cortex the patterns of this nerve activity are translated into images that represent the structure of the external world. Each globe is set in a bony protective socket (the orbit) (Fig. 19.1) within the skull and fitted with six muscles that provide the precise movement needed for the depth perception made possible by binocular vision, as well as for the coordinated tracking movements.

The globe (Fig. 19.2) is essentially composed of three concentric spheres or balls. The anterior one-sixth of each sphere is modified to permit the access of light, control the amount of it entering the system, and focus it on the light-sensitive lining. As with many organs, the basic pattern is most easily understood when it is studied during its development in the embryo before differentiation of the complex adult features has been completed.

Development (Fig. 19.3)

Each eye originates as a hollow, lateral outgrowth from the forebrain, the *optic vesicle*. It immediately comes into contact with the overlying ectoderm and, by invagination of its lateral portion, becomes a two-layered *optic cup*. The cavity of the optic vesicle is obliterated during cup formation, when the inner and outer layers come in contact. These two fused layers form the innermost of the three concentric spheres comprising the adult eyeball. Its different regions become retina, ciliary epithelium, and pigmented layers of the iris. The mesenchyme around the outer surface of the optic cup differentiates into two layers. That in contact with the cup becomes the richly vascular and pigmented *uvea*, the middle layer of the adult globe. Its different regions become choroid, ciliary body, and connective tissue of the iris.

The outer mesenchyme becomes a thick layer of dense connective tissue, the outermost of the concentric spheres of the globe. This tissue differentiates into the opaque white sclera posteriorly and the transparent cornea anteriorly.

Also anteriorly, between the inner and outer layers of mesenchyme coats (and therefore between the future cornea and outer surface of the iris), a fluid-filled cleft develops that becomes lined by a simple squamous epithelium. This is the *anterior chamber* of the eye. The mesenchyme of the posterior wall of this cleft at first covers both iris and pupil (the iridopupillary membrane). Parts of this persist to form the outer layer of the iris, but that portion over the pupil breaks down. Thus the anterior chamber becomes continuous, through the pupil, with the fluid-filled space between iris and lens, the *posterior chamber* (Fig. 19.4).

The ectoderm overlying the primitive optic vesicle thickens to become the lens placode. This placode also invaginates, closes over, and pinches free of the ectoderm to lie within the optic cup as the *lens vesicle*. The lens vesicle is converted to lens by the great elongation of the cells of its posterior wall. These extend forward as long fibers and make contact with the anterior wall, thus filling up the lumen of the vesicle. The anterior wall remains relatively unchanged and hence the anterior hemisphere of the lens is coated with a (cuboidal) *lens epithelium*. As the lens grows, new

fibers are added to its exterior at the equator by elongation of cells from the edge of the lens epithelium.

Adult Structure

Each of the components established by the developmental processes outlined above differentiates into the complex structure necessary for its adult function.

COATS (Fig. 19.5). The histologic organization of each of the three basic layers and its regional specializations will now be considered.

Tunica fibrosa. This tough, dense, connective tissue coat consists of two regions. The *sclera* covers the posterior five-sixths of the globe, and the *cornea* the anterior one-sixth.

Sclera. The most important function of this layer is probably the precise maintenance of the shape and rigidity of the eyeball as an optically effective chamber with constant dimensions. It is formed of intertwined and branching bundles and sheets of collagen fibers generally parallel to the surface and embedded in ground substance containing scattered fibroblasts. It is opaque, white in color, and about 0.5 mm thick. The extraocular muscles are inserted into it. Its outer surface is very loosely attached, by tenuous connective tissue fibers, to a sheath of orbital connective tissue (Tenon's capsule), within which the eyeball can be moved by the muscles. It is penetrated by the *vortex veins* behind the equator, and by posterior ciliary vessels and nerves. Instead of a single large opening posteriorly for passage of the optic nerve, here the sclera is perforated by numerous small openings through which nerve fibers leave in bundles. This perforated area is termed the lamina cribrosa.

Cornea (Fig. 19.6). The anterior one-sixth of the globe has a shorter radius of curvature than the rest and consequently bulges from

Fig. 19.1. Drawing of left *eye* and associated structures in situ, anterior view. Only two of the six extraocular muscles are shown.

Fig. 19.2. Diagram of horizontal section through the center of the right *eye*.

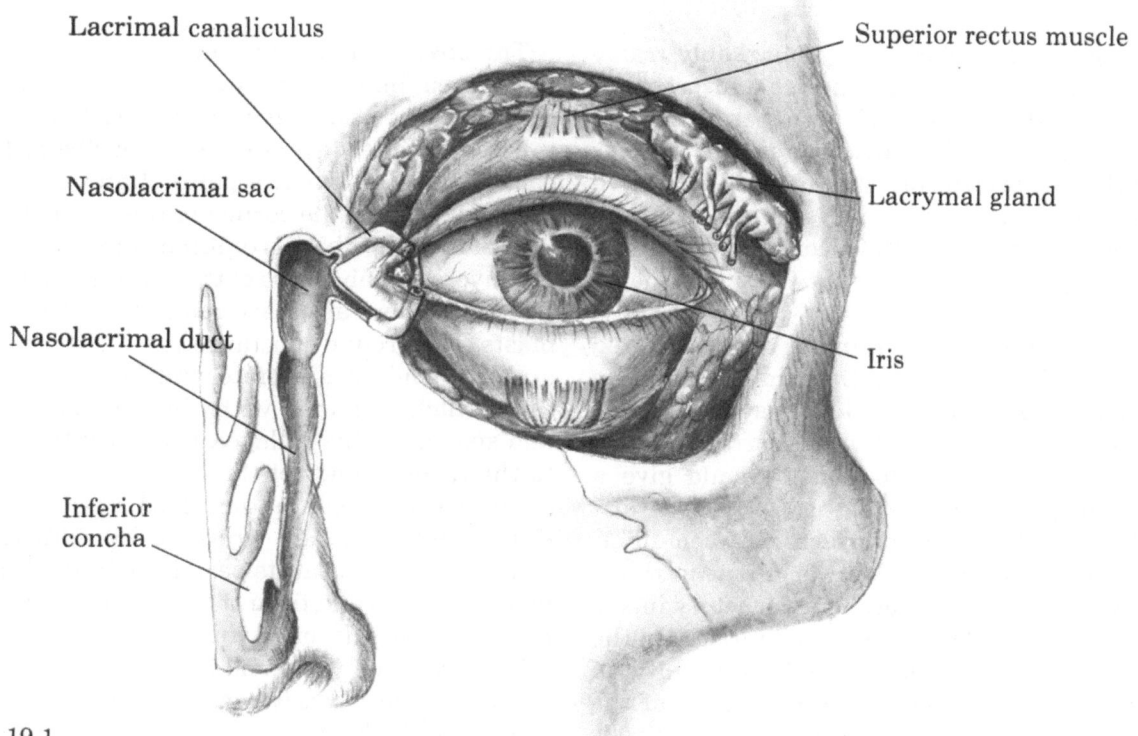

Lacrimal canaliculus

Nasolacrimal sac

Nasolacrimal duct

Inferior
concha

Superior rectus muscle

Lacrymal gland

Iris

19.1

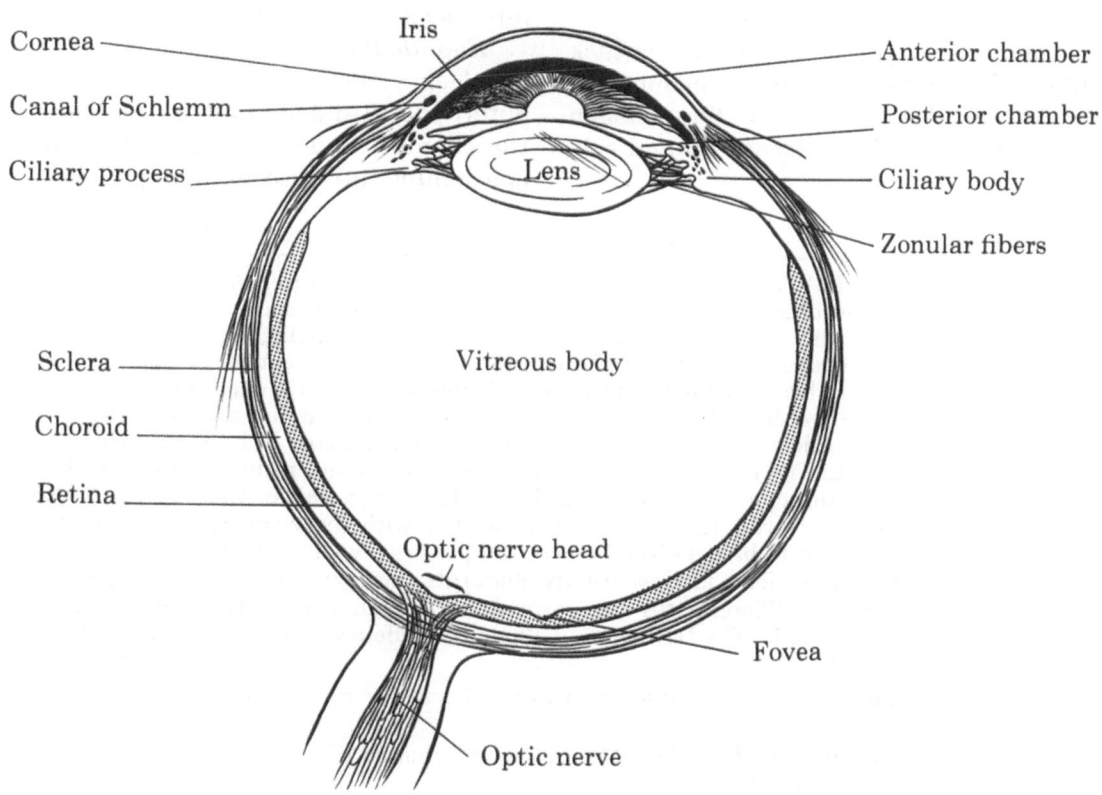

Cornea

Canal of Schlemm

Ciliary process

Iris

Anterior chamber

Posterior chamber

Ciliary body

Zonular fibers

Lens

Sclera

Choroid

Retina

Vitreous body

Optic nerve head

Fovea

Optic nerve

19.2

the general surface. It is remarkably transparent, with a smooth surface and precisely uniform thickness which permit transmission of clear sharp light patterns to the interior of the eye. It is the first surface with refractive properties; these contribute to image formation. It consists of a thick collagenous stroma with epithelia covering its inner and outer surfaces.

The *corneal epithelium* is nonkeratinized stratified squamous epithelium of unusually constant thickness (five to six layers of cells). The superficial layer of cells is extraordinarily smooth and even. Roughness would give a ground-glass effect and thus produce a loss of clarity. Since all interfaces between different media are refractive, variations in thickness would also produce unsatisfactory image transmission. Thus both characteristics of the epithelium, smoothness and uniformity of thickness, contribute to transparency of the cornea. Turnover time for the epithelial cells is about a week. Following local injury, as in abrasion, the epithelium regenerates quickly.

Bowman's membrane is an unusually thick (8–12 μm) homogenous basement membrane. It consists of a dense feltwork of fine collagen fibers embedded in a condensed ground substance.

The *stroma*, making up more than 90% of the cornea, imparts great strength and rigidity to this structure. It is composed of many precise, parallel layers of collagen fibers. In each layer all fibers are parallel and extend from one edge of the cornea to the other. The direction of the fibers is different in the different layers. All fibers are of the same diameter. Between layers are scattered flattened fibroblasts. The ground substance contains considerable chondroitin sulfate and keratan sulfate, which, together with the uniform size and spacing of the collagen fibers, contribute to the transparency of the cornea.

The cornea contains no blood vessels. Its nutritional needs are provided by diffusion from blood vessels at its periphery in the limbus (*see below*) and from the fluid in the anterior chamber. Although it is avascular it contains occasional lymphoid cells.

"Endothelial" basement (Descemet's) *membrane* is a thick (about 8 μm) basement membrane of uniform fine collagen fibers and some elastin, which supports the epithelium of the inner surface of the cornea.

"Endothelium." The epithelial covering of the deep surface of the cornea, the unfortunately so-called *endothelium*, faces the anterior chamber. It is a layer of simple squamous epithelium. Its cells contain more rough endo-

Fig. 19.3. Three stages in the *embryonic development of the eye.* **A:** Anterior view of the head of the embryo. The anterior portion of the left side of the embryo's head has been cut away to show optic vesicle bulging laterally from the brain and pushing out against the ectoderm. **B:** Enlargement of the left eye only. The vesicle has invaginated to form a double walled optic cup which is connected to brain by the optic stalk. The ectoderm has been induced by the cup to form a lens vesicle which invaginates and later pinches free to lie within the rim of the cup. **C:** The inner wall of the cup differentiates into retina, and nerve fibers grow back through the stalk to the brain. The outer wall of the cup will become the pigment layer. The cavity of the cup fills with the vitreous. The edge of the cup thins out to become iris. Cells of the posterior wall of the lens vesicle elongate to form lens fibers and eventually obliterate the cavity of the lens vesicle. Ectoderm over cup differentiates into corneal and conjunctival epithelium. (After Fig. 19.1 in Moore, K. The Developing Human. Philadelphia; W B Saunders, 1973.)

Fig. 19.4. Closeup cutaway drawing of *anterior portion of eye.*

Fig. 19.5. *Wall of the globe.* Sclera (S), choroid (C), and retina (R). ×85. (Courtesy of D. Johnson.)

Fig. 19.6. *Cornea* with epithelium (E) resting on Bowman's membrane (long arrow) on external surface. Descemet's membrane (short arrow) and endothelium (En) cover the internal surface. ×150. (Courtesy of D. Johnson.)

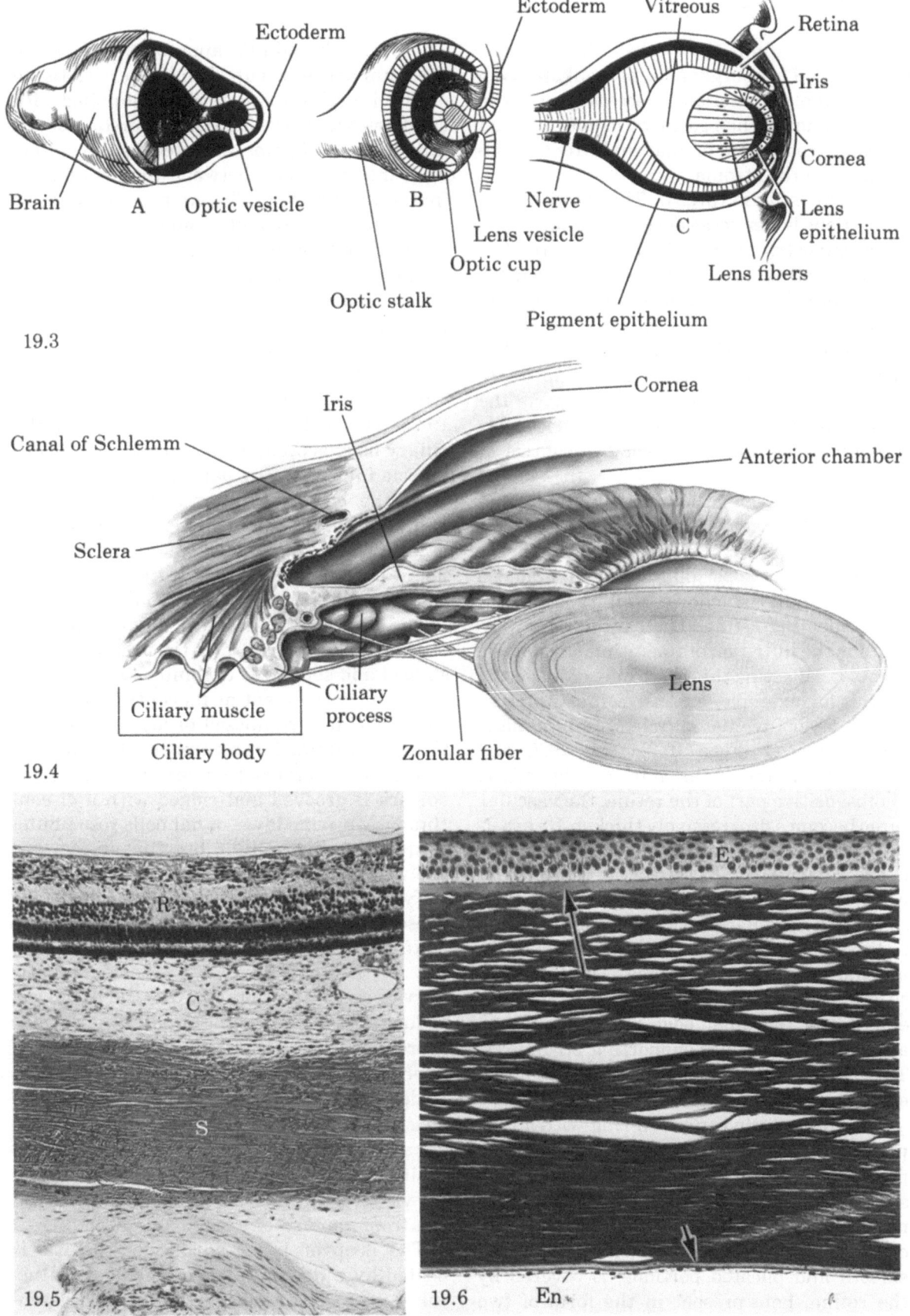

Ectoderm

Brain   A   Optic vesicle

Optic stalk

Ectoderm

B

Lens vesicle

Optic cup

Vitreous   Retina

Iris

Cornea

Nerve

C

Lens epithelium

Lens fibers

Pigment epithelium

19.3

Iris   Cornea

Canal of Schlemm

Anterior chamber

Sclera

Lens

Ciliary muscle   Ciliary process

Ciliary body

Zonular fiber

19.4

R

C

S

19.5

E

En

19.6

plasmic reticulum than other simple squamous cells. These organelles probably provide the synthetic functions necessary for the maintenance of the basement membrane and for the production of materials to be contributed to the stroma.

Tunica vasculosa (uvea). This middle layer of the globe is composed of richly vascularized, loose connective tissue (Fig. 19.5) with the full range of cell types usually found in such tissue, plus a large population of heavily pigmented cells. It is differentiated into three regions: the *choroid* (Fig. 19.5), which underlies the retina; the thickened ring-shaped *ciliary body,* which surrounds and supports the lens at its equator; and the *iris,* which forms the adjustable diaphragm for the control of pupillary size.

The *choroid* coats the outside of the retina and lines the inside of the sclera. Its rich vascular supply is organized such that the larger vessels lie more peripherally and a dense mesh of capillaries (choriocapillary layer) lies just under the retina. The choroid is important for the nutrition of the retina. Pathologic processes affecting this layer may damage the retina; for example, extensive inflammation of this layer (uveitis) may lead to blindness.

Ciliary body (Figs. 19.2, 19.4, 19.7, and 19.16). Beginning at the anterior edge of the photosensitive part of the retina, the vascular tunic becomes progressively thicker. Its greatest thickness is just deep to the limbus. This is the ciliary body. In section, it resembles a wedge lying against the inner surface of the sclera, with its sharp peripheral edge tapering to the choroid and its broad internal end facing the lens, iris, and cornea. The limbus is situated along the outer edge of the broad end. Along the inner edge of the broad end are attached the lens-supporting structures. The iris projects from the center of the broad end.

The ciliary body is a broad ring with a thin peripheral edge and a thicker inner edge. The posterior surface of the ring is relatively smooth over its peripheral two-thirds but has numerous radial ridges, the *ciliary processes,* on its inner third. This surface, both the smooth and plicated portions, is covered by the retina, here present in the form of two layers of cuboidal epithelium (Fig. 19.7b).

These are the adult's apposed two walls of the embryo's optic cup. The connective tissue of the ciliary processes is richly supplied with capillaries that provide the precursors for the fluid (*aqueous humor*) secreted by the epithelium into the space between limbus and iris (*posterior chamber*). The aqueous humor provides nutrients to, and removes wastes from, the lens and cornea, which are without blood supplies of their own. From the ciliary body between ciliary processes arise a web of countless, fine, strong inelastic fibers (*zonular fibers*) that are inserted into the capsule of the lens (*see below*). In aggregate these fibers constitute the *suspensory ligament* (Figs. 19.4 and 19.7a) of the lens. The central core of the ciliary body is occupied by bundles of smooth muscle innervated by parasympathetic fibers from the oculomotor nerve. Contraction of certain parts of this complex *ciliary muscle* (Fig. 19.7a) reduces tension on the zonular fibers and allows the lens to round up and thus change focus for near vision.

Iris (Fig. 19.8). The most anterior portion of the tunica vasculosa is the iris. It is disc-shaped and separates the anterior and posterior chambers except at its central aperture, the *pupil*. It is composed of loose connective tissue containing large numbers of pigmented cells and numerous blood vessels. Its anterior surface is grooved and ridged with a discontinuous covering layer of flat cells resembling a squamous epithelium, but that in fact are probably fibroblasts.

Two groups of smooth muscle fibers are present in the iris. A circular *pupillary sphincter* lies near the free margin of the pupil. It is controlled by parasympathetic nerves; its contraction narrows the pupil and reduces the amount of light entering the eye. More peripherally located, radially arranged fibers enlarge the pupil when they contract under sympathetic stimulation. These fibers constitute the *pupillary dilator* muscle. Balanced function of these two muscle groups maintains a pupillary diameter appropriate for visual needs and for protection of the retina from damage of excessive light.

The deep or inner surface of the iris is coated by a double layer of cuboidal epithelium, again representing the forward extension of the two layers of the retina already described over the ciliary body. It is heavily pigmented. Variation in number of pigment cells in the connective tissue of the iris is responsible for variation in eye color. If these cells are few in number, light passes through the overlying connective tissue and is reflected from the pigmented epithelium on the deep surface. In this situation the iris appears blue. Increasing amounts of connective tissue pigment produce green, gray, and brown eyes. In albinism, a condition in which nearly all pigment is absent, the characteristic pink color is produced by reflection of light from the blood vessels of the iris.

Tunica interna (retina). As stated in the section on its development, the internal layer of the wall of the globe is produced by apposition of the inner and outer layers of the wall of the embryonic optic cup. It is an outgrowth of the neural tube of the embryo and thus is an extension of the brain. The fibrous and vascular coats represent dura and arachnoid, respectively. The histologic structure of the retina differs in different regions. Two of these areas have already been mentioned. One of these is the double epithelial coating of the ciliary body (*pars ciliaris* of the retina) and the other, the heavily pigmented, light-reflecting, double epithelial layer that coats the posterior surface of the iris (*pars iridis*).

Pars optica. This portion of the retina is made up of two different layers, an outer *pigment layer* and an inner, photosensitive, *neural layer* (Fig. 19.9a). These are derived from the outer and inner layers of the embryonic optic cup. The remnant lumen of the optic vesicle (that is, the space between the two layers of the optic cup) becomes obliterated when neural and pigment layers become applied to each other. This is not a firm attachment, and the two layers may become separated to produce the serious problem of retinal detachment.

Pigment layer. This is a layer of simple cuboidal epithelium whose cells, except in albinos, are heavily pigmented. They rest on a thick basement membrane (Bruch's membrane), which separates them from the choroid and is unusual in having a network of elastic and reticular fibers embedded in its ground substance. The apical surface of each cell is provided with numerous microvilli and

with cylindrical, tubular extensions that fit over the ends of the photoreceptor cells of the neural layer (to be described shortly). A pigmented epithelial cell is far more complex than is suggested by its appearance under the light microscope. It has the arrangement of mitochondria and basal membrane folds characteristic of ion-pumping cells. It manufactures large quantities of melanin, which absorbs light and prevents light scattering, so that photons stimulate photoreceptors on only one passage through the light-sensitive cells. A major function recently discovered is the phagocytosis and lysosomal digestion of worn out light-sensitive discs discarded at the tips of the retinal rods (*see below*).

Neural layer. Although there are 10 visible layers in histologic sections of this photosensitive tissue, there are only three layers of nerve cells (Fig. 19.9b) concerned with the transduction, integration, and conduction of the light-generated impulse to the brain. These are (1) the layer of rods and cones (the photoreceptors), (2) the layer of bipolar cells, and (3) the layer of ganglion cells. The impulse reaching the brain is thus carried over a three-neuron chain.

Rods and cones. The rods contain long narrow ends and the cones shorter, tapering, cone-shaped ends. Both types are partly embedded in the apices of cells of the pigment epithelium. The light-sensitive end of each cell is connected to the cell body by a narrow, short stalk. The stalk has the structure of the cilium, with nine doublets of microtubules but without the central pair (see Chapter 2), and a basal body. The light-sensitive part is the much modified distal portion of the cilium. Each consists of a closely packed stack of membranous discs derived from precisely parallel infoldings of the plasmalemma. In the rods, these pinch off from the surface membrane and become enclosed within the cell, but in the cones they retain their connections to the cell surface. In the rods, the discs are formed near the cell body and incorporate the visual pigment rhodoposin. These discs gradually move distally, where the oldest ones are shed, or perhaps are "bitten off," and digested by the pigment cells (Fig. 19.10). About 90 sacs per cell per day are shed. Turnover requires 10–12 days. The impact of photons on these discs produces a change in the configuration of rhodoposin and initiates an action potential in the membrane of the rod by a process not yet well understood.

In the cones, the discs are not shed and they contain a variety of pigments sensitive to blue, green, and red light. The dimensions and relative numbers of rods and cones vary in different areas of the retina.

Bipolar cells. Each neuron of this layer has a short dendrite, the branches of which receive impulses from several photoreceptor cells. Thus some integration apparently occurs in the bipolar cell. Each bipolar cell has a short axon that synapses with the dendrites of the ganglion cells in the next layer.

Fig. 19.7. *Ciliary body.* **a:** With lens, suspensory ligament (zonular fibers) (arrows), iris (I), ciliary muscle (Cm) and filtration angle (F). ×35. (Courtesy of D. Johnson.) **b:** With its covering of two layers of epithelial cells, the deeper of which is obscured by its great quantity of pigment. ×125. (Courtesy of D. Johnson.)

Fig. 19.8. *Iris* with anterior (A) and posterior (P) chambers. ×35.

Fig. 19.9. *Retina.* **a:** Photomicrograph. ×225. (Courtesy of D. Johnson.) **b:** Simplified diagram of the three cell chain involved in the reception and transmission of visual information. The sketch is aligned with the photomicrograph (a) so as to show the location of these cell types in the appropriate layers of the retina and in contrast with the pigment epithelium below.

Fig. 19.10. A cell of the *pigment epithelium.* Its much folded basal plasmalemma rests on the thick Bruch's membrane overlying the capillary layer of the choroid. The stages in the phagocytic process, although actually randomly distributed, have been arranged to suggest the sequence of events that takes place in the phagocytosis, lysosomal digestion and passage into capillaries of old discs from the tips of the rods. Melanin granules are numerous.

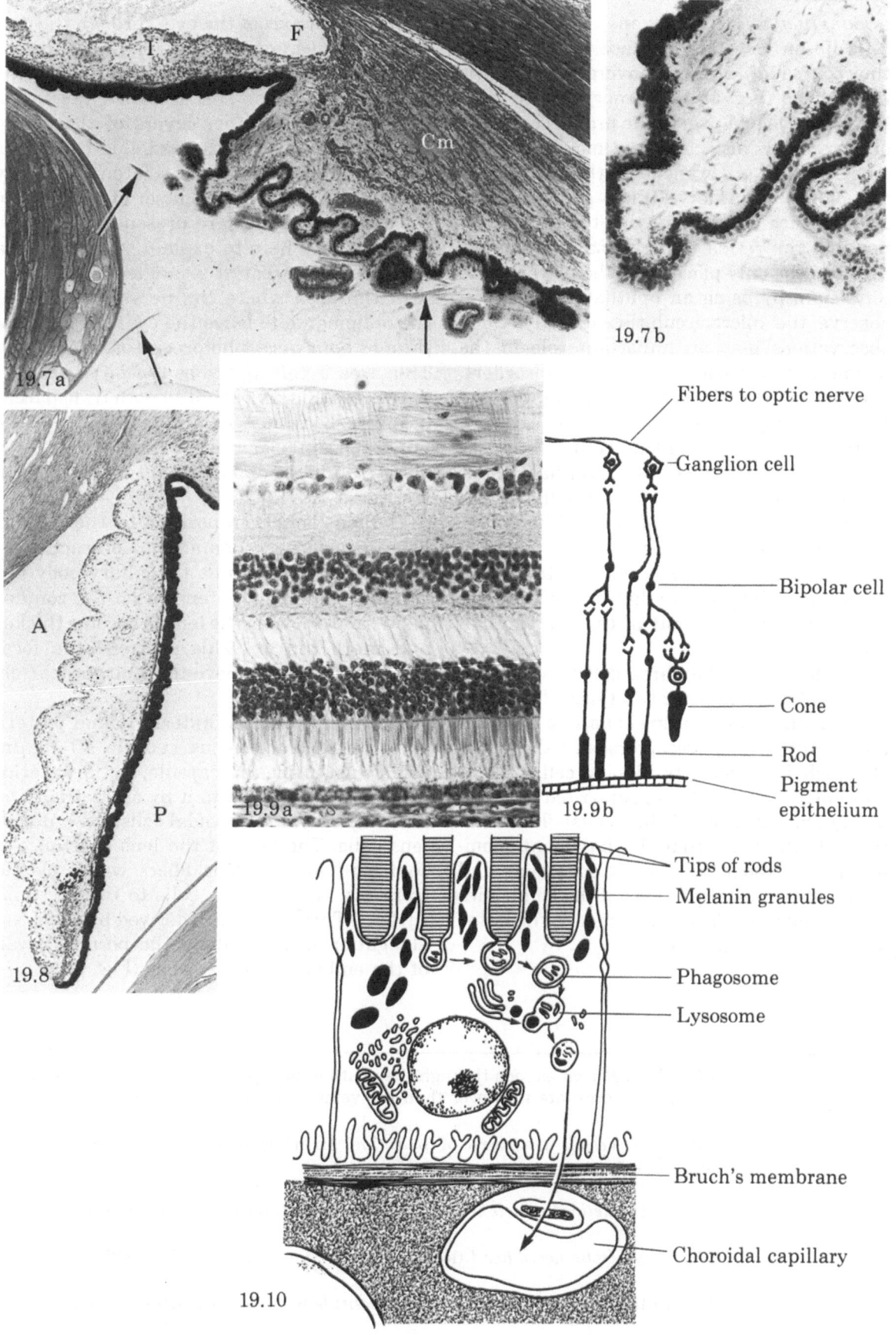

19.7a

F

I

Cm

19.7b

A

P

19.8

19.9a

Fibers to optic nerve

Ganglion cell

Bipolar cell

Cone

Rod

Pigment
epithelium

19.9b

Tips of rods

Melanin granules

Phagosome

Lysosome

Bruch's membrane

Choroidal capillary

19.10

Ganglion cells. The axons of these large cells lie on the inner surface of the retina; they course toward, and converge at, the optic nerve head (Fig. 19.14) through which they leave the eye and pass to the brain. This layer of nerve fibers also contains the retinal blood vessels, which are branches of the central vessels of the optic nerve (Figs. 19.11 through 19.13). Since all structures between the cornea and the retina are transparent, the eye provides the only place in the body where the physician, by using an ophthalmoscope, can observe the microcirculation directly. Such observations play an important role in the diagnosis of a variety of vascular disorders.

Light entering the eye impinges first on the layer of ganglion cell axons, passes through it and the ganglion cell layer itself, and so on through all the layers of the retina without producing a response, until it finally strikes the discs in the rods and cones. The action potential produced there then passes back through the three-neuron chain in the retina to the innermost layer, that of the ganglion cell axons, and then out of the eye through the optic nerve.

In addition to the three cell types of the neuron chain, there are two types of horizontally arranged integrating cells, one of which interconnects photoreceptors and the other of which interconnects bipolar cells. All of these neural elements are supported by irregularly shaped cells (Müller cells). These extend all the way from the basement membrane that separates the vitreous body and retina to the distal portions of the cell bodies of rods and cones. They are joined to the latter by junctional complexes.

The visual axis of the eye, through the center of cornea, pupil, and lens, also passes through a shallow pit in the retina at the back of the globe. This is called the fovea. In this area the inner layers of the retina are thinned out and the ganglion cell axons diverge to pass on either side on their way to the optic nerve. In the layer of photoreceptor cells, only cones are present here. These features may help to explain why the fovea is the area of greatest visual acuity.

In the area where the nerve fibers enter the optic nerve to leave the eye (the *optic papilla* or *optic disc*), photoreceptors are absent. This area is referred to as the *blind spot.*

THE LENS (Fig. 19.15) is a smooth transparent biconvex body just behind the iris and the pupil and anterior to the vitreous body. It is about 10 mm in diameter and 3.7–4.5 mm in thickness.

The lens is held in position by the zonular fibers (suspensory ligament). Contraction of the ciliary muscle pulls the ciliary body forward, slackening the tension on the zonular fibers, and allowing the lens to become thicker and more convex. This shortens the focal length, allowing the eye to focus on near objects.

The lens is covered anteriorly and posteriorly by a homogeneous capsule 10–18 μm thick. Just inside this capsule, on the anterior surface and attached to it by a basal lamina, is a single layer of cuboidal cells, the anterior lens cells. The bulk of the lens substance is composed of long lens fibers which extend from the anterior lens cells to the posterior surface. These fibers are derived by the great elongation of the cells of the posterior wall of the embryonic lens vesicle (Fig. 19.3C).

Fig. 19.11. *Retina* as seen through the ophthalmoscope. Fovea (F), optic nerve head (N). The arteries are narrower than the veins. (Courtesy of L. Rich.)

Fig. 19.12. *Vessels* in a spread of the retina. An artery is on the right. ×28. (Courtesy of D. Johnson.)

Fig. 19.13. *Retinal vessels with aneurysms.* ×85. (Courtesy of D. Johnson.)

Fig. 19.14. *Optic nerve head* (longitudinal section as in Fig. 19.2). ×85.

Fig. 19.15. *Lens, lens epithelium,* and *capsule* (C). ×560. (Courtesy of D. Johnson.)

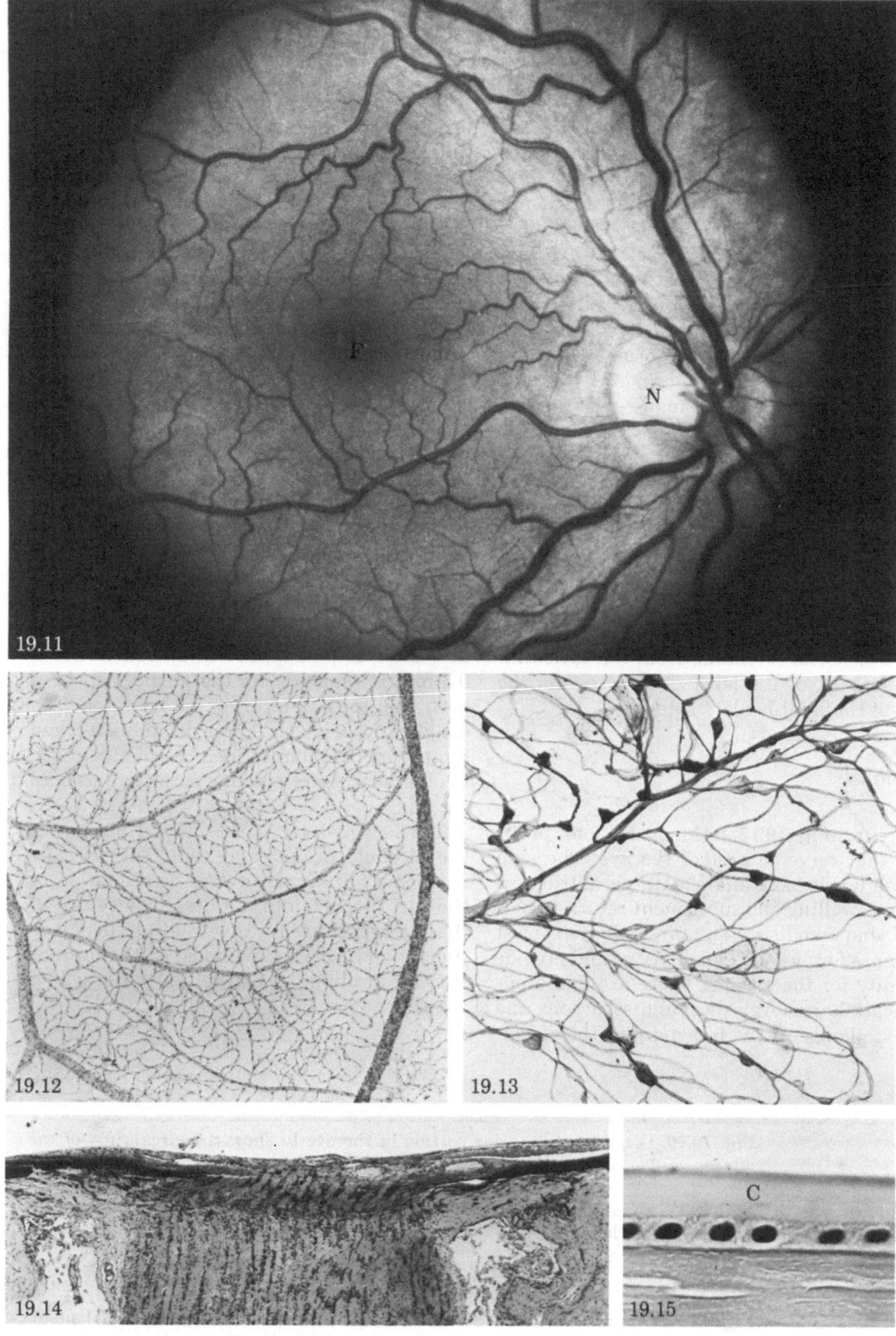

19.11

19.12

19.13

19.14

19.15

ANTERIOR AND POSTERIOR CHAMBERS (Figs. 19.4 and 19.16). The anterior chamber lies between the cornea and the iris and lens. The posterior chamber lies posterior to the iris and just anterior to the suspensory ligament of the lens. Both chambers are filled with a watery fluid, the aqueous humor, produced by filtration of blood from the ciliary processes. This fluid is drained from the anterior chamber at the angle formed by the cornea with the basal part of the iris. Here there is a series of labyrinthine spaces that drain into an irregular canal (the canal of Schlemm) that forms a complete ring around the lateral margin of the cornea. This canal is drained by small veins. Any obstruction to the drainage (Fig. 19.17a) of this humor results in an increase in intraocular pressure (Fig. 19.17b) called glaucoma.

VITREOUS BODY. This is a colorless, transparent, gelatinous mass filling the main cavity of the eye, between the lens and the retina. It is 99% water and contains polysaccharides and some collagen fibers randomly arranged. The hyaloid canal is a thin cylindrical network of fibrils extending from the optic disk to the back of the lens; this represents the site of the fetal hyaloid artery.

Adnexa

EYELIDS (Fig. 19.18) are movable folds of tissue that serve to protect the eye. The skin of the lids is loose and elastic, permitting extreme swelling and subsequent return to normal shape and size. The tarsal plates consist of dense fibrous and elastic tissue and provide rigidity for the eyelids. There are numerous delicate hairs (eyelashes) and sebaceous and sweat glands. At the free margins the epidermis becomes continuous with the epithelium of the palpebral conjunctiva.

The conjunctiva, covering the exposed surface of the globe (except for the cornea) and lining the deep surfaces of the lids, consists of a stratified columnar epithelium with scattered goblet cells on a delicate lamina propria. It is (unusual for epithelium) highly vascular. It also contains scattered lymphoid tissue.

THE LACRIMAL APPARATUS (Fig. 19.1) consists of the lacrimal gland, accessory glands, canaliculi, tear sac, and nasolacrimal duct. The lacrimal gland is a tear-secreting gland located in the anterior-superior temporal portion of the orbit. It consists of several separate glandular lobes with 6–12 excretory ducts connecting the gland to the conjunctival surface (superior conjunctival fornix). This is a tubuloalveolar gland with columnar serous cells with secretory granules, myoepithelial cells, and a basal lamina. The secretion of the gland passes down over the cornea and the conjunctiva, moistening their surfaces. The fluid drains into the lacrimal canaliculi through the lacrimal puncta, round apertures about 0.5 mm in diameter on the medial aspect of both the upper and lower lid margins. The canaliculi are about 1 mm in diameter and 8 mm long and join to form a common canaliculus just before opening into the lacrimal sac.

The lacrimal sac is the dilated portion of the lacrimal drainage system. The nasolacrimal duct is the downward continuation of the sac; it opens into the nasal cavity. All of these passages are lined with either nonkeratinizing stratified squamous epithelium or stratified columnar epithelium with goblet cells.

Fig. 19.16. Diagram of anterior portion of the eye to show the *circulation of the aqueous humor* (arrows).

Fig. 19.17. *Glaucoma.* **a:** Obliteration of the filtration angle (arrows) obstructing the canal of Schlemm (S) with adhesion of the iris to the cornea. ×35. **b:** Depression of the optic nerve head due to increased pressure in the globe. ×35. (Courtesy of D. Johnson.)

Fig. 19.18. *Eyelid.* Note hair follicles (H), glands (G) obscuring the tarsal plate, muscle (M), and conjunctival (concave) surface. ×7.5. (Courtesy of D. Johnson.)

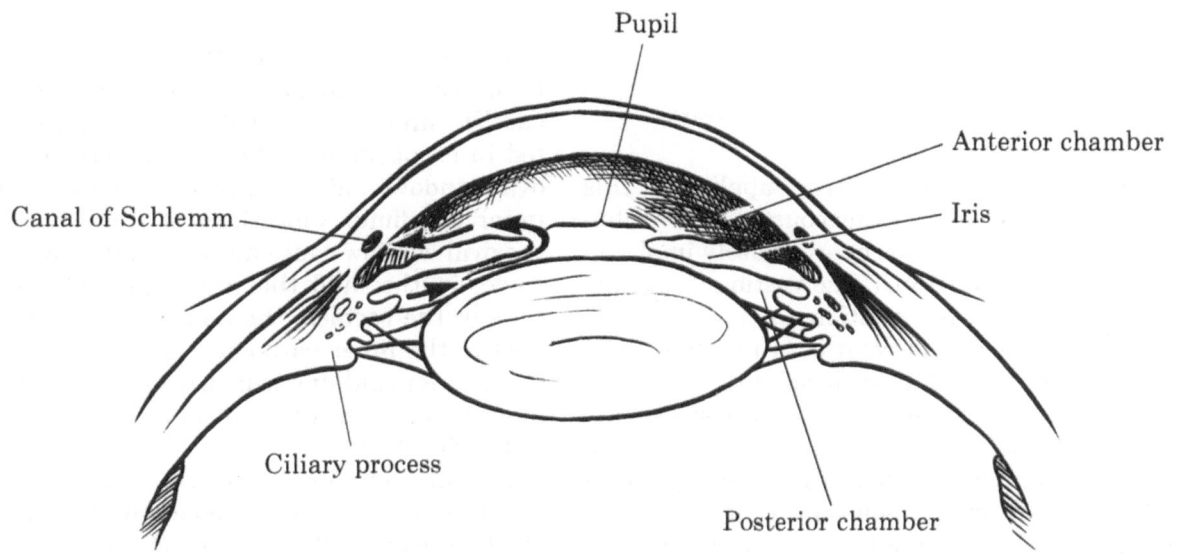

Pupil

Anterior chamber

Canal of Schlemm

Iris

Ciliary process

Posterior chamber

19.16

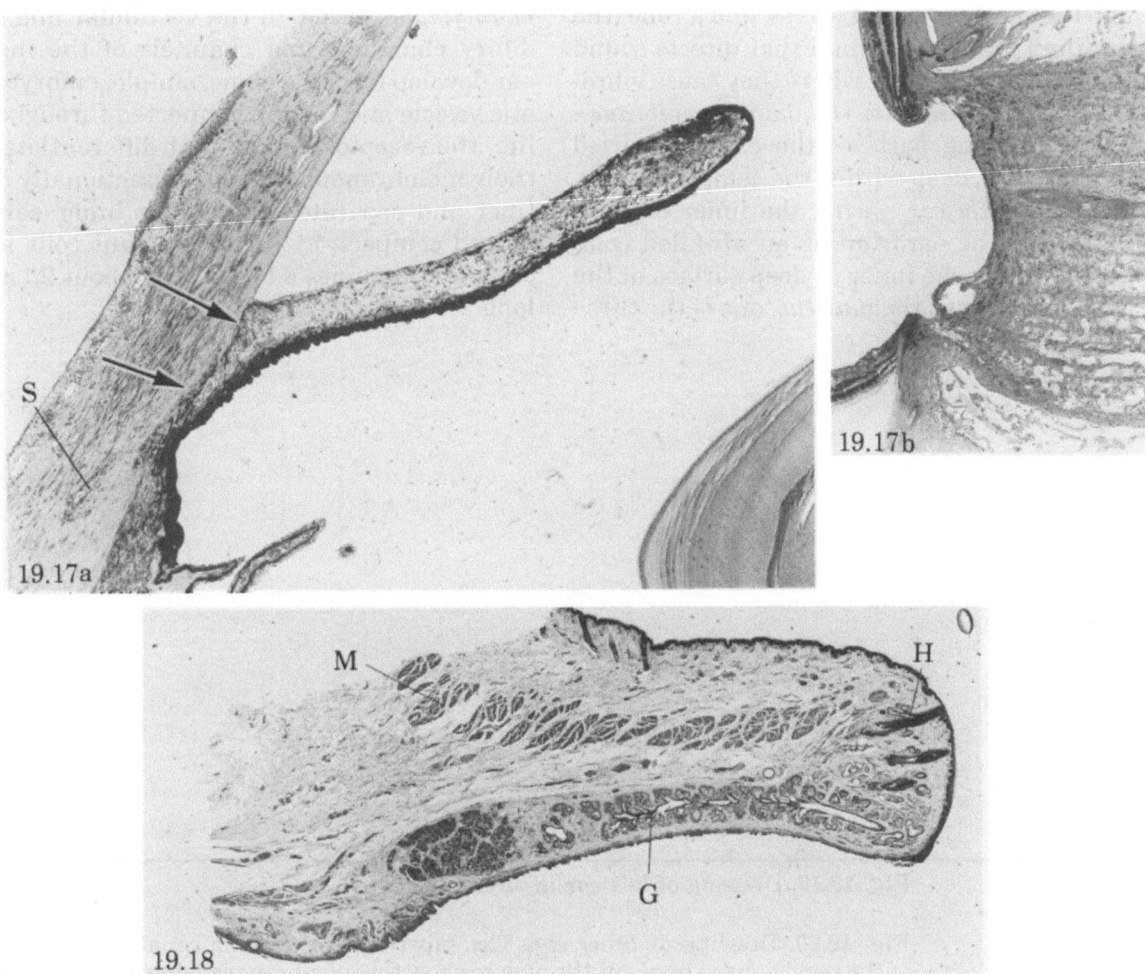

S

19.17a

19.17b

M

H

O

G

19.18

Ear

Overview (Fig. 19.19)

The two synonymous terms applied to this complex organ, the statoacoustic and vestibulocochlear apparatus, appropriately imply its two distinct functions. The vestibular component provides information to the CNS concerning linear and rotational movements of the head, as well as position with respect to gravity. The cochlear or acoustic components transmit sound waves from external air to an internal fluid system, where they produce movements in a membrane that are transduced to nerve impulses interpreted by the CNS as sound. The sensory cells in both acoustic and vestibular portions of the ear are mechanoreceptors.

The *external ear* consists of a skin-covered flap that gathers sound waves, and a tube (the *auditory meatus*) or canal that directs sound waves to its inner ear, where they cause vibrations in the *ear drum (tympanic membrane)*. The remaining parts of the ear are buried in chambers deep within the temporal bone.

The *middle ear,* facing the inner or deep surface of the eardrum, is an air-filled compartment. To the inner or deep surface of the drum is attached the *malleus,* one of the three minute bones (or *ossicles*) that transmit vibrations across the middle ear cavity to the inner ear. The innermost ossicle, the *stapes,* is situated in an opening in the bony labyrinth, the oval window, and is in direct contact with the inner ear fluid. Vibrations of the stapes in the oval window cause movement (a traveling wave) in the fluid that stimulates sensitive cells in the cochlea, the auditory or acoustic part of the inner ear. The vestibular part of the system contains cells sensory to inertial movements of the contained fluid rather than to its vibration.

The *inner ear* (Fig. 19.20) consists of a series of spaces and channels in bone, the *bony labyrinth,* filled with fluid, the *perilymph.* Within the bony labyrinth, and generally conforming to its shape, is suspended an interconnected series of membranous chambers and tubes, the *membranous labyrinth.* This is filled with *endolymph.* Although the vestibular and auditory chambers and channels of the inner ear develop from the same, simple, embryonic otic vesicle and remain connected throughout life, the receptor organs that differentiate in their membranous walls are functionally distinct and separate. The entire inner ear is indeed compact; by means of tight coils and circlets it occupies a space only about 20 mm long.

Fig. 19.19. Drawing of left *ear in situ.*

Fig. 19.20. Drawing of *inner ear.* The superior semicircular canal and two coils of the cochlea have been cut through to show the membranous labyrinth suspended inside the bony labyrinth. The inset (lower right) is an enlarged cross-section of one turn of the cochlea.

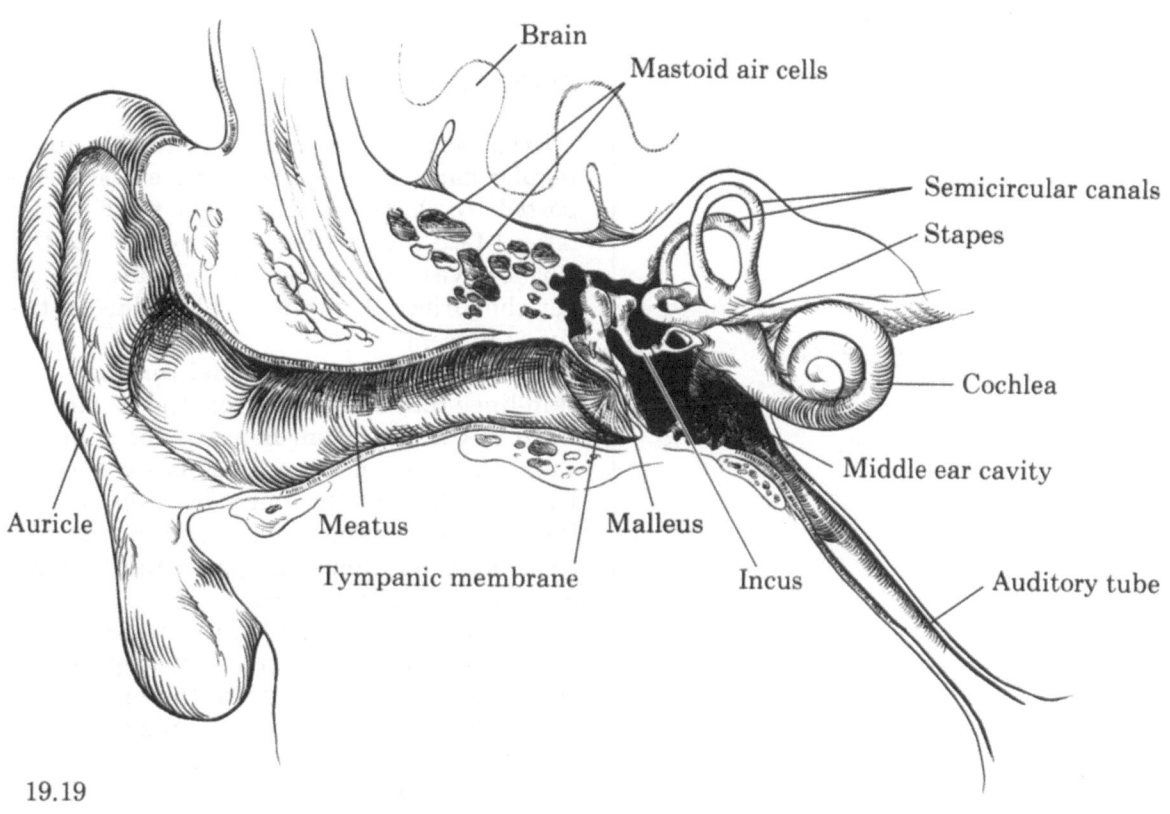

Brain

Mastoid air cells

Semicircular canals

Stapes

Cochlea

Middle ear cavity

Auricle

Meatus

Tympanic membrane

Malleus

Incus

Auditory tube

19.19

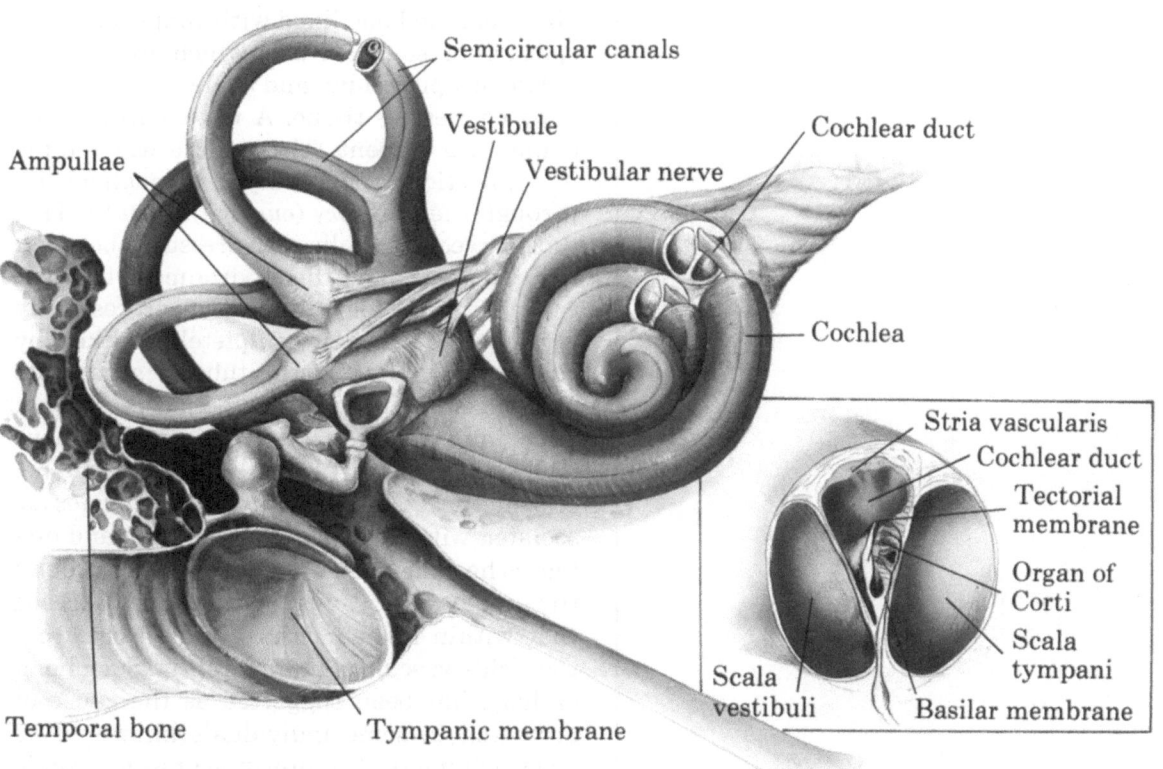

Semicircular canals

Vestibule

Vestibular nerve

Cochlear duct

Ampullae

Cochlea

Stria vascularis

Cochlear duct

Tectorial membrane

Organ of Corti

Scala tympani

Scala vestibuli

Basilar membrane

Temporal bone

Tympanic membrane

19.20

Auditory System

EXTERNAL EAR. The *auricle* (pinna) is an irregular flap of skin and connective tissue supported by elastic cartilage. On most of the lateral face the cartilage is very close to the surface with epidermis resting directly on perichondrium. Elsewhere subcutaneous tissue is present.

The external auditory canal (*meatus*) is a skin-lined tube extending from the surface inward to the ear drum. Beneath the skin the wall of its outer portion is composed of cartilage, and that of the inner or deep portion is of bone. Ceruminous glands, producing wax (cerumen), are numerous, particularly in the outer portion of the tube.

The *tympanic membrane* or eardrum stretches across the bottom or deep end of the canal, separating it from the middle ear cavity. Its outer surface is covered with skin similar to that lining the canal. This rests on a dense but well-vascularized fibroelastic membrane. Its deep surface, facing the tympanic cavity, is covered with simple cuboidal epithelium.

THE MIDDLE EAR (tympanic cavity) is an air-filled space in bone lined with simple cuboidal epithelium, some areas of which are ciliated. Between epithelium and bone is a layer of loose connective tissue. A few small mucous glands are present. The middle ear retains its connection to the pharynx throughout life through the *auditory* (*eustachian*) *tube*. This tube serves to equalize air pressures between the middle ear and the environment through the pharynx. This equalization process may be impaired or even completely blocked by edema in the wall of the tube or around its pharyngeal orifice if an infection is present. Such impairment is often painfully obvious in descent from altitude, as in an airplane, or sometimes during the pressure changes associated with underwater swimming and diving. When the pressure in the tissues around the middle ear cavity significantly exceeds that within it, hemorrhage may occur from the richly vascular lamina propria. Such hemorrhage has been suggested as the cause of drowning in some individuals known to be good swimmers. The presumed mechanism is irritation of the nearby vestibular apparatus by the hemorrhage, leading to disorientation sufficient to affect the adequacy of swimming movements.

From the posterior wall of the middle ear cavity a short narrow tunnel leads to another air-filled chamber slightly smaller than the tympanic cavity, the *mastoid antrum*. After birth numerous *mastoid air cells* sprout from the wall of this antrum, continuing to grow, branch, and rebranch until puberty.

The three ossicles of the tympanic cavity form a bridge across this cavity from the tympanic membrane to the oval window, one of two membranous partitions between the middle and inner ears. The joints between the ossicles make the bridge flexible. However, coupling is such that the chain almost moves as a whole. The last of these bones, the stapes, fits closely into the window frame. As indicated above, this arrangement delivers the sound-induced vibrations to the oval window. The intensity of the transmission of sound may be modified by the action of two small muscles, one of which alters the tension of the tympanic membrane (tensor tympani muscle), and the other of which modifies the movement of the stapes (stapedius muscle).

Anatomic characteristics of the middle ear as mentioned above—an air-containing space, largely confined within bone, but having openings connected to other passages—makes this a likely site for infection. The disease is otitis media—inflammation of the middle ear. It is painful, like any inflammatory process in a tight compartment, as well as serious. Infections of the middle ear that extend to the mastoid air cells may even have fatal results by extension into the cranial cavity.

AUDITORY PORTION OF INNER EAR (Figs. 19.21 through 19.28). The components of the inner ear concerned with hearing will be described in the sequence in which the traveling wave moves through the system.

Bony labyrinth. Vibrations of the stapes at the oval window are transmitted to the fluid contained within the vestibule, a chamber of the bony labyrinth filled with perilymph. Perilymph is a fluid similar, but not identical, to cerebrospinal fluid. Perilymphatic spaces may be connected with the subarachnoid space of the brain by a narrow channel, the perilymphatic duct, which is not always pat-

ent. From the vestibule, fluid movements are transmitted into the spiral portion of the bony labyrinth, the *cochlea*. The 2½ turns of this tapering spiral cavity are coiled around a central bony column, the *modiolus* (Fig. 19.21). The spiral lumen is divided by the membranous labyrinth (*see below*) such that vibrations in perilymph contained in one division, the *scala vestibuli*, are transmitted across the membranous labyrinth into the perilymph of the other division, the *scala tympani* (Figs. 19.20, 19.22 through 19.25). In passing from the scala vestibuli to the scala tympani, the vibrations of the perilymph initiate movement in the intervening membranous labyrinth. This movement produces deformation of stereocilia on sensory cells within the membranous labyrinth. The lower end of the scala tympani, at the base of the cochlea, terminates at the membrane covering the *round window*, through which vibrations are dissipated to the air of the middle ear.

Membranous labyrinth of the cochlea. This thin-walled membranous tube (the *cochlear duct*) is wound around the central screw-shaped modiolus and is attached to the sharp, bony, spiral shelf (the *osseous spiral lamina*). The cochlear duct is also attached to the outer wall of the bony labyrinth across from the spiral lamina by means of the connective tissue *spiral ligament*. The walls of the cochlear duct facing the scalae are flattened. Thus a cross-section of the cochlear duct approximates the form of an isosceles triangle with its base attached to the spiral ligament and outer bony wall, its apex attached to the spiral lamina, and each of its two sides facing a perilymphatic scala.

The stria vascularis (Fig. 19.24) occupies the lateral wall of the cochlear duct (the base of the triangle). It is composed of a vascularized, stratified, cuboidal epithelium. The stria vascularis is responsible for the maintenance of the high potassium (approximately 140 meq/l) and low sodium concentrations of the endolymph, which are probably accomplished by a sodium–potassium exchange pump in the epithelial cells. The organ of Corti will not operate without the high potassium concentration and the accompanying positive endocochlear potential, although the operative mechanisms are unclear at present.

Fig. 19.21. Scanning electron micrograph of *modiolus*. ×20. (Courtesy of C. Smith. From Smith CA. Structure of the cochlear duct. In Beagley H (ed). Audiology and Audiological Medicine. Oxford Press, New York, 1982.)

Fig. 19.22. Section of the *cochlea* close to the axis of the modiolus showing several sections of the coils with cochlear duct (scala media) (C) and auditory nerve (N). ×20. (Courtesy of C. Smith.)

Fig. 19.23. Transverse section of the *organ of Corti*. Note cochlear duct (C), tectorial membrane (T) resting on the hair cells (H), and stria vascularis (S). ×300. (Courtesy of C. Smith. From Smith CA. Structure of the cochlear duct. In Beagley H (ed). Audiology and Audiological Medicine. Oxford Press, New York, 1982).

Fig. 19.24. Electron micrograph of a section of the *stria vascularis* bordering the cochlear duct (C). This is one of the rare examples in the human body of a vascularized epithelium. Note vessels (V). About ×2000. (Courtesy of C. Smith.)

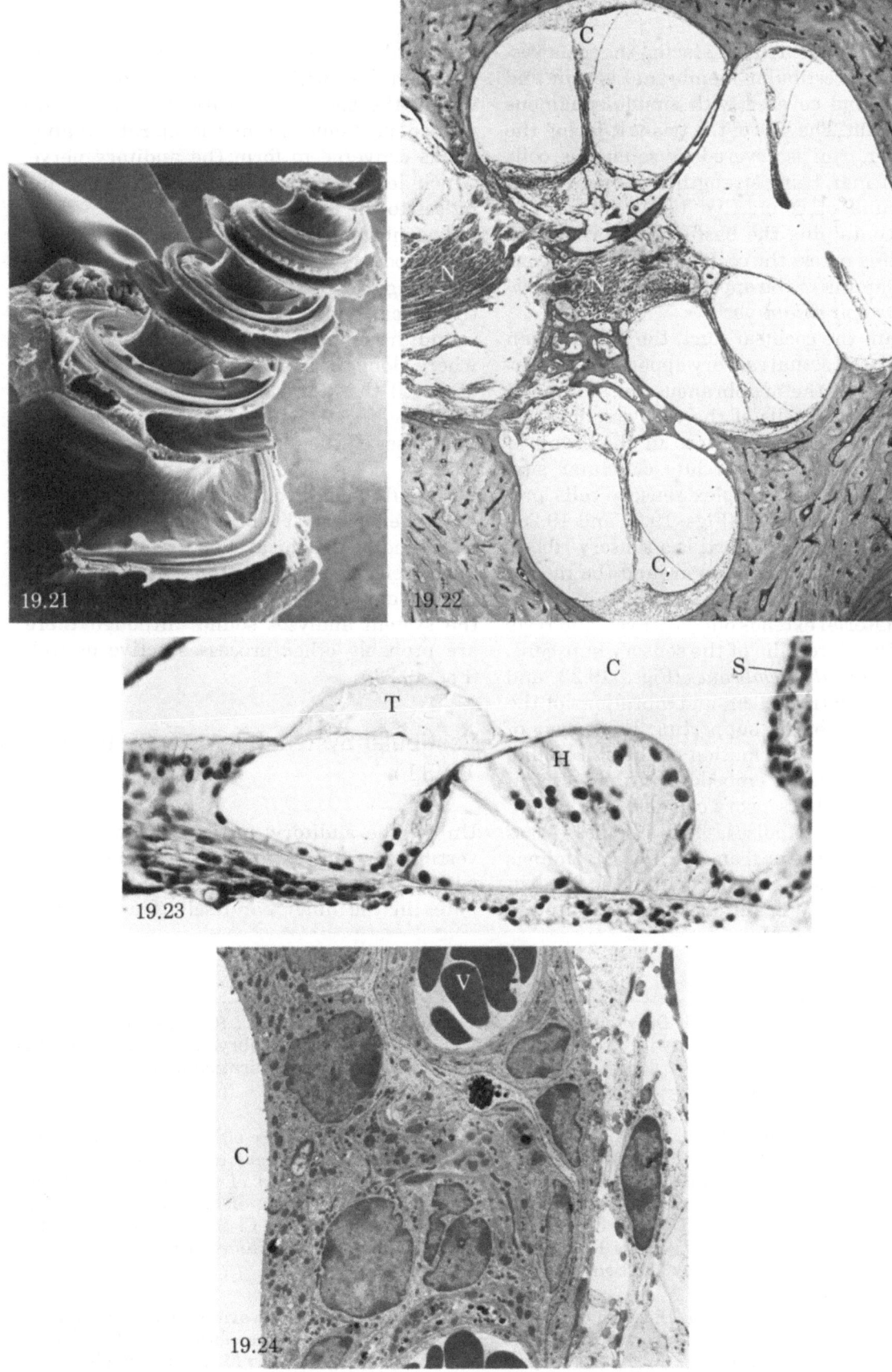

19.21

19.22

19.23

19.24

The side of the triangle facing the scala vestibuli (the vestibular membrane) is thin and delicate and covered with simple squamous epithelium. The side of the triangle facing the scala tympani is covered by squamous cells but is firmer, being strengthened by a *basilar membrane* of connective tissue fibers. The sheet containing the basilar membrane and extending across the cochlea from the osseous spiral lamina to the opposite wall is the *membranous spiral lamina.*

Within the cochlear duct, the spiral organ of Corti, the actual sensory apparatus of hearing, rests on the membranous spiral lamina. The epithelial cells of the cochlear duct are variable in form, but those in the organ of Corti are differentiated into columnar supporting cells and complex sensory cells provided with stereocilia (Figs. 19.25 and 19.26). In toto, the organ of Corti is a sensory ribbon wound like a spiral ramp around the modiolus. From its inner edge a shelf of fibro-gelatinous material extends outward over, and rests upon, the stereocilia of the sensory hair cells. This *tectorial membrane* (Figs. 19.23 and 19.25) is relatively firm and vibrations of the basilar membrane supporting the organ of Corti produce deformation of the stereocilia, some of which are embedded in the tectorial membrane. This sensory cell deformation initiates nerve impulses. The impulses pass along nerve fibers from peripheral endings around the hair cells to neurons located in a long spiral ganglion also arranged around

the cochlea within the modiolus. This spiral ganglion lies within a cavity that courses within the base of the thread of the screw-shaped modiolus. From the spiral ganglion axons converge to form the auditory nerve, which leaves the modiolus and carries impulses to the CNS.

The vibration of the stapes in the oval window produces a wave in the perilymph (the *traveling wave*) that moves from the base to the apical end of the cochlea. The driving sound frequency of the stapes determines where along the basilar membrane (and organ of Corti) the vibration will be greatest and the sensory cells will have adequate stimulation to set off the nerve fibers (Figs. 19.27 and 19.28).

High-frequency sound produces waves that have their greatest vibration in the lower or basal end of the spiral. Low frequencies produce their effective vibrations toward the upper end of the spiral. This is one way in which the system analyzes sound, although there are probably other processes active as well (Fig. 19.28).

Vestibular System (Figs. 19.29 through 19.31).

Unlike the auditory portion of the ear, the vestibular requires no anatomic connection with the exterior. Vestibular function originates in the inner ear itself. This function

Fig. 19.25. Drawing of a cross-section of the *cochlear duct* (Courtesy of C. Smith and F. Harwin. From Smith C.A. The inner ear: its embryological development and microstructure. In Tower D.B. (ed). Human Communication and Its Disorders, Vol. 3, pp 1–18. Raven Press, New York, 1975.)

Fig. 19.26. Scanning electron micrograph of the *sensory surface* of the *organ of Corti*. The apical ends of the cells are outlined by and covered with tiny scattered microvilli. The groups of sensory hairs on the three rows of outer (above) and one row of inner (below) hair cells can be seen. Each group of hairs arises from the apical end of one hair cell. About ×3000. (Courtesy of C. Smith. From Elias H. Pauly J.E., Burns R.E. Histology and Human Microanatomy, 4th ed, New York, John Wiley and Sons, 1978.)

Fig. 19.27. Diagram of *auditory function*. The traveling wave produced at the oval window moves toward the apex of the cochlea and produces vibrations in the basilar membrane. (Modified with permission from Fig. 21.4 in Barr M. The Human Nervous System. Hagerstown, Harper & Row, 1974.)

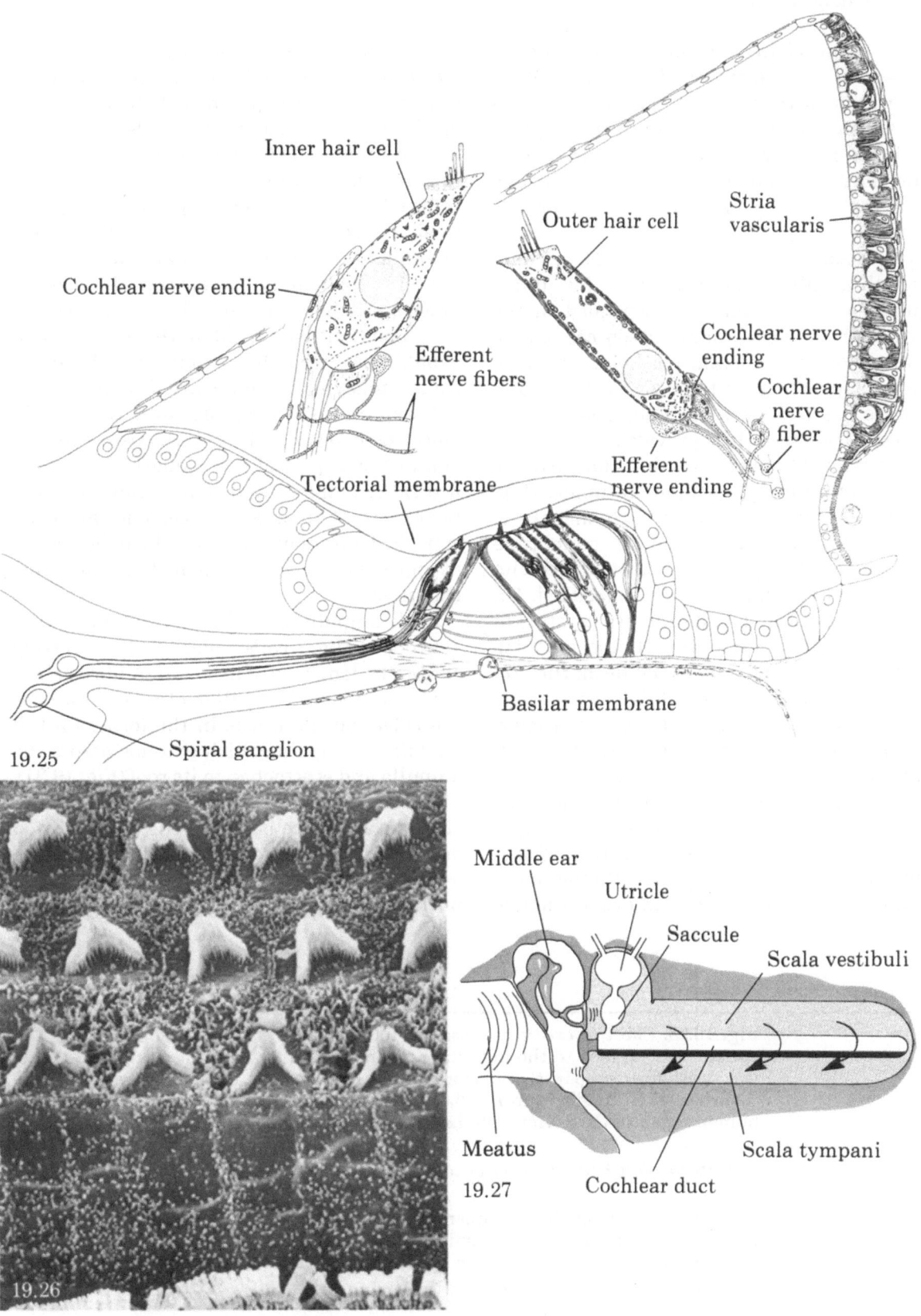

Inner hair cell

Cochlear nerve ending

Outer hair cell

Stria vascularis

Cochlear nerve ending

Cochlear nerve fiber

Efferent nerve fibers

Efferent nerve ending

Tectorial membrane

Basilar membrane

Spiral ganglion

19.25

19.26

Middle ear

Utricle

Saccule

Scala vestibuli

Meatus

19.27

Cochlear duct

Scala tympani

is one of providing information to the CNS concerning movements of the head and its orientation with respect to gravity. The important functional component in this apparatus is the membranous labyrinth and its content of endolymph. The bony labyrinth and perilymph supply only support and protection.

THE SACCULE AND UTRICLE (Fig. 19.29) are delicate, thin-walled chambers lined by simple squamous epithelium and suspended in the perilymph of the vestibule. Each contains a small plaque of columnar epithelium that includes supporting and sensory cells. These plaques are the *maculae*. Each sensory cell (hair cell) of a macula is provided with stereocilia (similar to long microvilli), and with one cilium containing its usual microtubules (Fig. 19.30). The free surface of each macula is coated with a fibro-gelatinous membrane (otolithic membrane) in which the stereocilia and cilia of the hair cells are embedded. On the surface of this membrane are crystals of calcium carbonate (otoliths). If the maculae are tilted by movements of the head, the otolithic membranes and crystals tend to slide downhill, thus bending the hairs and triggering nerve impulses. In addition, linear acceleration, as in an airplane takeoff, displaces the otolithic membrane posteriorly and initiates the appropriate nerve impulses.

SEMICIRCULAR CANALS AND AMPULLAE. Functions of these structures are: three-dimensional spatial orientation, and orientation as to angular acceleration and deceleration. Across the vestibule from the open basal end of the cochlea are openings of the bony labyrinth of the semicircular canals. The three canals are placed at right angles to each other in three different planes, one of which is horizontal. The other two are approximately vertical. Suspended in the perilymph of these channels are delicate, tubular, membranous semicircular canals. Except for the sensory neuroepithelial cells, their lining is of simple squamous epithelium. All of the membranous canals open into the utricle and share the same endolymph. There are five instead of the expected six openings into the utricle, since the two vertical canals share a common channel over part of their length. The canals are 12–22 mm long and about 1 mm in diameter except at their ampullae. The latter are spherical dilations, one of which is located at one end of each canal near its opening into the utricle.

Each ampulla contains a ridge (crista) of neuroepithelial cells placed transversely across the long axis of its canal. A fibro-gelatinous mass similar to that of a macula caps the ridge, but here it is in the form of a tall fin called a cupula, which extends across the ampulla and is attached to its roof (Fig. 19.31). In its base are embedded the stereocilia and cilia of the hair cells. When the head is tilted or rotated, a semicircular canal is turned like a wheel and the inertia of the endolymph pushes the cupula to one side or the other

---

Fig. 19.28. Effect of *excessive noise,* partial destruction of the organ of Corti. The patient was exposed to the high intensity noise of a sawmill for many years. This is a nerve fiber preparation demonstrating loss of nerve endings between arrows. (Courtesy of G. Bredberg in Bredberg G. Cellular pattern and nerve supply of the human organ of Corti. Acta Oto-Laryngol Suppl 236:1968.)

Fig. 19.29. *Vestibular portion* of inner ear.

Fig. 19.30. Scanning electron micrograph of the *hair cells of the saccular macula.* About ×3000. (Courtesy of C. Smith. From Smith C.A., Tanaka K. Some aspects of the structure of the vestibular apparatus. In Naunton RF (ed). The Vestibular System. New York, Academic Press, 1975.)

Fig. 19.31. Diagram of a *crista ampullaris.* Even slight movement of fluid in the canal moves the lower end of the cupula over the hair cells and initiates nerve impulses.

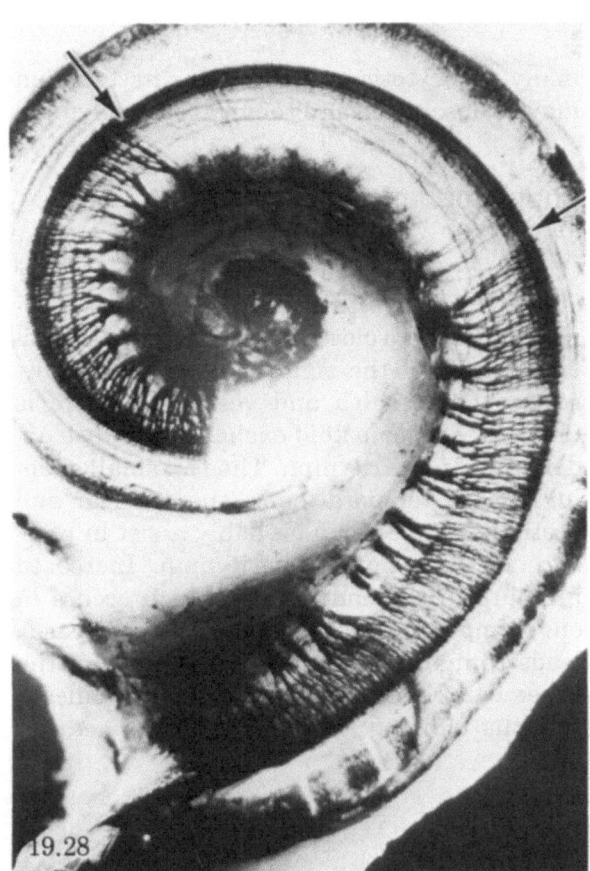

19.28

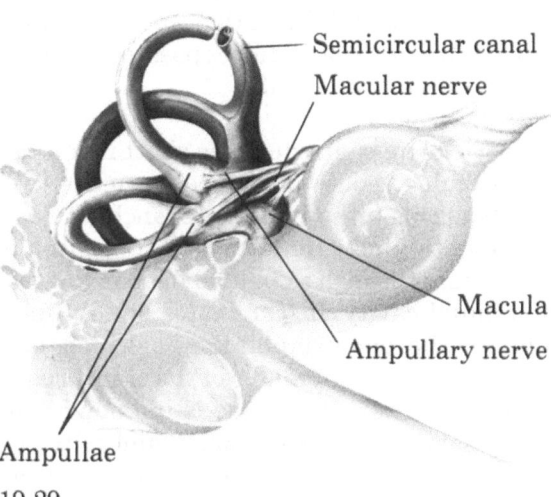

Semicircular canal

Macular nerve

Macula

Ampullary nerve

Ampullae

19.29

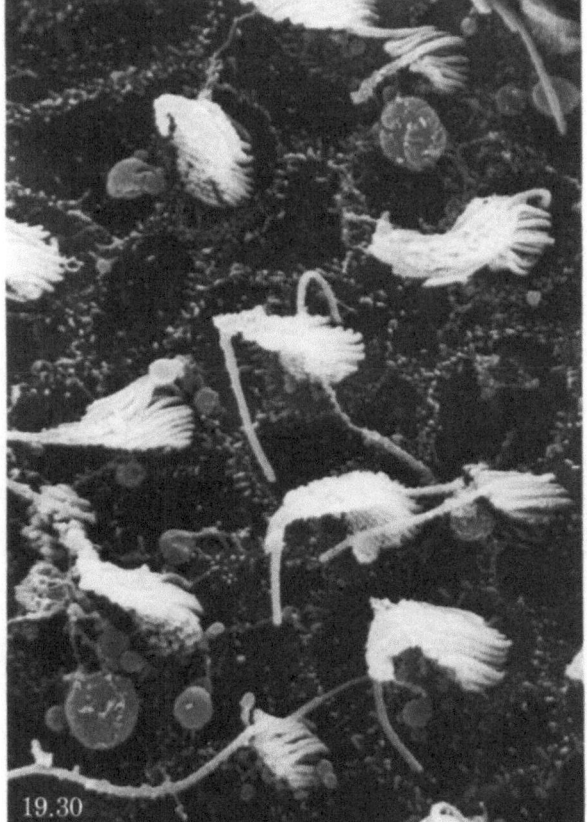

19.30

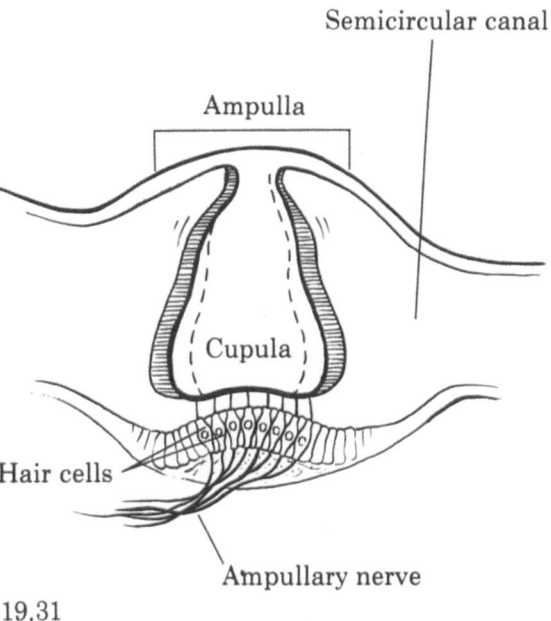

Semicircular canal

Ampulla

Cupula

Hair cells

Ampullary nerve

19.31

of its resting position. One theory (there are several) suggests that the base of the cupula slides across the hair cells. By this means even small head movements would be sufficient to produce hair cell deformation and to initiate nerve impulses. The impulses pass via the vestibular nerve to the CNS.

ENDOLYMPHATIC DUCT AND SAC. The saccule and utricle are connected by a short membranous tubule. About midway between the two chambers this tube gives off a branch (the endolymphatic duct) that leaves the vestibule and courses through a channel in bone toward the cranial cavity. It terminates blindly in a dilation, the endolymphatic sac, which lies just outside the dura mater of the cranial cavity. The function of this sac is unknown but it may serve as an expansion chamber to reduce pressure in the membranous labyrinth. However, it has been found to be lined by tall columnar epithelial cells, some of which are vacuolated and have apical microvilli and many pinocytotic vesicles. Thus its function may be absorption and removal of endolymph.

Endolymphatic Hydrops

Control of fluid balance within the inner ear (and especially within the membranous labyrinth, which is a closed epithelial tube) is critical because of the rigid bony case that surrounds the cochlea and vestibule. There is undoubtedly some fluid exchange between endolymph and perilymph. The two small openings in the temporal bone (the cochlear and vestibular aqueducts) probably assist in pressure equilibration in perilymph. Increased pressure in the endolymph, which occurs in endolymphatic hydrops (Meniere's disease), leads to malfunction of both portions of the inner ear. Symptoms are vertigo (dizziness), tinnitus (ringing in the ears), and hearing loss.

20 Recapitulation with Variations: "Play It Again, Sam"

Introduction

"There are more things in heaven and earth, Horatio, than are dreamt of in your philosophy."

(Hamlet, Act I, Scene V, lines 166–167, by William Shakespeare).

One cannot deny the fundamental interdependence of structure and function in biology and medicine. This is now a hoary and possibly boring adage. But is it also recognized that structure and function determine the characteristics of disease? Is it understood that diseases are experienced, measured, and classified as they are mainly because of the anatomic parts affected? The history of quackery depends largely on the lack of this perception. How else would anyone accept an elixir not only as a panacea—a cure for countless ills of all sorts—but also as a preventive against any disease? Yet, a little sensible reflection on the complexity and detailed specificity (that is, the fine anatomy and physiology) of the human body can prevent the frauds of quackery. Severed nerve fibers are not induced to regrow and to function normally again by the action of an odoriferous nostrum. Metastatic cancer will not be overcome by an extract of fruit pits. There is no advantage in overdosage with vitamins. The only likely victory over disease lies in seeing it for what it is and this means looking at it, possibly with old and simple tools or perhaps with new and subtle tricks. But look at it we must; otherwise we are only charlatans whether we admit it or not.

There is one more reason to study histology, a purely hedonistic reason—the beauty of it. If museums and art collections can be devoted largely or entirely to the external human form, which is so readily accessible to examination by anyone, how much greater is the value in the internal components of the body, particularly when magnified. Of course processing and staining also help in the study of tissues. The world of histology is truly a magnificent one. So let us consider it not as an ugly or maleficent ogre whose shadow, the final exam, darkens our lives and causes our subsequent and often permanent revulsion. Let us accept it as a valuable aid that may make our lives, and in them the science and the practice of medicine, more enjoyable as well as better understood.

We present these ideas at the end of our book rather than at the beginning because we think they may be an incentive to application and further study of this subject after completion of the course in histology. We intend them only to introduce concepts which extend from our basic subject of histology and which may play leading roles in subsequent courses.

The Concept of Normality

The physician should first identify and then treat disease. In order for one to make a diagnosis he or she must hold a clear concept of normality and of its range. It is not enough to know that the apex beat of the heart is normally most forceful to the left of the sternum. The doctor should be able to state how far to the left is acceptable; also in which intercostal space(s) the beat should be; and how forceful it should be and how different physiologic conditions may affect it. And regarding physical stature, is one man less normal than his brother because he is fatter? or shorter? or less muscular or less athletic? Clearly rigid limitations present some disadvantages. In histology, just as in physical examination, we are obliged to present not simply the single ideal normal but some range of what is acceptable.

The traditional concept of normal human biology ignores many variations in form and substance. Problems arise because there is no satisfactory definition of normal. When does one cross the border into disease? Students often recognize and appreciate this confusion. They can openly discuss such questions as: "Isn't baldness (or pulmonary anthracosis, solar tanning of skin, pregnancy, menopause) normal?"; "Is this about the usual degree of arteriosclerosis for a 70-year-old man?"; "Why do some children outgrow their hypersensitivities?"; "What is the prevalence of incidental malignancy or tuberculous Gohn complex?"; and ultimately, "What is normal, anyway?" (Fig. 20.1).

Aging

As histology represents structure in life we are obliged to recognize that this structure

---

Fig. 20.1. Histogram. Frequency distribution of hematocrit values in adult white females in the United States (1960–62). (From Miale, John B: Laboratory medicine: hematology, ed. 6, St Louis, 1982, The C. V. Mosby Co.; data from National Center for Health Statistics, 1967.)

Fig. 20.2. *Carcinoma of the prostate.* This is formed of small irregular glands. It was an incidental finding at the autopsy of a 66-year-old man. Concretions in nonmalignant glands are visible at left. ×85. (Courtesy of K. Schmidt.)

Fig. 20.3. Arteriosclerosis with *near occlusion* of the common iliac artery, a lesion often present in the elderly. ×7.5.

Fig. 20.4. *Lymph node in youth* is full, complete, and cellular and has germinal centers. ×20.

Fig. 20.5. *Lymph node in old age* is largely replaced with fat and has few and indistinct germinal centers. ×10.

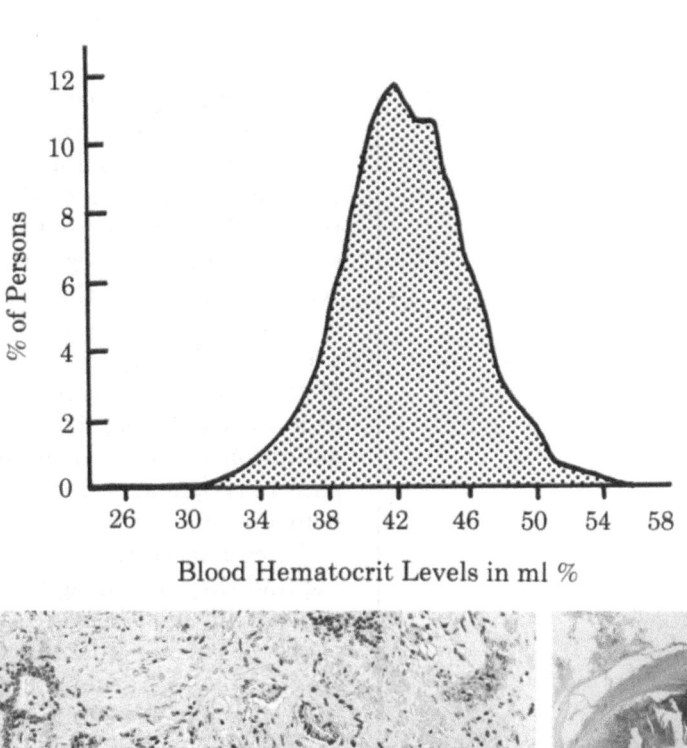

20.1

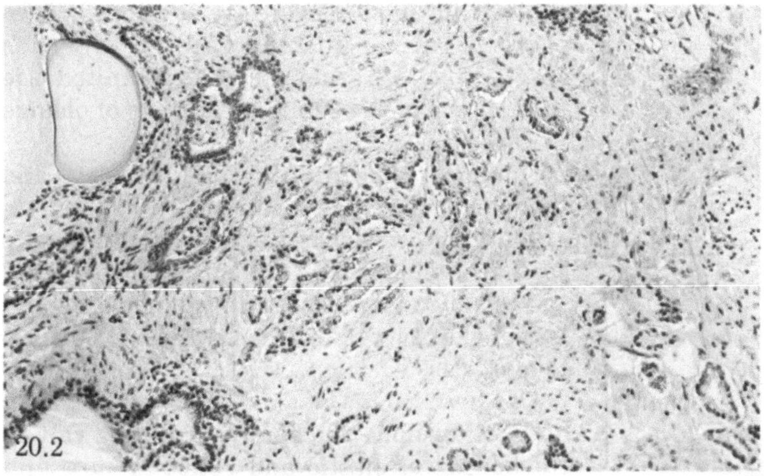

20.2

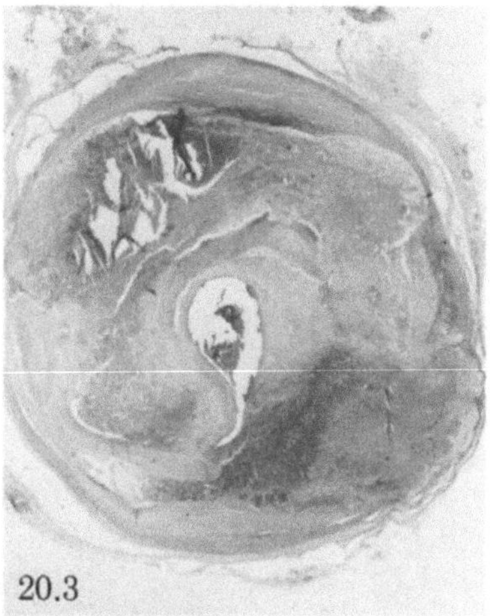

20.3

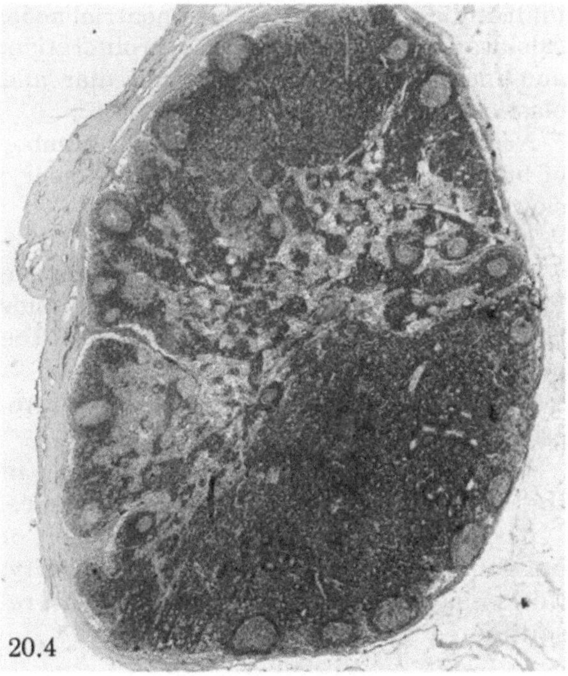

20.4

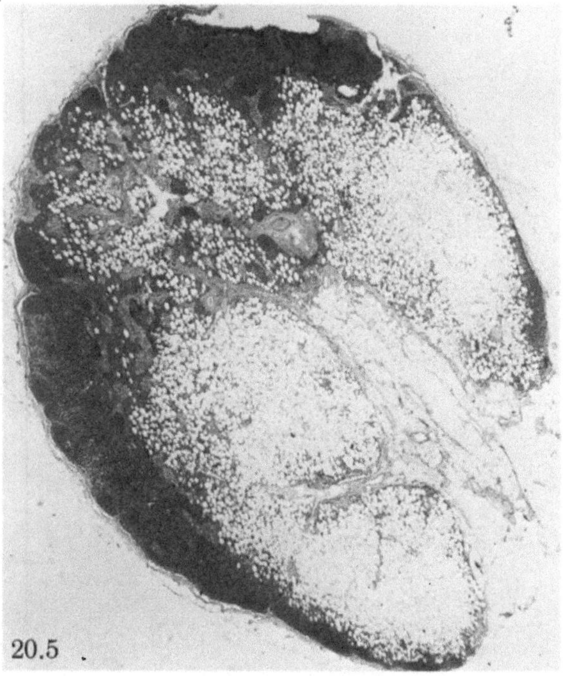

20.5

changes during the course of that life. A common term for this process is aging, but there are many concepts and connotations of that term. Some of these conflict. We know some things about aging and we can define it as the changes in biologic tissues that are the result of time and that are not attributable to overt disease. This definition includes every process in life that occurs after fertilization of the ovum. Generally the use of the term is more restricted. To some individuals the definition of aging includes only what happens to people older than they are. For others it means the changes that lead to death.

We can describe some of the changes of aging and they are being better defined as concepts of life and of disease are developed. However, we remain unable to specify why each species has a rather narrowly limited life span. Some of the common findings of old age in several species are:

Outward appearance: wrinkled, dry, and less elastic skin; gray hair.

Musculature: decreased muscular mass, strength, endurance, and agility.

Skeleton: stooped posture; calcification and loss of elasticity of ligaments and tendons; osteoporosis.

Cardiovascular system: increased rigidity and collagenous thickening of heart valves; thickening of elastic and reticular nets and infiltration of fat in and about sinoatrial node; calcification of media, elastic proliferation, and increase in collagen, in muscular and elastic arteries (Fig. 20.3).

Nervous system: decrease in total number of brain cells; failing of short-term memory; slower reaction time.

Eyes: presbyopia; cataracts.

Capacities for taste and smell: progressive loss with decrease in number of taste buds per papilla and in number of fibers in the olfactory nerves.

Auditory system: loss of hearing (higher frequencies first).

Vestibular system: degenerative changes in the inner ear, with disturbance of balance.

Respiratory system: decrease in numbers of pulmonary alveoli; decrease in vital capacity; thickening of respiratory membrane with resulting reduction of diffusing capacity.

Dental system: loss of teeth.

Gastrointestinal system: reduced gastrointestinal motility.

Renal system: reduction of glomerular filtration.

Prostate: hyperplasia and carcinoma (Fig. 20.2).

Reproductive organs, male and female: atrophy.

Endocrine system: decrease in production of TSH by the pituitary and decrease in the basal metabolic rate.

Adaptability: relative inability to adapt or respond to stress. This refers to regulation of temperature, blood pH, and serum glucose level, as well as to more complex human traits (*see later*).

Whether these changes result from age alone or from the accumulation of environmental influences is moot. The point is that appearances change with life (Figs. 20.4 through 20.7).

Variations in Cellular Growth

Atrophy and Hypertrophy

Another group of variations in histology centers about the range of cellular activity in certain tissues. One example concerns the size of cells. Consider the difference between the muscle cells in the biceps of a weight lifter and of a bookworm, to contrast two normal specimens. The two are different, not only by gross standards in vivo on "Muscle Beach," but of course also in functional ability. Histologically the difference is probably just as marked if accurately measured, but it is not so easily recognized by casual observation.

When the cell size exceeds the expected normal bounds (whatever *they* are), we refer to this as hypertrophy—enlargement of cells. We have already demonstrated this in smooth muscle of the pregnant uterus (Fig. 6.4). Pregnancy, though an extraordinary series of physiologic and anatomic changes, is still a "normal" event—which points up an interesting discrepancy of our system. Pathologic examples of hypertrophy occur in the myocar-dium as a result of obstructions of blood flow in, for example, stenosis of the aortic valve following rheumatic fever.

We refer to the condition in which cells are unduly small, because of either lack of use or lack of nutrition, as *atrophy*, which implies that these cells had been at one time within the normal range. In the postmenopausal endometrium and myometrium atrophy is common. In such a case this too has to be considered as a "physiologic" or normal event. For more severe, more easily recognized, and more important examples of atrophy, see the adrenal cortex after prolonged steroid therapy (Fig. 16.40) or striated muscle after interruption of its motor nerve supply.

Agenesis, Aplasia, and Hypoplasia

There are three terms referring to reduction in *numbers* of cells. *Agenesis* means a lack of formation of a structure or of a cell type; conventionally this is an inborn lack. *Aplasia* (a, lack of; plasia, forming or molding) implies a complete lack of any cellular reproduction (and therefore of cells, as in aplastic anemia). *Hypoplasia* means a number of cells that is less than normal—as may occur in any of the endocrine glands under appropriate conditions.

Hyperplasia

Hyperplasia denotes excessive numbers of cells, as in either endocrine or exocrine glands under appropriate stimulation, or in endothelial cells or fibroblasts, or some types of epithelial cells during inflammation and in simple healing. The healing fracture (Fig. 5.21) demonstrates this in respect to fibrous tissue, bone and cartilage.

Metaplasia

Metaplasia is the substitution of one type of adult tissue for another. The most common variety is squamous metaplasia, in which stratified squamous epithelium replaces simple or pseudostratified columnar. This occurs for the most part in bronchial epithelium and in endocervical epithelium of the uterus. It usually results because of chronic inflammation. Bony metaplasia of connective tissue may occur in areas of calcification. Cartilaginous metaplasia (Fig. 20.8) is a common component of certain epithelial tumors.

The process of metaplasia of any sort is an abnormal form of maturation, rather than a replacement of all the cells of the tissue. If the stimulus that has given rise to an instance of squamous metaplasia is removed, the process may reverse; that is, the normal columnar epithelium may in time reappear as the metaplastic squamous epithelium disappears.

Dysplasia

Dysplasia connotes a disorder of form, a more severe distortion than metaplasia. This may also be a reversible result of inflammation, but it can be a step in the development of malignancy. In simplest terms it is an intermediate, and potentially or theoretically reversible but abnormal, phase (Figs. 20.9 through 20.11).

Fig. 20.6. *Ovary from a 7-month-old girl,* with many active follicles, mostly primordial. ×37. (Courtesy of J. Rieke.)

Fig. 20.7. *Ovary, postmenopausal.* There are no follicles, and one corpus albicans (lower right). ×37.

Fig. 20.8. *Cartilaginous metaplasia* (arrows) in a pleomorphic adenoma (mixed tumor) of the parotid gland. ×85.

The following three photographs are from vaginal smears and at the same magnification, ×250. (Courtesy of E. Nassir.)

Fig. 20.9. *Normal vaginal smear.* The squamous epithelial cells are quite regular, with much cytoplasm and small nuclei.

Fig. 20.10. *Epithelial dysplasia,* an intermediate stage in the development of malignancy. There is more variation among the cells, many having an increased nuclear-cytoplasmic ratio.

Fig. 20.11. *Carcinoma of the uterine cervix.* Almost all of the cells are abnormal. They show more variation, as well as hyperchromatism and enlargement.

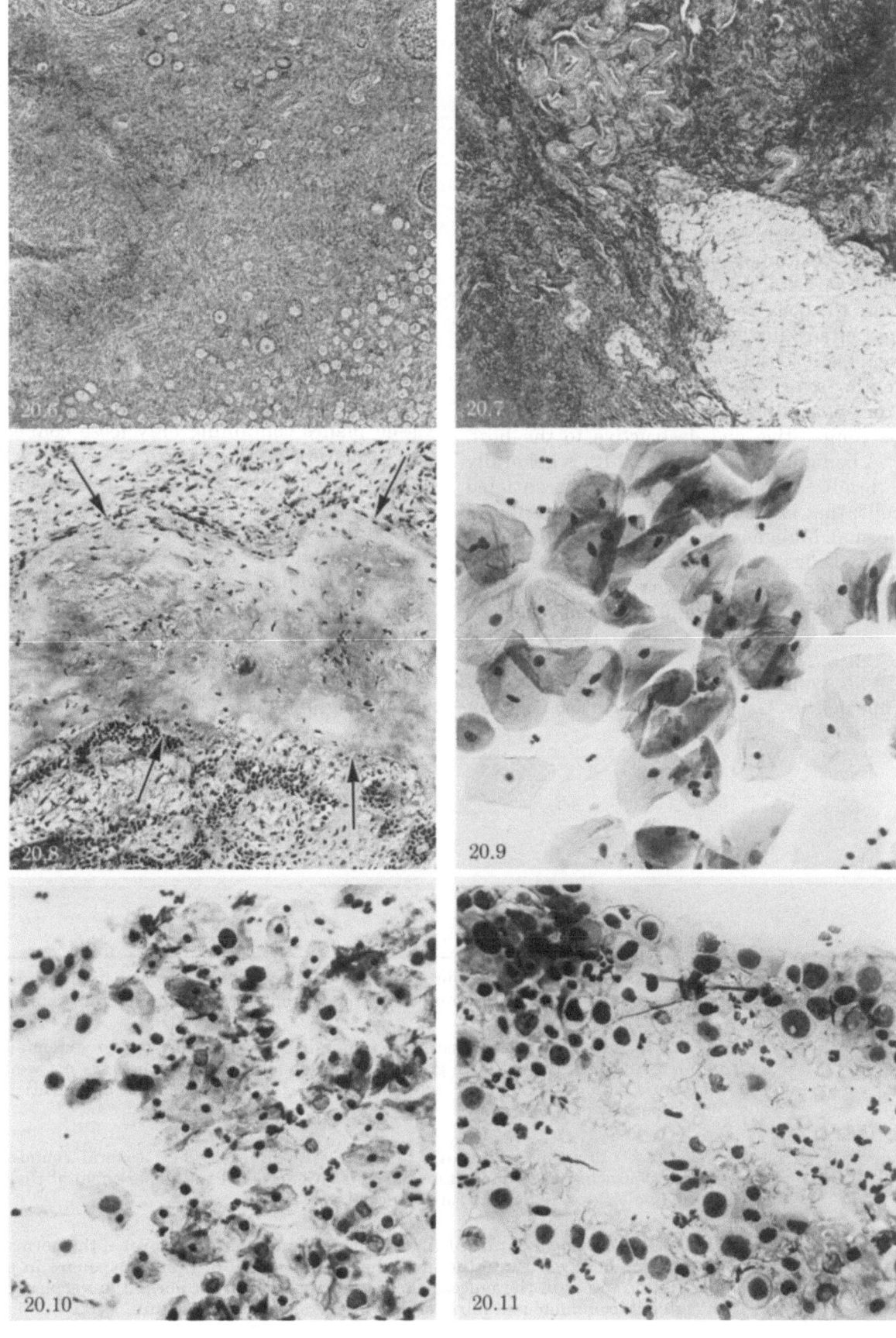

Neoplasia (Figs. 20.11 through 20.15)

Neoplasia (neo, new) is an autonomous cellular proliferation. A more specific definition is "an abnormal mass of tissue, the growth of which exceeds and is uncoordinated with that of the normal tissues and persists in the same excessive manner after cessation of the stimuli which evoke the change"* A neoplasm—or tumor—is therefore an autochthonous parasite, that is, a parasite originating from the body itself. It competes with its host and often kills him or her. Morphologically, neoplastic tissue usually resembles the normal more or less, but it is also likely to differ from normal in being less organized. It may be competitive and destructive to the host.

A benign neoplasm (Fig. 20.12) is generally a localized collection of well differentiated cells; that is, their individual form simulates normal. Malignant neoplasms (Fig. 20.13) will likely be less differentiated, thus more primitive in appearance, and less easily recognized as to their cell of origin. So it may become

difficult to decide on the basis of cellular growth pattern what tissue or organ is the site of origin of the primary malignancy. This is particularly true if it makes its presence known first in a site distant from that in which it arose.

The most significant expression of malignancy is invasiveness (Fig. 20.15). Tumor cell groups tend to infiltrate and replace other tissues. They may grow as solid, bulky masses along a broad front or as small islands more subtly scattered through a tissue. They may extend into cavities such as a pleural space or a capillary or venous channel, come loose from their attachments, travel to distant sites (Fig. 20.14), and continue to grow in these. Tissue planes containing only loose connective tissue are another route of spread. All such extensions may be referred to as *metastases.*

Cells shed from epithelial surfaces offer an easy and reliable source of diagnostic information. Individual normal epithelial cells, as well as malignant and dysplastic and inflammatory ones, all may be distinguished fairly reliably. The study of such specimens constitutes the field of exfoliative cytology (Figs. 20.9 through 20.11).

---

* From Willis RA The Spread of Tumors in the Human Body. London, Butterworth and Co., 1952.

Fig. 20.12. A *benign tumor,* fibroadenoma, of breast. This has a distinct border (arrows) around the entire tumor separating it from the surrounding fat. ×85.

Fig. 20.13. *Carcinoma* of breast. The tumor has an irregular border extending into fat. Although the cells are grouped in a glandular pattern, they are not well-differentiated and the "glands" have no lumen or other evidence of organization. ×85. (Courtesy of B. Harty.)

Fig. 20.14. *Carcinoma metastatic to lungs.* The lungs contain several rounded masses, characteristic of metastases (arrows). (Courtesy of the Department of Diagnostic Radiology, Oregon Health Sciences University.)

Fig. 20.15. *Carcinoma of the colon.* **a:** Tumor extends above the level of the normal mucosa and downward into the muscularis (arrow). ×5. **b:** From the square in **a.** Edge of the tumor in the mucosa shows the transition from normal to neoplastic, though still columnar and fairly orderly, hyperchromatic structure. ×100.

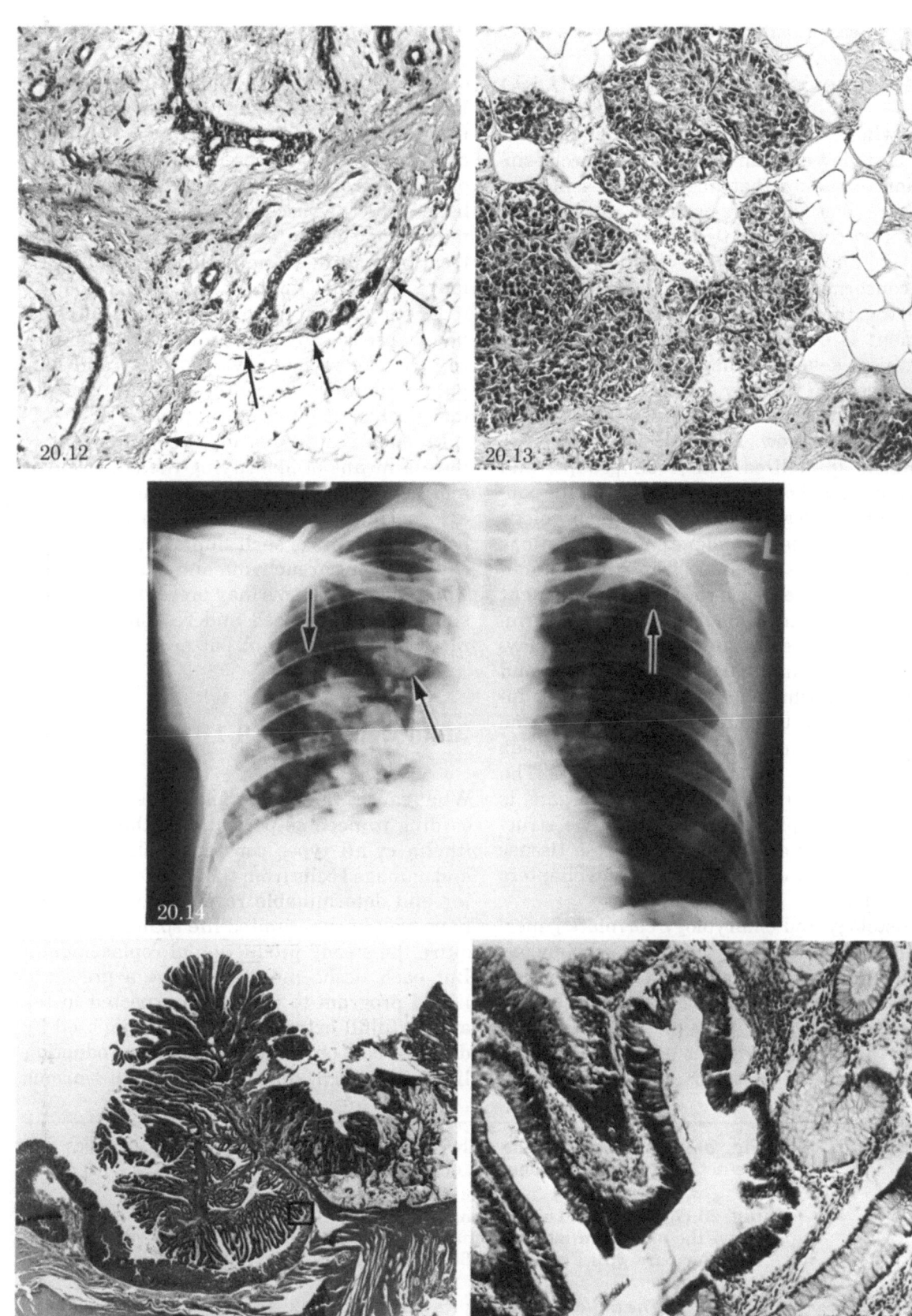

1,2,3,4,5,6,7,8,9,10,11,12,13,14,15,16,17,18,19,20

Histogenesis (Figs. 20.16 and 20.17)

"He who sees things from their beginning has the best view of them" (Aristotle). The classification of tissues that has been presented in the previous chapters is based, as is traditional with histology texts, on morphology—that is, appearance—alone. But as we must be concerned with predictable changes due to aging, the relationship of histology to development is even more important. The adult organism develops from a fertilized ovum, a single cell. In the tiny embryo certain primitive regions and structures take shape, change, and grow. Later these give rise to complex specialized cells, cell groups, and adult organs. For help in establishing the concepts of histology, a reference to embryology is needed in order to understand the functions and capabilities of tissues. The 2 mm human embryo has three basic recognized component layers: ectoderm, endoderm, and mesoderm. Each gives rise subsequently to many cell layers and anatomic structures (Figs. 20.16 and 20.17). Somewhat later but still early in intrauterine life these different layers become extensively rearranged and develop complex functional and anatomic relationships. The extension of blood vessels into all organs is just one example of this process. The structure of organs assembled from these tissues is the subject matter of most of the chapters of this book.

Histology and embryology correlate generally, although there are some inconsistencies. Thus ectoderm and endoderm supply epithelium, mainly for lining the digestive tube and for coating the skin, while mesoderm supplies everything else as well as a good deal of epithelium. This correlation with germ layers extends even into the field of tumor biology. For example, carcinomas that arise from epithelia are likely to metastasize via lymphatic channels, while sarcomas, which generally originate from connective tissue, muscle, or bone, take the vascular route. The difference may become important in selecting the proper treatment. It does the patient no good to remove regional lymph nodes in treatment of most sarcomas, but in many types of carcinoma (breast, thyroid, or lip, for example), resection of regional lymph nodes and lymphatic channels in continuity with the primary tumor is often recommended.

In some cases it is not only important to have a means of identifying the embryologic and the histologic cell type of a tumor; it may also be important to be able to distinguish between tumors of such similar-appearing tissues as liver parenchyma and adrenal cortex. These two neoplasms may present themselves similarly but proceed and respond to treatment in quite different patterns.

Stem Cells (Fig. 20.18)

What causes tissues to replace themselves according to need as perfectly as they do? Epithelia of all types constantly shed mature and damaged cells from their surfaces at regular and determinable rates. Blood cells also have well-known limited life spans. These require the steady production of replacements. But each tissue must also have a preestablished program to replace unexpected losses and to fulfill extra requirements imposed by disease. Not only must there be production lines in which cells pass through various

Fig. 20.16. *Histogenesis.* The embryonic origins of the main adult cell types and the detailed path of development of one group, the blood cells.

Fig. 20.17. *Fetal gut.* This section, transversely through the thorax of an embryo, shows the undifferentiated structure of the esophagus (above) and the trachea (below). Compare with Fig. 12.16. ×85.

Fig. 20.18. *The cell cycle.* This figure from Chapter 2 is repeated here to illustrate the stem cell concept. For a cell population to maintain itself, not all products of mitosis can be permitted to progress to end cells. At least one product of division must retain its potential to recycle. This implies a permanent population of undifferentiated cells.

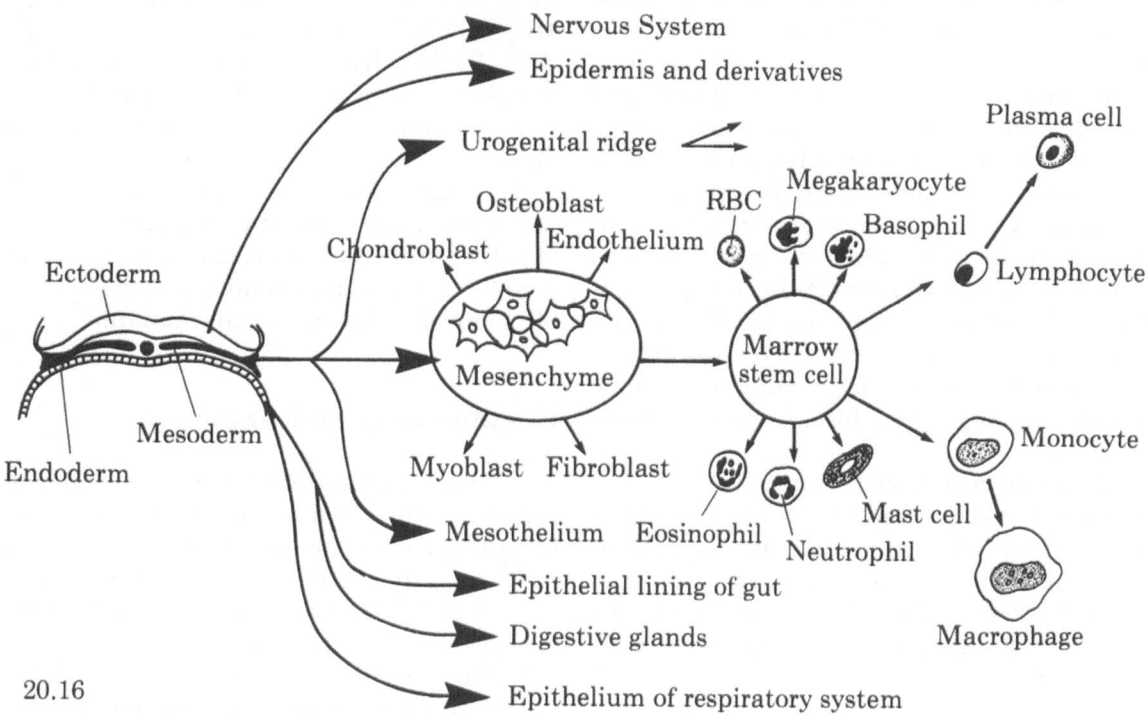

20.16

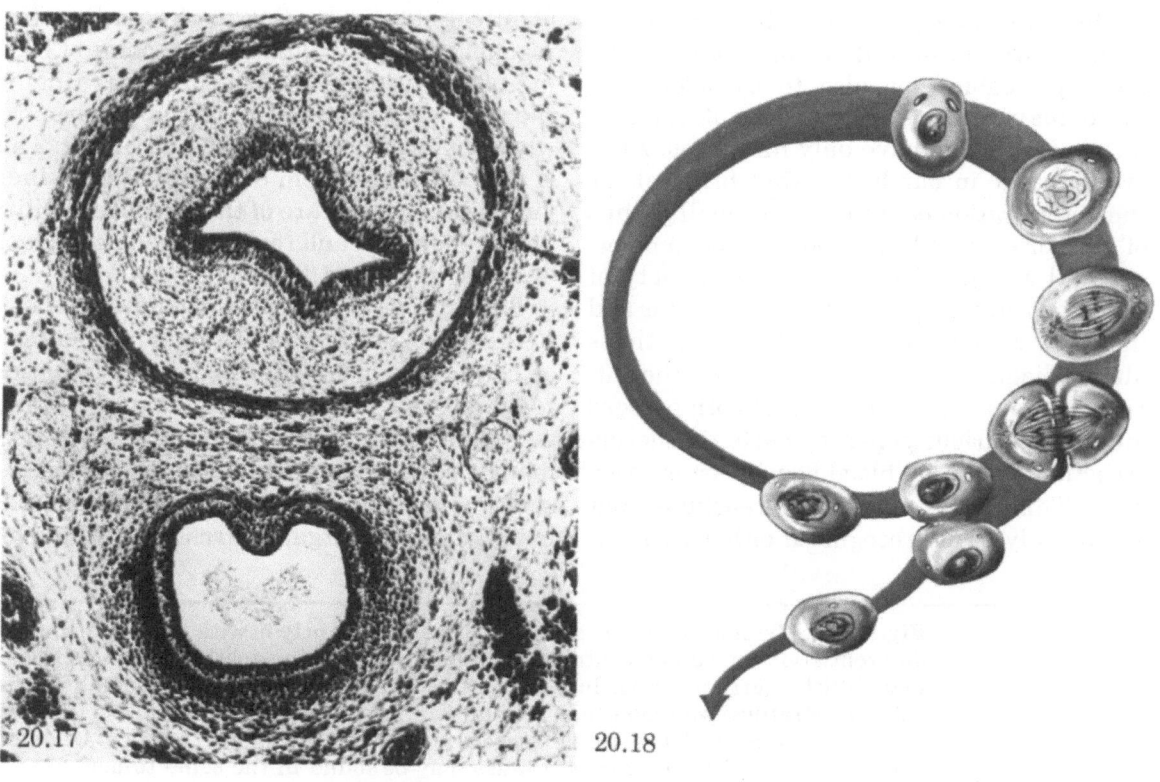

20.17

20.18

stages to the mature product, but there must also be replacement of the individual parent or progenitor cells themselves. In other words, some progenitors must be able to divide into two or more cells, one of which may mature and at least one of which becomes another progenitor. Also there must be opportunity for increase in the frequency of divisions and the means of controlling the production so as to maintain a dynamic equilibrium. Mechanisms of this system, and specifically the signals that turn on and off the division rates, are understood only in their most elementary aspects, although the subject has drawn much attention.

The occurrence of such tumors as teratomas and teratocarcinomas—that is, tumors with a variety of differentiated tissues representing more than a single germ layer—suggests the persistence in the adult of totipotent cells from the embryo, perhaps even germ cells (Fig. 20.19).

Degeneration and Necrosis

Death and dying, as we are reminded by Shakespeare and Kubler-Ross, are part of life. Nothing in biology is static. It behooves us to recognize not only that many of our cells are replaceable, but also to consider that there may be a finite number of replacements—even cats have only nine lives. Also, events occur in our bodies that bring about the deterioration or the death of small groups of cells or even of large segments of some organs all at once. There is a large variety of infectious organisms capable of doing this and in many strange and interesting, sometimes almost diagnostic, patterns. However, the outright champion killer disease, of both persons and their various separate parts, is the obstruction of arterial blood flow by arteriosclerosis. This causes a series of reactions that are usually easily recognized either by gross

or microscopic examination. These are collectively called ischemic necrosis, or infarcts (Fig. 20.20). (Ischemia means lack of blood supply, necrosis means death of cells or tissues, and infarct is an area of ischemic necrosis).

There are of course also instances of degeneration or deterioration of individual cells or of cell groups from numerous causes. Besides simple aging and ischemia, a large number of chemical substances come to mind.

Regeneration and Repair

Not all cell populations have the remarkable regenerative capacity of epithelium and erythrocytes. At the opposite extreme are the neurons. All of these are formed approximately by the time of birth and no multiplication or replacement of them can occur after this. In general, the tissues that are better able to regenerate are composed of more primitive and less specialized cells.

The subject of regeneration cannot be dealt with adequately without considering differentiation. Removal of a limb of a frog tadpole may be followed by faultless regrowth of an identical substitute. But in the mature frog regeneration occurs only to the point of healing of the wound. Clearly there is a time in the life of every tissue which determines whether its loss will be made up or not. This is part of the problem of aging. Elderly individuals are well aware of their reduced ability for regeneration and repair as well as the lack of other important functions (sob!).

The capacity of tissues to regenerate is basic to the subject of wound healing and therefore of concern, not only in terms of adaptation to simple loss of an organ by trauma or surgery, but more importantly in the development of and adjustment to many diseases—such as arteriosclerosis, infarction of the heart and other organs, cirrhosis of the liver

---

Fig. 20.19. *Teratocarcinoma*, a tumor of germ cell origin with multiple lines of differentiation. **a:** Tumor contains identifiable developing tooth (T), bone (B), and hair follicles (arrows). ×35. **b:** Bone and loose pigmented tissue resembling iris. ×250. **c:** Stratified squamous epithelium (E) with keratin, smooth muscle (M), and possible sweat ducts (D). ×150. **d:** Nervous (cerebral) gray matter. ×250. **e:** Undifferentiated cells. ×250. All of these tissues may be found in the same tumor.

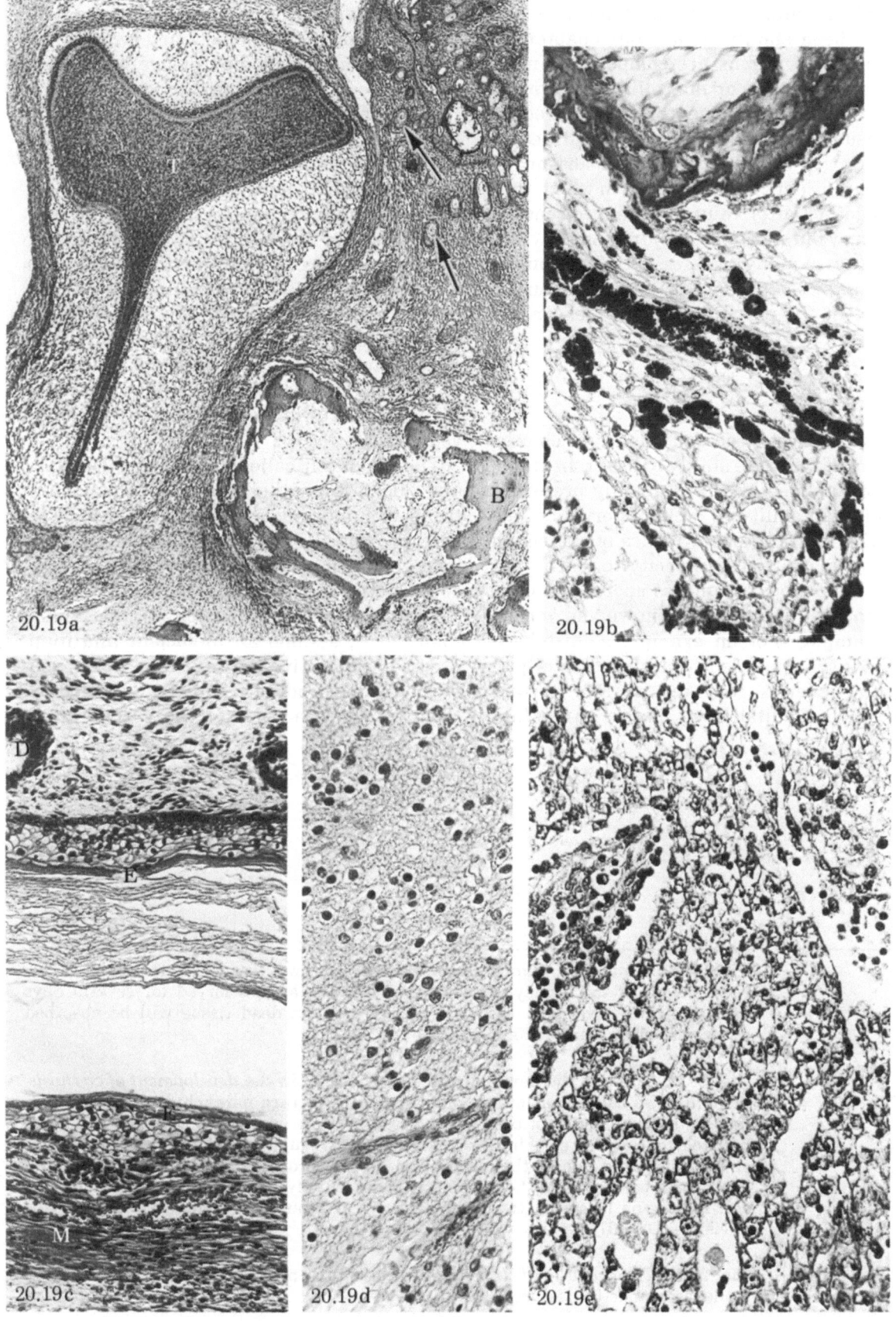

20.19a

20.19b

20.19c

20.19d

20.19e

and inflammatory conditions of many tissues. As has been shown in previous chapters of this book, all organs are composed of more than one cell type or noncellular substance. These different components in any one structure usually have different innate abilities for regeneration and the presence or absence of disease may depend on the ways in which they act together after injury. In fact, disease is not injury but *reaction* to injury and the characteristics of many diseases, both functionally and anatomically, depend heavily upon responses of the particular cells which are affected.

Adaptation

One of the most basic and important characteristics of life is the ability to adapt. In extension of this idea, we have already presented loss of adaptability as a characteristic of aging. The most obvious evidence of this aging process relates to the capacity to learn—not just school subjects but also sports and communication, for some well-known and verifiable examples. For an example in histology, consider the changes in the structure of pulmonary arteries that result from certain types of congenital heart disease. An infant was born with a large opening between the aorta and main pulmonary artery. She survived childhood, but died at age 46 because of this defect. The opening caused an equalization of pressure in the two large arteries. For her entire life systolic pressure in the pulmonary artery was 100 mm Hg or more—70 mm Hg higher than normal. The establishment of an unusually high resistance in this system was necessary to equalize flow in these two arterial systems. A unidirectional shunt, as would have resulted if the pulmonary artery pressure had been normal, would have caused heart failure and a much earlier death. The distortions seen in these pulmonary arteries may be thought of as part of the tradeoff—pulmonary arteriosclerosis in exchange for 46 years of life.

The condition called cirrhosis (Figs. 20.21 and 20.22) is another example of a biologic tradeoff. Following multiple insults or a severe, prolonged, or repeated damage, the liver in regenerating itself is forced into a disordered pattern. Liver cells, no longer having a normal scaffold on which to reestablish themselves, assume an inefficient and inappropriate collective arrangement. This usually happens gradually and the distorted architecture is the price of the regeneration.

Fig. 20.20. Border of a *renal infarct*. The more normal tissue is to the right. Structural details of the kidney, as with other tissues, are preserved for several days after the cells have died. Eventually, however, the dead tissue will be absorbed and replaced by scar. ×120.

Fig. 20.21. This and the next figure show two stages in the *development of cirrhosis*, including the deleterious effects of scar. In this picture parenchymal distortion is moderate. Some bands of connective tissue have nearly surrounded the nodule of hepatocytes (N). The cells have regenerated in irregular pattern so that the central vein is displaced out of this cell group. It has probably been incorporated into one of the portal tracts. Consequently blood supply to hepatocytes is inefficient, as they are no longer in the ideal pathway. A group of degenerated hepatocytes is visible (D). ×37.

Fig. 20.22. The *endstage of cirrhosis*, nodules of parenchyma (N) completely isolated by dense connective tissue. ×37.

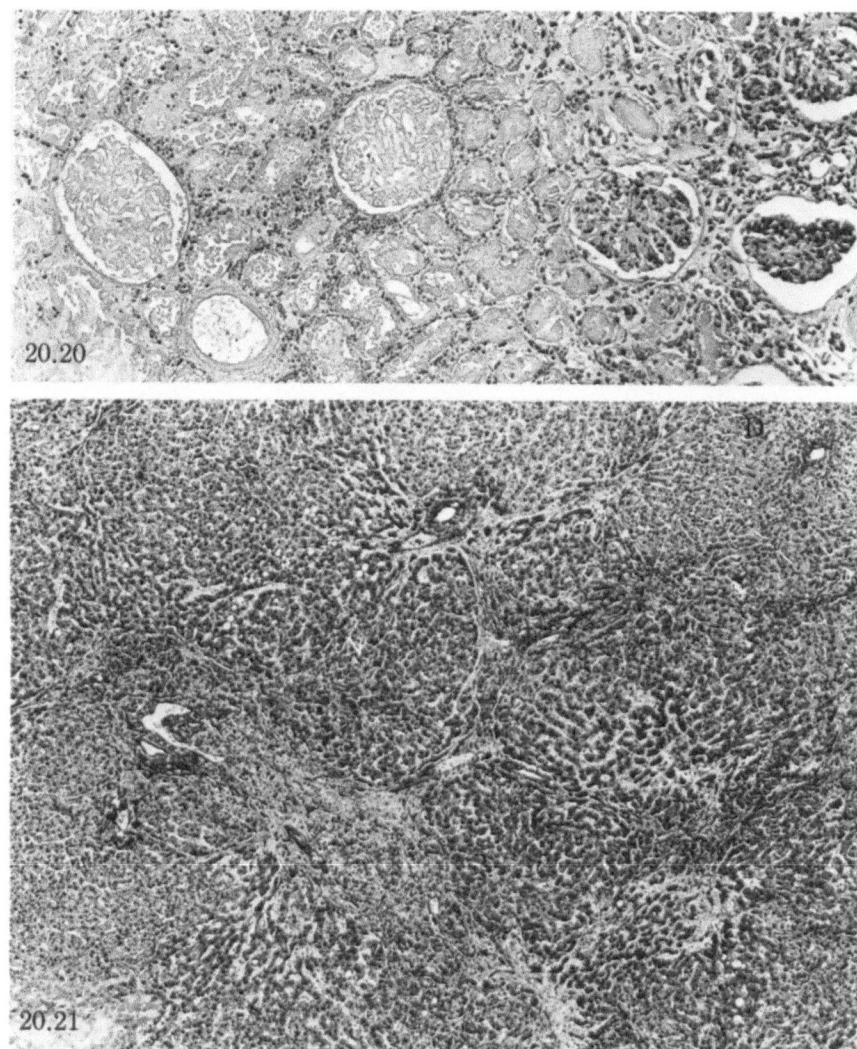

20.20

20.21

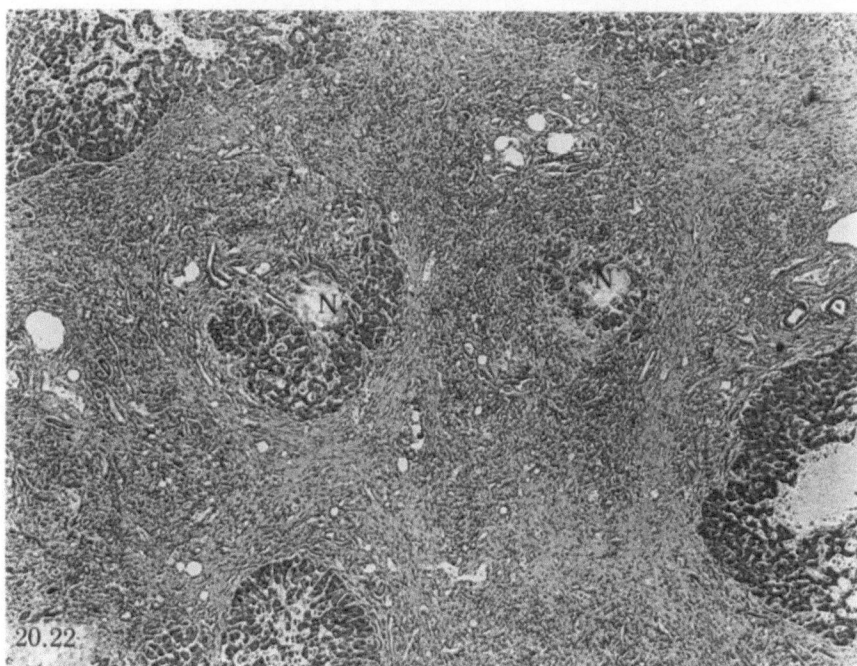

20.22

Other Useful Books

Dictionaries:

Dorland's Illustrated Medical Dictionary, 26th ed. Philadelphia: Saunders, 1981.

Melloni's Illustrated Medical Dictionary. Baltimore: Williams and Wilkins, 1979.

Stedman's Illustrated Medical Dictionary, 24th ed. Baltimore: Williams and Wilkins, 1982.

Textbooks: Histology and Cytology

Arey LB: Human Histology, 4th ed. Philadelphia: Saunders, 1974.

Bloom W, Fawcett DW: A Textbook of Histology, 10th ed. Philadelphia: Saunders, 1974.

Borysenko M, Borysenko J, Beringer T, Gustafson A: Functional Histology. A Core Text. Boston: Little, Brown, 1979.

Copenhaver WM, Kelly DE, Wood RL: Bailey's Textbook of Histology, 17th ed. Baltimore: Williams and Wilkins, 1978.

Cowdry EV: A Textbook of Histology, 4th ed. Philadelphia: Lea and Febiger, 1950.

Dyson RD: Cell Biology. A Molecular Approach, 2nd ed. Boston: Allyn and Bacon, 1978.

Elias H, Pauly JE, Burns ER: Histology and Human Microanatomy, 4th ed. New York: John Wiley and Sons, 1978.

Fawcett DW: The Cell, 2nd ed. Philadelphia: Saunders, 1981.

Gardner DL, Dodds TC: Human Histology, 3rd ed. New York: Churchill Livingstone, 1975.

Ham AW, Cormack DH: Histology, 8th ed. Philadelphia: Lippincott, 1979.

Junqueira LC, Carneiro J: Basic Histology, 3rd ed. Los Altos: Lange Medical Publications, 1980.

Leeson TS, Leeson CR: Histology, 4th ed. Philadelphia: Saunders, 1981.

Lentz, TL: Cell Fine Structure. Philadelphia: Saunders, 1971.

Rhodin JAG: Histology, A Text and Atlas. New York: Oxford University Press, 1974.

Williams PL, Warwick R: Gray's Anatomy, 36th English edition. Philadelphia: Saunders, 1980.

Weiss L, Greep ROO: Histology, 4th ed. New York: McGraw-Hill, 1977.

Wheater PR, Burkitt HG, Daniels VG: Functional Histology. Edinburgh: Churchill Livingstone, 1979.

Textbooks: Pathology

Anderson WAD, Kissane JM: Pathology, 7th ed. St. Louis: Mosby, 1977.

Anderson WAD, Scotti TM: Synopsis of Pathology, 10th ed. St. Louis: Mosby, 1980.

Golden A: Pathology. Understanding Human Disease. Baltimore: Williams and Wilkins, 1982.

King D, Geller LM, Krieger P, Silva F, Lefkowitch JH: A Survey of Pathology. New York: Oxford University Press, 1976.

Robbins SL, Cotran RS: Pathologic Basis of Disease, 2nd ed. Philadelphia: Saunders, 1979.

Rosai J, Ackerman L: Ackerman's Surgical Pathology, 6th ed. St. Louis: Mosby, 1980.

Smith C: Core Pathology. Fundamental Concepts and Principles. Oradell, New Jersey: Medical Economics, 1981.

Willis RA: Pathology of Tumours, 4th ed. New York: Appleton-Century-Crofts, 1967.

Textbooks: Embryology

Arey LB: Developmental Anatomy, 7th ed. Philadelphia: Saunders, 1974.

Balinsky, BI: An Introduction to Embryology, 5th ed. Philadelphia: Holt, Rinehart and Winston, 1981.

Corliss EC: Patten's Human Embryology. Elements of Clinical Development. New York: McGraw-Hill, 1976.

Langman J: Medical Embryology, 4th ed. Baltimore: Williams and Wilkins, 1981.

Atlases

Curran RC: Color Atlas of Histopathology, 2nd ed. New York: Oxford University Press, 1972.

Di Fiore MSH: Atlas of Human Histology, 5th ed. Philadelphia: Lea and Febiger, 1981.

Fujita T, Tanaka K, Tokunaga J: SEM Atlas of Cells and Tissues, 2nd ed. Tokyo and New York: Igaku-Shoin, 1981.

Gasser RF: Atlas of Human Embryos. Hagerstown, Maryland: Harper and Row, 1975.

Hammarsen F: Histology. Baltimore, Munich: Urban and Schwarzenburg, 1980.

Kessel RG, Kardon RH: Tissues and Organs. A Text-Atlas of Scanning Electron Microscopy. San Francisco: WH Freeman, 1979.

Leeson TS, Leeson RC: A Brief Atlas of Histology. Philadelphia: Saunders, 1979.

O'Rahilly R: A Color Atlas of Human Embryology. Philadelphia: Saunders, 1975.

Reith EJ, Ross MH: Atlas of Descriptive Histology, 3rd ed. Hagerstown, Maryland: Harper and Row, 1977.

Rhodin JAG: An Atlas of Histology. New York: Oxford University Press, 1975.

Sandritter W: Color Atlas of Histopathology, 6th ed. Chicago: Yearbook Medical Publishers, 1979.

Methods for Microscopy

Chayen J, Bitensky L, Butcher RG: Practical Histochemistry. London: John Wiley and Sons, 1973.

Feteanu A: Labeled Antibodies in Biology and Medicine. Tunbridge Wells, Kent, England: Abacus Press and New York: McGraw-Hill, 1978.

Hayat MA: Principles and Techniques of Electron Microscopy. Biological Applications. Vols. 1, 2, 3. New York: Van Nostrand Reinhold, 1970.

Hamashima Y: Immunohistopathology. Tokyo: Igaku-Shoin and Philadelphia: Lippincott, 1976.

Luna L: Manual of Histologic Staining Methods of the Armed Forces Institute of Pathology, 3rd ed. New York: McGraw-Hill, 1968.

Galigher AE, Kozloff EN: Essentials of Practical Microtechnique, 2nd ed. Philadelphia: Lea and Febiger, 1971.

Pearse AGE: Histochemistry. Theoretical and Applied, Vol. 1, 4th ed, 1980. Vol., 2, 3rd ed, 1972. New York: Churchill Livingstone.

Preece A: A Manual for Histologic Technicians, 2nd ed. Boston: Little, Brown, 1965.

Troyer H: Principles and Techniques of Histochemistry. Boston: Little, Brown, 1980.

Trump BR, Jones RT: Diagnostic Electron Microscopy. Vol. 1. New York: John Wiley and Sons, 1978.

Index